HANDBOOK OF INFANT BIOPSYCHOSOCIAL DEVELOPMENT

Contributors

Iryna Babik, PhD, Physical Therapy Department, University of Delaware, Newark, Delaware

Patricia J. Bauer, PhD, Department of Psychology, Emory University, Atlanta, Georgia

Martha Ann Bell, PhD, Department of Psychology, Virginia Polytechnic Institute and State University, Blacksburg, Virginia

Marc H. Bornstein, PhD, Child and Family Research, Eunice Kennedy Shriver National Institute of Child Health and Human Development, Bethesda, Maryland

Kristin A. Buss, PhD, Department of Psychology, The Pennsylvania State University, University Park, Pennsylvania

Susan D. Calkins, PhD, Department of Human Development and Family Studies and Department of Psychology, University of North Carolina at Greensboro, Greensboro, North Carolina

Julie M. Campbell, PhD, Department of Psychology, University of North Carolina at Greensboro, Greensboro, North Carolina

Sunghye Cho, MS, Department of Psychology, The Pennsylvania State University, University Park, Pennsylvania

John Colombo, PhD, Schiefelbusch Institute for Life Span Studies and Department of Psychology, University of Kansas, Lawrence, Kansas

Brian Crosby, PhD, Department of Psychology, The Pennsylvania State University, University Park, Pennsylvania

Mary Dozier, PhD, Department of Psychological and Brain Sciences, University of Delaware, Newark, Delaware

Ruth Feldman, PhD, Department of Psychology, Bar-Ilan University, Ramat Gan, Israel

About the Editor

Susan D. Calkins, PhD, is the Bank of America Excellence Professor in the Department of Human Development and Family Studies and the Department of Psychology at the University of North Carolina at Greensboro, where she directs the Child and Family Research Network. Dr. Calkins conducts longitudinal studies of the biological, psychological, and social processes that influence emotional development from infancy through young adulthood.

KH

© 2015 The Guilford Press
A Division of Guilford Publications, Inc.
370 Seventh Avenue, Suite 1200, New York, NY 10001
www.guilford.com

Printed in the United States of America

This book is printed on acid-free paper.

Last digit is print number: 9 8 7 6 5 4 3 2 1

Library of Congress Cataloging-in-Publication Data is available from the publisher.

ISBN 978-1-4625-2212-5

5/9/16

HANDBOOK OF
Infant Biopsychosocial Development

Edited by

Susan D. Calkins

THE GUILFORD PRESS
New York   London

specific biological and genetic techniques and measures will learn much from the individual chapters within each section. The hope is that, with the help of this volume and the contributors' discussions of current research studies and findings, principles of a biopsychosocial perspective can be integrated into the thinking and perhaps the approach taken by scientists and practitioners alike.

In considering the work presented in this volume, it is important to keep in mind that just as infant development is the consequence of many interacting influences and forces, so too is the science of that development. The work presented in this volume is the product of both the contributors and several influential scientists whose research laid the groundwork for the field as it exists today. Although each of the contributors could name his or her own sources of influence and inspiration, mine include (in addition to Gilbert Gottlieb) Dante Cicchetti, Martha Cox, Tony DeCasper, Alison Fleming, Nathan Fox, Megan Gunnar, Steve Porges, Arnold Sameroff, Steve Suomi, and many others whose work and ideas—and their willingness to share both—are the foundation of my own. I am grateful to have had the opportunity to learn from all of them.

Contents

PART V. THE FUTURE OF INFANCY RESEARCH

PART I

SETTING THE STAGE

CHAPTER 1

Introduction to the Volume

Seeing Infant Development through a Biopsychosocial Lens

Susan D. Calkins

The Biopsychosocial Lens: Conceptual Integration across Domains of Infant Functioning

The development of the human infant from a seemingly passive, dependent, and immature organism at birth to—within a span of 2 to 3 very short years—a walking, talking, seemingly independent person, is a truly remarkable process. The effort to understand these rapid changes has been the domain of infancy researchers for more than 100 years. However, late in the 20th century, the world of infancy research entered an exciting and somewhat intellectually and methodologically challenging era. The introduction of sophisticated technology, providing access to genetic and physiological processes, allowed scientists to study developmental changes that were hard to access observationally. Ultimately, this led to a more integrated view of human development that incorporated the multiple biological and behavioral factors that conspired, in sometimes unknown ways, to produce unique developmental processes and pathways. Changes in the way scientists thought about development shifted rapidly and substantially from a purely maturational perspective (growth causes change) to an environmental perspective (family causes change) to a biological perspective (development is gene driven), and finally to variations on the interactionist theme: nature (genes and biology) and nurture (families, peers, and culture) interacted in complex ways to produce a range of developmental outcomes.

Clearly, the recent interactionist perspectives hold the most promise for understanding how biology, behavior, and environment all contribute to

3

developmental outcomes. As such, the aim of this volume is to present recent, novel, and paradigm-shifting work that has viewed infant development through a *biopsychosocial* lens. This lens offers a unique perspective on a period of life characterized by rapid changes across different domains of function, broadly characterized as biological, psychological, and social. And, this perspective has implications for how we think about, study, and analyze the data we collect about infants in these different domains.

The conceptual integration of biological, behavioral, and social levels of analysis (Gottlieb, 2007) has been referred to in various ways, including *developmental science* (Cairns, Elder, & Costello, 1996) and *developmental* or *dynamic systems theory* (Lewkowicz, 2011; Lickliter, 2008). Regardless of the label, these approaches articulate clear support for a unique perspective on development, one that gives greater acknowledgment of the complex and reciprocal, rather than prescriptive, role of biological processes in transactional models of development (Calkins, 2011; Sameroff, 2010). The biopsychosocial perspective aims to account for the *processes* and *mechanisms* responsible for growth and change in structure and functioning in children, within the context of families and the broader social context, and with an appreciation of the contribution of underlying biological processes.

The articulation of the basic principles of the biopsychosocial approach was stimulated by several landmark studies of genetic and biological processes in humans and animals. This work led to reformulations of developmental theory and, eventually, a movement toward empirical designs and analytical techniques crafted specifically to reveal the dynamic nature of early development. Thus, the biopsychosocial lens we rely on in this volume provides scholars of infancy with a view of development that crosses multiple levels within and between individuals. The focus of the work in this volume varies considerably from chapter to chapter; as a whole, the work presented here encompasses the genetic, neural, physiological, psychological, familial, and contextual levels of individual functioning, and together yield a richer understanding of the daunting complexity of human infants and their worlds.

Emergence of the Biopsychosocial Perspective in the Study of Infancy

The contemporary study of infant development has yielded remarkable growth in our understanding of the very early emerging skills and abilities of young children. Historically, efforts to study human infants viewed them as somewhat passive creatures whose development depended largely on the maturation of the brain and on the interventions of others. Soon, however, clever research methodologies evolved for studying the appearance and development of skills in humans lacking the linguistic skills to reveal their cognitive and social knowledge. These methodologies capitalized on the primitive abilities of infants—looking, sucking, and motor movement—to infer skills and knowledge that ranged from the perceptual to the social. In this way, science began to view infants as active participants in their own development, capable of using their social environments to facilitate subsequent learning and skill development. A large body of infancy research conducted throughout the latter half of the 20th century adopted this perspective and focused on identifying patterns of abilities and developments in the broad domains of emotion and cognition, as well on studying the significance of individual differences in these domains for later functioning, adaptation, and mental health (cf. Bremner & Fogel, 2004).

Two significant changes in the field of child development in the late 20th and early 21st centuries, one conceptual and one methodological, again altered our view of infancy, this time to one that acknowledged the complex interactions among the child's biology, his or her behaviors, and his or her environment (Gottlieb, 2007; Sameroff, 2010; Shonkoff, 2010). First, the field of psychology more broadly, and developmental psychology in particular, began to concede that the "nature–nurture" debate was irrelevant, because the partitioning of genetic and environmental influences in development was likely impossible given their interdependence (Lewkowicz, 2011; Meaney, 2010). Instead, the field began to embrace a more complex view of development that considered how dimensions of both nature and nurture dynamically interact across time. The movement toward this perspective was precipitated by studies of the role of genes in human and animal behavioral and biological phenomena that illuminated the complex ways that genes and environments both participate in the developmental process.

The first such investigations were done with nonhuman animals and retrospective studies of human adults. For example, several pioneering animal studies focused on the serotonin transporter gene. A repeat length polymorphism in the promoter region of this gene (*5-HTTLPR*) has been shown to affect the rate of serotonin uptake and may play a role in a range of problematic behavioral outcomes, including aggression. This work revealed that rhesus monkeys that were raised by peers, rather than mothers, exhibited more behavioral and physiological problems (alcohol consumption, poor stress reactivity), and deficits in self-regulation (impulsivity, inappropriate aggression, orienting problems, risk taking) if they possessed the risk allele of the serotonin transporter-linked promoter region (*5-HTTLPR*; s/s or s/l) instead of the nonrisk allele (l/l). These findings suggest that the risk allele of the serotonin transporter gene was only predictive of maladaptive outcomes for monkeys in poor-quality rearing environments. For those monkeys that experienced a natural and supportive mother–infant relationship, there was no effect of genotype (Barr et al., 2004; Bennett et al., 2002; Champoux et al., 2002; Suomi, 2006).

Similarly, in two influential studies of gene–environment (G–E) interactions in human adults, Caspi and colleagues (2002) found that early adverse experience alone did not predict adult psychopathology. As with the animal studies described previously, adults carrying the risk (s/s or s/l) allele of serotonin were more likely to be depressed when they experienced stressful life events than adults without the short allele or those with the short allele who did not experience stressful life events (Caspi et al., 2002). In a second study, they found that childhood maltreatment alone did not predict antisocial behavior in adulthood, but rather that there was a significantly higher chance of developing later antisocial behavior for those individuals who possessed the risk allele of the functional polymorphism of the monoamine oxidase A (*MAOA*) gene and also experienced maltreatment (Caspi et al., 2003).

The study of G–E interaction suggests that the environment in which genes are expressed alters behavioral outcomes. However, the characterization of this interaction is far from simple and the mechanisms through which development occurs are quite complex. For example, other animal work demonstrates quite convincingly that the effect of the environment occurs at both the biological and behavioral levels. For example, Meaney and colleagues have studied the rearing experience of rat pups and its role in the development of the hypothalamic–pituitary–adrenocortical (HPA) axis, which is principally involved in the behavioral response to stress (Meaney, 2010). Rat mothers naturally differ in the amount of "licking and grooming" (LG) caregiving behaviors they provide their pups; high amounts of these behaviors appear to influence the development of the rat pup's developing stress system. Rat pups of low-LG mothers that are cross-fostered with high-LG mothers become themselves less stress reactive, both physiologically and behaviorally, suggesting that the environmental exposure to different caregiving experiences alters the expression of genes that are implicated in the development of the stress system (Champagne et al., 2008; Meaney, 2010).

These influential studies of the dynamic influences across genetic, physiological, and behavioral levels has guided recent work in the field of infant development. In one such study, researchers examined the effect of the dopamine receptor gene D2 (*DRD2*) on infant physiological responses to stress over the first year of life in the context of infants' experiences with caregivers (Propper et al., 2008). Infants possessing the *taq*1 A1 polymorphism of *DRD2*, associated with impulse-control problems and sensation-seeking behaviors, who were also exposed to sensitive maternal caregiving over the first year of life, exhibited a more optimal and expected cardiac response to stress at 12 months of age, comparable to the cardiac reactivity of those infants possessing the nonrisk version of the gene. Infants without the risk allele displayed typical and effective cardiac response to stress regardless of whether mothers were sensitive, suggesting that the caregiving environment may, in fact, be less important for their regulatory outcomes.

So, as the scientific understanding of human genetic and psychobiological processes has grown, scholars have come to abandon the notion that development is gene driven and instead have adopted an appreciation of reciprocal processes at all levels of development. This perspective has led to a shift in focus in the field of developmental psychology, and in the study of infant development in particular, that has influenced our attempts to understand and study *how* specific behavioral developments emerge and influence infant development and functioning, as well as how those developments feedback to influence both biological and social processes. Scientists have come to view development as a fundamentally *dynamic process* involving transactions between the child and his or her environment that influence children's development, and the behavior of those who comprise their environment, at multiple biological and behavioral levels (e.g., Blair, 2002; Calkins, 2011; Lewkowicz, 2011).

Empirical Implications of a Biopsychosocial Perspective

According to the biopsychosocial perspective, the child's biology, behavior, and social environment are changing one another continually over the course of development. This view of development has emerged because the science of development, and the empirical work that investigates these processes, has become much more interdisciplinary in nature and begun to incorporate biological constructs and principles, as well as empirical measures and findings, from the fields of genetics, neuroscience, comparative psychology, psychobiology, and psychophysiology. This interdisciplinary nature of the perspective has led to new challenges in the study of infant development.

Understanding development in such a comprehensive and transactional way implies that investigators adopt a multilevel perspective, and perhaps as well, to actually study development across different levels of influences, ranging from the genetic to the social (Gottlieb, 2007). This multilevel perspective led to a critical empirical shift in the way development is studied both in the laboratory and in the field. Over the last several years, multilevel empirical approaches to the study of infant development have proliferated. Investigators traditionally interested in a specific behavioral phenomenon such as temperament, memory, or attachment began to view these behaviors as embedded in a complex system of biological and social processes. And, as this volume reflects, the work that has emerged has surveyed a diversity of specific indicators of these processes, often using longitudinal designs to study children and their environments over time.

One area of growth in this work has been the specification of what constitutes "environment." Although the term often applies to the family environment, more recently, we have begun to broaden and deepen our understanding of this term, describing the family and its functioning at a more micro level, and going beyond the family to the larger social and cultural world in which the child and the family are embedded. Moreover, when considering G–E interaction, the environment consists of everything from the cellular to the social. Indeed, as Shanahan and Hofer (2005) noted, the *E* in *G–E* might best be conceptualized as *exposure*, a term that highlights the range of processes that may alter the pathway initiated by the gene's cellular action at biological and behavioral levels across development.

In addition to the challenges of design and choice of methods that are inherent in work addressing biopsychosocial processes, analytical challenges are substantial as well. The models that have been proposed are often depicted in ways that visually represent the various levels and their interdependence, but the translation of these models to statistical analysis has been slower in emerging. Much of the early work on infant development relied on relatively simplistic correlations and regressions to examine longitudinal developmental associations. Cutting-edge research driven by theoretical models designed to capture the multiple levels of functioning and how these levels change over time requires appropriately sophisticated analytical techniques.

The analytic landscape is rapidly evolving in an effort to meet this need and new advanced statistical techniques are being developed for both person- and variable-centered analyses. Within variable-centered approaches, techniques such as repeated measures analysis of variance and regression analyses have been overshadowed by growth curve modeling, path analyses, and time series analyses, with the goal of describing the trajectories of change in variables that are central to infant functioning and identifying multiple predictors of deviation from those trajectories (Laursen & Hoff, 2006). Researchers have also begun to use more person-centered approaches including profile or class analyses to address questions regarding group or individual differences in patterns of development across time and associations among variables at multiple levels of child functioning. Measurement challenges are associated with these techniques, but nevertheless, they offer a means through which researchers can examine trajectories and complex associations among behavioral constructs of interest. A key point here is that, often, developmental pathway models, which are clearly well suited to the longitudinal study of infant development, predated the statistical techniques to test them (Curran & Willoughby, 2003). Nevertheless, the ongoing development and refinement of statistical methods to test such models is key to further advances in this area.

The adoption of a biopsychosocial perspective on infant development has produced a corpus of work that is rich, though often challenging to integrate, a consequence that may be largely a function of its relative youth compared with the larger body of more traditional developmental research. Importantly, though, these studies routinely reveal a complexity in development that has changed the way we think about development in general and that have motivated efforts to identify specific pathways to optimal versus compromised outcomes in childhood. Moreover, studying development across levels of biology, behavior, and environment provides us with insight into the more *proximal* developmental mechanisms and processes that affect both infant development and the environments in which infants develop, and that can help us to identify critical points of entry for early intervention and prevention. In short, a biopsychosocial lens on development holds the promise of advancing the theoretical, empirical, analytical, and translational agenda of the field of infancy.

Overview of This Volume

The goal of this volume is to provide a selective review of current, cutting-edge work that assesses infant functioning across different biological, behavioral, and/or contextual levels to inform our understanding of development. The authors selected for inclusion in this volume are each conducting research from within a biopsychosocial perspective, incorporating into their work at least two levels of analysis, from the genetic to the environmental. As is clear from the work presented in this volume, integrating this perspective into their work has challenged infancy researchers to grapple with complex conceptual, empirical, and analytical problems. Many questions remain about how best to consider how these transactional processes operate across time and context; how to measure and analyze biological, behavioral, and social processes that may be difficult to disentangle; and how to translate those findings into strategies to positively influence outcomes for young children. Nevertheless, clear from this volume is that these challenges are being met and the field of infancy is quickly evolving to reflect the rapid pace of empirical and analytical advances. In adopting a multilevel approach—a biopsychosocial approach—this volume will provide a conceptual, empirical, and translational road map for research on infant development in the 21st century.

REFERENCES

Barr, C. S., Newman, T. K., Shannon, C., Parker, C., Dvoskin, R. L., Becker, M. L., et al. (2004). Rearing condition and rh5-HTTLPR interact to influence limbic–hypothalamic–pituitary–adrenal axis response to stress in infant macaques. *Biological Psychiatry, 55*(7), 733–738.

Bennett, A. J., Lesch, K. P., Heils, A., Long, J. C., Lorenz, J. G., Shoaf, S. E., et al. (2002). Early experience and serotonin transporter gene variation interact to influence primate CNS function. *Molecular Psychiatry, 7*(1), 118–122.

Blair, C. (2002). School readiness: Integrating cognition and emotion in a neurobiological conceptualization of children's functioning at school entry. *American Psychologist, 57*, 111–127.

Bremner, J. G., & Fogel, A. (2004). *Blackwell handbook of infant development.* Oxford, UK: Wiley Blackwell.

Cairns, R. B., Elder, G. H., & Costello, E. J. (Eds.). (1996). *Developmental science.* Cambridge, UK: Cambridge University Press.

Calkins, S. D. (2011). Caregiving as coregulation: Psychobiological processes and child functioning. In A. Booth, S. McHale, & N. Lansdale (Eds.), *Biosocial foundations of family processes* (pp. 49–59). New York: Springer.

Caspi, A., McClay, J., Moffitt, T., Mill, J., Martin, J., Craig, I. W., et al. (2002). Role of genotype in the cycle of violence in maltreated children. *Science, 297*(5582), 851–854.

Caspi, A., Sugden, K., Moffitt, T. E., Taylor, A., Craig, I. W., Harrington, H., et al. (2003). Influence of life stress on depression: Moderation by a polymorphism in the 5-HTT gene. *Science, 301*(5631), 386–389.

Champagne, D. L., Bagot, R. C., van Hasselt, F., Ramakers, G., Meaney, M. J., de Kloet, E., et al. (2008). Maternal care and hippocampal plasticity: Evidence for experience-dependent structural plasticity, altered synaptic functioning, and differential responsiveness to glucocorticoids and stress. *Journal of Neuroscience, 28*(23), 6037–6045.

Champoux, M., Bennett, A., Shannon, C., Higley, J. D., Lesch, K. P., & Suomi, S. J. (2002). Serotonin transporter gene polymorphism, differential early rearing, and behavior in rhesus monkey neonates. *Molecular Psychiatry, 7*, 1058–1063.

Curran, P. J., & Willoughby, M. T. (2003). Implications of latent trajectory models for the study of developmental psychopathology. *Development and Psychopathology, 15*(3), 581–612.

Gottlieb, G. (2007). Probabilistic epigenesis. *Developmental Science, 10*, 1–11.

Laursen, B. & Hoff, E. (2006). Person-centered and variable-centered approaches to longitudinal data. *Merrill–Palmer Quarterly, 52*, 377–389.

Lewkowicz, D. J. (2011). The biological implausibility of the nature–nurture dichotomy and what it means for the study of infancy. *Infancy, 16*, 331–367.

Lickliter, R. (2008). Developmental dynamics: The new view from the life sciences. In A. Fogel, B. J. King, & S. G. Shanker (Eds.), *Human development in the twenty-first century: Visionary ideas from systems scientists* (pp. 11–17). Cambridge, UK: Cambridge University Press.

Meaney, M. (2010). Epigenetics and the biological definition of gene x environment interactions. *Child Development, 81*, 49–71.

Propper, C., Moore, G., Mills-Koonce, R., Halpern, C., Hill, A., Calkins, S., et al. (2008). Gene–environment contributions to the development of vagal tone. *Child Development, 79*, 1378–1395.

Sameroff, A. (2010). A unified theory of development: A dialectic integration of nature and nurture. *Child Development, 81*, 6–22.

Shanahan, M. J., & Hofer, S. (2005). Social context in gene–environment interactions: Retrospect and prospect. *Journal of Gerontology, 60B*, 65–76.

Shonkoff, J. (2010). Building a new biodevelopmental framework to guide the future of early childhood policy. *Child Development, 81*, 49–71, 357–367.

Suomi, S. J. (2006). Risk, resilience, and gene environment interactions in rhesus monkeys. *Annals of New York Academy of Sciences, 1094*(1), 52–62.

CHAPTER 2

Gilbert Gottlieb and the Biopsychosocial Perspective on Developmental Issues

Timothy D. Johnston

Gilbert Gottlieb's developmental research, both empirical and theoretical, provides much of the foundation for the biopsychosocial approach represented in this volume. This brief chapter summarizes the salient features of Gottlieb's contributions to developmental theory under three broad headings:

1. The perspective of probabilistic epigenesis.
2. The importance of multiple levels of analysis.
3. The diverse roles of experience in development.

All three contributions derived from Gottlieb's empirical research on the development of species recognition in ducklings (see Gottlieb, 1971, 1997, for summaries), from which he drew general theoretical insights that apply to both human and nonhuman behavioral development.

The Perspective of Probabilistic Epigenesis

Along with many other developmentalists, Gottlieb rejected the idea that different behaviors can be given categorically distinct developmental explanations. In particular, he rejected the classification of behaviors, or features of behavior, as either innate (genetically determined) or acquired (experientially determined). One of the strongest influences on Gottlieb's thinking about development was the work of Zing-Yang Kuo who, beginning in the 1920s, published a series of articles questioning the explanatory utility of the concept of instinct. Like some other writers of the period, Kuo was reacting to the widespread use of instinct in psychology to explain almost any animal or human behavior that was not clearly the result of learning and experience. William James, in his seminal textbook of psychology (James, 1890, Ch. 10), listed over 20 human instincts to explain a wide range of human behaviors. Subsequently, the social psychologist William McDougall (1908) developed his hormic psychology, a general account of animal and human behavior in which a carefully elaborated theory of instinct played a central role. Kuo's first paper (1921), written while he was an undergraduate student at the University of California at Berkeley, was one of the earliest to criticize the unrestrained use of instinct as an explanation for behavior and gave rise to what became known as the anti-instinct movement. Kuo also conducted extensive experimental studies of development in nonhuman animals, and devised a technique for visualizing the embryonic behavior of ducklings, allowing him to trace the developmental origins of behavior into prenatal life. In 1963, Gottlieb invited Kuo to visit his laboratory in Raleigh, North Carolina, and started a long series of experiments on the prenatal origins of behavior in several species, primarily the mallard duck (*Anas platyrhynchos*).

Mallard ducklings show a strong and selective approach response to a particular call, the maternal assembly call, uttered by the mother duck. This response is seen most readily shortly after hatching, when the mother gives the call to lead her brood off the nest. The fact that the response appears very soon after hatching and occurs without any prior exposure to the call (which is not given by nesting females), diagnoses it as innate or instinctive according to the conventional definitions, and to the distinction between innate and learned behavior. However, Gottlieb's experimental research demonstrated that the ducklings' response to the maternal call is not independent of experience, as the diagnosis of innateness implies. During the last few days of incubation before hatching, the embryonic duckling pushes its bill into the airspace at the blunt end of the egg and begins to emit vocalizations (see Gottlieb, 1997, p. 22, Fig. 2.2). Using a devocalization procedure developed with John Vandenbergh (Gottlieb & Vandenbergh, 1968), Gottlieb was able to show that prenatal auditory exposure to those self-produced vocalizations is both necessary and sufficient for the selective postnatal response to the maternal call to develop normally. This experimental finding led him to articulate a view of behavioral development that was grounded in Kuo's anti-instinct writings, and that he refined and elaborated over the subsequent decades. The general perspective, which also owes much to other writers (see below), goes under various names, including interactionism, transactionalism, and dynamic systems theory, but Gottlieb referred to it as *probabilistic epigenesis*. Let's briefly examine the historical background to this theoretical viewpoint.

At the beginning of the 20th century, the designation of certain behaviors in both animals and humans as instinctive was quite unproblematic. The term was applied to behavior that appears in a more or less fully developed form without the need for experience and is performed without the need for volition or conscious control. As noted above, turn-of-the-century psychologists freely invoked instinct to explain numerous behaviors that seemed to share these characteristics. Many of them drew on Darwin's theory of evolution by natural selection to justify their application of instinct to both humans and nonhumans, and this seemed to ground the concept firmly in an important body of emerging biological theory. Instincts were explained by reference to evolutionary mechanisms and, in consequence, seemed not to require any particular developmental explanation. They were thought to appear in a predetermined way, the outcome of internal maturational processes that could perhaps be explained in physiological or anatomical terms, but required no special attention from psychologists.

The anti-instinct movement, of which Kuo was an important architect (see Bernard, 1921; Carmichael, 1925; Dunlap, 1919, 1922; Tolman, 1922, for other early contributions), gained traction primarily by questioning the explanatory adequacy of instinct. As Kuo (1924) pointed out, a psychology of instinct is a "finished psychology." It purports to explain but all it really does is to label, and having labeled certain behaviors as instinctive, we seem to be under no obligation to provide any further explanation. Kuo objected that, to the contrary, all behaviors have a developmental history and the psychologist who wishes to explain the development of behavior must also explain the development of instincts. But how? Kuo and his fellow anti-instinctivists had no good answer to this question and so by default, instinct continued to be widely accepted as an explanation for behavior through the first half of the 20th century. Especially important in the development of mid-20th-century instinct theory was the work of European ethologists such as Konrad Lorenz (1935, 1937, 1956).

Lorenz and his colleagues articulated a theory of instinct that was firmly grounded in evolutionary biology and drew on extensive observations and experiments on behavior in a wide variety of animal species, mostly under natural conditions in the field. To these elements, which had been in place in the biological study of behavior since the late 19th century (Richards, 1987), Lorenz added a high degree of theoretical precision and eventually, and most important, an apparent explanation for the development of instinct by reference to significant contemporary advances in genetics (Lorenz, 1965). The distinction between the phenotype (the discernible appearance of an organism) and the genotype (the composition of its hereditary material) had been understood since early in the century (Johannsen, 1909), but it was not until the elucidation of the structure of deoxyribonucleic acid (DNA) by Watson and Crick (1953) that it became possible to understand in outline how the hereditary material might specify phenotypic characters, including behavior. Asserting a strict separation between acquired and instinctive behavior, Lorenz attributed the former straightforwardly to learning and other experiential mechanisms (such as imprinting) and explained the development of instincts as a process of maturation under the control of genetic information.

In Lorenz's writing, maturation (often "strictly determined maturation") involves the passive and predetermined unfolding of fixed genetic information that directly and precisely specifies the organization of instinctive behavior. Lorenz consistently insisted on a strict separation between acquired and instinctive behavior, and on the strict specification of the latter by the genes. His theoretical views elicited significant criticism, especially from a group of American comparative psychologists with whom Gottlieb was closely associated, most notably T. C. Schneirla (1949, 1956, 1966) and Daniel S. Lehrman (1953, 1970). Their argument was that behavior cannot be neatly divided into the mutually exclusive categories of learned and instinctive, and that Lorenz's claim that the genes directly specify some aspects of the behavioral phenotype seriously misrepresents the nature of development. Lehrman's criticism was especially clearly stated and influential (Silver & Rosenblatt, 1987; Johnston, 2001) and presaged many of the features that Gottlieb would later incorporate into his theory of probabilistic epigenesis. Lehrman (1953) described several experimental results showing important roles for experience in the development of behavior that are not readily diagnosed as instances of learning, showing that the contributions of experience are more complex than can be captured by the distinction between learned and innate behavior. Echoing Kuo, he wrote, "To say of a behavior that it develops by maturation is tantamount to saying that the obvious forms of learning do not influence it, and that we therefore do not consider it necessary to investigate its ontogeny further" (Lehrman, 1953, pp. 344–345).

One of Lehrman's important insights was to recognize the logical inadequacy of the isolation or deprivation experiment that Lorenz and others proposed as the best experimental tool for identifying innate or instinctive behaviors. In the deprivation experiment, an animal is raised in conditions that deprive it of any opportunity to learn or to practice a particular behavior. If, despite the lack of such opportunity, the behavior nonetheless appears in its usual form, it can be reliably diagnosed as innate, the result of genetically determined maturation. Lehrman (1953) pointed out that although one can deprive an animal of some experiences in the course of rearing, it is impossible to deprive it of all sensory stimulation—the animal must be reared in *some* environment and be exposed to *some* stimulation. In particular, he noted, the animal will always be exposed to stimulation produced by its own activity and such self-produced stimulation may well contribute to the development of behavior that appears even after rearing in very deprived conditions. Both the idea that experience may play more roles in development than those identified by various forms of learning and the potential importance of self-stimulation to development became important elements of Gottlieb's theory of probabilistic epigenesis (see further below).

A key idea in probabilistic epigenesis is the importance of bidirectional interactions in development. Whereas predetermined epigenesis (i.e., Lorenz's "strictly determined maturation") postulates unidirectional causation in the pathway from genes to behavior, probabilistic epigenesis inserts bidirectional relationships. Gottlieb first introduced the developmental importance of bidirectional interactions in a chapter on prenatal behavior published in 1970 (although written several years earlier, in 1965; see Gottlieb, 1997, p. 13, footnote). He drew on a number of experiments to illustrate how embryonic behavior is not only affected by developing anatomical structures but can itself influence the development of those structures. Rather than conceiving of the relationship between structure and function (which includes both overt behavior and physiological activity) as predetermined and unidirectional (structure → function), Gottlieb argued that it should be viewed as probabilistic and bidirectional (structure ↔ function). He chose the term *probabilistic* in this context to recognize the fact that "the behavioral development of individuals within a species does not follow an invariant or inevitable course, and, more specifically, that the sequence or outcome of individual behavioral development is probable (with respect to norms) rather than certain" (Gottlieb, 1970, p. 123). Thus, whereas adherents of the predetermined view hold that if a behavior develops prenatally at all, it will develop in only a single determinate way, the probabilistic view maintains that modifications in function may produce variations in structural, and thus in subsequent functional, development.

Although in this chapter Gottlieb (1970) was writing specifically about prenatal behavior, the domain in which he carried out the great majority of his own experimental work, in his later writings he applied his analysis to behavior across the entire lifespan. The very stable and highly constrained world of the embryo tends to restrict naturally occurring variation in experiential input to development, making it easy to overlook (from a probabilistic perspective) the developmental contributions of that experience. Furthermore, behaviors that appear very early in postnatal life, immediately after birth or hatching, have been taken as innate or instinctive precisely because there seems to have been no opportunity for experience to play any role in their development. The manipulation of prenatal experience thus provides especially potent evidence to support a probabilistic view of development in general.

The Importance of Multiple Levels of Analysis

The idea that developmental analysis must involve multiple levels of explanation is integral both to probabilistic epigenesis and to the biopsychosocial approach represented by the contributions to this volume. Gottlieb clearly articulated such multilevel thinking in several of his theoretical publications, arguing in particular that bidirectional interactions among genetic, neural, behavioral, and environmental influences are pervasive in development and must be investigated empirically and incorporated into our explanations.

Gottlieb's (1970) initial conception of probabilistic epigenesis dealt only with two levels of analysis: the structural (anatomical) composition of the organism and the functional (physiological, behavioral) activity made possible by that structure. For behavior, neural structure and function is especially important, but Gottlieb, like Kuo and Lehrman before him, also acknowledged the importance of taking non-neural structures into account when considering the development of behavior. Lehrman (1953, p. 344) had suggested that the gradual improvement of pecking accuracy in young chicks may be influenced as much by the animal's growing muscular strength and stability as it is by either practice or a mysterious underlying maturational process. In a similar vein, one of Gottlieb's examples of the reciprocal interactions of structure and function was the finding that immobilization of the joints of the legs causes anatomical malformations in chick embryos (Drachman & Sokoloff, 1966). More recently, Thelen and her colleagues have demonstrated the importance of physical growth for understanding the development of locomotion in human infants (Thelen, 1995; Thelen, Kelso, & Fogel, 1987).

According to predetermined epigenesis, anatomical structure arises through a maturational process that is controlled by the genes. Gottlieb's (1970) initial explication of probabilistic epigenesis made no direct mention of genetic influences in development, but by 1971 his depictions of epigenesis began to include a recognition of the genes as precursors of structural maturation. Interestingly, his initial depiction of the genetic contribution (Gottlieb, 1971, p. 6) showed the relationship between genes and structure as unidirectional, whereas the other relationships are bidirectional. However, subsequent formulations consistently include a bidirectional arrow between genes and structure (e.g., Gottlieb, 1976a, 1983, 1992, 1997):

genes ↔ structural maturation ↔ function

Gottlieb had long suspected that gene activity is itself susceptible to developmental influences. In his 1976 *Psychological Review* article (Gottlieb, 1976a, p. 219) he hinted that such influences probably occur and, although he provided no direct evidence, he apparently felt sufficiently sure that they do occur to use a bidirectional arrow, with its implication of reciprocal causal influence. It is apparent, however, that Gottlieb's belief that bidirectional influences are pervasive in development and include the genes long predates that publication. In a short essay written just a few years before his death (Gottlieb, 2001, pp. 45–46), he relates how in the mid-1960s he tried to persuade a neurobiologist colleague to compare the ribonucleic acid (RNA) and protein composition of neurons in the brains of normal and devocalized ducklings, showing that his emerging probabilistic viewpoint readily allowed him to imagine that reciprocal interactions would be found at all levels of analysis of the developing organism. By this time, there were a few scattered results in the experimental literature demonstrating that experience could affect RNA and protein diversity (Hydén & Egyházi, 1962, 1964; Rose, 1967), and by the late 1970s an established literature was beginning to emerge (e.g., Grouse, Schrier, Bennett, Rosenzweig, & Nelson, 1978; Rosenzweig & Bennett, 1978; Uphouse & Bonner, 1975). It was becoming clear that gene activity is not autonomous, as implied by Lorenz's (1965) idea of strictly determined maturation caused by the genes, but is itself modified by physiological events, some of which are responses to sensory stimulation.

The inclusion of bidirectional influences affecting the genes extended the levels of analysis encompassed by Gottlieb's theoretical views and, most important, made the genes integral components of the developing system, rather than allowing them to stand outside the process of developmental change as a kind of "unmoved mover." It is interesting that writers who have objected to the learned-innate distinction, in part by pointing out roles for experience that are not clearly instances of learning, have often been accused of de-emphasizing, or even ignoring, the role of genetic influences and espousing a radical kind of environmentalism (see, e.g., the reactions to Lehrman's critique of Lorenz, discussed in Johnston, 2001). It is, of course, true that biopsychologists like Schneirla and Lehrman had little to say in detail about how the genes might influence development and more to say about the contributions of experience. Remember that Lehrman published his critique of Lorenz in the same year in which James Watson and Francis Crick published their paper proposing the double-helical structure of the DNA molecule (Watson & Crick, 1953). The study of molecular genetics was itself in an early embryonic phase at that time and there was simply very little information available about gene function. Once the information did start to become available, Gottlieb readily incorporated it into his probabilistic thinking about development.

The term *function* in Gottlieb's various depictions of probabilistic epigenesis requires some unpacking. It encompasses both physiological function and overt behavior (Gottlieb, 1970) and also includes experience (Gottlieb, 1997, p. 90). Experience, in turn, may be produced either by the organism itself (as in the prenatal self-stimulation that Gottlieb studied in his experiments with ducklings), or by the external environment. Components of the environment can be classified in a number of different ways. Gottlieb himself (e.g., 1992, p. 186) referred to physical, social, and cultural components, but other kinds of classification are possible and, indeed, the distinctions among these three categories are far from clear. Is the auditory environment of a human infant growing up in a French-speaking community physical, social, or cultural? The answer is, of course, "all three," and whether the focus should be on physical, social, or cultural descriptors of the environment depends on the interests of the investigator and the questions being investigated.

The difficulty inherent in describing "the environment" highlights an interesting theoretical challenge for multilevel approaches to developmental analysis, which I call the problem of taxonomic incompatibility between levels. That is, descriptors that apply at one level often do not map cleanly on to descriptors at some other level. This problem is most evident when we consider genetic contributions to the development of behavior, and it has consistently bedeviled attempts to clarify our thinking about that issue. We now clearly understand, in a way that we did not during much of the period when theoretical ideas about behavioral development were taking shape, that genes are molecules, and what they do is to regulate the production of other molecules, specifically messenger RNA (mRNA) and thus, indirectly, proteins. Behavior, of course, is not made up of molecules and mapping the molecular taxonomy of the genes on to the distinctly nonmolecular taxonomy of behavior has been, to put it mildly, problematic. One very influential mapping strategy has been via the concept of information. In response to Lehrman's (1953) criticism that neither genes nor environment alone could be said to determine or specify behavior directly, Lorenz (1965) reframed his position in terms of the *information for* behavior. Information, he said, could come either from the genes (in which case the behavior is innate) or from the environment (in which case the behavior is acquired). Although the information metaphor seems to solve the problem of taxonomic incompatibility by using a language that can be applied to different levels of analysis, it is in fact deeply flawed (see Oyama, 1985, 2000; Johnston, 1987) and has created serious problems for developmental theory.

Although Gottlieb's own experimental work focused primarily on the developmental effects of self-produced physical (auditory) stimulation (Gottlieb, 1971), he saw the multilevel approach to development as essential to the full understanding of developmental processes across the entire lifespan. Indeed, he conducted experiments with colleagues examining the effects of the postnatal social environment on the malleability of auditory preferences in ducklings (e.g., Gottlieb, 1991c, 1997). His theoretical writings show that he expected a fully multilevel approach to be the only viable approach to a complete developmental analysis. This recognition was a logical consequence of his probabilistic approach, not merely an incidental feature of probabilistic epigenesis. The essence of the probabilistic approach is that developmental causes do not act in isolation; rather, they interact in a reciprocal fashion, as shown by the bidirectional arrows in Gottlieb's depictions. It is obviously important from that perspective to ensure that one has considered all the possible interactions that might affect the development of the behavior under consideration. Hence, a multilevel approach is required to encompass as many factors on as many levels as necessary to the complete analysis.

The Diverse Roles of Experience in Development

Given the focus of Gottlieb's experimental research on experiential contributions to development, it is not surprising that he devoted careful attention to the question of how those contributions should be classified and understood. For a good part of the 20th century, the paradigm for understanding experiential contributions to development was provided by the various theories of learning that made up much experimental psychological research. The nature of those theories changed over time, from John B. Watson's (1924) classical behaviorism, through various versions of neobehaviorism, to the more cognitive theories that became prevalent after about 1960. However, so long as the distinction between innate and acquired behavior was considered to be productive, it was widely accepted that the development of innate behaviors would be explained by genetic mechanisms and the development of acquired behaviors by the mechanisms of learning. Learning, however it was conceived in detail, thus defined the role that experience plays in behavioral development.

Schneirla and Lehrman, in their criticisms of the traditional conception of development, both pointed out the limitations inherent in defining experience as synonymous with learning. Both of them wanted to expand the concept of experience to include a much wider range of influences. As discussed above, Lehrman (1953) paid special attention to the logical weaknesses of the deprivation experiment in his critique of Lorenz's theory of instinct. He pointed out that no experiment can deprive an animal of all experience and that the most one can conclude from a deprivation experiment is that the particular experiences that have been excluded do not play a role in the development of any behavior that appears normally. A deprivation experiment may provide grounds to rule out a role for learning in the development of some behavior but, said Lehrman, it does not rule out a role for experience. His analysis gave special weight to the need for a more nuanced taxonomy of experiential effects on behavioral development than simply "learning" or "not learning."

Gottlieb's own research provided a rich source of data on which to base such a taxonomy. In his studies of the mallard duckling's response to the maternal call, Gottlieb found that ducklings that are deprived of the experience of hearing their own embryonic calls (by devocalizing them and rearing them in isolated, sound-proofed incubators) do not show the species-typical response to the maternal call after hatching. However, if a recording of the embryonic call is played to these devocalized ducklings at the appropriate time during incubation, the postnatal response to the maternal call is reinstated. These two results show that prenatal exposure to the embryonic call is both necessary and sufficient for the normal postnatal development of the specific response to the maternal call (see Gottlieb, 1971).

Gottlieb's experiments revealed yet another important feature of the developmental role of this prenatal self-produced experience. The embryonic duckling demonstrates a specific response to the maternal call even *before* it begins emitting calls in the egg around day 22 of incubation. Naturally, the behavior used to demonstrate this specificity differs between the prenatal and postnatal periods. After hatching, response specificity is shown by locomotor approach behavior in a choice test. However, before hatching, the embryo periodically engages in bill-clapping, a behavior that is specifically inhibited by playing a recording of the maternal call. Thus, the specificity of response appears before the embryo begins to makes its own calls, and hearing the (self-produced) embryonic call is necessary to *maintain* that specificity into postnatal life.

Maintenance is one of three roles of experience that Gottlieb proposed in subsequent theoretical papers (Gottlieb, 1976a, 1976b, 1981). The other two are *facilitation* and *induction*. Facilitation is demonstrated when the behavior does develop in the absence of the facilitating experience, but its development is delayed so that it appears later in life than normal. Induction is perhaps the most familiar role of experience and is demonstrated when the behavior does not develop at all in the absence of the inducing experience. In most conventional examples of learning, experience plays an inductive role. Aslin (1981) later added two roles to Gottlieb's classification. One of the these, *attunement*, is best understood as a refinement of facilitation and occurs when a behavior reaches a less fully developed state (on some metric or other) than normal in the absence of the attuning experience. To use Aslin's own example, attunement is shown if a specific level of perceptual acuity develops when the attuning experience is available, but a lower level of acuity develops when that experience is withheld. Aslin's second additional role, which he called *maturation*, is shown when the behavior develops similarly with or without exposure to the experience. However, this really amounts to a demonstration that the experience in question plays no role in the development of a specific behavior.

One of Gottlieb's most distinctive but often overlooked theoretical contributions is his recognition that important experiential contributions may not always be obviously related to the behavior in whose development they play a role. In many cases where the development of behavior depends on experience, there is what might be called a *rational relationship* (Johnston, 1997) between the behavior and the experience that is (perhaps only putatively) required for its development. Thus, for example, it makes rational sense that the development of species-specific song in the chaffinch might depend on hearing the song of adult birds or that accuracy of pecking in gull chicks might improve with practice, and indeed both of these possibilities have been empirically verified (by Thorpe, 1958, and Hailman, 1967, respectively). It also seems rationally plausible that a duckling might have to hear the maternal call of its species while still in the egg in order to show a selective attraction to the call after hatching, even though that turns out not to be the case. But there is no obvious reason for supposing a priori that the duckling should have to hear its own calls in order to demonstrate this specificity after hatching. This is what Gottlieb (1981, 1992; see Miller, 1997) called a nonobvious role for experience in development.

Gottlieb's experimental work, like Schneirla's and Lehrman's, was based in naturalistic observations of his subjects' behavior (Gottlieb, 1971, Ch. 1). In this respect, if not in many others, their approach was in agreement with ethologists like Lorenz, and stood in contrast to much of the prevailing work in experimental psychology, which favored highly simplified, artificial conditions for the study of learning. This ecological approach encouraged an inventory of possible influences on development drawn from observation and relatively unconstrained by a priori theoretical expectations. That is one reason Gottlieb was open to the possibility of nonobvious developmental relationships, which emerge most readily when one focuses on what *might* empirically occur in the developing system, rather than on what *ought* rationally to occur from some specific theoretical perspective.

Conclusion

In this chapter I have limited my attention to the major elements of Gottlieb's theoretical approach to behavioral development, but it should be noted that his work addressed a wider range of topics as well. His experimental work concerned prenatal and early postnatal development in ducklings, but he applied his theoretical perspective to human development as well (e.g., Gottlieb, 1983, 1991b). Indeed, the chapters in this volume show the extent to which the biopsychosocial approach to human development has been influenced by Gottlieb's probabilistic epigenesis. He was critical of the nondevelopmental approach of much behavioral genetics (Gottlieb, 1995) and was deeply interested in the relationship between development and evolutionary change, which he explored in a monograph (Gottlieb, 1992) and in several articles (Gottlieb, 1987, 1991a, 2002; Johnston & Gottlieb, 1990). These wider writings all incorporate, in one way or another, his theoretical perspective on development, with its emphasis on probabilistic epigenesis, multiple levels of analysis, and a diversity of roles for experience in the development of behavior.

REFERENCES

Aslin, R. (1981). Experiential influences and sensitive periods in perceptual development: A unified model. In R. N. Aslin, J. R. Alberts, & M. R. Petersen (Eds.), *Development of perception* (Vol. 1, pp. 5–44). New York: Academic Press.

Bernard, L. L. (1921). The misuse of instinct in the social sciences. *Psychological Review, 28,* 96–119.

Carmichael, L. (1925). Heredity and environment: Are they antithetical? *Journal of Abnormal and Social Psychology, 20,* 245–260.

Drachman, D. B., & Sokoloff, L. (1966). The role of movement in embryonic joint development. *Developmental Biology, 14,* 401–420.

Dunlap, K. (1919). Are there any instincts? *Journal of Abnormal Psychology, 14,* 307–311.

Dunlap, K. (1922). The identity of instinct and habit. *Journal of Philosophy, 19,* 85–94.

Gottlieb, G. (1970). Conceptions of prenatal behavior. In L. R. Aronson, E. Tobach, D.

S. Lehrman, & J. S. Rosenblatt (Eds.), *Development and evolution of behavior: Essays in memory of T. C. Schneirla* (pp. 111–137). San Francisco: Freeman.

Gottlieb, G . (1971). *Development of species identification in birds: An inquiry into the prenatal determinants of perception.* Chicago: University of Chicago Press.

Gottlieb, G. (1976a). Conceptions of prenatal development: Behavioral embryology. *Psychological Review, 83,* 215–234.

Gottlieb, G. (1976b). The roles of experience in the development of behavior and the nervous system. In G. Gottlieb (Ed.), *Studies on the development of behavior and the nervous system: Vol. 3. Neural and behavioral specificity* (pp. 25–54). New York: Academic Press.

Gottlieb, G. (1981). Roles of early experience in species-specific perceptual development. In R. N. Aslin, J. R. Alberts, & M. R. Petersen (Eds.), *Development of perception* (Vol. 1, pp. 5–44). New York: Academic Press.

Gottlieb, G. (1983). The psychobiological approach to developmental issues. In P. H. Mussen (Ed.), *Handbook of child psychology: Vol. II. Infancy and developmental psychobiology* (pp. 1–26). New York: Wiley.

Gottlieb, G. (1987). The developmental basis of evolutionary change. *Journal of Comparative Psychology, 101,* 262–271.

Gottlieb, G. (1991a). Behavioral pathway to evolutionary change. *Rivista di Biologia, 84,* 385–409.

Gottlieb, G. (1991b). Epigenetic systems view of human development. *Developmental Psychology, 27,* 33–34.

Gottlieb, G. (1991c). Social indication of malleability in ducklings. *Animal Behavior, 41,* 953–962.

Gottlieb, G. (1992). *Individual development and evolution: The genesis of novel behavior.* New York: Oxford University Press.

Gottlieb, G. (1995). Some conceptual deficiencies in "developmental" behavior genetics. *Human Development, 38,* 131–141.

Gottlieb, G. (1997). *Synthesizing nature–nurture: Prenatal roots of instinctive behavior.* Mahwah, NJ: Erlbaum.

Gottlieb, G. (2001). A developmental psychobiological systems view: Early formulation and current status. In S. Oyama, P. E. Griffiths, & R. D. Gray (Eds.), *Cycles of contingency: Developmental systems and evolution* (pp. 41–54). Cambridge, MA: MIT Press.

Gottlieb, G. (2002). Developmental–behavioral initiation of evolutionary change. *Psychological Review, 109,* 211–218.

Gottlieb, G., & Vandenbergh, J. G. (1968). Ontogeny of vocalization in duck and chick embryos. *Journal of Experimental Zoology, 168,* 307–326.

Grouse, L. D., Schrier, B. K., Bennett, E. L., Rosenzweig, M. R., & Nelson, P. G. (1978). Sequence diversity studies of rat brain RNA: Effects of environmental complexity in rat brain RNA diversity. *Journal of Neurochemistry, 30,* 191–203.

Hailman, J. P. (1967). The ontogeny of an instinct: The pecking response in chicks of the laughing gull (*Larus atricilla* L.). *Behaviour, 15*(Suppl.), 1–159.

Hydén, H., & Egyházi, E. (1962). Nuclear RNA changes of nerve cells during a learning experiment in rats. *Proceedings of the National Academy of Sciences, 48,* 1366–1373.

Hydén, H., & Egyházi, E. (1964). Changes in RNA content and base composition in cortical neurons of rats in a learning experiment involving transfer of handedness. *Proceedings of the National Academy of Sciences, 52*, 1030–1035.

James, W. (1890). *Principles of psychology.* New York: Holt.

Johannsen, W. (1909). The genotype conception of heredity. *American Naturalist, 45*, 129–159.

Johnston, T. D. (1987). The persistence of dichotomies in the study of behavioral development. *Developmental Review, 7*, 149–182.

Johnston, T. D. (1997). Comment on Miller. In C. Dent-Read & P. Zukow-Goldring (Eds.), *Evolving explanations of development: Ecological approaches to organism–environment systems* (pp. 509–513). Washington, DC: American Psychological Association.

Johnston, T. D. (2001). Towards a systems view of development: An appraisal of Lehrman's critique of Lorenz. In S. Oyama, P. E. Griffiths, & R. D. Gray (Eds.), *Cycles of contingency: Developmental systems and evolution* (pp. 15–23). Cambridge, MA: MIT Press.

Johnston, T. D., & Gottlieb, G. (1990). Neophenogenesis: A developmental theory of phenotypic evolution. *Journal of Theoretical Biology, 147*, 471–495.

Kuo, Z.-Y. (1921). Giving up instincts in psychology. *Journal of Philosophy, 18*, 645–664.

Kuo, Z.-Y. (1924). A psychology without heredity. *Psychological Review, 31*, 427–448.

Lehrman, D. S. (1953). A critique of Konrad Lorenz's theory of instinctive behavior. *Quarterly Review of Biology, 28*, 337–363.

Lehrman, D. S. (1970). Semantic and conceptual issues in the nature–nurture problem. In L. R. Aronson, E. Tobach, D. S. Lehrman, & J. S. Rosenblatt (Eds.), *Development and evolution of behavior: Essays in memory of T. C. Schneirla* (pp. 17–52). San Francisco: Freeman.

Lorenz, K. Z. (1935). Der Kumpan in der Umwelt des Vogels. *Journal für Ornithologie, 83*, 137–213, 289–413.

Lorenz, K. Z. (1937). Uber die Bildung des Instinktbegriffes. *Naturwissenschaften, 25*, 289–300, 307–318, 324–331.

Lorenz, K. Z. (1956). The objectivistic theory of instinct. In P. P. Grassé (Ed.), *L'Instinct dans le comportement des animaux et de l'homme* (pp. 51–76). Paris: Masson.

Lorenz, K. Z. (1965). *Evolution and modification of behavior.* Chicago: University of Chicago Press.

McDougall, W. (1908). *Introduction to social psychology.* London: Methuen.

Miller, D. B. (1997). The effects of nonobvious forms of experience on the development of instinctive behavior. In C. Dent-Read & P. Zukow-Goldring (Eds.), *Evolving explanations of development: Ecological approaches to organism–environment systems* (pp. 457–507). Washington, DC: American Psychological Association.

Oyama, S. (1985). *The ontogeny of information: Developmental systems and evolution.* Cambridge, UK: Cambridge University Press.

Oyama, S. (2000). *The ontogeny of information: Developmental systems and evolution* (2nd ed.). Durham, NC: Duke University Press.

Richards, R. J. (1987). *Darwin and the emergence of evolutionary theories of mind and behavior.* Chicago: University of Chicago Press.

Rose, S. P. R. (1967). Changes in visual cortex on first exposure of rats to light: Effect on incorporation of tritiated lysine into protein. *Nature, 215,* 253–255.

Rosenzweig, M. R., & Bennett, E. L. (1978). Experiential influences of brain anatomy and brain chemistry in rodents. In G. Gottlieb (Ed.), *Early influences* (pp. 289–327). New York: Academic Press.

Schneirla, T. C. (1949). Levels in the psychological capacities of animals. In R. W. Sellars, V. J. McGill, & M. Farber (Eds.), *Philosophy for the future* (pp. 243–286). New York: Macmillan.

Schneirla, T. C. (1956). Interrelationships of the "innate" and the "acquired" in instinctive behavior. In P. P. Grassé (Ed.), *L'Instinct dans le comportement des animaux et de l'homme* (pp. 387–452). Paris: Masson.

Schneirla, T. C. (1966). Behavioral development and comparative psychology. *Quarterly Review of Biology, 41,* 283–302.

Silver, R., & Rosenblatt, J. S. (1987). The development of a developmentalist: Daniel S. Lehrman. *Developmental Psychobiology, 20,* 563–570.

Thelen, E. (1995). Motor development: A new synthesis. *American Psychologist, 50,* 79–95.

Thelen, E., Kelso, J. A. S., & Fogel, A. (1987). Self-organizing systems and infant motor development. *Developmental Review, 7,* 39–65.

Thorpe, W. H. (1958). The learning of song patterns by birds, with especial reference to the song of the chaffinch, *Fringilla coelebs. Ibis, 100,* 535–570.

Tolman, E. C. (1922). Can instincts be given up in psychology? *Journal of Abnormal and Social Psychology, 17,* 139–152.

Uphouse, L. L., & Bonner, J. (1975). Preliminary evidence for effects of environmental complexity on hybridization of rat-brain RNA to rat unique DNA. *Developmental Psychobiology, 8,* 171–178.

Watson, J. B. (1924). *Behaviorism.* New York: Norton.

Watson, J. D., & Crick, F. H. C. (1953). A structure for deoxyribose nucleic acid. *Nature, 171,* 737–738.

PART II

PERCEPTUAL AND COGNITIVE PROCESSES

CHAPTER 3

Introduction to Part II

Bringing the Field of Infant Cognition and Perception toward a Biopsychosocial Perspective

Martha Ann Bell

Infant behavior is complicated and requires a multilevel approach to understand its developmental course. The biopsychosocial perspective can provide that multilevel conceptualization of infant cognitive and perceptual development. Indeed, the socioemotional and adversity/risk literatures focused on infant development have been enthusiastic about embracing the biopsychosocial perspective (e.g., Calkins, Propper, & Mills-Koonce, 2013). As a result, these areas are making great strides in moving away from the nature–nurture polarity that has ruled the field of developmental psychology for too many years. The area of cognition and perception, however, is still mired in the muck of the nature–nurture debate. The chapters in this section represent research that is the exception to the nature–nurture division. The field of infant cognition and perception in general is still very much divided into researchers who espouse a maturational perspective of cognitive development, those who embrace a nativist point of view, and those like the authors of these chapters who are focused on a multilevel approach that incorporates complex biological processes situated in a rich, complex social environment.

In this section overview, I first focus on long-standing concerns in the field, including the popular points of view that attempt to enhance infant cognition by ascribing adult-like explanations to simple infant behaviors or attempt to reduce infant behaviors to maturation in brain circuits. I then focus on two areas of research where biopsychosocial models influence how we think about infant cognitive development. The ideas I present here are not new and they are not mine. I reference liberally from some of the many writings and conferences presentations by Lickliter (2012, 2013; Lickliter & Honeycutt, 2003, 2013), and the commentaries by Lewkowicz (2011), Oakes (2009), and Haith (1998). I follow the writing of Michel and Moore in their book *Developmental Psychobiology* (1995, Ch. 8, "Cognitive Development") in focusing on nativism and brain maturation as points of concern in infant cognition and perception research. I am grateful to all these developmentalists for nudging me toward a more biopsychosocial perspective in my own research.

Cute Baby Tricks and Rich Interpretation

In 2013, I attended a symposium at the meeting of the International Society for Developmental Psychobiology (ISDP) titled "Communicating Developmental Psychobiology." The opening remarks to the symposium were thought provoking and should impress upon developmental scientists the need to take care with our interpretation of what we see infants do. In brief, infant behavior is complicated. Simple explanations are typically embraced by parents and the general public and are highlighted in the media. But simple explanations do not accurately depict complex behaviors of complex systems (Montgomery-Downs, 2013). In other words, few aspects of development are black and white; there are multiple shades of gray (Hayne, 2013).

A perspective on infant cognition that has a firm hold on a small, but vocal, portion of the field is an area that is typically described as nativism. These researchers hold firm to the notion that infants are born with modules that address core knowledge, including number (e.g., Wynn, 1992), physical reasoning (e.g., Baillargeon & Graber, 1987; Spelke, 1998), and moral thought and action (e.g., Hamlin, Wynn, & Bloom, 2007). The research methods used by nativists are intriguing; a developmental colleague many years ago said to me that the nativist methodology is a great example of "cute baby tricks." Indeed, Haith (1998) wrote over 15 years ago of his concern that much of infant cognition was in the head of the researcher rather than in the head of the infant. He coined the phrase "rich interpretation" to describe the tendency of infant researchers to ignore basic developmental processes and suggest instead that infants are capable of cognitive processes that even older children cannot accomplish.

Like many of us who do cognition and perception research with infants, researchers from the nativism perspective rely on infant looking time as the variable of interest because infants cannot tell us what they think or understand (Haith, 1998; Newcombe, 2014). The problem becomes that measuring how long infants look at one stimulus versus how long they look at a different stimulus relegates complex infant cognitive processes to a very simple infant behavior. Using that simple behavior to conclude that infants look longer at a particular stimulus because of its perceptual features is very appropriate (e.g., Bogartz, Shinskey, & Speaker, 1997; Scarf, Imuta, Colombo, & Hayne, 2012). Using that simple behavior to conclude that "babies are smarter than we think" or "infants are little scientists" may be appealing to parents and the general public and make for popular media sound bites, but it discounts developmental processes acquired through interaction with a complex environment (Haith, 1998; Newcombe, 2014). It also ignores the biopsychosocial perspective that bidirectional changes occur across developmental time in genetic, neural, behavioral, and environmental levels of analysis.

In reaction to nativism, it is not enough to focus solely on what infants learn from the environment in our study of infant development. Lewkowicz (2011) has emphasized that the nature–nurture debate, or the innate–acquired debate, that is engaged in by some researchers focused on infant cognition and perception is no long scientifically interesting. He advocates abandoning the "origins" question and focusing instead on the mechanisms associated with development, including organismic and environmental variables (Sameroff, 2010). Similarly, Spencer and colleagues (2009) state that the nativist–empiricist debate distracts attention away from a more systems view of development that emerges through cascades of interactions across multiple levels of causation.

Lickliter has written and spoken passionately about the need to move away from our foundational dichotomies of biological–environmental, innate-learned, heredity–development, and nativist–empiricist, and view development as a process that is situated, contingent, and experience dependent (Lickliter, 2012; Lickliter & Honeycutt, 2013). At the 2013 ISDP symposium I previously mentioned, Lickliter proposed three main points to focus our thinking so that we take development seriously (Lickliter, 2013; Lickliter & Honeycutt, 2003). First, we need to acknowledge that development is complicated and remember that complexity is not simplicity in disguise. If the cognitive or perceptual outcome is in place before the process begins, then we do not need "development." Other than the "rich interpretation" associated with nativist conclusions, this is perhaps the most striking point of core knowledge; if much cognitive knowledge is already in place from early infancy, then what actually develops? Second, we need to remember that development is historical. Behaviors have a history that influences their emergence and maintenance. We need to remember that there are nested levels of time: real time, developmental time, and evolutionary time. Finally, development is situated. It is situated physically, biologically, and socially. Development does not reside in the genes or in the environment, but emerges from the relational dynamics of a brain in a body in a complicated social environment (Lickliter, 2013).

Arguments for and against cute baby tricks and rich interpretation actually hinder rather than promote advances in behavioral sciences (Lickliter & Honeycutt, 2013) and focus attention away from developmental processes (Spencer et al., 2009). Infant brains have an "expectancy" of having experience for learning about the physical world (Newcombe, 2014); the expectant brain and a sociocultural context interact in complex ways in the progressive emergence of increasingly complex cognitive systems (Michel & Moore, 1995). The biopsychosocial perspective encompasses these multilevel processes.

Brains and Maturation and Reductionism

Another problem trend in the area of infant cognition and perception, and one to which I have contributed, is the use of brain maturation as an explanation for cognitive change (e.g., Bell & Fox 1992; Cuevas, Bell, Marcovitch, & Calkins, 2012). Although most developmentalists reject nativism and argue that it is necessary to integrate physiological and experiential factors to comprehend development, it is often the case that biology and experience are separated and brain growth alone is allowed to account for developmental change in behavior (Michel & Moore, 1995). A biopsychosocial perspective is not compatible with the notion that internal and external determinants operate separately in development (Michel & Moore, 1995).

The foundation view of classic developmental cognitive neuroscience research is that maturation of specific brain areas determines an infant's cognitive behaviors and knowledge (Michel & Moore, 1995). Much of this literature is based on comparing infant behavior with that of brain-damaged adults and brain-lesioned monkeys, as well as brain-intact infant monkeys (e.g., Diamond, 1990). Human infants perform like infant monkeys or brain-lesioned adult monkeys on various reaching and grasping tasks, with the explanation being lack of brain maturation for human infants. Thus, human infant brain immaturity is likened to adult human and adult monkey brain damage. Clearly, there is great value to considering information about the development of the nervous system when studying cognitive and perceptual development. But the nervous system of the infant is not an incomplete or immature version of the adult nervous system. The development of a neural structure allows it to be incorporated into the neural system, which may contribute to additional cognitive and perceptual experiences than the ones of interest in a specific research study (Michel & Moore, 1995). These additional other experiences will likely contribute to the behavior of interest, leading us back to our original premise that infant behavior is complicated and, thus, explanations of cognitive development that rely solely on maturation are less than satisfactory.

Because infant behavior is so complicated, much of the research in the field of infant cognition and perception has focused on very specific behaviors in an attempt to understand how these processes develop. Oakes (2009) has written eloquently about this "Humpty Dumpty problem" in infant cognitive development and the great need to put all these infant cognitive and perceptual abilities back together again to learn how they work jointly in development. In reality, this reductionism is not a problem specific to infant cognitive development; it also is evident in much of the work from a cognitive or cognitive neuroscience framework.

Another concern with the tradition of reductionism is that much of the study of individual infant cognitive and perceptual skills has been done by assessing infants' responses to arbitrary stimuli in the research lab. We do this in an attempt to isolate potential mechanisms of the behavior of interest, but in doing so we ignore the important fact that biopsychosocial systems interact together over development (Lickliter & Honeycutt, 2013). The end result, as Oakes (2009) notes, is that we know very little about mechanisms of developmental change regarding infant cognition and perception. Developmental changes in one cognitive ability likely contribute to changes in another cognitive skill, making it critical to study the codevelopment of different cognitive skills. In essence, what is required is a multilevel approach that is situated physically, biologically, and socially.

As I have written in the paragraphs above, the field of infant cognition and perception has been much slower to embrace a biopsychosocial perspective than have the fields of infant socioemotional development and infant adversity/risk. As noted by Michel and Moore (1995), attempts to simplify complicated infant cognitive behaviors have resulted in less than desirable representations of cognitive development. There are some areas of infant cognitive research, however, where biopsychosocial models are beginning to be used. These areas of research are changing our ways of thinking about infant cognitive development.

Positive Parents and Infant Brains

The view that nurturing and supportive maternal responses are vital for healthy psychosocial growth is incorporated into classic psychological theories (Thompson, 2006). The caregiving environment has been given an essential role in an infant's socioemotional development; however, little attention has been given to the role of that same caregiving environment to the development of infant cognition. Colombo and Saxon (2002) have proposed, however, that infant cognitive status (e.g., length of attention or ability to remember over a length of time) interacts with some aspect of caregiver interaction across development. Over time, these interactive processes influence the child's cognitive outcome. Similarly, it may be that by supporting infants in the development of attentional skill, in part to relieve early infant distress for example (Ruff & Rothbart, 1996), caregivers are contributing to the attentional skills associated with later cognitive processing. Thus, caregiver behavior may be essential for cognition as it is for socioemotional development, although how this is manifested is unknown.

Empirical evidence for the argument that parenting behaviors have an effect on children's brain development typically has focused on maltreated children (see reviews by Belsky & de Haan, 2011; Hughes, 2011). Maltreatment, however, is not the only contributor to less than optimal brain development. The prefrontal dopamine system associated with cognitive processes can be affected by environmental variations that are not as extreme as maltreatment (Diamond, 2011). Indeed, there are some reports that maternal caregiving behaviors during early childhood are associated with early childhood cognitive behaviors in normative samples. Research by Hughes and Ensor (2009), for example, indicates that maternal behaviors such as scaffolding and planning, as well as the level of family chaos, were predictive of children's cognitive abilities at age 4. Hammond, Muller, Carpendale, Bibok, and Liebermann-Finestone (2012) also report associations between maternal scaffolding and children's cognitive abilities at age 4.

There have been recent empirical reports that the caregiving environment during infancy contributes to the development of cognitive behaviors associated with frontal functioning during toddlerhood and early childhood. Bernier, Carlson, and Whipple (2010) reported that maternal sensitivity, mind–mindedness, and autonomy support, measured when infants were 12 and 15 months of age, predicted toddler cognition both 6-months and 1-year later, with autonomy support emerging as the strongest predictor. The authors speculated that responsive parenting could be the mechanism for promoting cognitive development through its effects on neurological development. It is generally accepted that early experiences play a role in brain development, as environmental experiences shape the synaptic pruning and cultivation that occur in infancy (e.g., Greenough, Black, & Wallace, 1987). Bernier and colleagues (2010) suggested that responsive parenting in infancy may promote cognitive development indirectly, by supporting optimal neural development, and directly, by providing an appropriate social environment to observe and practice positive regulatory strategies associated with cognition.

The work by Bernier and colleagues also examined the effects of maternal behaviors during infancy on child cognitive development up to age 3 (Bernier et al., 2010; Matte-Gagne & Bernier, 2011). In our own work (Kraybill & Bell, 2013), we extended the length of time that maternal behaviors affect child cognition. We measured mother's positive affect during her interactions with her 10-month-old infant and demonstrated that this maternal behavior was correlated with cognitive skills several years later at ages 4 and 6, in early childhood and early middle childhood, respectively. We also demonstrated that measures of infant frontal electrophysiology (the electroencephalogram, [EEG]) likewise predicted cognitive skills at these older ages (Kraybill & Bell, 2013).

What may be most intriguing is that we can find no empirical data in the literature demonstrating that parenting behaviors during infancy are associated with infant cognition in normative samples. Perhaps this means that "time" is a critical aspect of the mechanism by which parenting behaviors impact cognitive development. Indeed, if the biopsychosocial perspective involves a multilevel approach with bidirectional influences over time, then we may need to discover the best ruler and the best clock (i.e., Fischer & Rose, 1994) in order to assess the influence of parent behaviors on infant cognitive development.

Cascades and Systems Beyond Infancy

Infant cognitive behavior is complicated. Researchers of infant cognition and perception work to understand the complex associations among multiple levels of biology, behavior, social environment, and other aspects of infant development, without getting mired in the muck of rich interpretation and simple maturational explanations. At the same time, there is great appreciation that these infant cognitive behaviors, based many times on simple looking time measures, have great predictive value for later, more sophisticated cognitive skills. Various measures of infant information processing (e.g., speed of habituation, visual recognition memory, looking time) are related to cognitive development in childhood (e.g., Bornstein & Sigman, 1986; Colombo, 1993: Cuevas & Bell, 2014), early adolescence (Rose, Feldman, & Jankowski, 2012), and even to intelligence in adulthood (Fagan, Holland, & Wheeler, 2007). This longitudinal process is often conceived of as a "developmental cascade" if there are assessments across multiple ages, where structures, functions, or processes in the individual child demonstrate a unique longitudinal pattern (Bornstein, Hahn, & Suwalsky, 2013).

The most intriguing longitudinal studies, however, are those that have a more biopsychosocial perspective and include not only infant endogenous factors but also exogenous factors such as parenting behaviors, parent education, and home environment. Although sometimes referred to as encompassing a "systems" perspective in the literature (e.g., Bornstein, Hahn, & Wolke, 2013), we can conceptualize the multilevel interactions from a biopsychosocial point of view. Here are two examples of recent studies.

Bornstein and colleagues (2013) reported that information-processing efficiency during infancy was related to general mental development during toddlerhood, which was related to intelligence during middle childhood, which was in turn related to academic achievement during adolescence. Importantly, maternal education level contributed to academic achievement either directly or indirectly through its influence on toddler and middle childhood cognitive measures. In this model, maternal education was the only social or environmental factor that contributed to child cognitive development, although mothers reported on their parenting behaviors during the infancy portion of the study; the home environment was assessed by the research team during the infancy portion of the study as well. The impact of maternal education did not receive much attention in the discussion of the findings, however.

Our research team focused on the cognitive development of children at ages 24, 36, and 48 months, and examined three aspects of the caregiving environment at 10, 24, and 35 months: maternal education, maternal cognition, and maternal parenting behaviors (Cuevas et al., 2014). The cognitive processes we examined were those associated with complex processing, rather than more simple-looking behaviors. In thinking about potential mechanisms, we turned to the conceptual framework suggested by Calkins (2011) concerning the multiple biological and behavioral levels at which caregiving affects children. Calkins has noted that maternal caregiver behavior must be regulated within the caregiver, so as to affect her own behavior, and that caregiver behavior must also be regulatory between the caregiver and the child. We found that maternal cognition and maternal caregiving during infancy provide unique information about child cognitive development during toddlerhood and early childhood. Maternal caregiving also mediated the effects of maternal cognition on child cognitive development. These associations were evident even after controlling for the effects of maternal education. Although our assessments of cognition did not include infancy, it was the caregiving measures during infancy that affected later child cognitive development. The biopsychosocial aspects of our study are evident in our focus on cognitive development situated within developmental time and within a social environment.

Conclusion

Infant cognition and perception are complicated and considering infant behaviors within a biopsychosocial framework makes infant cognition appear even more complex. To adopt a nativistic or maturational framework or to reduce complex cognitive processes into individual component behaviors in order to simply infant cognition may be appealing on the surface. This attempt at simplification, however, fails to capture an informative view of infant cognition and perception. It fails to capture the biopsychosocial view that cognition is the consequence of the complex, multileveled, inseparable physical, biological, and social environments with which the infant interacts during development. The biopsychosocial perspective presents a comprehensive view of infancy. The chapter authors in this infant cognition and perception section highlight the value of such a perspective in studying the complicated behaviors of a complex system.

ACKNOWLEDGMENTS

The writing of this chapter was supported by Grant No. HD049878 from the Eunice Kennedy Shriver National Institute of Child Health and Human Development (NICHD). The content is solely the responsibility of the author and does not necessarily represent the official views of the NICHD or the National Institutes of Health. Conversations with Leigh Bacher, Kimberly Cuevas, and Amy Learmonth at the 2013 meeting of the International Society for Developmental Psychobiology were instrumental in shaping my thinking about how to focus these introductory remarks to Part II of this handbook.

REFERENCES

Baillargeon, R., & Graber, M. (1987). Where is the rabbit?: 5.5-month-old infants' representation of the height of a hidden object. *Cognitive Development, 2,* 375–392.

Bell, M. A., & Fox, N. A. (1992). The relations between frontal brain electrical activity and cognitive development during infancy. *Child Development, 63,* 1142–1163.

Belsky, J., & de Haan, M. (2011). Annual research review: Parenting and children's brain development: The end of the beginning. *Journal of Child Psychology and Psychiatry, 52,* 409–428.

Bernier, A., Carlson, S. M., & Whipple, N. (2010). From external regulation to self-regulation: Early parenting precursors of young children's executive functioning. *Child Development, 81,* 326–339.

Bogartz, R. S., Shinskey, J. L., & Speaker, C. (1997). Interpreting infant looking. *Developmental Psychology, 33,* 408–422.

Bornstein, M. H., Hahn, C.-S., & Suwalsky, J. T. D. (2013). Physically developed and exploratory young infants contribute to their own long-term academic achievement. *Psychological Science, 24,* 1906–1917.

Bornstein, M. H., Hahn, C.-S., & Wolke, D. (2013). Systems and cascades in cognitive development and academic achievement. *Child Development, 84,* 154–162.

Bornstein, M. H., & Sigman, M. D. (1986). Continuity in mental development from infancy. *Child Development, 57,* 251–274.

Calkins, S. D. (2011). Caregiving as coregulation: Psychobiological processes and child functioning. In A. Booth, S. M. McHale, & N. S. Landale (Eds.), *Biosocial foundations of family processes* (pp. 49–59). New York: Springer.

Calkins, S. D., Propper, C., & Mills-Koonce, W. R. (2013). A biopsychosocial perspective on parenting and developmental psychopathology. *Development and Psychopathology, 25,* 1399–1414.

Colombo, J. (1993). *Infant cognition: Predicting later intellectual functioning.* Newbury Park, CA: Sage.

Colombo, J., & Saxon, T. F. (2002). Infant attention and the development of cognition: Does the environment moderate continuity? In H. E. Fitzgerald, K. H. Karraker, & T. Luster (Eds.), *Infant development: Ecological perspectives* (pp. 35–60). Washington, DC: Garland Press.

Cuevas, K., & Bell, M. A. (2014). Infant attention and early childhood executive function. *Child Development, 85,* 397–404.

Cuevas, K., Bell, M. A., Marcovitch, S., & Calkins, S. D. (2012). Electroencephalogram and heart rate measures of working memory at 5 and 10 months. *Developmental Psychology, 48,* 907–917.

Cuevas, K., Deater-Deckard, K., Watson, A. J., Kim-Spoon, J., Morasch, K. C., & Bell, M. A. (2014). What's mom got to do with it?: Contributions of maternal executive function and caregiving to the development of executive function across early childhood. *Developmental Science, 17*, 224–238.

Diamond, A. (1990). The development and neural bases of memory functions as indexed by the AB and delayed response tasks in human infants and infant monkeys. In A. Diamond (Ed.), *The development and neural bases of higher cognitive functions* (pp. 267–317). New York: New York Academy of Sciences Press.

Diamond, A. (2011). Biological and social influences on cognitive control processes dependent on prefrontal cortext. In O. Braddick, J. Atkinson, & G. Innocenti (Eds.), *Progress in brain research* (Vol. 189, pp. 319–340). Burlington, MA: Academic Press.

Fagan, J. F., Holland, C. R., & Wheeler, K. (2007). The prediction, from infancy, of adult IQ and achievement. *Intelligence, 35*, 225–231.

Fischer, K. W., & Rose, S. P. (1994). Dynamic development of coordination of components in brain and behavior: A framework for theory and research. In G. Dawson & K. W. Fischer (Eds.), *Human behavior and the developing brain* (pp. 3–66). New York: Guilford Press.

Greenough, W. T., Black, J. E., & Wallace, C. S. (1987). Experience and brain development. *Child Development, 58*, 539–559.

Haith, M. M. (1998). Who put the cog in infant cognition?: Is rich interpretation too costly? *Infant Behavior and Development, 21*, 167–179.

Hamlin, J. K., Wynn, K., & Bloom, P. (2007). Social evaluation by preverbal infants. *Nature, 450*, 557–559.

Hammond, S. I., Muller, U., Carpendale, J. I., Bibok, M. B., & Liebermann-Finestone, D. P. (2012). The effects of parental scaffolding on preschoolers' executive function. *Developmental Psychology, 48*, 271–281.

Hayne, H. (2013, November). Communicating developmental psychobiology to the government. In H. E. Montgomery-Downs (Chair), *Communicating developmental psychobiology*. Symposium conducted at the annual meeting of the International Society for Developmental Psychobiology, San Diego, CA.

Hughes, C. (2011). Changes and challenges in 20 years of research into the development of executive functions. *Infant and Child Development, 20*, 251–271.

Hughes, C. H., & Ensor, R. A. (2009). How do families help or hinder the emergence of early executive function? In C. Lewis & J. I. M. Carpendale (Eds.), Social interaction and the development of executive function. *New Directions in Child and Adolescent Development, 123*, 35–50.

Kraybill, J. H., & Bell, M. A. (2013). Infancy predictors of preschool and post-kindergarten executive function. *Developmental Psychobiology, 55*, 530–538.

Lewkowicz, D. J. (2011). The biological implausibility of the nature–nurture dichotomy and what it means for the study of infancy. *Infancy, 16*, 331–367.

Lickliter, R. (2012). Exploring the dynamics of development and evolution: Comment on Blair and Raver (2012). *Developmental Psychology, 48*, 658–661.

Lickliter, R. (2013, November). Communicating developmental psychobiology to nativists. In H. E. Montgomery-Downs (Chair), *Communicating developmental psychobiology*. Symposium conducted at the annual meeting of the International Society for Developmental Psychobiology, San Diego, CA.

Lickliter, R., & Honeycutt, H. (2003). Developmental dynamics: Toward a biologically plausible evolutionary psychology. *Psychological Bulletin, 129*, 819–835.

Lickliter, R., & Honeycutt, H. (2013). A developmental evolutionary framework for psychology. *Review of General Psychology, 17*, 184–189.

Matte-Gagne, C., & Bernier, A. (2011). Prospective relations between maternal autonomy support and child executive functioning: Investigating the mediating role of child language ability. *Journal of Experimental Child Psychology, 110*, 611–625.

Michel, G. F., & Moore, C. L. (1995). *Developmental psychobiology: An interdisciplinary science.* Cambridge MA: MIT Press.

Montgomery-Downs, H. E. (2013, November). Introduction. In H. E. Montgomery-Downs (Chair), *Communicating developmental psychobiology.* Symposium conducted at the annual meeting of the International Society for Developmental Psychobiology, San Diego, CA.

Newcombe, N. (2014). Exploring infant cognition. *Observer, 27*(10).

Oakes, L. M. (2009). The "Humpty Dumpty problem" in the study of early cognitive development. *Perspectives on Psychological Science, 4*, 352–358.

Rose, S. A., Feldman, J. F., & Jankowski, J. J. (2012). Implications of infant cognition for executive functions at age 11. *Psychological Science, 23*, 1345–1355.

Ruff, H. A., & Rothbart, M. K. (1996). *Attention in early development: Themes and variations.* New York: Oxford University Press.

Sameroff, A. (2010). A unified theory of development: A dialectic integration of nature and nurture. *Child Development, 81*, 6–22.

Scarf, D., Imuta, K., Colombo, M., & Hayne, H. (2012). Social evaluation or simple association?: Simple associations may explain moral reasoning in infants. *PLoS ONE, 7*, e42698.

Spelke, E. S. (1998). Nativism, empiricism, and the origins of knowledge. *Infant Behavior and Development, 21*, 181–200.

Spencer, J. P., Blumberg, M. S., McMurray, B., Robinson, S. R., Samuelson, L. K., & Tomblin, J. B. (2009). Short arms and talking eggs: Why we should no longer abide the nativist–empiricist debate. *Child Development Perspectives, 3*, 79–87.

Thompson, R. A. (2006). The development of the person: Social understanding, relationships, self, conscience. In W. Damon & R. M. Lerner (Series Eds.) & N. Eisenberg (Vol. Ed.), *Handbook of child psychology: Vol. 3. Social, emotional, and personality development* (6th ed., pp. 24–98). New York: Wiley.

Wynn, K. (1992). Addition and subtraction by human infants. *Nature, 358*, 749–750.

CHAPTER 4

A Biopsychosocial Perspective on Looking Behavior in Infancy

Lisa M. Oakes

The goal of this chapter is to understand the development of attention, considering a biospsychosocial perspective. Historically, in the field of infancy, *looking* and *attending* have been equated. Rather than considering looking as a measure of attentional processes, infancy research has drawn conclusions about attention from patterns of looking. For example, studies examined stimulus factors that influence infants' looking (or attention); how looking (or attention) changed over trials, with familiarity, and across development; and hypotheses were generated about what factors underlie attention getting (i.e., the latency to look) versus attention holding (i.e., the duration of looking). This literature has yielded significant understanding into the factors that contribute to looking behavior in infancy, and how looking behavior changes with development. However, conclusions about the underlying attentional processes from such studies are indirect, and are probably incomplete. We know that adults frequently covertly shift their attention in the absence of eye movements, and that looking and attention are not the same thing. We know little about covert shifts of attention in prelinguistic infants, although some work examining event-related potentials (ERPs) and looking behavior suggest that young infants also can covertly shift attention (Richards, 2000, 2001). More problematic, however, is that in the infant literature *attention* is not often thought of as a *process*; rather, *looking* is an outcome measure. This contrasts with an enormous literature on the processes by which the direction of visual attention and gaze is controlled in adults. To be clear, outcome measures can inform us about process, but deeper understanding into attention in infancy—and how it relates to attention at different points in development—is gained by thinking about attentional processes.

This chapter examines the development of visual attention processes—and looking behavior—as influenced by multiple factors. Visual attention development will be best understood by considering how these multiple factors operate together. Infants' developing attentional processes are determined by (1) the neuroanatomical structures involved in controlling eye movements, attention, and visual perception; (2) cognitive developmental changes in memory, perceptual abilities, and so on; and (3) the infants' social history, and what events, objects, and people have been encountered (and looked at) before. In other words, looking behavior develops and changes as a function of developmental changes in the underlying biological, cognitive, and social systems that contribute to attentional processes.

This approach contrasts with the large body of research studying and measuring infants' looking behavior in which looking behavior is considered a *tool* for answering questions about other topics. This study of looking behavior has been extremely important in our understanding of cognitive development. In my own lab, for example, we have used infants' looking behavior as a tool for understanding infants' visual causal perception (Oakes, 1994), object categorization (Oakes & Ribar, 2005), and visual short-term memory (Oakes, Baumgartner, Barrett, Messenger, & Luck, 2013). The body of work relying on looking as a tool has underlying assumptions (both tested and untested) that infants' looking is determined by stimulus properties, such as the novelty or complexity of the stimulus (Cohen, DeLoache, & Rissman, 1975; Fantz & Fagan, 1975; Martin, 1975); by infants' surprise or recognition that an outcome is unexpected (Baillargeon, 1987a; Needham, Baillargeon, & Kaufman, 1997; Wilcox, Schweinle, & Chapa, 2003); or by a drive to acquire information or form representations (Colombo & Mitchell, 2009). Although foundational work examined the bases of infants' looking behavior, with only a few exceptions most researchers relying on visual attention and looking in infants are more concerned with looking as a *measure* or *indicator* of cognitive processes, than as looking (and visual attention) as a process to be studied.

The framework adopted here is based on the assumption that cognitive development reflects learning and development at multiple levels. Therefore, this chapter considers how looking time and attentional processes reflect the interaction of neuroanatomical changes, the infants' history in terms of everyday interactions with people and things, and cognitive developmental changes. The general framework derives from the argument that much of the field of infant cognitive development suffers from the "Humpty Dumpty problem" (Oakes, 2009). That is, researchers have tended to study cognitive abilities in isolation (i.e., breaking cognition into pieces), rather than examining how multiple abilities codevelop or operate together in development (i.e., putting the pieces back together again). In the present case, the focus is on the development of a single broad process—infants' visual attention (although there are many different specific behaviors related to this process)—with an eye to the multiple levels or factors that contribute to development.

Historical Perspectives on the Study of Looking Time or Visual Attention in Infancy

As a first step, we consider how visual attention has been studied in infancy. Historically, the study of visual attention in infancy was the same as the study of infant looking. Researchers asked questions about how long infants looked, where they looked (when given a choice), how fast they looked, and so on. Experiments provided descriptions of how infants' looking, including habituation and novelty preference, varies with age and the stimulus presented (Colombo & Mitchell, 2009; Ruff & Rothbart, 1996). Some programs of research attempted to uncover the mechanisms of these developmental changes. For example, based both on observed changes in looking behavior and our limited understanding of the development of the neuroanatomical structures thought to subserve visual attentional networks, researchers speculated that changes in control of looking shifts reflect the development from attentional control primarily by subcortical structures to increasing involvement of cortical structures (Johnson, 1990). Other researchers explored mechanisms external to the infant, such as how parental interactions with infants facilitate and encourage infants' visual attention and looking behaviors (Landry & Chapieski, 1988; Landry, Chapieski, & Schmidt, 1986; Landry, Garner, Swank, & Baldwin, 1996). Finally, some researchers have examined the connection between cognitive-processing and looking behaviors, attributing developmental changes in looking to developmental changes in cognitive abilities (Cohen, 1998).

All this work on infants' looking time originated with the pioneering work of Fantz (1958, 1964), using the apparatus depicted in Figure 4.1. Based on work with chimpanzees, Fantz created this apparatus in which infants were placed in front of a chamber, and two images were presented directly in their line of sight. The observer recorded both the direction of the infants' looking (i.e., to the left or right picture) and how long the infants looked. Using procedures like this, Fantz and his colleagues made numerous observations that shaped our understanding of the origins and early development of visual ability, perception, and cognition. A primary question addressed in these early studies was whether infants had pattern vision, questioning conventional wisdom at the time that pattern vision emerged with learning. Fantz and his colleagues (Fantz, 1963; Fantz & Nevis, 1967) examined visual preference of infants between birth and 6 months of age for black-and-white patterns, faces, checkerboards, stripes, shapes, and other stimuli; demonstrated that infants perceive patterns from birth; and that their pattern perception develops over the first postnatal months.

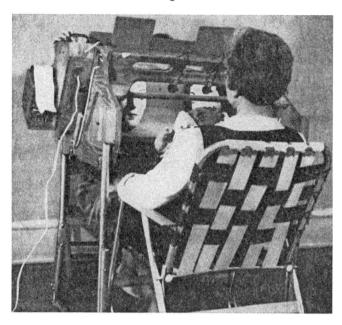

FIGURE 4.1. The infant visual preference procedure developed by Fantz. From Fantz and Nevis (1967). Copyright 1967 by Wayne State University Press. Reprinted by permission.

On the basis of such studies, Fantz and Nevis (1967) argued that the infant visual system is characterized by "selectivity for patterns" consistent with evidence from nonhuman animals that the visual system responds more strongly to perceptual input rather than unpatterned light. Further work revealed that not only do infants selectively attend to some stimuli over others, but that their looking at stimuli reflected the relative familiarity or novelty of the stimulus. In an extremely important study, Fantz (1964) presented infants with pairs of stimuli over a series of trials. One of the stimuli remained the same from trial to trial; the other stimulus in each pair was different on each trial. All infants started out at approximately 50%, which indicates looking equally at the two items. But, infants 2 months and older gradually shifted more and more of their looking toward the new stimulus on each trial, reducing the proportion of their looking devoted to the unchanging stimulus. Fantz (1964) concluded that this pattern indicated "perception, recognition, and satiation of interest in a particular pattern" (p. 669).

This foundational study led to an explosion of studies examining infants' changing looking as a function of familiarization. The data from one such study are presented in Figure 4.2. In this study, Pancratz and Cohen (1970) presented 4-month-old infants with a single colored shape (e.g., a green circle, a blue triangle) on a series of trials. Infants' looking on each trial was recorded, and the total looking duration on each block of two trials is presented in Figure 4.2. The bottom line is that infants' looking systematically decreased as the stimulus

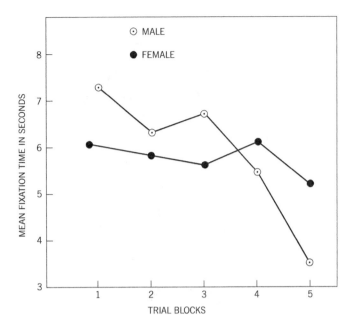

FIGURE 4.2. Decrease in looking time by 4-month-old infants across trials as observed by Pancratz and Cohen (1970). From Pancratz and Cohen (1970). Copyright 1970 by Elsevier. Reprinted by permission.

became familiar over those blocks. Studies like this opened the door for using this procedure (or a variation) to study many aspects of infants' memory, perception, and other cognitive abilities. These studies conducted in the 1960s and 1970s established that infants' visual preferences could be measured by simply recording their looking behavior, and that we can understand something about infants' attentional, perceptual, and cognitive processes by examining differences in looking. Decades later we see the legacy of this discovery. Infants' looking behavior is widely used in the field not to only understand perception, memory, and attention but also to draw conclusions about infants' inferences, reasoning, and beliefs. Looking has been used to probe infants' understanding of the emotional states, motivations, and goals of actors. More recently, the availability of automatic infrared eye trackers has allowed researchers to dive even deeper into how infants think, learn, and attend.

Initially, Fantz's seminal work was used to identify the factors that control infants' looking behaviors. Studies revealed that infants looked longer at complex than at simple stimuli, at least if the complex stimuli did not exceed some difficult to define maximum level of complexity (Brennan, Ames, & Moore, 1966; Greenberg & O'Donnell, 1972; Hunter, Ames, & Koopman, 1983). Moreover, the observation that infants' looking changes over familiarization led to the procedures designed to uncover limits and characteristics of memory processes (Cohen, DeLoache, & Pearl, 1977; Cohen et al., 1975; Cohen & Gelber,

1975; Fagan, 1970, 1971, 1972, 1973, 1977b; McCall, 1973; McCall, Kennedy, & Dodds, 1977; Rose, Gottfried, Mello-Carmina, & Bridger, 1982).

This body of work as a whole reveals several important facts about infants' looking. First, from a young age, infants' looking is not random. Infants have *preferences*—that is, they look at some stimuli more than at others. Of course, we are unable to determine whether or not such biases reflect voluntary processes (and our current understanding of brain development would suggest that in the first few months after birth such preferences reflect involuntary processes), but evidence of visual preferences results show that infants' looking—and attention—is systematic.

The second fact revealed by this body of work is that infants' looking—and visual attention—changes over development. An example of development is illustrated in Figure 4.3. These data come from a study comparing looking patterns by infants of several different ages to the same stimuli (Martin, 1975). In general, this study reveals that—consistent with the data from a number of studies—given the same stimuli and experimental procedures, older infants look for shorter durations than do younger infants, older infants' looking duration habituates more quickly, and visual preferences for novelty become more robust over age (see Colombo & Mitchell, 2009; Rose, Feldman, & Jankowski, 2004, for a review). Thus, infants' visual attention and looking behavior change over developmental time. What such findings do not reveal is *why* infants' looking behavior changes. Each type of change may reflect changes in neuroanatomical structures, cognitive processing, or social influences on looking.

The field was only beginning to scratch the surface in our understanding of the processes of attention in infancy, and how they develop, when a strong interest emerged in the 1980s on using infants' looking as a tool to understand other aspects of cognition. The work demonstrating that looking time reflected (in part) infants' memory and preference for novelty allowed researchers to examine other aspects of infants' cognitive processing based on their looking behavior. Researchers began to use looking time measures to ask how infants' categorized stimuli (Strauss, 1979; Younger, 1985), whether they recognized that objects maintain their physical properties when hidden (Baillargeon, 1987b), and whether they were sensitive to physical constraints in the world (Spelke, Kestenbaum, Simons, & Wein, 1995). Clever experimental designs allowed researchers to analyze looking patterns and draw conclusions about the development of perceptual, memory, and cognitive abilities in infancy. Indeed, this tradition continues as researchers use looking time to uncover developmental changes in visual short-term memory abilities (Ross-Sheehy, Oakes, & Luck, 2003), the features used in object individuation (Wilcox, 1999), and sensitivity to numerical information (Cordes & Brannon, 2009), to name just a few domains of inquiry. With the introduction of eye trackers, experimental designs have emerged that allow us to ask other kinds of questions, for example, questions about the kinds of expectations infants form for sequences of events

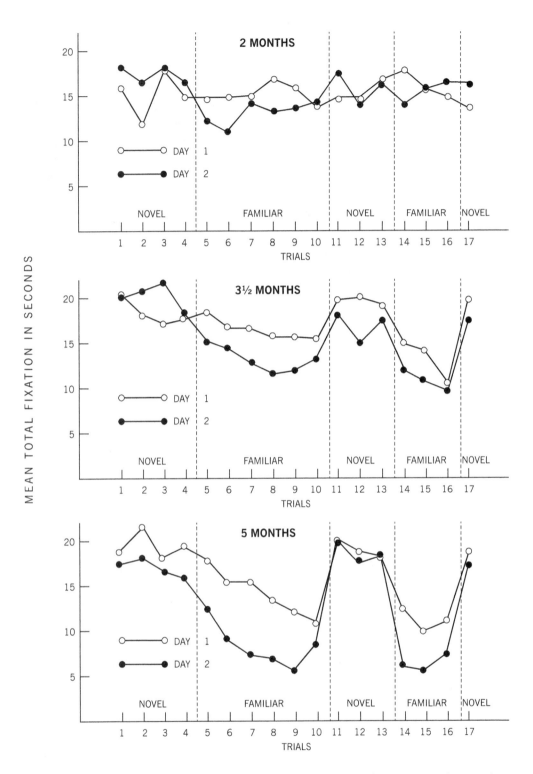

FIGURE 4.3. Data reported by Martin (1975) on looking patterns by 2-, 3.5-, and 5-month-old infants over repeated trials with the same novel and familiar stimuli on different testing days. From Martin (1975). Copyright 1975 by the American Psychological Association. Reprinted by permission.

(Kirkham, Slemmer, Richardson, & Johnson, 2007) or the actions of other people (Gredebäck, Stasiewicz, Falck-Ytter, Rosander, & von Hofsten, 2009). The point is that looking time has been an important tool for understanding basic cognitive development, and researchers have discovered ways to make inferences about other abilities from infants' looking patterns. However, the rise in interest in using looking as a tool has meant that there has been relatively less focus on the factors that contribute to the development of looking—and visual attention—itself.

To be clear, it is not that this question was completely abandoned. Some researchers have used careful experimental designs, novel tasks, and nonlooking measures, to provide some understanding of developmental change in visual attention itself. For example, researchers measuring heart rate (Richards, 1989; Richards & Casey, 1992) or behavioral and facial expression changes (Oakes & Tellinghuisen, 1994; Ruff, 1986) have shown that infants' looking at a target actually reflects different levels of attentional engagement or arousal, or attentional state. Others have used marker tasks, or tasks for which the neural substrates have been identified in adults through lesions and imaging, to understand infants' visual attention (Harman, Posner, Rothbart, & Thomas-Thrapp, 1994). One problem with such an approach is that it is impossible to design a task for infants that truly has all the elements of the adult version of the task, and this raises the possibility that a slight task variation may result in different processes being assessed.

Thus, there does exist a body of work aimed at understanding the development of visual attention itself—that is, studies that have explored the processes of attention, and not only studies that have used looking behavior as a tool. This work has provided a deeper understanding into the nature of visual attention itself and has yielded understanding into the general development of infants' visual attention.

What Is *Attention*?

Before exploring what is known about the development of visual attention in infancy, we must be clear what is meant by the term *attention*. Although William James (1890) famously said that "Everyone knows what attention is," more recent discussions have made it clear that the term *attention* is used to refer to a number of different interrelated processes (see, e.g., Chun, Golomb, & Turk-Browne, 2011; Luck & Vecera, 2002). Indeed, an influential volume of essays on attention in the 1980s was entitled *Varieties of Attention* (Parasuraman & Davies, 1984). Thus, one problem with studying attention is that there is no single way it has been defined. The term *attention* is often used to describe situations when there is more information available than can be processed or when decisions must be made about which of several available dimensions should be used to make distinctions among items. Thus attention is involved in *selecting* information for processing, *inhibiting* responding to nonselected or irrelevant information, and *maintaining* focus on the relevant information. Casually, we may ask a child to "pay attention," roughly meaning to stay on-task and to ignore distractions. We may also be frustrated by a spouse's ability to focus his or her attention so deeply on the newspaper that he or she does not realize that children are asking for the milk to be passed. We may also talk about what captures our attention—how features of the world are difficult to ignore and what we find compelling. Considered together, these examples illustrate that attention is not a unified concept, and that the phrase *visual attention* may mean different things in different contexts.

Several different theoretical accounts or taxonomies of attention have been proposed. In an influential model, Posner and Petersen (Petersen & Posner, 2012; Posner & Petersen, 1990) described distinct networks for three aspects of attention: *alerting*, *orienting*, and *control*. These networks are involved in different attentional functions and they are each subserved by different neural structures. The alerting attentional network is involved in the system's ability to *sustain* attention, and involves (at least in adults) frontal and parietal brain regions. This network is involved in the ability to maintain an attentional state for a period of time. The orienting attentional network is involved in the *selection* of information to process, either by selecting a location in space or by selecting a particular type of information; this network involves either a dorsal stream set of connections including frontal eye fields and the intraparietal sulcus or a more ventral stream set of connections involving the temporoparietal junction and the ventral frontal cortex. The *executive attentional network* is involved in *switching*, *inhibiting*, and general top-down control of attention, and involves frontal cortices and the anterior cingulate cortex.

Attention in Infancy

All of these aspects of attention develop during infancy, and developmental changes in sustained attention, selective attention, and attentional control are reflected in the duration of infants' looking at stimuli, their preference to look at some stimuli over others, their latency to look at a stimulus, and so on. It also seems clear, however, that looking behaviors (such as durations, switching, and latency) reflect multiple systems—that is, there is no single indicator of attentional alerting, orienting, or control. When shown a pair of stimuli presented side by side, for example, the duration of infants' looking to one of the stimuli reflects their ability to sustain attention to the preferred stimuli, to inhibit responding to the nonpreferred stimuli, and to select one stimulus to be the focus of attention. Moreover, their cognitive processing of each stimulus, the meaning of the stimuli for the infant, and their past experience with items like the stimuli all may contribute to their behavior in this context.

Nevertheless, Posner and Petersen's taxonomy is useful for describing developmental changes in infancy in attention, and can provide a framework for understanding the factors that contribute to those developmental changes. For example, because the parietal and frontal brain regions involved in sustained attention in adults (Posner & Petersen, 1990) are poorly developed early in infancy, alerting—and sustained attention—are mediated mainly by subcortical structures such as the superior colliculus (Colombo, 2001). But it is not the case that these processes are nonfunctioning early in infancy. Richards and colleagues (reviewed in Richards & Casey, 1992) measured heart rate changes during infants' looking, and have identified several heart rate-defined attentional phases during a look that presumably reflect different levels of attentional engagement, or different levels of arousal. In particular, the period of sustained attention, indicated by a sustained decrease in heart rate, is similar to Posner and Petersen's alerting attentional processes. During sustained attention (as defined by a decrease in heart rate), infants are less easily distracted by other stimuli (Richards, 1997b) and they learn more about stimuli they view during sustained attention (compared with stimuli they view during other heart rate-defined attentional phases; Richards, 1997a). Thus, this phase of attention seems to reflect when infants are maintaining an engaged attentional state.

Although sustained attention is observed in very young infants, it undergoes substantial development over the course of infancy. For example, changes in the cardiac response during sustained attention changes over the first 5 or 6 months suggest increasing engagement during sustained attention (Casey & Richards, 1988). Beyond 6 months, infants' ability to sustain attention continues to develop in terms of increased endogenous control of attention (see Colombo, 2001). For example, using a *distraction* procedure, my colleagues and I observed an increase in development over infants' endogenous control of attention between 6 and 10 months (Oakes, Kannass, & Shaddy, 2002). In this study, infants' were observed playing with (and attending to) an attractive, colorful, multipart target (a toy that was affixed to a suction cup on a high-chair tray) in the presence of a distractor (a colorful, blinking light presented on a nearby TV screen, accompanied by a sound). In this context, infants are generally more resistant to distraction—and thus more deeply engaged attentionally—when judged to be in a focused or concentrated state (i.e., looking at the toy with signs of concentration, such as furrowed brow and slowed motor movements) than when judged to be in a more casual attentional state (i.e., looking at the toy with a relaxed facial expression; Oakes & Tellinghuisen, 1994), and after they have been looking at the target for relatively longer periods of time (Oakes, Ross-Sheehy, & Kannass, 2004). As evidence of increasing endogenous control over attention, we found in this context an increase over age in infants' ability to effectively moderate their resistance to distraction as a function of the importance of maintaining attention to the toys (Oakes et al., 2002). Following familiarization with two toys, 9- and 10-month-old infants were slower to look at a distractor when they were investigating never-before-seen toys than when they were investigating the toys explored during the familiarization phase. At 6 months, infants' latencies to look at the distractor were the same for relatively familiar and relatively novel toys. We concluded that this developmental shift reflected, at least in part, infants' emerging endogenous control over attentional state. Thus, there appear to be changes in cortical control over and engagement in the alerting attention network in the second half of the first postnatal year.

Changes during infancy from involuntary control to more voluntary control also can be seen in selective attention. Young infants are often described as completely stimulus driven. From the first weeks after birth, infants have the ability to attend selectively—when presented with two stimuli, side by side, infants show a preference for (i.e., look at more) one stimulus (Fantz, 1963). Thus, they can look at (select) one stimulus and inhibit moving their gaze toward the other. But, this selectivity in early infancy seems to be involuntary. Dannemiller (1998, 2000) found, for example, that infants younger than 4 months are automatically drawn to look at moving or red targets. In other words, young infants have little control over the stimulus to which they attend; instead, some stimulus characteristics seem to automatically capture their attention. Such selection appears to rapidly become under more cortical control. For example, Mondloch and colleagues (1999) demonstrated that whereas newborn infants' preferences to look at faces appears to be determined by subcortical structures, by 6 weeks infants' preference to look at faces appears to be determined by developing cortical structures.

Additional understanding of the development of early selection and orienting comes from examination in infants of phenomena observed in adults. One phenomenon is *inhibition of return* (IOR). Although the onset of a stimulus at a location initially biases the system to orient toward that location, once a location is attended there is a tendency for the system to avoid returning attention to that location (Klein, 2000). This tendency to inhibit refocusing attention to a previously attended location presumably reflects the system's apparent interest in novelty, and perhaps the drive to search the environment efficiently. Because IOR is thought to involve the superior colliculus (Klein, 2000), this aspect of orienting should be present early in infancy. Indeed, IOR has been observed in newborn infants (Simion, Valenza, Umiltà, & Barba, 1995; Valenza, Simion, & Umiltà, 1994), although dramatic changes in IOR have been observed between 3 and 6 months of age (Clohessy, Posner, Rothbart, & Vecera, 1991). Changes over this time period may reflect changes in neural connectivity that controls IOR, such as connections to and from the superior colliculus, or the difficulties of measuring precisely these behaviors in young infants (i.e., differences in findings may reflect differences in testing procedures, stimuli, and so on). It is clear that at least later in infancy, IOR is related to broader attentional mechanisms; Markant and Amso (2013) observed selective learning in a context that elicited IOR. That is, using an IOR procedure to manipulate the location of infants' selective attention, Markant and Amso found that 9-month-old infants learned more about items presented at the attended location than at items presented at the unattended location.

A second phenomenon is *gaze shifting* when two stimuli compete for attention. Much of our understanding of infants' ability to engage in gaze shifting comes from studies using a *gap-overlap procedure*. In this task, infants' attention is drawn to a central point via an interesting fixation stimulus. At some point, a new stimulus is presented in the periphery, and infants' latency to look at that new stimulus is recorded. In "gap" trials, the central stimulus is removed before the peripheral stimulus is presented—thus, there is no competition for attention. In "overlap" trials, the peripheral stimulus is presented while the infant is still fixating on the central stimulus, and thus the infant must disengage from one stimulus to orient to the other. In the first few postnatal months, infants' exhibit "sticky fixations," and have difficulty disengaging from the central stimulus to the simultaneously presented peripheral stimulus (Hood, 1995), consistent with earlier observations that young infants engage in "obligatory attention" (Stechler & Latz, 1966) and are apparently unable to voluntarily look away from a stimulus. Thus, for very young infants, competition for attention presents a difficult problem. This difficulty may reflect a bias against responding when the infant is engaged on a stimulus (Richards, 1997b); the inability to disengage, or break fixation, to the central stimulus (Hood, 1995); or problems with initiating an eye movement while looking at a central stimulus (Johnson, 1990).

Infants' ability to shift to the peripheral stimulus develops rapidly (Hunnius & Geuze, 2004), and by 6 months, infants' responding in the overlap trials looks similar to that of adults (Csibra, Tucker, & Johnson, 1998). To be clear, both 6-month-old and adult fixation is somewhat "sticky" in the overlap condition—they are slower to orient to the peripheral stimulus in the overlap trials than in the gap trials. But they disengage much more quickly than do younger infants. It is noteworthy that in older infants, the nature of the central stimulus can influence infants' responding in this task. For example, when the central stimulus is a human face, the affect depicted by that face (e.g., fearful vs. happy) determines how "sticky" fixation is in 7-month-old infants (Peltola, Leppänen, Palokangas, & Hietanen, 2008). Thus, infants' orienting, selection, and disengagement undergoes significant changes in the first 6 postnatal months, but factors such as the type of stimuli can induce differences in behavior even beyond this period.

Finally, our findings with the distraction procedure described earlier also reveal developmental changes in selection and orienting (Oakes et al., 2002, 2004; Oakes & Tellinghuisen, 1994). Recall that in our procedure we assess infants' response to a distractor as they play with and attend to a toy, affixed to a specific location on a high-chair tray. In general, 9- and 10-month-old infants are more resistant to distraction than are 6- to 7-month-old infants (Oakes et al., 2002; Oakes & Tellinghuisen, 1994), suggesting that these older infants could better *maintain* their selection of and orienting to the central target (in this case a colorful, complex, multipart toy) in the face of a (less informative) distractor. Thus, in this context inhibiting responding to the distractor is the more effective strategy for learning about the objects. The point is that the ability to selectively maintain attention to a target or shift attention to a new target develops across the first year.

These examples illustrating developmental changes in sustained and selective attention also reveal significant changes in attentional *control*. In the first postnatal months, attention is externally controlled: infants' attentional fixation seems obligatory (Stechler & Latz, 1966) and automatically orient toward some stimuli over others (Dannemiller, 1998, 2000). But, as is evident from the developmental changes described in this section, over the first 12 months infants increasingly become able to voluntarily control their attention. Over the first 6 months infants' level of engagement during sustained attention increases (Casey & Richards, 1988); by 6 months infants' gaze shifting when stimuli compete for attention looks adult-like (Csibra et al., 1998; Hunnius & Geuze, 2004); and between 6 and 10 months infants become increasingly able to resist distraction, particularly when attention is actively engaged in learning new information (Oakes et al., 2002).

Clearly, no task engages a single attention network, and none of these attentional processes operates in isolation. In a crowded visual scene, orienting and selection may involve disengagement. Top-down control may interact with the salience of particular features to determine where infants attend. The *interaction* of these different attentional processes determines where infants look, how long they look, how quickly they look, and so on. Thus, infants' looking behavior provides a window to these attentional processes, but understanding infants' attention from their looking requires carefully considering the multiple attentional processes that must be involved.

The following sections provide a discussion of the factors that contribute to these developments. As described earlier, the present framework is that the development of each of these processes reflect multiple factors interacting together. Thus, the final section presents a framework for understanding these developmental changes by considering the interaction of these multiple factors.

Biological, Psychological, and Social Influences on Attention Development

As described at the start of this chapter, we understand the development of attention—and cognitive processes more generally—as the result of multiple interacting factors. Just as developmental changes in visual attention behaviors and looking do not reflect the development of only one of the systems described in the previous section, those developmental changes do not reflect *only* biological *or* cognitive *or* social factors. Rather, we argue that during infancy, attentional processes develop through the interaction of such factors. The following sections describe the role of each of these types of factors.

Biological Factors That Contribute to Changes in Visual Attention

Neuroanatomical factors contribute to the development of attention networks. That is, developmental changes in infants' looking behaviors reflect, at least in part, the development of the neuroanatomical pathways involved in maintaining sustained attention, orienting and selecting, and controlling attention. Of course, these are not the only biological factors that contribute to infants' visual attention and looking behavior. At the most fundamental level, infants' visual behavior is constrained by the immaturity of the retina, including changes in the number, efficiency, and distribution of the photoreceptors. At birth, the peripheral parts of the retina resemble those of an adult, but the macula is very immature—the cells are immature, there are fewer of them, and their organization is different (Abramov et al., 1982). Moreover, even the neurotransmitting properties of these neurons in the newborn's retina are much less effective than those of an adult (Hollyfield, Frederick, & Rayborn, 1983). As a result, the weeks and months after birth are characterized by dramatic changes in vision as the retina becomes able to transmit more information about light to the parts of the brain that process such information. Indeed, during this period there are rapid changes in visual acuity and contrast sensitivity (see Banks & Dannemiller, 1987, for a review). These profound changes in what the infants can actually see most certainly contribute to the development of looking and visual attention in the first months of life.

In addition, infants' visual attention and looking behavior develop as a function of the maturation of brain regions involved in controlling eye movements, processing information from the retinas, and integrating different types of information. Researchers who study visual attention in adults examine the *cognitive neuroscience* of attention—the goal of this body of work is to understand brain–behavior relations. Developmental changes in infants' visual behavior must reflect (at least in part) the development of those brain–behavior relations. Indeed, we can generally characterize much of the changes in visual attention as reflecting a general shift to increasing cortical control of or engagement in visual attention, as cortical regions involved in vision and visual attention develop (Atkinson & Braddick, 2012; Johnson, 1990).

Consider the visual behavior of a newborn infant. At birth, infants exhibit visual preferences and saccadic pursuit tracking, likely controlled by the superior colliculus and the connections between the superior colliculus and the lateral geniculate nucleus (see Johnson, 2010, for a review). Recall that IOR can be observed in newborn infants (Valenza et al., 1994). IOR is thought to be a function of the superior colliculus because patients with damage to the superior colliculus do not show IOR and patients with cortical damage but an intact superior colliculus do show IOR (Klein, 2000). Thus, the developmental status of subcortical structures at birth allows newborn infants to engage in some visual attention processes, but they are unable to coordinate motor and visual abilities, resulting in what Atkinson (2000) refers to as "crude orienting."

Cortical control over visual behavior begins to develop rapidly, and we see many changes in visual behavior over the first postnatal year (and beyond) that likely reflect this increasing cortical control. For example, oculomotor control is achieved both by the superior colliculus and the frontal eye fields (Johnson, 1995). Developmental changes in the middle temporal area, and the magnocellular pathway allow smooth pursuit tracking by 2 months, and development by 4 months in the frontal eye fields and parvocellular pathway allow more anticipatory visual tracking (see Johnson, 1990, for a discussion). Moreover, changes in shifts of attention and inhibition of automatic saccades are likely due to maturation and connectivity of the frontal eye fields, and increasing engagement by cortical structures (Hood & Atkinson, 1993). However, subcortical structures—and the connections and communication between those structures and cortical structures—continue to develop. Thus, it is important not to oversimplify the developmental trajectory as visual attention being fully subcortically controlled to visual attention being fully cortically controlled (Johnson, 1990).

Consider as an example the changes in the *gap-overlap* task described earlier. Six-month-old infants (and adults) are faster to look at the peripheral stimulus in gap trials (when the central stimulus is removed before the onset of the peripheral stimulus) than in the overlap trials (when the central stimulus remains on when the peripheral stimulus is presented), indicating that attention operates differently when there is and is not competition. However, the ability to disengage or shift attention in the overlap trials—and thus how "sticky" the fixations to the target are—develops considerably over the first postnatal months. Infants 3 months and younger have extreme difficulty disengaging from a central target to shift fixation to a peripheral target, exhibiting much longer latencies to look to the peripheral than do older infants (Hood, 1995). This high level of stickiness is also seen in Balint's syndrome patients, adults who have bilateral legions in the parietal lobes (Culham, 2002). Therefore, young infants' difficulty in coping with competition for attention in the gap trials may reflect an immaturity in parietal regions (although such development is also likely influenced by continued development of subcortical structures, as well as developing connections between cortical and subcortical structures). Indeed, existing evidence suggests dramatic changes in the parietal cortex during the first 6 postnatal months (Chugani, 1998; Deoni et al., 2011).

What is clear from the discussion thus far is that it would be a mistake to think about these three attention networks—and the neuroanatomical structures that support them—as developing in a rigid sequence. Instead, in any given context, these networks operate together and developmental changes in multiple cortical regions have a profound effect on how infants orient, sustain, and control attention.

Visual Attention and Cognitive Abilities

Developmental changes in infants' visual attention and visual behavior do not only reflect neuroanatomical changes. A primary goal of early studies on infants' looking behavior was to understand the role of cognitive processes on visual attention. Specifically, questions were asked about how basic information processing and memory determined where and how long infants looked. And, a very large body of literature shows a connection between infants' looking and cognitive processes. Early on, this connection was explained using a model based on Sokolov's comparator model (Cohen, 1973; Colombo & Mitchell, 2009). According to this approach, when infants attend to a stimulus (i.e., look at it) they form a memory for that stimulus. When they next encounter an item, they compare the stored information with the currently available information. If there is a match, the infant will be less interested than if there is a mismatch. Thus, looking is explicitly described as a function of how much what infants are looking at matches a previously formed memory, and thus reflects cognitive processing. This view has been challenged over the years (see Colombo & Mitchell, 2009, for a review). But it is widely accepted that infants' looking time is related to their memory processes.

The general finding that infants prefer to look at novel stimuli than familiar stimuli supports this conclusion. Fagan (1972, 1977a) took advantage of this fact about infants' looking, and developed a "novelty preference" procedure to study the development of memory in infants. In this task, infants are not habituated, but they are given a standard familiarization period with a stimulus (e.g., they are shown an image of a face for 20 seconds). Following this familiarization period, infants are shown a pair of stimuli—the now-familiar stimulus with a novel stimulus. The logic is that if infants could form a memory for the familiar stimulus in the time allowed during familiarization, then they should show a preference for (i.e., look longer at) the novel stimulus. Studies using this procedure have revealed significant insight into the development of memory in human infants—for example, older infants can form memories more quickly than do younger infants (Rose et al., 1982), and infants require more time to form memories of complex images than to form memories of simpler images (Fagan, 1974).

Thus, infants' looking behavior is *qualitatively* related to cognitive processes—if they remember they show a novelty preference. However, looking measures and cognitive abilities are also *quantitatively* related. For example, individual differences in the *strength* of infants' novelty preference at 5 to 7 months predicts their verbal IQ at 4 to 7 years (Fagan & McGrath, 1981). Infants born prematurely and those born at term (at least between 5 and 7 months of age, corrected age for preterm infants) show weaker novelty preferences than do infants born at term (see, e.g., Rose, Feldman, McCarton, & Wolfson, 1988). Such findings suggest that infants' looking time provides insight into how effective they are as information processors, and that there is a fairly direct relation between infants' looking behavior and their cognitive processes.

The assumption of such a quantitative relation between looking and cognitive abilities underlies work by Colombo and his colleagues (Colombo, Mitchell, Coldren, & Freeseman, 1991) comparing learning by infants who are *long lookers* to learning by infants who are *short lookers*. In this work, infants' baseline level of looking is determined in a neutral pretest, and then their learning of some new stimulus is assessed. Longer looking during this pretest is assumed to reflect generally slower or less efficient processors of visual information. Therefore, longer-looking infants should show different learning than do shorter-looking infants. Indeed, results from a number of studies reveal that long- and short-lookers learn differently about visually presented information (Colombo et al., 1991; Jankowski, Rose, & Feldman, 2001). Thus, infants' looking behavior appears to be a function, at least in part, of underlying cognitive processes.

Other work has attempted to understand infants' ongoing cognitive processes by interrupting those processes after different amounts of looking. The logic is that if we interrupt infants early in their looking, they will have engaged in less learning or processing, and thus they will have less fully encoded, processed, represented, and so on, the stimuli. If we allow them more time to look at the familiar stimuli, they will have engaged in more learning or processing, and thus they will have more fully encoded, processed, and represented those stimuli. Hunter, Ross, and Ames (1982), for example, showed that infants exhibited a preference for *familiarity* when their habituation was interrupted, but they showed the expected preference for novelty when they were allowed to become fully habituated. Rose and her colleagues (1982) showed that infants' novelty preference in the novelty preference procedure was a function of their study time; more robust novelty preferences were observed when infants were given more time to study stimuli than when they were given less time to study those stimuli. Roder, Bushnell, and Sasseville (2000) systematically examined changes in novelty and familiarity preferences over time by assessing infants' novelty preference on a series of successive trials in which a familiar stimulus was paired with a different novel stimulus. On early trials (when infants had looked at the familiar stimulus for shorter durations), infants showed a *familiarity preference*, and on later trials (after more time looking at the familiar stimulus) infants showed a *novelty preference*.

Horst, Oakes, and Madole (2005) explicitly examined the changing nature of infants' representations of a collection of items by examining how they responded to different kinds of novelty following varying amounts of study time. We habituated 10-month-old infants to a category of items—for example, four objects that were all acted on in the same way (e.g., squeezed), and made the same sound when acted on (e.g., squeaked), but looked different (e.g., purple and round, pink and oblong). Following different amounts of accumulated looking to the familiar stimulus set, we measured infants' interest in novel items that differed in appearance and/or function. We assumed that infants were engaged in actively learning about, forming representations of, and categorizing the items during their looking, and that infants would have learned more deeply after accumulating more looking than after accumulating less looking. We found that infants' pattern of novelty preferences differed as a function of the amount of time they looked at the familiar stimuli, suggesting that the processes of learning, representing, and categorizing the stimuli influenced the duration of looking.

Such findings about the connection between infants' looking and their cognitive processing provide the foundation of Cohen's (1998) information-processing theory of infants' looking. In this view, infants' looking is a function of the number of "units" of information infants are processing—when stimuli or situations present more units of information to infants, they look for longer durations. Thus, infants look longer at complex stimuli than at simple stimuli because presumably complex stimuli have more units. In addition, because with age infants become able to process stimuli in larger "chunks" (and thus the same stimuli have fewer units to process for older infants than for younger infants), the duration of looking to any given stimulus should decrease with age. Theories like this suggest a very direct relation between infants' looking and their cognitive processes.

In recent years, the availability of automatic eye trackers have allowed researchers to attempt to make even stronger links between looking behavior and cognitive processes. For example, Kirkham and colleagues (2007) examined infants' learning of spatiotemporal sequences (i.e., where shapes appeared sequentially in different locations in a predictable pattern). A series of studies using habituation showed the discriminations infants could make between familiar and novel sequences. Using an eye tracker, Kirkham and colleagues evaluated infants' *learning* of the sequences by examining their eye movements to predictable and unpredictable locations. The logic was that where infants looked—and how quickly they moved their eyes to those locations—provided insight into their anticipations for the sequences, reflecting their memory for consistent sequences.

Other work has examined infants' gaze patterns in the absence of learning, with the assumption that those gaze patterns provide insight into learning in other contexts. For example, we have conducted studies examining infants' looking at the diagnostic (head) regions of images of dogs and cats (Hurley & Oakes, 2015; Kovack-Lesh, McMurray, & Oakes, 2014). Four-month-old infants who have pets at home show stronger biases to look at the head regions of images of dogs and cats than do 4-month-old infants who do not have pets at home. We use this pattern to help understand other findings that 4-month-old infants with pets show more sophisticated learning of images of dogs and cats than do 4-month-old infants without pets (Kovack-Lesh, Horst, & Oakes, 2008; Kovack-Lesh, Oakes, & McMurray, 2012). The point is that infants' gaze patterns are thought to reflect the strategies infants use to acquire information about visual stimuli and to learn about those stimuli.

In summary, infants' looking behavior seems to be closely tied to cognitive processes. Infants' looking provides insight into their learning, memory, and representation of an event or object. Thus, any explanation of infants' looking that ignores the role of cognitive processes will be incomplete.

The Influence of Social Factors on Attention

Attention—as is true for all cognitive abilities—develops in a social context. Indeed, one aspect of attention that develops during infancy, and plays a critical role in social and linguistic development, is joint attention, or the process by which two people (usually caregiver and infant) share attention to the same object, event, or person (Grossmann & Johnson, 2010; Scaife & Bruner, 1975). But more broadly, infants' attentional abilities develop as they look at and interact with human faces; look at and inspect objects in their environment; and experience competition for attention in contexts such as playgroups, cluttered day care settings, zoos, homes with pets and siblings, outdoor playgrounds, and so on. Such experiences must influence infants' developing visual attention. They provide a context for the infant to practice attentional abilities. Contexts challenge infants' abilities to maintain their attention, orient and select, and control their attentional processes. Some experiences directly shape infants' developing attention abilities. What is clear is that infants' everyday experiences are other factors that contribute to the development of attention.

There is some evidence that infants' attention is directly shaped by their social interactions. For example, infants' attention to toys is different during independent play and during play with a caregiver (Landry & Chapieski, 1988; Landry et al., 1986; Lawson, Parrinello, & Ruff, 1992); infants engage in more sophisticated or focused attention during social interactions than when playing alone. For example, Landry and Chapieski (1988) observed that 6-month-old infants looked at toys more and investigated more toys when interacting with their mothers than when playing alone. Moreover, the particular strategies mothers adopted shaped infants' attention to toys in these interactions (Landry et al., 1996). Of course, conclusions about direction of effect are difficult to draw; other work has shown that infants' visual engagement at one time point predicts mothers' interactional style at a later time point (Sigman & Beckwith, 1980), consistent with the possibility that caregivers are not scaffolding infants' attention but rather are reacting responsively to individual differences in infants' attentional styles and developmental levels. But such findings suggest a connection between attention and social interactions.

Other work suggests a more indirect, and potentially profound, effect on infants' developing visual attention. Specifically, infants' social experiences—at least as construed as their everyday experience looking at, visually inspecting, and orienting toward objects, people, and actions—provide them with opportunities to use, adapt, and develop their visual attention abilities. Everyday experiences provide the input to the visual system, the contexts in which to engage and disengage visual attention, the objects to maintain a sustained attention toward, conflict that requires control over attention, and so on. It would not be surprising, therefore, if those experiences shaped the development of visual attention in important ways.

In fact, infants' visual attention does reflect their everyday experience. By 3 months, infants look longer at faces that are from a familiar race than at faces that are from a novel race (Kelly, Liu, et al., 2007; Kelly et al., 2005); newborns do not show such preferences (Kelly et al., 2005). Thus, infants come to prefer to look at faces that are like those that they have been viewing, inspecting, and orienting toward during the first postnatal weeks. Such preferences are probably related to the cognitive processes influencing attention described in the previous section: when encountering novel faces in an experimental setting, infants are likely comparing those faces to their representations of previously encountered faces, and their visual preferences are likely related to the fact that it is easier for them to process information about new faces that are similar to their past experience than about new faces that are different from their past experience.

However, this development of preferring to look at relatively familiar stimuli also suggests that through the daily experience of looking at, visually inspecting, and orienting to objects, actions, and people in their environment infants *learn* how to attend to and learn about those types of objects, actions, and people in their environment. They learn what features of human faces are most diagnostic; they learn where to look when viewing a human performing common actions (such as picking up and moving objects); and they anticipate the outcomes of events by directing their gaze to where the action will appear, rather than remaining focused on where the action had occurred (such as looking at the edge of an occluder where an object is expected to emerge).

Consider recent findings on infants' visual inspection of human faces. We used an eye-tracking procedure to examine developmental changes between 4 and 12 months of age in how infants scan faces (Oakes & Ellis, 2013). Younger and older infants scanned upright faces differently—younger infants were narrower in their scanning, focusing their gaze on the eye region more than did older infants, whereas older infants scanned more features in the internal region, focusing on the eyes, nose, and mouth. Although it is likely that development of cortical control over eye movements and other attentional processes and infants' cognitions about how to learn about faces contribute to such findings, these results also suggest that there are changes due to differences in *experience*. This is particularly clear when we consider infants' scanning of *inverted* faces. We observed no change in scanning of inverted faces; across the ages tested, infants focused narrowly on the eye region. Thus, the changes in scanning we observed for upright faces do not simply reflect maturation of the neural structures that underlie the attention networks, or infants' basic cognitive abilities. Rather, changes in infants' scanning changes differently reflected how the particular stimuli made contact with their previous experience. In this case, we observed different developmental trajectories for infants' visual inspection of faces in the more familiar upright orientation than for their visual inspection of faces in the less familiar inverted orientation.

The point is that comparison of infants' visual inspection of relatively familiar (upright faces) and relatively unfamiliar (inverted faces) stimuli suggests that experience and knowledge help infants to learn how to attend to stimuli. When they are younger, inexperienced, and naïve, infants engage in less sophisticated scanning patterns, perhaps reflecting immature orienting, selection, and control networks. With age, experience, and knowledge, scanning patterns change, perhaps reflecting more mature orienting, selection, and control networks.

This general conclusion is supported by evidence of infants' visual inspection of own- and other-race faces. In particular, Asian and White 3- to 10-month-old infants show different developmental changes in scanning of own- versus other-race faces (Liu et al., 2011; Wheeler et al., 2011). Both groups of infants changed their scanning of own-race faces relative to their scanning of other-race faces, suggesting that increased experience with a particular type of face induced infants to look differently at faces similar to those familiar faces and faces different from those familiar faces. Interestingly, although both White infants and Asian infants shifted their scanning of own-race versus other-race faces, the pattern was different for the two groups. Specifically, White infants looked increasingly at the eyes of own-race faces (Wheeler et al., 2011), whereas Asian infants decreased their looking to the internal features of other-race (White) faces (Liu et al., 2011). Such differences may reflect infants' increasing awareness of cultural expectations for mutual gaze during interpersonal interactions, or they may reflects infants' learning of which features are most diagnostic for discriminating faces from their own race. In addition, these differences in face scanning may underlie developmental differences in infants' ability to discriminate and remember other and own-race faces (Kelly et al., 2009; Kelly, Quinn, et al., 2007).

We have observed similar differences for how infants with and without pets scan images of dogs and cats like those depicted in Figure 4.4 (Hurley & Oakes, 2015; Kovack-Lesh et al., 2014). In these studies, 4-month-old infants with pets at home had stronger biases to look at the heads and faces of dog and cat images than did 4-month-old infants without pets at home. This difference is particularly interesting given findings that infants can distinguish between

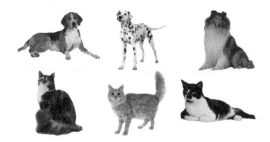

FIGURE 4.4. Examples of the type of stimuli used in studies comparing visual attention to images of cats and dogs by infants with and without pet experience. From Kovack-Lesh, Horst, and Oakes (2008). Copyright 2008 by the International Society on Infant Studies. Reprinted with permission from John Wiley & Sons, Inc.

images of dogs and cats based only on information in the head and face region (Quinn & Eimas, 1996; Spencer, Quinn, Johnson, & Karmiloff-Smith, 1997). When infants are shown images of dogs and cats without head and face regions, in contrast, they are unable to discriminate between those images. Thus, the finding that infants with pets have a stronger bias to look at the head and face regions of images of dogs and cats (Hurley & Oakes, 2015; Kovack-Lesh et al., 2014) suggests that infants with pets attend more to the most informative regions of the images than do infants without pets. Infants' everyday experience appears to contribute to the development of infants' ability to orient to and select features of items when engaged in visual inspection.

Such everyday experiences also appear to influence infants' ability to select among multiple available items and deal with competition for attention. Kovack-Lesh et al. (2014) assessed 4-month-old infants' attention when presented with *pairs* of cats and dogs, allowing us to understand more about the relation in a more challenging context. For example, we analyzed infants' gaze transitions and found that infants with pets had more *within-animal* transitions (i.e., shifting their gaze from one part of an animal to a different part of that same animal) than did infants without pets. This may indicate that infants with pets were better able in this context to maintain their attention to one item in the face of distraction (i.e., the presence of the other animal). In addition, infants with pets not only looked more at the heads than did infants without pets, but when shifting their glance from one animal to the other, infants with pets were more likely to shift to or from the head region. That is, their comparisons of the two animals were more likely to involve the head regions than were the comparisons by the infants without pets. These gaze-shift data may reveal that at 4 months infants have better attentional control when viewing relatively familiar items than when viewing less familiar items.

Taken as a whole, the work described in this section illustrates the role of everyday interactions on infants' developing attention. Infants learn about familiar items, and their attentional behaviors differ when the targets of attention are more or less familiar. This suggests that changes in orienting, selection, control, and so on are not solely a function of neuroanatomical development or increasing cognitive capabilities, but that they are also a function of the ways in which infants have used those attentional behaviors in their interactions with the objects, people, animals, and so on in their environment.

Putting It All Together: A Framework for Understanding Infants' Attention

The previous sections described the separate influences of biological, cognitive, and social factors on infants' looking and visual attention. However, our view is that these factors *together* determine how infants' visually attend, and how visual attention develops, and none of these factors actually operate in isolation. Looking behavior at any given moment reflects, at least in part, influences of one factor as mediated by another factor. Daily experience with animals, for example, makes images of animals easier to process. Thus, differences in looking behavior toward images of cats and dogs between infants with and without pets likely reflects how daily experience contributes to infants' learning and memory of such stimuli, and it is impossible to isolate the influence of either factor.

Our conceptual framework is depicted in Figure 4.5. (Note, in this framework, we use the broad term *attentional processes* to refer to the processes subserved by the subcortical and cortical systems described earlier.) Several features of this conceptual framework are important. First, multiple factors contribute to infants' looking behavior. As described in previous sections—and as depicted in Pathways 1, 2, and 3—we can conceptualize direct influences of daily experience, attentional processes, and other cognitive processes (such as memory, learning, etc.) on infants' looking behavior. Solid lines in this figure represent such effects. The previous sections described the influences on looking and visual attention as depicted by these solid lines.

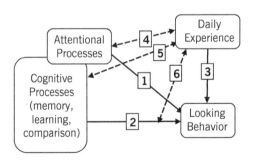

FIGURE 4.5. A conceptual model for how factors contribute to infants' looking. Adapted from Kovack-Lesh, McMurray, and Oakes (2014). Copyright 2014 by the American Psychological Association. Adapted by permission.

However, it is unlikely that any of these factors directly influences looking without the contribution of the other factors. As described above, daily
experience with some types of objects (animals, faces of particular races, etc.)
may make those objects easier to process—infants may form memories and
representations of relatively familiar objects more quickly than relatively novel
objects, infants may have developed strategies for how to deploy their attention to the most meaningful parts of relatively familiar objects. Any observed
effect of daily experience, therefore, actually reflects, at least in part, the effect
of such experience on cognitive and attentional processes that contribute to
visual attention. The *dotted* pathways in Figure 4.5 (Pathways 4, 5, and 6) represent the types of bidirectional relations we propose. Not only will infants'
daily experiences shape the attentional strategies infants use, their use of those
attentional strategies will shape those interactions. For example, cultures (and
parents) differ in whether during a mutual gaze one looks in the eyes of the
other person (Anzures, Quinn, Pascalis, Slater, & Lee, 2013; Fu, Hu, Wang,
Quinn, & Lee, 2012). Infants in different cultures may therefore learn from
face-to-face interactions to focus more on the eye regions or the nose regions of
faces during such interactions. Moreover, what infants learn about faces from
visual inspection of faces will differ depending on the particular strategy they
adopt—infants who come to look more at the eye region will learn more (in the
future) about the eyes of faces than will infants who come to look more at the
nose region. The point is that attention and learning are ultimately a function of
how these two influences operate together and shape each other.

The existing literature demonstrates such bidirectional relations. Recall that
4-month-old infants with pets show a stronger bias to look at the heads of dogs
and cats than do infants without pets (Hurley & Oakes, 2015; Kovack-Lesh et
al., 2014), showing that attentional control, selection, and so on are influenced
by what infants have learned about how to look at images of animals. Even 4-
and 6-month-old infants who do not have pets show a bias to look at the head
regions of images of animals (Hurley & Oakes, 2015; Kovack-Lesh et al., 2014;
Quinn, Doran, Reiss, & Hoffman, 2009), demonstrating that young infants can
and do find the diagnostic regions of these images even when they do not have
relevant experience. But infants show a *stronger bias* at 4 months if they had a
pet at home. It is not simply that infants look longer or faster at relatively familiar stimuli, but they deploy their attention differently depending on their past
experience with similar items. Their past experience seems to help them *learn
how to attend* to those stimuli.

Looking behavior also reflects bidirectional relations between attentional
and other cognitive processes. In Figure 4.5, these two boxes overlap, illustrating the connection between these two factors. Attentional processes are cognitive abilities, but we have also talked about them here as separate processes. Just
as infants' looking behavior is not a pure reflection of their everyday experiences, looking behaviors that seem to reflect attention or other cognitive processes (such as memory, comparison, or categorization) almost certainly reflect

this intersection between mulitple processes. Consider two looking behaviors described in earlier sections: disengagement in the gap-overlap procedure and long- versus short-looking. Earlier, attention switching and disengagement in the gap-overlap procedure was discussed in terms of neuroanatomical development; once cortical structures involved in shifting attention, oculomotor control, and disengagement are developed, infants show adult-like responding in this task (by 6 months). Long- versus short looking, in contrast, was discussed in terms of speed of processing; infants who are long lookers are assumed to be slower or less efficient processors than infants who are short lookers. Thus, these two measures of attentions were discussed in terms of *either* attentional processes *or* other cognitive processes. However, these two aspects of looking behavior are likely influenced by attention *and* other cognitive processes.

Indeed, Frick and colleagues found that individual differences in looking behavior (long- vs. short-lookers) was related to disengagement in gap trials of the gap-overlap task (Frick, Colombo, & Saxon, 1999). They argue that some of the variability in the length of infants' looking reflects development of the neural attentional systems involved in disengagement. That is, whether infants were short- or long lookers reflected disengagement processes, as well as other cognitive processes such as processing speed. Thus, looking behavior that is taken to reflect speed of processing actually reflects a combination of processing speed and disengagement, as well as other factors and processes. Similarly, although looking behavior in the gap-overlap task can be taken as reflecting disengagement, evidence shows that other processes are involved. Peltola and colleagues (2008) found that when the central stimulus in a gap-overlap task was a face, 7-month-old infants had more difficulty disengaging from fearful faces than from happy or neutral faces. Although this effect does not directly assess the role of cognitive processing on infants' disengagement, it does suggest that how quickly infants shift their gaze from the central to the peripheral stimulus reflects not only attentional processes but also infants' psychological processing of the central stimulus (in this case, the familiarity or emotional significance of the faces). Moreover, these processes may truly have bidirectional influences on looking behavior. Long lookers may have more difficulty disengaging because they are slower at processing the target of fixation—that is, disengagement may be determined, in part, by the processing of the target stimulus. It is also possible that disengagement processes operate differently when the fixation target is more familiar, more emotionally demanding, and so on. The networks in the brain are engaged in multiple tasks, and it is not surprising that behavior reflects bidirectional influences of these processes.

Finally, Pathway 6 suggests a different kind of interaction among these influences on infants' looking behavior. Specifically, at any given moment infants may use attentional strategies that reflect cognitive influences on attention or basic attentional abilities (e.g., engaging and disengaging in competing stimuli in ways that allow comparison of those stimuli), but those attentional strategies operate differently—and be more or less effective—depending on the interaction between infants' past experience and the stimuli being attended to at that moment. For example, in two separate investigations we found that only 4-month-old infants who had pets at home *and* who engaged in more comparison during testing learned about the series of cats presented during familiarization (Kovack-Lesh et al., 2008, 2012). Infants who did not have pets and infants who had pets but exhibited low levels of comparison did not show evidence of learning. This raises the possibility that when infants engage in a more sophisticated learning strategy (in this case, looking back and forth between two simultaneously presented stimuli), they learn more when using this strategy with relatively familiar stimuli than when using it with less familiar stimuli. That is, attentional engagement, selection, orienting, and so on may be more effective when the to-be-learned stimuli are related to one's past experience (and thus, one has *learned how to learn* about those items) than when the to-be-learned stimuli are more distant from one's past experience.

The framework described here addresses the "Humpty Dumpty problem" (Oakes, 2009) in the study of infant visual attention. Rather than studying looking as reflecting either attentional processes and networks or cognitive processes or social factors and everyday interactions, this framework illustrates how looking behavior reflects the interaction of those factors. Importantly, this framework also provides a direction for future research. Although some understanding can be gained by studying biological, cognitive, and social factors on the development of visual attention, a full understanding can only be gained by studying how these factors interact. That is, by building on previous work examining isolated components of visual attention, we can begin to understand how attention and looking behavior reflects how those components work together. For example, future work might ask how social interactions scaffold infants' attention, facilitating development of infants' ability to sustain attention. Or work may be conducted examining how disengagement processes are influenced by the psychological processes engaged by the central target. The goals of such work would be to understand how multiple factors together determine behavior, and how attention is the result of such interactions and relations among processes.

Summary

We take the perspective that infants' looking and the direction and duration of infants' looking at any given moment reflects the interaction among infants' existing knowledge or history, their ability to learn about the stimuli, and their basic attentional skills. This is a biopsychosocial perspective in that it reflects the interaction among biological factors (i.e., neural pathways that control attention), psychological processes (i.e., basic cognitive development), and social factors (i.e., the infants' history with objects, events, and people). Development of infants' looking behavior cannot be reduced to any one of these factors, but reflects, instead, developmental changes at multiple levels and changes in the interactions among these factors with development. Continued understanding of this development requires that future research focuses on these interactions. That is, it is important to understand attentional processes in the context of social interactions, considering the demands on cognitive resources, as well as what is known about developing cortical control of attentional processes. In addition, it must be recognized that there is no "pure" influence of maturing brain regions on attentional processes, and that such influences also reflect the infant's history of social interactions and use of attentional processes in conjunction with other cognitive processes. Addressing such questions requires thinking carefully about the stimuli used to assess attentional processes, as well as ways to examine these developing questions in methods other than presenting computer-generated stimuli to infants and measuring looking behavior. Traditional stimuli and methods will continue to yield insight into this development, but deeper understanding will be gained by adapting stimuli and methods in a way that allows us to consider the interactions among these multiple factors and how they work together to influence and determine the development of visual behaviors.

REFERENCES

Abramov, I., Gordon, J., Hendrickson, A., Hainline, L., Dobson, V., & Labossiere, E. (1982). The retina of the newborn human infant. *Science, 217*, 265–267.

Anzures, G., Quinn, P. C., Pascalis, O., Slater, A. M., & Lee, K. (2013). Development of own-race biases. *Visual Cognition, 21*, 1165–1182.

Atkinson, J. (2000). *The developing visual brain.* Oxford, UK: Oxford University Press.

Atkinson, J., & Braddick, O. (2012). Visual attention in the first years: Typical development and developmental disorders. *Developmental Medicine and Child Neurology, 54*, 589–595.

Baillargeon, R. (1987a). Object permanence in 3½- and 4½-month-old infants. *Developmental Psychology, 23*, 655–664.

Baillargeon, R. (1987b). Young infants' reasoning about the physical and spatial properties of a hidden object. *Cognitive Development, 2*, 179–200.

Banks, M. S., & Dannemiller, J. L. (1987). Infant visual psychophysics. In P. Salapatek & L. B. Cohen (Eds.), *Handbook of infant perception* (Vol. 1, pp. 115–184). New York: Academic Press.

Brennan, W., Ames, E., & Moore, R. (1966). Age differences in infants' attention to patterns of different complexities. *Science, 49*, 354–356.

Casey, B. J., & Richards, J. E. (1988). Sustained visual attention in young infants measured with an adapted version of the visual preference paradigm. *Child Development, 59*, 1514–1521.

Chugani, H. T. (1998). A critical period of brain development: Studies of cerebral glucose utilization with PET. *Preventative Medicine, 27,* 184–188.

Chun, M. M., Golomb, J. D., & Turk-Browne, N. B. (2011). A taxonomy of external and internal attention. *Annual Review of Psychology, 62,* 73–101.

Clohessy, A. B., Posner, M. I., Rothbart, M. K., & Vecera, S. P. (1991). The development of inhibition of return in early infancy. *Journal of Cognitive Neuroscience, 3,* 345–350.

Cohen, L. B. (1973). A two-process model of infant attention. *Merrill-Palmer Quarterly, 19,* 157–180.

Cohen, L. B. (1998). An information processing approach to infant perception and cognition. In F. Simion & G. Butterworth (Eds.), *The development of sensory, motor, and cognitive capacities in early infancy: From sensation to perception* (pp. 277–300). Hove, UK: Psychology Press.

Cohen, L. B., DeLoache, J. S., & Pearl, R. A. (1977). An examination of interference effects in infants' memory for faces. *Child Development, 48,* 88–96.

Cohen, L. B., DeLoache, J. S., & Rissman, M. W. (1975). The effect of stimulus complexity on infant visual attention and habituation. *Child Development, 46,* 611–617.

Cohen, L. B., & Gelber, E. R. (1975). Infant visual memory. In L. B. Cohen & P. Salapatek (Eds.), *Infant perception: From sensation to cognition: Vol. I. Basic visual processes* (pp. 347–404). New York: Academic Press.

Colombo, J. (2001). The development of visual attention in infancy. *Annual Review of Psychology, 52,* 337–367.

Colombo, J., & Mitchell, D. W. (2009). Infant visual habituation. *Neurobiology of Learning and Memory, 92,* 225–234.

Colombo, J., Mitchell, D. W., Coldren, J. T., & Freeseman, L. J. (1991). Individual differences in infant visual attention: Are short lookers faster processors or feature processors? *Child Development, 62,* 1247–1257.

Cordes, S., & Brannon, E. M. (2009). Crossing the divide: Infants discriminate small from large numerosities. *Developmental Psychology, 45,* 1583–1594.

Csibra, G., Tucker, L. A., & Johnson, M. H. (1998). Neural correlates of saccade planning in infants: A high-density ERP study. *International Journal of Psychophysiology, 29,* 201–215.

Culham, J. C. (2002). Parietal cortex. In L. Nadel (Ed.), *Encyclopedia of cognitive science* (Vol. 3, pp. 451–457). Houndmills, UK: Macmillan.

Dannemiller, J. L. (1998). A competition model of exogenous orienting in 3.5-month-old infants. *Journal of Experimental Child Psychology, 68,* 169–201.

Dannemiller, J. L. (2000). Competition in early exogenous orienting between 7 and 21 weeks. *Journal of Experimental Child Psychology, 76,* 253–274.

Deoni, S. C. L., Mercure, E., Blasi, A., Gasston, D., Thomson, A., Johnson, M., et al. (2011). Mapping infant brain myelination with magnetic resonance imaging. *Journal of Neuroscience, 31,* 784–791.

Fagan, J. F. (1970). Memory in the infant. *Journal of Experimental Child Psychology, 9,* 217–226.

Fagan, J. F. (1971). Infants' recognition memory for a series of visual stimuli. *Journal of Experimental Child Psychology, 11,* 244–250.

Fagan, J. F. (1972). Infants' recognition memory for faces. *Journal of Experimental Child Psychology, 14,* 453–476.

Fagan, J. F. (1973). Infants' delayed recognition memory and forgetting. *Journal of Experimental Child Psychology, 16,* 424–450.

Fagan, J. F. (1974). Infant recognition memory: The effects of length of familiarization and type of discrimination task. *Child Development, 45,* 351–356.

Fagan, J. F. (1977a). An attention model of infant recognition. *Child Development, 48,* 345–359.

Fagan, J. F. (1977b). Infant recognition memory: Studies in forgetting. *Child Development, 48,* 68–78.

Fagan, J. F., & McGrath, S. K. (1981). Infant recognition memory and later intelligence. *Intelligence, 5,* 121–130.

Fantz, R. L. (1958). Pattern vision in young infants. *Psychological Record, 8,* 43–47.

Fantz, R. L. (1963). Pattern vision in newborn infants. *Science, 140,* 296–297.

Fantz, R. L. (1964). Visual experience in infants: Decreased attention familiar patterns relative to novel ones. *Science, 146,* 668–670.

Fantz, R. L., & Fagan, J. F. (1975). Visual attention to size and number of pattern details by term and preterm infants during the first six months. *Child Development, 46,* 3–18.

Fantz, R. L., & Nevis, S. (1967). Pattern preferences and perceptual–cognitive development in early infancy. *Merrill-Palmer Quarterly: Journal of Developmental Psychology, 13,* 77–108.

Frick, J. E., Colombo, J., & Saxon, T. F. (1999). Individual and developmental differences in disengagement of fixation in early infancy. *Child Development, 70,* 537–548.

Fu, G., Hu, C. S., Wang, Q., Quinn, P. C., & Lee, K. (2012). Adults scan own- and other-race faces differently. *PlOS ONE, 7,* e37688.

Gredebäck, G., Stasiewicz, D., Falck-Ytter, T., Rosander, K., & von Hofsten, C. (2009). Action type and goal type modulate goal-directed gaze shifts in 14-month-old infants. *Developmental Psychology, 45,* 1190–1194.

Greenberg, D. J., & O'Donnell, W. J. (1972). Infancy and the optimal level of stimulation. *Child Development, 43,* 639–645.

Grossmann, T., & Johnson, M. H. (2010). Selective prefrontal cortex responses to joint attention in early infancy. *Biology Letters, 6,* 540–543.

Harman, C., Posner, M. I., Rothbart, M. K., & Thomas-Thrapp, L. (1994). Development of orienting to locations and objects in human infants. *Canadian Journal of Experimental Psychology, 48,* 301–318.

Hollyfield, J. G., Frederick, J. M., & Rayborn, M. E. (1983). Neurotransmitter properties of the newborn human retina. *Investigative Ophthalmology and Visual Science, 24,* 893–897.

Hood, B. M. (1995). Shifts of visual attention in the human infant: A neuroscience approach. In C. Rovee-Collier & L. P. Lipsitt (Eds.), *Advances in infancy research* (Vol. 9, pp. 163–216). Norwood, NJ: Ablex.

Hood, B. M., & Atkinson, J. (1993). Disengaging visual attention in the infant and adult. *Infant Behavior and Development, 16,* 405–422.

Horst, J. S., Oakes, L. M., & Madole, K. L. (2005). What does it look like and what can it do?: Category structure influences how infants categorize. *Child Development, 76*, 614–631.

Hunnius, S., & Geuze, R. H. (2004). Gaze shifting in infancy: A longitudinal study using dynamic faces and abstract stimuli. *Infant Behavior and Development, 27*, 397–416.

Hunter, M. A., Ames, E. W., & Koopman, R. (1983). Effects of stimulus complexity and familiarization time on infant preferences for novel and familiar stimuli. *Developmental Psychology, 19*, 338–352.

Hunter, M. A., Ross, H. S., & Ames, E. W. (1982). Preferences for familiar or novel toys: Effects of familiarization time in 1-year-olds. *Developmental Psychology, 18*, 519–529.

Hurley, K. B., & Oakes, L. M. (2015). Experience and distribution of attention: Pet exposure and infants' scanning of animal images. *Journal of Cognition and Development, 16*(1), 11–30.

James, W. (1890). *The principles of psychology* (Vol. 1). New York: Holt.

Jankowski, J. J., Rose, S. A., & Feldman, J. F. (2001). Modifying the distribution of attention in infants. *Child Development, 72*, 339–351.

Johnson, M. H. (1990). Cortical maturation and the development of visual attention in early infancy. *Journal of Cognitive Neuroscience, 2*, 81–95.

Johnson, M. H. (1995). The inhibition of automatic saccades in early infancy. *Developmental Psychobiology, 28*, 281–291.

Johnson, M. H. (2010). *Developmental cognitive neuroscience*. Oxford, UK: Wiley.

Kelly, D. J., Liu, S., Ge, L., Quinn, P. C., Slater, A. M., Lee, K., et al. (2007). Cross-race preferences for same-race faces extend beyond the African versus Caucasian contrast in 3-month-old infants. *Infancy, 11*, 87–95.

Kelly, D. J., Liu, S., Lee, K., Quinn, P. C., Pascalis, O., Slater, A. M., et al. (2009). Development of the other-race effect during infancy: Evidence toward universality? *Journal of Experimental Child Psychology, 104*, 105–114.

Kelly, D. J., Quinn, P. C., Slater, A. M., Lee, K., Ge, L., & Pascalis, O. (2007). The other-race effect develops during infancy: Evidence of perceptual narrowing. *Psychological Science, 18*, 1084–1089.

Kelly, D. J., Quinn, P. C., Slater, A. M., Lee, K., Gibson, A., Smith, M., et al. (2005). Three-month-olds, but not newborns, prefer own-race faces. *Developmental Science, 8*, F31–F36.

Kirkham, N. Z., Slemmer, J. A., Richardson, R., & Johnson, S. P. (2007). Location, location, location: Development of spatiotemporal sequence learning in infancy. *Child Development, 78*, 1559–1571.

Klein, R. M. (2000). Inhibition of return. *Trends in Cognitive Sciences, 4*, 138–147.

Kovack-Lesh, K. A., Horst, J. S., & Oakes, L. M. (2008). The cat is out of the bag: The joint influence of previous experience and looking behavior on infant categorization. *Infancy, 13*, 285–307.

Kovack-Lesh, K. A., McMurray, B., & Oakes, L. M. (2014). Four-month-old infants' visual investigation of cats and dogs: Relations with pet experience and attentional strategy. *Developmental Psychology, 50*, 402–413.

Kovack-Lesh, K. A., Oakes, L. M., & McMurray, B. (2012). Contributions of attentional style and previous experience to 4-month-old infants' categorization. *Infancy, 17,* 324–338.

Landry, S. H., & Chapieski, M. L. (1988). Visual attention during toy exploration in preterm infants: Effects of medical risk and maternal interactions. *Infant Behavior and Development, 11,* 187–204.

Landry, S. H., Chapieski, M. L., & Schmidt, M. (1986). Effects of maternal attention-directing strategies on preterms' response to toys. *Infant Behavior and Development, 9,* 257–269.

Landry, S. H., Garner, P. W., Swank, P. R., & Baldwin, C. D. (1996). Effects of maternal scaffolding during joint toy play with preterm and full-term infants. *Merrill–Palmer Quarterly, 42,* 177–199.

Lawson, K. R., Parrinello, R., & Ruff, H. A. (1992). Maternal behavior and infant attention. *Infant Behavior and Development, 15,* 209–229.

Liu, S., Quinn, P. C., Wheeler, A., Xiao, N., Ge, L., & Lee, K. (2011). Similarity and difference in the processing of same- and other-race faces as revealed by eye tracking in 4- to 9-month-olds. *Journal of Experimental Child Psychology, 108,* 180–189.

Luck, S. J., & Vecera, S. P. (2002). Attention. In H. Pashler & S. Yantis (Eds.), *Steven's handbook of experimental psychology: Vol. 1. Sensation and perception* (3rd ed., pp. 235–286). Hoboken, NJ: Wiley.

Markant, J., & Amso, D. (2013). Selective memories: Infants' encoding is enhanced in selection via suppression. *Developmental Science, 16,* 926–940.

Martin, R. M. (1975). Effects of familiar and complex stimuli on infant attention. *Developmental Psychology, 11,* 178–185.

McCall, R. B. (1973). Encoding and retrieval of perceptual memories after long-term familiarization and the infant's response to discrepancy. *Developmental Psychology, 9,* 310–318.

McCall, R. B., Kennedy, C. B., & Dodds, C. (1977). The interfering effect of distracting stimuli on the infant's memory. *Child Development, 48,* 79–87.

Mondloch, C. J., Lewis, T. L., Budreau, D. R., Maurer, D., Dannemiller, J. L., Stephens, B. R., et al. (1999). Face perception during early infancy. *Psychological Science, 10,* 419–422.

Needham, A., Baillargeon, R., & Kaufman, L. (1997). Object segregation in infancy. In C. Rovee-Collier & L. P. Lipsitt (Eds.), *Advances in infancy research* (Vol. 11, pp. 1–44). Greenwich, CT: Ablex.

Oakes, L. M. (1994). The development of infants' use of continuity cues in their perception of causality. *Developmental Psychology, 30,* 748–756.

Oakes, L. M. (2009). The "Humpty Dumpty problem" in the study of early cognitive development: Putting the infant back together again. *Perspectives on Psychological Science, 4,* 352–358.

Oakes, L. M., Baumgartner, H. A., Barrett, F. S., Messenger, I. M., & Luck, S. J. (2013). Developmental changes in visual short-term memory in infancy: Evidence from eye-tracking. *Frontiers in Psychology, 4,* 697.

Oakes, L. M., & Ellis, A. E. (2013). An eye-tracking investigation of developmental changes in infants' exploration of upright and inverted human faces. *Infancy, 18,* 134–148.

Oakes, L. M., Kannass, K. N., & Shaddy, D. J. (2002). Developmental changes in endogenous control of attention: The role of target familiarity on infants' distraction latency. *Child Development, 73,* 1644–1655.

Oakes, L. M., & Ribar, R. J. (2005). A comparison of infants' categorization in paired and successive presentation familiarization tasks. *Infancy, 7,* 85–98.

Oakes, L. M., Ross-Sheehy, S., & Kannass, K. N. (2004). Attentional engagement in infancy: The interactive influence of attentional inertia and attentional state. *Infancy, 5,* 239–252.

Oakes, L. M., & Tellinghuisen, D. J. (1994). Examining in infancy: Does it reflect active processing? *Developmental Psychology, 30,* 748–756.

Pancratz, C. N., & Cohen, L. B. (1970). Recovery of habituation in infants. *Journal of Experimental Child Psychology, 9,* 208–216.

Parasuraman, R., & Davies, D. R. (Eds.). (1984). *Varieties of attention.* London: Academic Press.

Peltola, M. J., Leppänen, J. M., Palokangas, T., & Hietanen, J. K. (2008). Fearful faces modulate looking duration and attention disengagement in 7-month-old infants. *Developmental Science, 11,* 60–68.

Petersen, S. E., & Posner, M. I. (2012). The attention system of the human brain: 20 years after. *Annual Review of Neuroscience, 35,* 73–89.

Posner, M. I., & Petersen, S. E. (1990). The attention system of the human brain. *Annual Review of Neuroscience, 13,* 25–42.

Quinn, P. C., Doran, M. M., Reiss, J. E., & Hoffman, J. E. (2009). Time course of visual attention in infant categorization of cats versus dogs: Evidence for a head bias as revealed through eye tracking. *Child Development, 80,* 151–161.

Quinn, P. C., & Eimas, P. D. (1996). Perceptual cues that permit categorical differentiation of animal species by infants. *Journal of Experimental Child Psychology, 63,* 189–211.

Richards, J. E. (1989). Development and stability in visual sustained attention in 14, 20, and 26 week old infants. *Psychophysiology, 26,* 422–430.

Richards, J. E. (1997a). Effects of attention on infants' preference for briefly exposed visual stimuli in the paired-comparison recognition-memory paradigm. *Developmental Psychology, 33,* 22–31.

Richards, J. E. (1997b). Peripheral stimulus localization by infants: Attention, age, and individual differences in heart rate variability. *Journal of Experimental Psychology: Human Perception and Performance, 23,* 667–680.

Richards, J. E. (2000). Localizing the development of covert attention in infants with scalp event-related potentials. *Developmental Psychology, 36,* 91–108.

Richards, J. E. (2001). Cortical indexes of saccade planning following covert orienting in 20-week-old infants. *Infancy, 2,* 135–157.

Richards, J. E., & Casey, B. J. (1992). Development of sustained visual attention in the human infant. In B. A. Campbell, H. Hayne, & R. Richardson (Eds.), *Attention and information processing in infants and adults: Perspectives from human and animal research* (pp. 30–60). Hillsdale, NJ: Erlbaum.

Roder, B. J., Bushnell, E. W., & Sasseville, A. M. (2000). Infants' preferences for familiarity and novelty during the course of visual processing. *Infancy, 1,* 491–507.

Rose, S. A., Feldman, J. F., & Jankowski, J. J. (2004). Infant visual recognition memory. *Developmental Review, 24,* 74–100.

Rose, S. A., Feldman, J. F., McCarton, C. M., & Wolfson, J. (1988). Information processing in seven-month-old infants as a function of risk status. *Child Development, 59*, 589–603.

Rose, S. A., Gottfried, A. W., Mello-Carmina, P., & Bridger, W. H. (1982). Familiarity and novelty preferences in infant recognition memory: Implications for information processing. *Developmental Psychology, 18*, 704–713.

Ross-Sheehy, S., Oakes, L. M., & Luck, S. J. (2003). The development of visual short-term memory capacity in infants. *Child Development, 74*, 1807–1822.

Ruff, H. A. (1986). Components of attention during infants' manipulative exploration. *Child Development, 57*, 105–114.

Ruff, H. A., & Rothbart, M. K. (1996). *Attention in early development*. New York: Oxford University Press.

Scaife, M., & Bruner, J. S. (1975). The capacity for joint visual attention in the infant. *Nature, 253*, 265–266.

Sigman, M., & Beckwith, L. (1980). Infant visual attentiveness in relation to caregiver–infant interaction and developmental outcome. *Infant Behavior and Development, 3*, 141–154.

Simion, F., Valenza, E., Umiltà, C., & Barba, B. D. (1995). Inhibition of return in newborns is temporo-nasal asymmetrical. *Infant Behavior and Development, 18*, 189–194.

Spelke, E. S., Kestenbaum, R., Simons, D. J., & Wein, D. (1995). Spatiotemporal continuity, smoothness of motion and object identity in infancy. *British Journal of Developmental Psychology, 13*, 113.

Spencer, J., Quinn, P. C., Johnson, M. H., & Karmiloff-Smith, A. (1997). Heads you win, tails you lose: Evidence for young infants categorizing mammals by head and facial features. *Early Development and Parenting, 6*, 113–126.

Stechler, G., & Latz, E. (1966). Some observations on attention and arousal in the human infant. *Journal of the American Academy of Child Psychiatry, 5*, 517–525.

Strauss, M. S. (1979). Abstraction of prototypical information by adults and 10-month-old infants. *Journal of Experimental Psychology: Human Learning and Memory, 5*, 618–632.

Valenza, E., Simion, F., & Umiltà, C. (1994). Inhibition of return in newborn infants. *Infant Behavior and Development, 17*, 293–302.

Wheeler, A., Anzures, G., Quinn, P. C., Pascalis, O., Omrin, D. S., & Lee, K. (2011). Caucasian infants scan own- and other-race faces differently. *PLoS ONE, 6*, e18621.

Wilcox, T. (1999). Object individuation: Infants' use of shape, size, pattern, and color. *Cognition, 72*, 125–166.

Wilcox, T., Schweinle, A., & Chapa, C. (2003). Object individuation in infancy. In H. Hayne & J. W. Fagen (Eds.), *Progress in infancy research* (Vol. 3, pp. 193–243). Mahwah, NJ: Erlbaum.

Younger, B. A. (1985). The segregation of items into categories by 10-month-old infants. *Child Development, 56*, 1574–1583.

CHAPTER 5

Biopsychosocial Perspectives on the Development of Attention in Infancy

John Colombo and Brenda Salley

Attention is a core concept in psychology, and a fundamental component in information-processing models for human cognition. For the most part, within the field of early cognitive development, attention was primarily used as a means to study other cognitive mechanisms or processes, such as recognition memory or the nature of representation. Beginning in the 1980s, however, attention became a topic of study in its own right, owing to the convergent use of behavioral and psychophysiological measures in the study of infants' responses to stimuli (Richards, 1989), and to reports suggesting that measures of attention in infancy were modestly predictive of intellectual and language outcomes in later childhood (Bornstein & Colombo, 2012). In the field of education, attention was rarely considered as a construct worthy of study in and of itself , except in cases when attentional deficits interfered with learning (Barkley, 1997) or presented a marker for potential psychopathology (Walsh, Elsabbagh, Bolton, & Singh, 2011). However, in the last decade, attention (sometimes under the guise of even less well-specified constructs such as "engagement" or even "mindfulness") has come to the fore in the field of education as measures of attention have been found to be predictive of various forms of achievement (Sarver et al., 2012). As we have noted elsewhere (Colombo, Kannass, Walker, & Brez, 2012), among the more salient reasons for this is confusion in professional and academic circles about what attention actually is, about its functions or products, or how to translate basic findings to more applied contexts.

John Colombo and Brenda Salley share primary authorship on this chapter.

In keeping with the theme of this volume, the purpose of this chapter is to examine the construct of attention in the context of its psychological, biological, and social attributes, with primary emphasis on its relevance for human infancy. We present an organizational framework for considering different *varieties of attention* (James, 1890), and then briefly review the concomitant variety of biological mechanisms that presumably contribute to these forms of attentional function. Finally, in consideration of the social context of attention, we turn to examine the nature and impact of an emergent literature on *social attention* in development, and review the nature of attention as employed in social contexts or with "social" stimuli, with an eye toward understanding whether this form of attention might represent an independent or dissociable form of the construct.

Attention: Functions and Forms

More than a century ago, William James (1890) articulated *selection* as the central concept of the construct of attention, and it is probably safe to characterize attention as the mechanism through which an organism (presumably besieged by innumerable environmental inputs) selects a stimulus or stimulus property for processing or action. Over the past century, the nature of that selection has been debated on two fronts. One concerns the question of whether selection of some inputs categorically excludes other inputs (Broadbent, 1958; Cherry, 1953) or whether it merely emphasizes some inputs while still allowing others to enter the information-processing system (LaBerge, Carlson, Williams, & Bunney, 1997; Treisman & Gelade, 1980). A second debate concerns whether there is a single attentional channel (Gladstones, Regan, & Lee, 1989; Welford, 1959) or whether attentional resources are distributed more widely or as discrete or modular channels (Wickens, 1991). While these issues have largely been pursued within studies of adults and older children, they are relevant to infancy in that they bear on the proposed existence of specialized modules for processing in early infancy, such as for the processing of faces (Scherf & Scott, 2012) or other social stimuli as discussed later in this chapter.

As with most constructs in the behavioral sciences, attention may be measured at different levels of the organism. At the behavioral level, sensory receptors are directed toward the stimulus that is being attended to; this level of measurement is reflected in many paradigms used in infancy, including habituation (Colombo & Mitchell, 2009), gap-overlap tasks (Blaga & Colombo, 2006; Frick, Colombo, & Saxon, 1999), and eye-tracking technologies (Oakes, 2012). Attention may also be measured in infancy through bodily responses such as heart rate (Colombo et al., 2010), respiration (Richards, 2010), or pupil dilation (Jackson & Sirois, 2009), or through brain measures such as electroencephalography (Bell & Wolfe, 2007) or evoked potentials (Reynolds, Courage, & Richards, 2010).

The Functions of Attention

At this point, we look to review the fundamental *functions* of attention; in other words, we attempt to address the question of what attention *does* for human cognitive activity. Simply stated, we posit that attention increases the probability of learning. As decades of work on implicit learning show (Perruchet & Pacton, 2006), learning can certainly occur in the absence of attention, even in human infants (Aslin & Newport, 2012). However, events learned in such ways may require extended exposures before being acquired; we would propose that attention accelerates or raises the probability that acquisition will occur quickly. The question remains, however, as to how this efficiency is realized. This question may be partially answered by considering the effects of attention on processing and representation of cognition at the neural level.

Attention Raises Stimulus Gain

Data from electrophysiology and neuroimaging have long suggested that the neural representation of an attended stimulus in the brain is enhanced, relative to an unattended stimulus (Hillyard, Vogel, & Luck, 1998). Such enhancement might be attributable to an amplification of the intensity or magnitude of the neural representation of the attended stimulus (Hernandez-Peon, 1966), or to the suppression of other irrelevant stimulus representations or random ambient noise (Neill & Westberry, 1987). In any case, attention appears to increase the *gain* of the stimulus for the organism (Borji & Itti, 2014; Eldar, Cohen, & Niv, 2013). Indeed, much of infant attention research has capitalized on the widely cited orienting reflex (Sokolov, 1958, 1960), which involves the dampening of internal physiological mechanisms and autonomic output (Stekelenburg & Van Boxtel, 2001), including lowered heart rate (Graham & Clifton, 1966), slowed breathing (Denot-Ledunois, Vardon, Perruchet, & Gallego, 1998), increased motoric inhibition (Lawler, Obrist, & Lawler, 1975), and even slowed metabolic activity (Vanduffel, Tootell, & Orban, 2000). The ultimate consequence of increases in stimulus gain would be enhanced probability for that stimulus or event to be learned or acted upon.

Attention Promotes Coordinated Neural Activity

A related consequence of attention appears to be that it increases the likelihood of coordinated or synchronous neural activity within (Steinmetz, Roy, Fitzgerald, Hsiao, Johnson, et al., 2000) and across different (Albright, Jessell, Kandel, & Posner, 2000) areas of the brain. Such coordinated activity is likely fundamental to several critical functions in human behavior, ranging from the initiation of action (Rao et al., 1997) to the processes that underlie various forms of associative learning (Engel & Singer, 2001) and memory (Klimesch,

Freunberger, Sauseng, & Gruber, 2008). Indeed, several prominent authors have speculated that neural synchrony provides the basis for higher-order cognitive abilities, including the formation of neurocognitive networks (Bressler & Tognoli, 2006; Fries, 2005) that underlie the development of semantic memory.

The Forms of Attention

Given the myriad functions and broad conceptualizations presented for the construct of attention, there has been no shortage of proposals seeking to organize attentional processes into a working taxonomy. Such a taxonomy would have important implications for those of us who study attention in infants, and so we briefly review such efforts here.

One classic neuroscience-based model (Posner & Petersen, 1990) characterized attention in terms of three processes: (1) orienting to sensory events, (2) detection of signals, and (3) maintenance of a vigilant state. This model has been recently updated (Petersen & Posner, 2012) to reflect more generalized functions that include (1) alerting, (2) orienting, and (3) executive processes, bringing it into line with an earlier, more developmentally focused proposal (Ruff & Rothbart, 1996) that characterized attention as being reducible to a (1) attentional state, (2) selectivity, and (3) higher-order control. Our own group (Colombo, 2001; Colombo et al., 2012) has posited a model of infant attention involving four distinct phenomena: (1) alertness, (2) visuospatial orienting, (3) object-centered attention, and (4) endogenous attention. In recent years, however, we have been working to simplify and reduce this framework further; this chapter provides an opportunity for us to explicate an integrative framework that may serve to capture the scope of the construct adequately for developmental inquiry. The model (see Table 5.1) is based on the factorial crossing of two parameters that are described more fully in the following section: the form of attention (state vs. selection) and the path through which each form can be evoked (exogenous vs. endogenous). The cell contents provided in Table 5.1 are not meant to be exhaustive or comprehensive, but rather are meant to illustrate the potential utility of the framework.

Common to all of the models of attention discussed above are (1) a general *state* of readiness for external stimulation (e.g., alertness) and (2) a more targeted *process* that selects a specific stimulus or stimulus feature for emphasis or

TABLE 5.1. A Conceptual Framework for Attentional Processes

	Path of activation	
Form	Exogenous	Endogenous
Attentional state	Stimulus-driven arousal	Vigilance
Selective process	Attentional capture	Executive attention

processing (e.g., orienting). We posit these as two dissociable forms of attention: an *attentional state* that encompasses phenomena such as alertness, arousal, or vigilance; and an attentional *process* that reflects processes such as attentional capture, spatial orienting, and object-based attention. Both types of attention have been studied extensively in human infants. In the following sections, we outline the neural systems underlying these processes and their developmental course in infancy.

The Attentional State

Two neural systems that project from the brain stem or midbrain to cortical target areas appear to be critical to the basic state of alertness or readiness (Hasselmo, 1995). The grounding of the attentional state to systems originating in the brain stem is consistent with historical connections drawn between attention and phenomena such as the sleep–wake continuum, autonomic function, and arousal; it is also consistent with the use of vital functions such as respiration, heart rate, and pupil dilation as convergent measures of attention or attentional load.

NEURAL BASIS

One of the brain stem systems is characterized predominantly by the neurotransmitter norepinephrine (NE). This pathway originates in the locus coeruleus and projects to numerous targets in the cortex, limbic system, and cerebellum (Chamberlain, Muller, Blackwell, Robbins, & Sahakian, 2006) and appears to be fundamentally integral to the generation of the attentional state (Aston-Jones, Rajkowski, & Cohen, 1999; Chamberlain & Robbins, 2013). A second system is characterized by the predominance of acetylcholine (ACh); this system projects from brain stem nuclei to target populations of neurons in the frontal lobe (Bloem, Poorthuis, & Mansvelder, 2014). Among the functions of this system is the coordination or enhancement of coordinated (i.e., synchronous) firing across large populations of cells (Grossberg & Versace, 2008; Picciotto, Higley, & Mineur, 2012), which may provide the neural basis for many forms of associative learning (see below).

DEVELOPMENT

These ascending systems develop prenatally, but the attentional state appears to emerge late in the last trimester and develop quite rapidly during the early postnatal months. The argument for this is based on three points. First, the appearance of organized sleep–wake states in fetuses and very premature infants is fragile (Nijhuis, Prechtl, Martin, & Bots, 1982); for example, extremely premature infants tend to show nondifferentiated or indistinct behavioral states.

Second, the alert state is seen less than 10% of the time in newborns, with sleep states predominating during the perinatal period (Peirano, Algarin, & Uauy, 2003). Finally, the alert state emerges fairly rapidly during the first month, and becomes more common between 8 and 12 weeks of age (Colombo & Horowitz, 1987); this emergence of the alert state is coincident with an increase in visual attention seen between birth and 8–10 weeks of age on most laboratory tasks that employ visual fixation (Colombo, 2001, 2002).

Selective Processes

While the functions of the ascending NE and ACh pathways from the brain stem appear to map roughly onto the appearance of the attentional state, the selective processes that are manifest through fundamental components of visual attention are linked to two systems involving cortical-to-cortical pathways. These systems are identified in different ways by different authors (Colombo, 1995; Duncan, 1993; Petersen & Posner, 2012; Ruff & Rothbart, 1996), and systems are likely not as independent as initially proposed (Milner & Goodale, 2008). However, the descriptions of these systems and their functional characteristics generally converge, and so the consideration of selective processes in terms of the dorsal and ventral attentional streams remain a broadly used means for conceptualizing selective attention for the field of cognitive neuroscience.

NEURAL BASIS

The anatomy of the dorsal and ventral streams has been described elsewhere (Breitmeyer, 2014), but is reviewed briefly here. The *dorsal stream* projects from the retinal ganglia to the lateral geniculate nucleus of the thalamus; at the lateral geniculate, the dorsal stream is associated with layers of large cells (*magnocellular* layers) from which it projects to the visual cortex and then to the parietal lobe, where it receives input from a second pathway that runs from the retina to the superior colliculus of the brain stem. The advantage of this attentional system is that it does not require much light to function and that it responds very quickly, which makes it very sensitive to motion. However, the system is limited in that it can only process coarse visual input (e.g., large figures with high contrast). As such, the dorsal stream contributes to the perception of movement and analysis of the spatial ("where") aspects of vision. Some models (Posner & Petersen, 1990) suggest that the parietal areas are involved in the engagement (i.e., "locking in") and disengagement (i.e., "letting go") of attention to specific spatial locations. Like the dorsal stream, the *ventral stream* projects from the retina to a layer of small cells (*parvocellular* layers) in the lateral geniculate pathway and then to the visual cortex and then ultimately to the temporal lobe. The ventral stream responds more slowly than the dorsal stream and requires more light to function, but it is capable of processing the finer detailed features of objects within the visual field ("what"), and is adjacent to areas associated with memory and visual recognition.

DEVELOPMENT

In previous reviews (Colombo, 1995, 2001), we have presented evidence that the functions associated with these selective streams emerge from approximately 3 to 10 months of age; although the development of the selective processes continue well past infancy (Booth et al., 2003), the fundamental components allowing for selective attention are clearly present by the end of the first postnatal year. We have posited, however, that the development of infant attention during that first year might be best characterized by an understanding of the interaction among these somewhat distinct dorsal versus ventral streams and their relative immaturity during that time. Interestingly, although functions associated with the systems emerge by the end of the first year, they may have slightly different developmental courses; development of the ventral pathway may be sooner, given that pathways associated with the parvocellular visual system appear to develop earlier than those associated with the magnocellular visual system (Hickey, 1977; Hickey & Peduzzi, 1987). This pattern of development is consistent with observations that very early (or less mature) forms of infant attention would be focused on distinct object features/details (a parvocellular/ventral function), and that the emergence of attentional disengagement (a magnocellular/dorsal function) would be a later-developing phenomenon (Colombo, 2001, 2002, 2004; Hunnius, Geuze, & van Geert, 2006).

Exogenous and Endogenous Attention

Along with a consideration of two basic forms of attention, the model we present here also includes a factor that captures whether the forms are activated or evoked through events external to the organism (typically considered to be reflexive/involuntary and bottom-up in nature) or by endogenous demands (typically considered as voluntary and top-down in nature). Attention may be evoked by particular stimulus properties or bodily conditions (Hopfinger & Ries, 2005; Klein & Dick, 2002); among the terms used for this include *attentional capture* (Bacon & Egeth, 1994; Yantis & Hillstrom, 1994) and *exogenous attention* (Fuller & Carrasco, 2006). Alternatively, the organism may bring itself to an attentional state or may engage selective processes for goal-related or other motivational purposes; this has been called *executive attention* (Kane & Engle, 2002; Posner & DiGirolamo, 1998) or *endogenous attention* (Chong, Tadin, & Blake, 2005; Colombo & Cheatham, 2006). Evidence exists to suggest that the same underlying neural structures are activated for both reflexive and controlled or voluntary forms of attention (Corbetta et al., 1998); this is consistent with the notion that the two forms of attention are constants, regardless of the means by which they are evoked or activated.

Exogenous Attention

As noted above, exogenously driven forms of attention are conceptualized as being driven or evoked from the bottom-up, and so are likely to have their origin in sensory events (stimulus onsets and offsets, or other stimulus parameters) that activate attentional processes. In reality, the study of exogenous attention constitutes a large part of the early literature on human infant perception and cognition, which examined the effect of stimulus parameters such as luminance (Berlyne, 1958), contour (Spears, 1966), contour density (McCarvill & Karmel, 1976), complexity (McCall & Kagan, 1967), spatial frequency (Banks & Ginsburg, 1985), motion (Dannemiller, 1994), and various definitions of salience (Kaldy, Blaser, & Leslie, 2006) as determinants of visual behavior (i.e., orienting). Presumably, such exogenous effects are driven by stimulation from sensory systems through which attentional state or selective processes are activated. Dannemiller conducted numerous studies of exogenous orienting in infants during the late 1990s and 2000s, and developed a series of formal models for the phenomenon primarily in 3- to 4-month-old infants (Dannemiller, 1998, 2000). Most extant models of infant attention posit that exogenous attentional processes exist from birth and dominate attentional processes until about 4–6 postnatal months (Colombo, 2001; Johnson, 1994).

Endogenous Attention

Explication of the top-down regulation that characterizes endogenous attention, however, has been a topic of particular interest in the last decade. It is widely accepted that endogenous functions are regulated through frontal lobe structures (Miller & Cohen, 2001; Reynolds & Chelazzi, 2004), and it is likely that endogenous attention is a product of the integration of lower-order attentional components with working memory (Kane & Engle, 2002; Kane, Poole, Tuholski, & Engle, 2006). Indeed, endogenous control of the dorsal and ventral pathways is likely mediated through anatomical links to frontal areas (Colombo & Cheatham, 2006), which would allow for these attentional systems to be coordinated with other cognitive functions (Chica, Bartolomeo, & Lupianez, 2013; Tallon-Baudry, 2012). This proposal for the emergence of endogenous attention is consistent with more generalized models of the neural bases for higher-order cognitive activity (e.g., executive function), in which frontal areas serve to integrate input from other areas that mediate more fundamental functions (Banich, 2009; Miller & Cohen, 2001).

DEVELOPMENT

Although some accounts contend that attention is purposeful and voluntary even in newborns (Haith, 1980), more recent models find evidence for the emergence of voluntary attentional processes no earlier than 4 months (Colombo, 2001; Johnson, 1994) with robust emergence of coordination between memory and attention only after 6 months (Bell & Fox, 1992; Cuevas & Bell, 2011; Diamond, 1998; Oakes, Kannass, & Shaddy, 2002; Wolfe & Bell, 2007). The development of integrative functions that presumably provide the basis for the higher-order cognitive abilities seen in executive function (Banich, 2009), the establishment of semantic networks (Colombo & Cheatham, 2006), and more endogenous regulatory functions (Kraybill & Bell, 2013; Posner & Rothbart, 2000; Rueda, Posner, & Rothbart, 2005) likely emerge with maturation of frontal function beginning late in the first year and predominate behavioral development into the second and third years. This scenario has clear implications for our understanding of the emergence of attentional disorders, as well as for the search for early markers for such disorders.

Attention in Social and Nonsocial Contexts

Earlier in the chapter, we alluded to long-standing controversies over the presence of multiple channels for attention; in the developmental literatures, this debate has been largely manifest in discussions about the presence of separate channels for processing information that is social versus nonsocial in nature. This debate, particularly within a developmental context, has important implications for the architecture of cognition and translational efforts in understanding and intervening in areas of developmental disabilities. In the following sections, we review the extant literature pertaining to the construct of *social attention*.

Contextual Effects in Early Cognition

The attention processes described above unfold within a multimodal context that is both dynamic and complex, with multiple streams of information competing for attentional resources. Traditionally, infant research has almost exclusively considered the nonsocial context in the measurement of various aspects of attention regulation, using standard laboratory tasks (e.g., habituation, visual preference) that involved static and well-controlled stimuli (e.g., geometric patterns and objects). Within the infant social development literature, however, attention has been incorporated as a means through which infants process streams of information in dyadic interactions with an engaged partner (e.g., joint attention, social referencing). Consequently, there has been grow-ing interest in (and use of) the term *social attention* (e.g., Frank, Vul, & Saxe, 2012; Freeth, Foulsham, & Kingstone, 2013; Laidlaw, Risko, & Kingstone, 2012). The presence of this construct leads to the question of whether the social context differentially influences the activation of attention processes, and/or whether attentional forms may differ in the context of social and nonsocial streams of information.

Social Attention

Although the term *social attention* has appeared with increasing regularity in recent years, it is currently used as an umbrella term for a constellation of behaviors that involve some form of attention to other people. This ranges from attention in the form of social communication activity to more traditional mea-sures of attention orienting to people. Social attention has primarily emerged as a nonspecific reference for social dysfunction in autism spectrum disorder (Chawarska, Macari, & Shic, 2012; Dawson et al., 2004), as well as a slightly more specific definition of, or synonym for, joint attention (Mundy et al., 2007). Though basic developmental research has long considered early attention prefer-ences (e.g., early preference for viewing face stimuli), only recently has this been reframed as social attention (see, e.g., Perra & Gattis, 2010). Presently, there is no consensus on how the term *social attention* should be defined or mea-sured (although, see Birmingham & Kingstone, 2009; Risko, Laidlaw, Freeth, Foulsham, & Kingstone, 2012, for related discussions).

Does the Social Context Really Matter?

Only a limited number of studies yield findings that examine the question of whether the (social or nonsocial) context matters for attention regulation—in terms of developmental course, individual differences, and/or developmental outcomes. Contextual variants of attention regulation are briefly highlighted next, as appearing within both the general developmental and clinical litera-tures.

Attention to People

Early developmental observations have provided considerable evidence for the relevance of social information for infants, including the early preference for attending to faces and face-like configurations (Johnson, Dziurawiec, Ellis, & Morton, 1991), and early emerging skills for processing information from faces including sensitivity to eye contact, direction of gaze, and emotional expression (Cohn & Tronick, 1983; Farroni, Csibra, Simion, & Johnson, 2002; Farroni,

Massaccesi, Pividori, & Johnson, 2004). Studies that have directly considered attention in the context of both social and nonsocial information point to developmental changes in attention to social information during the first few months of life and underscore the importance of ecological paradigms.

Most often, infants have been presented with an array of images (usually photographs of people and objects displayed together on a single screen) in order to record their visual attention (e.g., first fixation, duration of looking, number of fixations). Generally speaking, young infants look equally to face and object displays early in the first year of life, whereas older infants and adults look more to faces, even when faces were not the most salient items in the display in terms of contrast and luminance (Di Giorgio, Turati, Altoe, & Simion, 2012; Gluckman & Johnson, 2013). This developmental pattern of increased attention to social information has been demonstrated for dynamic (i.e., movie) events as well (Frank, Vul, & Johnson, 2009).

Another avenue for characterizing contextual influences on attention is through the use of habituation paradigms, which reflect attention-processing efficiency. Almost without exception, early and recent studies of infant visual habituation have used *either* a nonsocial class of stimuli, such as geometric forms or checkerboards (e.g., Shaddy & Colombo, 2004) and objects/nonsocial scenes (e.g., Miller, 1972) *or* a social class of stimuli, such as photographs of faces (Gaither, Pauker, & Johnson, 2012); studies that have presented both classes of stimuli are limited by methodological limitations for this specific question (Pecheux & Lecuyer, 1983). Thus, while it is possible that some babies might differentially acquire information in contexts that may be primarily characterized as social or nonsocial (e.g., infants might attend more or less efficiently in one context versus another, perhaps because one type of information is more reinforcing or salient), this has not been directly examined.

Some developmentalists have argued that the majority of behavioral and neuroimaging studies to date have examined social attention in the lab by presenting faces in isolation, and thus may have promoted the overestimation of the degree to which we look at others' eyes and the degree to which we look where others are looking (Birmingham & Kingstone, 2009; Kingstone, 2009; Risko et al., 2012). Indeed, when attention is measured in various real-world settings, looking behavior is not straightforward, and likely varies as a function of the particulars of the social context. For example, in a live context, adults looked less often to another person while sitting in a waiting room, but looked more often to another person during a question-and-answer situation; the opposite pattern was observed during a videotaped condition (Freeth et al., 2013). Such differences are intriguing and further underscore the importance of exploring the nuances of individual differences in attention regulation in a real-world context.

Attention to Social Cues

Beyond looking at people, one particularly important component of adaptive social exchange involves attending to the cues of another person (e.g., head turns, gaze shifts, points). Early in the first months of life infants begin to share eye-to-eye gaze with a parent and within the first year also begin to follow a parent's gaze direction to look toward an object or event. A distinct body of research has been devoted to understanding the gaze-following processes, including the variety of social cues and combinations of cues that shift attention and their developmental course (see Frischen, Bayliss, & Tipper, 2007, for a review). It has been well established that adults and children both shift attention in response to cues with social relevance (e.g., eyes) *and* cues that do not have obvious inherent social valence, such as arrows (e.g., Senju, Tojo, Dairoku, & Hasegawa, 2004). Though it appears reasonable that social cues are unique in their attention-directing salience, the extent to which attention is differentially cued by socially relevant stimuli remains a matter of debate.

Ultimately, these early gaze-following skills support the emergence of more sophisticated attention coordination (joint attention) behavior. Infants begin to direct the attention of others for purely social purposes, a behavior that theoretically involves foundational attentional regulation processes (e.g., orienting, disengagement, and shifting in the context of people and objects; Mundy, Sullivan, & Mastergeorge, 2009). This triadic coordination of attention with another person *and* another object/event is considered critical for social cognitive and language development (see Meindl & Cannella-Malone, 2011, for a review).

THE SOCIAL PARTNER

As the critical component of the social context, we contend that the social partner may provide unique information that influences the development of basic attention skills (i.e., attentional state, orienting, endogenous attention). In comparison to nonsocial sources of information, other social agents provide access to relevant cues in an interactive context that is contingent and dynamic, which in turn may serve to recruit and organize attention. For example, parents provide critical word-learning opportunities by labeling objects that their child is attending to during joint attention episodes; and mothers who follow their children's focus of attention have children with larger vocabularies, compared with mothers who redirect their children's focus of attention (Tomasello & Todd, 1983). Other variations in the social context, such as rates of contingent responses between caregivers and infants have been linked to linguistic measures (Goldstein & Schwade, 2008). Furthermore, evidence from behavioral and neurobiological studies indicates that social experiences during infancy have an important and lasting impact on how social–perceptual information is processed and may be important for the development of brain networks that are involved in processing social stimuli and language development (Mills & Conboy, 2009).

Social Attention in Atypical Development

Thus far we have discussed attention patterns for typically developing individuals, but studies of atypical development provide critical insight for understanding contextual influences on attention regulation. Populations with differences in attentional processes related to the social context discussed here include individuals with autism spectrum disorder (ASD), Williams syndrome (WS), attention-deficit/hyperactivity disorder (ADHD), and premature infants.

AUTISM SPECTRUM DISORDER

ASD is diagnosed based on the presence of deficits in social communication and the presence of restricted interests/repetitive behaviors. Differences in attention to social aspects of the environment include deficits in joint attention, both in following the attention cues of others and directing the attention of others (Meindl & Cannella-Malone, 2011). The latter, deficits in initiating joint attention (sometimes used interchangeably with "social attention") are considered a hallmark characteristic of core ASD manifestations in social communication. Evidence suggests that early disruption in basic attention regulation may be a key contribution to later deficits in joint attention. Notable differences have been observed in basic attentional networks (i.e., alerting, orienting, and executive control networks), including dysregulation in arousal systems, impaired novelty processing, slowed attention disengagement and shifting, and deficits in executive control on complex tasks (see Keehn, Muller, & Townsend, 2013, for a recent review). Differences in visual attention and orienting are perhaps the earliest and most consistent symptoms of ASD (Zwaigenbaum et al., 2005). These include deficits in orienting to and processing social information, such as reduced preference for human speech (Kuhl, Coffey-Corina, Padden, & Dawson, 2005), preference for dynamic geometric images over dynamic social images (Pierce, Conant, Hazin, Stoner, & Desmond, 2011), atypical face scanning, recognition and attention to faces and eyes in laboratory settings (Chawarska & Shic, 2009; Chawarska & Volkmar, 2007; Jones & Klin, 2013), and decreased attention toward people versus objects in naturally occurring settings (Maestro et al., 2005).

Differences in shifting and disengaging attention are also evident among individuals with ASD. For example, infants with ASD most often shift attention between an object and another object, in comparison to typically developing and developmentally delayed infants who most often shift between an object and a person (Swettenham et al., 1998). Furthermore, infants at risk for autism, young children diagnosed with autism, and low-functioning adults with ASD take longer to disengage from a central target to orient toward a peripheral event (i.e., a visual orienting task designed to examine automatic attention shifting), when compared with controls (Elsabbagh et al., 2009; Kawakubo, Maekawa, Itoh, Hashimoto, & Iwanami, 2004; Landry & Bryson, 2004). Generally speaking, such differences in shifting and disengaging attention suggest impairments in the development of brain areas involved in the orienting network. In particular, activities that require the dynamic, reflexive modulation of attention (e.g., rapid alerting, orienting, disengaging, and shifting attention; in contrast to more effortful sustained attention processes) appear to be more impaired, while more effortful attention processes may be more intact (Townsend, Keehn, & Westerfield, 2012). In sum, these results provide convincing evidence for core differences in attention regulation among individuals with autism.

WILLIAMS SYNDROME

In contrast to ASD, individuals with WS display exaggerated bias *toward* social information. WS is a rare genetic disorder that involves the striking combination of mild to moderate learning disability alongside relative proficiency in language and hypersocial behavior. Individuals with WS display more frequent and prolonged fixation to faces (i.e., atypical visual orienting and disengagement) when viewing photographs and movies of social scenes (Riby & Hancock, 2008, 2009). During social interaction, individuals with WS are highly focused on the other person, often to the exclusion of any coordinated attention sharing with respect to objects or events (Laing et al., 2002). In other words, although WS may represent the opposite side of the continuum of social interest in comparison to ASD, the profile of attention engagement and regulation skill nonetheless results in significant functional social impairment.

ATTENTION-DEFICIT/HYPERACTIVITY DISORDER

ADHD involves deficits in sustained attention and other executive function impairments (e.g., deficits in response inhibition, working memory, temporal processing). ADHD is diagnosed based on behavioral symptoms of inattention, hyperactivity, and impulsivity, but individuals often present with corresponding social skill impairments, which may in fact be among the more debilitating consequences when present. Although the majority of spatial cueing studies do not indicate orienting deficits in ADHD (Huang-Pollock & Nigg, 2003), one recent study has found evidence suggesting the possibility of an attentional impairment in responding to socially relevant information. When compared with typically developing counterparts who shifted attention in response to both social (eyes) and nonsocial (arrows) cues, children and adolescents with ADHD displayed orienting responses only to nonsocial stimuli (Marotta et al., 2013).

PRETERM INFANTS

Similar to other groups with differences in basic attention skills, preterm infants also display difficulties in the context of social interaction, as these infants are at risk for compromised visual processing and tend to have less optimal visual attention abilities (e.g., orienting and sustained attention; van de Weijer-Bergsma, Wijnroks, & Jongmans, 2008). During mother–infant interactions preterm infants avert gaze more often and for longer periods and make fewer social bids to regain attention during a still-face procedure (De Schuymer, De Groote, Striano, Stahl, & Roeyers, 2011; Harel, Gordon, Geva, & Feldman, 2011). Preterm infants who more often averted gaze during a social context also displayed less mature attention skills in a nonsocial context, in that they were slower to disengage and shift attention in a competition paradigm (De Schuymer, De Groote, Desoete, & Roeyers, 2012). Similar to other clinical populations, early differences in attention regulation in preterm infants may have a downstream impact on the dynamic regulation of attention during social exchange with others.

The Social Brain

Within social neuroscience, there has been a growing interest in the specific network of brain areas referred to as the "social brain" that may be preferentially involved in processing social information. The social brain is generally considered to include the superior temporal sulcus (STS), the fusiform gyrus, the amygdala, the prefrontal cortex (PFC), and the mirror neuron system (Johnson, 2010). This is relevant for atypically developing populations, who may have disruptions to the social brain network (through combined interactions of experience and neural development) that result in failures or delays in specialization of cortical structures, which in turn produce downstream functional impairments in social communication. For example, individuals with autism are hypothesized to have early brain abnormalities (e.g., decreased activity in the fusiform face area, underactivity in the STS and amygdala) that disrupt early social attention and do not allow them to accrue necessary social experiences for real-world functional social communication (Shultz, Chawarska, & Volkmar, 2006).

Summary

Overall, there is considerable evidence indicating that social cues may engage behavioral and neural mechanisms in a way that is at least distinct from nonsocial cues. Although a handful of basic attention studies have considered this question, the methodologies used were not intended to tease apart the nature of social and nonsocial contextual influences on attention regulation. The majority of behavioral evidence comes from studies of atypical attention in clinical populations. Identifying differences in attentional processes under these contextual variations has the potential to offer a rich source of evidence that is relevant for both typical and atypical developmental pathways.

Overall Summary and Future Directions

Our objective in writing this chapter was to summarize the topic of attentional development from the viewpoint of behavioral, neural, and social perspectives. We have proposed a simplified framework for considering the many varieties of attention that may be found in the literature and the probable functions of attention within the general scope of cognitive development and learning. We briefly reviewed the major neural systems that contribute to attention and its development, with references to the emergence of the developmental state, selective processes, and the coordination of attention with other functions that serve higher-order cognitive development in toddlerhood and early childhood. A comprehensive understanding of the interplay of these attentional systems will be necessary for successful translational efforts in early identification, early intervention, and for the creation of conditions that contribute to optimal development. This survey of the development of attention suggests a number of important areas for work in the next decade. Clearly, there is more work to be done in the basic understanding of the neural bases of attention in human infants; as evidenced by even this brief review, the extant models are subject to revision and correction and can only be regarded as speculative. Certain specific topics for inquiry, however, appear to have potential for significant impact in the developmental sciences and beyond. The emergence of endogenous function late in the first year is seemingly well documented, but a question remains as to whether exogenous forms of attention seen earlier in the first year contribute to more executive forms of attention. Evidence from older predictive studies (Colombo, Shaddy, Richman, Maikranz, & Blaga, 2004) has been suggestive of this, but recent data (Cuevas & Bell, 2014) present stronger evidence for this case. Another potential avenue for inquiry is whether environmental manipulations of attention (e.g., attention training, exogenous induction of attention) that have proven to be fruitful with older children (Tang & Posner, 2009) might be relevant to infants, as some data suggest (Wass, Porayska-Pomsta, & Johnson, 2011); such an avenue would have implications for typically developing infants and clinical populations (Whalen, Schreibman, & Ingersoll, 2006).

Finally, we addressed the emergent debate over the existence of a specific form of *social attention*; while the definitive critical studies for establishing attentional processes that are qualitatively directed toward or affected by social targets and contexts are yet to be conducted, the extant evidence suggests that this may be a productive path for the future. To advance this line of research, it is necessary to shift toward a more precise use of the term *social attention*, a move that will be possible with systematic examination of the equivalence of social stimuli utilized within and across studies, as well as comparison of their approximation to real social interaction (Risko et al., 2012). Continued work focused on understanding brain areas and neural circuits that are preferentially active while negotiating aspects of the social environment will also be a critical area of inquiry, alongside examination of the specific motivational value of social stimuli. Articulating the nature of attention to social events has the potential to inform early identification and intervention efforts for young children with delayed and disordered development.

ACKNOWLEDGMENTS

This work was supported in part by Grant Nos. P30HD02528, R01HD047315, and K99HD075886; Brenda Salley was also initially supported by Grant No. T32HD057844.

REFERENCES

Albright, T. D., Jessell, T. M., Kandel, E. R., & Posner, M. I. (2000). Neural science: A century of progress and the mysteries that remain. *Cell, 100,* S1–S55.

Aslin, R. N., & Newport, E. L. (2012). Statistical learning: From acquiring specific items to forming general rules. *Current Directions in Psychological Science, 21*(3), 170–176.

Aston-Jones, G., Rajkowski, J., & Cohen, J. (1999). Role of locus coeruleus in attention and behavioral flexibility. *Biological Psychiatry, 46*(9), 1309–1320.

Bacon, W. F., & Egeth, H. E. (1994). Overriding stimulus-driven attentional capture. *Perception and Psychophysics, 55*(5), 485–496.

Banich, M. T. (2009). Executive function: The search for an integrated account. *Current Directions in Psychological Science, 18*(2), 89–94.

Banks, M. S., & Ginsburg, A. P. (1985). Infant visual preferences: A review and new theoretical treatment. *Advances in Child Development and Behavior, 19,* 207–246.

Barkley, R. A. (1997). Behavioral inhibition, sustained attention, and executive functions: Constructing a unifying theory of ADHD. *Psychological Bulletin, 121*(1), 65–94.

Bell, M. A., & Fox, N. A. (1992). The relations between frontal brain electrical activity and cognitive development during infancy. *Child Development, 63*(5), 1142.

Bell, M. A., & Wolfe, C. D. (2007). Changes in brain functioning from infancy to early childhood: Evidence from EEG power and coherence during working memory tasks. *Developmental Neuropsychology, 31*(1), 21–38.

Berlyne, D. E. (1958). The influence of the albedo and complexity of stimuli on visual fixation in the human infant. *British Journal of Psychology, 49,* 315–318.

Birmingham, E., & Kingstone, A. (2009). Human social attention: A new look at past, present, and future investigations. *Annals of the New York Academy of Sciences, 1156,* 118–140.

Blaga, O. M., & Colombo, J. (2006). Visual processing and infant ocular latencies in the overlap paradigm. *Developmental Psychology, 42*(6), 1069–1076.

Bloem, B., Poorthuis, R. B., & Mansvelder, H. D. (2014). Cholinergic modulation of the medial prefrontal cortex: The role of nicotinic receptors in attention and regulation of neuronal activity. *Frontiers in Neural Circuits, 8*, 16.

Booth, J. R., Burman, D. D., Meyer, J. R., Lei, Z., Trommer, B. L., Davenport, N. D., et al. (2003). Neural development of selective attention and response inhibition. *Neuroimage, 20*(2), 737–751.

Borji, A., & Itti, L. (2014). Optimal attentional modulation of a neural population. *Frontiers in Computational Neuroscience, 8*, 14.

Bornstein, M. H., & Colombo, J. (2012). Infant cognitive functioning and mental development. In S. Pauen (Ed.), *Early childhood development and later outcome* (pp. 118–147). Cambridge, UK: Cambridge University Press.

Breitmeyer, B. G. (2014). Contributions of magno- and parvocellular channels to conscious and non-conscious vision. *Philosophical Transactions of the Royal Society B–Biological Sciences, 369*(1641), 11.

Bressler, S. L., & Tognoli, E. (2006). Operational principles of neurocognitive networks. *International Journal of Psychophysiology, 60*(2), 139–148.

Broadbent, D. (1958). *Perception and communication.* Elmsford, NY: Pergamon Press.

Chamberlain, S. R., Muller, U., Blackwell, A. D., Robbins, T. W., & Sahakian, B. J. (2006). Noradrenergic modulation of working memory and emotional memory in humans. *Psychopharmacology, 188*(4), 397–407.

Chamberlain, S. R., & Robbins, T. W. (2013). Noradrenergic modulation of cognition: Therapeutic implications. *Journal of Psychopharmacology, 27*(8), 694–718.

Chawarska, K., Macari, S., & Shic, F. (2012). Context modulates attention to social scenes in toddlers with autism. *Journal of Child Psychology and Psychiatry, and Allied Disciplines, 53*(8), 903–913.

Chawarska, K., & Shic, F. (2009). Looking but not seeing: Atypical visual scanning and recognition of faces in 2- and 4-year-old children with autism spectrum disorder. *Journal of Autism and Developmental Disorders, 39*(12), 1663–1672

Chawarska, K., & Volkmar, F. (2007). Impairments in monkey and human face recognition in 2-year-old toddlers with autism spectrum disorder and developmental delay. *Developmental Science, 10*(2), 266–279.

Cherry, E. C. (1953). Some experiments on the recognition of speech, with one and two ears. *Journal of the Acoustical Society of America, 25*(5), 975–979.

Chica, A. B., Bartolomeo, P., & Lupianez, J. (2013). Two cognitive and neural systems for endogenous and exogenous spatial attention. *Behavioural Brain Research, 237*, 107–123.

Chong, S. C., Tadin, D., & Blake, R. (2005). Endogenous attention prolongs dominance durations in binocular rivalry. *Journal of Vision, 5*(11), 1004–1012.

Cohn, J. F., & Tronick, E. Z. (1983). Three-month-old infants' reaction to simulated maternal depression. *Child Development, 54*, 185–193.

Colombo, J. (1995). On the neural mechanisms underlying developmental and individual differences in visual fixation in infancy: Two hypotheses. *Developmental Review, 15*(2), 97–135.

Colombo, J. (2001). The development of visual attention in infancy. *Annual Review of Psychology, 52*, 337–367.

Colombo, J. (2002). Infant attention grows up: The emergence of a developmental cognitive neuroscience perspective. *Current Directions in Psychological Science, 11*(6), 196–200.

Colombo, J. (2004). Visual attention in infancy: Process and product in early cognitive development. In M. I. Posner (Ed.), *Cognitive neuroscience of attention* (pp. 329–341). New York: Guilford Press.

Colombo, J., & Cheatham, C. L. (2006). The emergence and basis of endogenous attention in infancy and early childhood. *Advances in Child Development and Behavior, 34*, 283–322.

Colombo, J., & Horowitz, F. D. (1987). Behavioral state as a lead variable in neonatal research. *Merrill-Palmer Quarterly, 33*(4), 423–437.

Colombo, J., Kannass, K. N., Walker, D., & Brez, C. D. (2012). The development of attention in infancy and early childhood: Implications for early childhood and early intervention. In S. L. Odom, E. Pungello, & N. Gardner-Neblett (Eds.), *Revisioning the beginning: The implications of developmental and health science for infant/toddler care and poverty* (pp. 21–48). New York: Guilford Press.

Colombo, J., & Mitchell, D. W. (2009). Infant visual habituation. *Neurobiology of Learning and Memory, 92*(2), 225–234.

Colombo, J., Shaddy, D. J., Anderson, C. J., Gibson, L. J., Blaga, O. M., & Kannass, K. N. (2010). What habituates in infant visual habituation?: A psychophysiological analysis. *Infancy, 15*(2), 107–124.

Colombo, J., Shaddy, D. J., Richman, W. A., Maikranz, J. M., & Blaga, O. M. (2004). The developmental course of habituation in infancy and preschool outcome. *Infancy, 5*(1), 1–38.

Corbetta, M., Akbudak, E., Conturo, T. E., Snyder, A. Z., Ollinger, J. M., Drury, H. A., et al. (1998). A common network of functional areas for attention and eye movements. *Neuron, 21*(4), 761–773.

Cuevas, K., & Bell, M. A. (2011). EEG and ECG from 5 to 10 months of age: Developmental changes in baseline activation and cognitive processing during a working memory task. *International Journal of Psychophysiology, 80*(2), 119–128.

Cuevas, K., & Bell, M. A. (2014). Infant attention and early childhood executive function. *Child Development, 85*(2), 397–404.

Dannemiller, J. L. (1994). Reliability of motion detection by young infants measured with a new signal-detection paradigm. *Infant Behavior and Development, 17*(1), 101–105.

Dannemiller, J. L. (1998). A competition model of exogenous orienting in 3.5-month-old infants. *Journal of Experimental Child Psychology, 68*(3), 169–201.

Dannemiller, J. L. (2000). Competition in early exogenous orienting between 7 and 21 weeks. *Journal of Experimental Child Psychology, 76*(4), 253–274.

Dawson, G., Toth, K., Abbott, R., Osterling, J., Munson, J., Estes, A., et al. (2004). Early social attention impairments in autism: Social orienting, joint attention, and attention to distress. *Developmental Psychology, 40*(2), 271–283.

De Schuymer, L., De Groote, I., Desoete, A., & Roeyers, H. (2012). Gaze aversion during social interaction in preterm infants: A function of attention skills? *Infant Behavior and Development, 35*(1), 129–139.

De Schuymer, L., De Groote, I., Striano, T., Stahl, D., & Roeyers, H. (2011). Dyadic and triadic skills in preterm and full term infants: A longitudinal study in the first year. *Infant Behavior and Development, 34*(1), 179–188.

Denot-Ledunois, S., Vardon, G., Perruchet, P., & Gallego, J. (1998). The effect of attentional load on the breathing pattern in children. *International Journal of Psychophysiology, 29*(1), 13–21.

Di Giorgio, E., Turati, C., Altoe, G., & Simion, F. (2012). Face detection in complex visual displays: An eye-tracking study with 3- and 6-month-old infants and adults. *Journal of Experimental Child Psychology, 113*(1), 66–77.

Diamond, A. (1998). Understanding the A-not-B error: Working memory vs. reinforced response, or active trace vs. latent trace. *Developmental Science, 1*(2), 185–189.

Duncan, J. (1993). Coordination of what and where in visual attention. *Perception, 22*(11), 1261–1270.

Eldar, E., Cohen, J. D., & Niv, Y. (2013). The effects of neural gain on attention and learning. *Nature Neuroscience, 16*(8), 1146–1236.

Elsabbagh, M., Volein, A., Holmboe, K., Tucker, L., Csibra, G., Baron-Cohen, S., et al. (2009). Visual orienting in the early broader autism phenotype: Disengagement and facilitation. *Journal of Child Psychology and Psychiatry, 50*(5), 637–642.

Engel, A. K., & Singer, W. (2001). Temporal binding and the neural correlates of sensory awareness. *Trends in Cognitive Sciences, 5*(1), 16–25.

Farroni, T., Csibra, G., Simion, F., & Johnson, M. H. (2002). Eye contact detection in humans from birth. *Proceedings of the National Academy of Sciences of the United States of America, 99*(14), 9602–9605.

Farroni, T., Massaccesi, S., Pividori, D., & Johnson, M. H. (2004). Gaze following in newborns. *Infancy, 5*(1), 39–60.

Frank, M. C., Vul, E., & Johnson, S. P. (2009). Development of infants' attention to faces during the first year. *Cognition, 110*(2), 160–170.

Frank, M. C., Vul, E., & Saxe, R. (2012). Measuring the development of social attention using free-viewing. *Infancy, 17*(4), 355–375.

Freeth, M., Foulsham, T., & Kingstone, A. (2013). What affects social attention? Social presence, eye contact and autistic traits. *PLoS ONE, 8*(1), e53286.

Frick, J. E., Colombo, J., & Saxon, T. F. (1999). Individual and developmental differences in disengagement of fixation in early infancy. *Child Development, 70*(3), 537–548.

Fries, P. (2005). A mechanism for cognitive dynamics: Neuronal communication through neuronal coherence. *Trends in Cognitive Sciences, 9*(10), 474–480.

Frischen, A., Bayliss, A. P., & Tipper, S. P. (2007). Gaze cueing of attention: Visual attention, social cognition and individual differences. *Psychological Bulletin, 133*(4), 694–724.

Fuller, S., & Carrasco, M. (2006). Exogenous attention and color perception: Performance and appearance of saturation and hue. *Vision Research, 46*(23), 4032–4047.

Gaither, S. E., Pauker, K., & Johnson, S. P. (2012). Biracial and monoracial infant own-race face perception: An eye tracking study. *Developmental Science, 15*(6), 775–782.

Gladstones, W. H., Regan, M. A., & Lee, R. B. (1989). Division of attention: The single-channel hypothesis revisited. *Quarterly Journal of Experimental Psychology Section A: Human Experimental Psychology, 41*(1), 1–17.

Gluckman, M., & Johnson, S. P. (2013). Attentional capture by social stimuli in young infants. *Frontiers in Psychology, 4,* 527.

Goldstein, M. H., & Schwade, J. A. (2008). Social feedback to infants' babbling facilitates rapid phonological learning. *Psychological Science, 19*(5), 515–523.

Graham, F. K., & Clifton, R. K. (1966). Heart-rate change as a component of orienting response. *Psychological Bulletin, 65*(5), 305–320.

Grossberg, S., & Versace, M. (2008). Spikes, synchrony, and attentive learning by laminar thalamocortical circuits. *Brain Research, 1218,* 278–312.

Haith, M. (1980). *Rules that babies look by.* Hillsdale, NJ: Erlbaum.

Harel, H., Gordon, I., Geva, R., & Feldman, R. (2011). Gaze behaviors of preterm and full-term infants in nonsocial and social contexts of increasing dynamics: Visual recognition, attention regulation, and gaze synchrony. *Infancy, 16*(1), 69–90.

Hasselmo, M. E. (1995). Neuromodulation and cortical function: Modeling the physiological basis of behavior. *Behavioural Brain Research, 67*(1), 1–27.

Hernandez-Peon, R. (1966). Physiological mechanisms in attention. In R. W. Russel (Ed.), *Frontiers in physiological psychology* (pp. 121–147). New York: Academic Press.

Hickey, T. L. (1977). Postnatal development of the human lateral geniculate nucleus: Relationship to a critical period for the visual system. *Science, 198,* 836–838.

Hickey, T. L., & Peduzzi, J. D. (1987). Structure and development of the visual system. In L. B. Cohen & P. Salapatek (Eds.), *Handbook of infant perception* (pp. 1–42). New York: Academic Press.

Hillyard, S. A., Vogel, E. K., & Luck, S. J. (1998). Sensory gain control (amplification) as a mechanism of selective attention: Electrophysiological and neuroimaging evidence. *Philosophical Transactions of the Royal Society of London Series B: Biological Sciences, 353*(1373), 1257–1270.

Hopfinger, J. B., & Ries, A. J. (2005). Automatic versus contingent mechanisms of sensory-driven neural biasing and reflexive attention. *Journal of Cognitive Neuroscience, 17*(8), 1341–1352.

Huang-Pollock, C. L., & Nigg, J. T. (2003). Searching for the attention deficit in attention deficit hyperactivity disorder: The case of visuospatial orienting. *Clinical Psychology Review, 23*(6), 801–830.

Hunnius, S., Geuze, R. H., & van Geert, P. (2006). Associations between the developmental trajectories of visual scanning and disengagement of attention in infants. *Infant Behavior and Development, 29*(1), 108–125.

Jackson, I., & Sirois, S. (2009). Infant cognition: Going full factorial with pupil dilation. *Developmental Science, 12*(4), 670–679.

James, W. (1890). *Principles of psychology.* New York: Holt.

Johnson, M. H. (1994). Visual attention and the control of eye movements in early infancy. In C. Umilta & M. Moscovitch (Eds.), *Attention and performance XV: Conscious and nonconscious information processing* (pp. 291–310). Cambridge, MA: MIT Press.

Johnson, M. H. (2010). Understanding the social world: A developmental neuroscience approach. In S. D. Calkins & M. A. Bell (Eds.), *Child development at the intersection of emotion and cognition: Human brain development* (pp. 153–174). Washington, DC: American Psychological Association.

Johnson, M. H., Dziurawiec, S., Ellis, H., & Morton, J. (1991). Newborns' preferential tracking of face-like stimuli and its subsequent decline. *Cognition, 40,* 1–19.

Jones, W., & Klin, A. (2013). Attention to eyes is present but in decline in 2–6-month-old infants later diagnosed with autism. *Nature, 504*(7480), 427–431.

Kaldy, Z., Blaser, E. A., & Leslie, A. M. (2006). A new method for calibrating perceptual salience across dimensions in infants: The case of color vs. luminance. *Developmental Science, 9*(5), 482–489.

Kane, M. J., & Engle, R. W. (2002). The role of prefrontal cortex in working-memory capacity, executive attention, and general fluid intelligence: An individual-differences perspective. *Psychonomic Bulletin and Review, 9*(4), 637–671.

Kane, M. J., Poole, B. J., Tuholski, S. W., & Engle, R. W. (2006). Working memory capacity and the top-down control of visual search: Exploring the boundaries of "executive attention." *Journal of Experimental Psychology: Learning, Memory, and Cognition, 32*(4), 749–777.

Kawakubo, Y., Maekawa, H., Itoh, K., Hashimoto, O., & Iwanami, A. (2004). Spatial attention in individuals with pervasive developmental disorders using the gap overlap task. *Psychiatry Research, 125,* 269–275.

Keehn, B., Muller, R. A., & Townsend, J. (2013). Atypical attentional networks and the emergence of autism. *Neuroscience and Biobehavioral Reviews, 37*(2), 164–183.

Kingstone, A. (2009). Taking a real look at social attention. *Current Opinion in Neurobiology, 19*(1), 52–56.

Klein, R. M., & Dick, B. (2002). Temporal dynamics of reflexive attention shifts: A dual-stream rapid serial visual presentation exploration. *Psychological Science, 13*(2), 176–179.

Klimesch, W., Freunberger, R., Sauseng, P., & Gruber, W. (2008). A short review of slow phase synchronization and memory: Evidence for control processes in different memory systems? *Brain Research, 1235,* 31–44.

Kraybill, J. H., & Bell, M. A. (2013). Infancy predictors of preschool and post-kindergarten executive function. *Developmental Psychobiology, 55*(5), 530–538.

Kuhl, P. K., Coffey-Corina, S., Padden, D., & Dawson, G. (2005). Links between social and linguistic processing of speech in preschool children with autism: Behavioral and electrophysiological measures. *Developmental Science, 8*(1), F1–F12.

LaBerge, D., Carlson, R. L., Williams, J. K., & Bunney, B. G. (1997). Shifting attention in visual space: Tests of moving-spotlight models versus an activity-distribution model. *Journal of Experimental Psychology: Human Perception and Performance, 23*(5), 1380–1392.

Laidlaw, K. E., Risko, E. F., & Kingstone, A. (2012). A new look at social attention: Orienting to the eyes is not (entirely) under volitional control. *Journal of Experimental Psychology: Human Perception and Performance, 38*(5), 1132–1143.

Laing, E., Butterworth, G., Ansari, D., Gsodl, M., Longhi, E., Panagiotaki, G., et al. (2002). Atypical development of language and social communication in toddlers with Williams syndrome. *Developmental Science, 5,* 233–246.

Landry, R., & Bryson, S. E. (2004). Impaired disengagement of attention in young children with autism. *Journal of Child Psychology and Psychiatry, 45*(6), 1115–1122.

Lawler, K. A., Obrist, P. A., & Lawler, J. E. (1975). Cardiac and somatic responses during attention. *Psychophysiology, 12*(2), 230–231.

Maestro, S., Muratori, F., Cavallaro, M. C., Pecini, C., Cesari, A., Paziente, A., et al. (2005). How young children treat objects and people: An empirical study of the first year of life in autism. *Child Psychiatry and Human Development, 35*(4), 383–396.

Marotta, A., Casagrande, M., Rosa, C., Maccari, L., Berloco, B., & Pasini, A. (2013). Impaired reflexive orienting to social cues in attention deficit hyperactivity disorder. *European Child and Adolescent Psychiatry, 23*(8), 649–657.

McCall, R. B., & Kagan, J. (1967). Attention in the infant: Effects of complexity, contour, perimeter, and familiarity. *Child Development, 38*(4), 939–952.

McCarvill, S. L., & Karmel, B. Z. (1976). A neural activity interpretation of luminance effects on infant pattern preferences. *Journal of Experimental Child Psychology, 22*(3), 363–374.

Meindl, J. N., & Cannella-Malone, H. I. (2011). Initiating and responding to joint attention bids in children with autism: A review of the literature. *Research in Developmental Disabilities, 32*(5), 1441–1454.

Miller, D. J. (1972). Visual habituation in the human infant. *Child Development, 43*(2), 481–493.

Miller, E. K., & Cohen, J. D. (2001). An integrative theory of prefrontal cortex function. *Annual Review of Neuroscience, 24*, 167–202.

Mills, D., & Conboy, B. T. (2009). Early communicative development and the social brain. In M. de Haan & M. R. Gunnar (Eds.), *Handbook of developmental social neuroscience* (pp. 175–206). New York: Guilford Press.

Milner, A. D., & Goodale, M. A. (2008). Two visual systems re-viewed. *Neuropsychologia, 46*(3), 774–785.

Mundy, P., Block, J., Delgado, C., Pomares, Y., Van Hecke, A. V., & Parlade, M. V. (2007). Individual differences and the development of joint attention in infancy. *Child Development, 78*(3), 938–954.

Mundy, P., Sullivan, L., & Mastergeorge, A. M. (2009). A parallel and distributed-processing model of joint attention, social cognition and autism. *Autism Research, 2*(1), 2–21.

Neill, W. T., & Westberry, R. L. (1987). Selective attention and the suppression of cognitive noise. *Journal of Experimental Psychology: Learning Memory and Cognition, 13*(2), 327–334.

Nijhuis, J. G., Prechtl, H. F. R., Martin, C. B., Jr., & Bots, R. S. G. M. (1982). Are there behavioural states in the human fetus? *Early Human Development, 6*(2), 177–195.

Oakes, L. M. (2012). Advances in eye tracking in infancy research. *Infancy, 17*(1), 1–8.

Oakes, L. M., Kannass, K. N., & Shaddy, D. J. (2002). Developmental changes in endogenous control of attention: The role of target familiarity on infants' distraction latency. *Child Development, 73*(6), 1644–1655.

Pecheux, M. G., & Lecuyer, R. (1983). Habituation rate and free exploration tempo in 4-month-old infants. *International Journal of Behavioral Development, 6*(1), 37–50.

Peirano, P., Algarin, C., & Uauy, R. (2003). Sleep–wake states and their regulatory mechanisms throughout early human development. *Journal of Pediatrics, 143*(4), S70–S79.

Perra, O., & Gattis, M. (2010). The control of social attention from 1 to 4 months. *British Journal of Developmental Psychology, 28*(4), 891–908.

Perruchet, P., & Pacton, S. (2006). Implicit learning and statistical learning: One phenomenon, two approaches. *Trends in Cognitive Sciences, 10*(5), 233–238.

Petersen, S. E., & Posner, M. I. (2012). The attention system of the human brain: 20 years after. *Annual Review of Neuroscience, 35*, 73–89.

Picciotto, M. R., Higley, M. J., & Mineur, Y. S. (2012). Acetylcholine as a neuromodulator: Cholinergic signaling shapes nervous system function and behavior. *Neuron, 76*(1), 116–129.

Pierce, K., Conant, D., Hazin, R., Stoner, R., & Desmond, J. (2011). Preference for geometric patterns early in life as risk factor for autism. *Archives of General Psychiatry, 68*(1), 101–109.

Posner, M. I., & DiGirolamo, G. J. (1998). Conflict, target detection, and cognitive control. In R. Parasuraman (Ed.), *The attentive brain* (pp. 401–423). Cambridge, MA: MIT Press.

Posner, M. I., & Petersen, S. E. (1990). The attention system of the human brain. *Annual Review of Neuroscience, 13*, 25–42.

Posner, M. I., & Rothbart, M. K. (2000). Developing mechanisms of self-regulation. *Development and Psychopathology, 12*(3), 427–441.

Rao, S. M., Harrington, D. L., Haaland, K. Y., Bobholz, J. A., Cox, R. W., & Binder, J. R. (1997). Distributed neural systems underlying the timing of movements. *Journal of Neuroscience, 17*(14), 5528–5535.

Reynolds, G. D., Courage, M. L., & Richards, J. E. (2010). Infant attention and visual preferences: Converging evidence from behavior, event-related potentials, and cortical source localization. *Developmental Psychology, 46*(4), 886–904.

Reynolds, J. H., & Chelazzi, L. (2004). Attentional modulation of visual processing. *Annual Review of Neuroscience, 27*, 611–647.

Riby, D. M., & Hancock, P. J. (2008). Viewing it differently: Social scene perception in Williams syndrome and autism. *Neuropsychologia, 46*(11), 2855–2860.

Riby, D. M., & Hancock, P. J. (2009). Looking at movies and cartoons: Eye-tracking evidence from Williams syndrome and autism. *Journal of Intellectual Disability Research, 53*(2), 169–181.

Richards, J. E. (1989). Sustained visual-attention in 8-week-old infants. *Infant Behavior and Development, 12*(4), 425–436.

Richards, J. E. (2010). The development of attention to simple and complex visual stimuli in infants: Behavioral and psychophysiological measures. *Developmental Review, 30*(2), 203–219.

Risko, E. F., Laidlaw, K., Freeth, M., Foulsham, T., & Kingstone, A. (2012). Social attention with real versus reel stimuli: Toward an empirical approach to concerns about ecological validity. *Frontiers in Human Neuroscience, 6*, 143.

Rueda, M. R., Posner, M. I., & Rothbart, M. K. (2005). The development of executive attention: Contributions to the emergence of self-regulation. *Developmental Neuropsychology, 28*(2), 573–594.

Ruff, H. A., & Rothbart, M. K. (1996). *Attention in early development: Themes and variations.* Oxford, UK: Oxford University Press.

Sarver, D. E., Rapport, M. D., Kofler, M. J., Scanlan, S. W., Raiker, J. S., Altro, T. A., et al. (2012). Attention problems, phonological short-term memory, and visuospatial short-term memory: Differential effects on near- and long-term scholastic achievement. *Learning and Individual Differences, 22*(1), 8–19.

Scherf, K. S., & Scott, L. S. (2012). Connecting developmental trajectories: Biases in face processing from infancy to adulthood. *Developmental Psychobiology, 54*(6), 643–663.

Senju, A., Tojo, Y., Dairoku, H., & Hasegawa, T. (2004). Reflexive orienting in response to eye gaze and an arrow in children with and without autism. *Journal of Child Psychology and Psychiatry, 45*(3), 445–458.

Shaddy, D. J., & Colombo, J. (2004). Developmental changes in infant attention to dynamic and static stimuli. *Infancy, 5*(3), 355–365.

Shultz, T. R., Chawarska, K., & Volkmar, F. (2006). The social brain in autism: Perspectives from neuropsychology and neuroimaging. In S. O. Moldin & J. R. Rubenstein (Eds.), *Understanding autism: From basic neuroscience to treatment* (pp. 323–348). Boca Raton, FL: CRC Press.

Sokolov, E. N. (1958). *Perception and the conditioned reflex.* Oxford, UK: Publishing House, Moscow University.

Sokolov, E. N. (1960). Neural model of the stimulus and the orienting reflex. *Voprosy Psychologii, 4,* 61–72.

Spears, W. C. (1966). Visual preference in the four-month old infant. *Psychonomic Science, 4*(6), 237–238.

Steinmetz, P. N., Roy, A., Fitzgerald, P. J., Hsiao, S. S., Johnson, K. O., & Niebur, E. (2000). Attention modulates synchronized neuronal firing in primate somatosensory cortex. *Nature, 404*(6774), 187–190.

Stekelenburg, J. J., & Van Boxtel, A. (2001). Inhibition of pericranial muscle activity, respiration, and heart rate enhances auditory sensitivity. *Psychophysiology, 38*(4), 629–641.

Swettenham, J., Baron-Cohen, S., Charman, T., Cox, A., Baird, G., Drew, A., et al. (1998). The frequency and distribution of spontaneous attention shifts between social and nonsocial stimuli in autistic, typically developing and nonautistic developmentally delayed infants. *Journal of Child Psychology and Psychiatry, 39*(5), 747–753.

Tallon-Baudry, C. (2012). On the neural mechanisms subserving consciousness and attention. *Frontiers in Psychology, 3,* 11.

Tang, Y. Y., & Posner, M. I. (2009). Attention training and attention state training. *Trends in Cognitive Sciences, 13*(5), 222–227.

Tomasello, M., & Todd, J. T. (1983). Joint attention and lexical acquisition style. *First Language, 4,* 197–212.

Townsend, J., Keehn, B., & Westerfield, M. (2012). "Abstraction of mind": Attention in autism. In M. Posner (Ed.), *Cognitive neuroscience of attention* (Vol. 2, pp. 357–373). New York: Guilford Press.

Treisman, A. M., & Gelade, G. (1980). Feature-integration theory of attention. *Cognitive Psychology, 12*(1), 97–136.

van de Weijer-Bergsma, E., Wijnroks, L., & Jongmans, M. J. (2008). Attention development in infants and preschool children born preterm: A review. *Infant Behavior and Development, 31*(3), 333–351.

Vanduffel, W., Tootell, R. B. H., & Orban, G. A. (2000). Attention-dependent suppression of metabolic activity in the early stages of the macaque visual system. *Cerebral Cortex, 10*(2), 109–126.

Walsh, P., Elsabbagh, M., Bolton, P., & Singh, I. (2011). In search of biomarkers for autism: Scientific, social and ethical challenges. *Nature Reviews Neuroscience, 12*(10), 603–612.

Wass, S., Porayska-Pomsta, K., & Johnson, M. H. (2011). Training attentional control in infancy. *Current Biology, 21*(18), 1543–1547.

Welford, A. T. (1959). Evidence of a single-channel decision mechanism limiting performance in a serial reaction task. *Quarterly Journal of Experimental Psychology, 11*(4), 193–210.

Whalen, C., Schreibman, L., & Ingersoll, B. (2006). The collateral effects of joint attention training on social initiations, positive affect, imitation, and spontaneous speech for young children with autism. *Journal of Autism and Developmental Disorders, 36*(5), 655–664.

Wickens, C. D. (1991). Processing resources and attention. In D. L. Damos (Ed.), *Multiple-task performance* (pp. 3–34). London: Taylor and Francis.

Wolfe, C. D., & Bell, M. A. (2007). The integration of cognition and emotion during infancy and early childhood: Regulatory processes associated with the development of working memory. *Brain and Cognition, 65*(1), 3–13.

Yantis, S., & Hillstrom, A. P. (1994). Stimulus-driven attentional capture: Evidence from equiluminant visual objects. *Journal of Experimental Psychology: Human Perception and Performance, 20*(1), 95–107.

Zwaigenbaum, L., Bryson, S., Rogers, T., Roberts, W., Brian, J., & Szatmari, P. (2005). Behavioral manifestations of autism in the first year of life. *International Journal of Developmental Neuroscience, 23*(2–3), 143–152.

CHAPTER 6

The Development and Brain Mechanisms of Joint Attention

Stefanie Hoehl and Tricia Striano

Infants are social beings from early on. Soon after birth newborns attend specifically to other people and start communicating with them through the imitation of facial gestures (Johnson, Dziurawiec, Ellis, & Morton, 1991; Meltzoff & Moore, 1977). Within the first weeks, infants develop expectations about others' behavior in turn-taking conversations and become upset when their caregiver does not respond to their communicative bids (Tronick, Als, Adamson, Wise, & Brazelton, 1978). Abilities relating to perceiving, understanding, and interacting with other people are all aspects of social cognition (Striano & Reid, 2006). Social cognition allows predicting others' actions, learning from them, and collaborating with them. Thus, it underlies the development of human culture, which is inconceivable without cooperation and social learning (Csibra & Gergely, 2011; Tomasello, Carpenter, Call, Behne, & Moll, 2005).

One important aspect of social cognition is joint attention. Joint attention is the ability to focus attention at something in the environment together with someone else while at the same time being aware of sharing attention (Schilbach et al., 2010; Striano, Reid, & Hoehl, 2006). As such, it involves monitoring an interactive partner's attention in relation to the self, an external event or object, and the interactive partner's attention toward the same event or object (Striano & Stahl, 2005). Joint attention can be achieved either by following another person's attention focus to something in the environment (i.e., responding to joint attention) or by actively directing others' attention (i.e., initiating joint attention), though in a natural interaction both partners may take turns in directing the other's attention.

Infants' ability to engage in triadic (person–object–person) joint attention interactions is related to later language development (Baldwin, 1995; Brooks & Meltzoff, 2005), intention-based imitation, and use of mental state language (Kristen, Sodian, Thoermer, & Perst, 2011). Therefore, some researchers have suggested that joint attention is one of the building blocks of social cognition upon which other complex skills, like understanding others' mental states, are developed (Baron-Cohen, 1994; Barresi & Moore, 1993).

In this chapter we provide an overview on the development of joint attention in infancy. Starting with a sensitivity for direct eye contact and rudimentary gaze cueing in newborns (Farroni, Csibra, Simion, & Johnson, 2002; Farroni, Massaccesi, Pividori, & Johnson, 2004), infants become able to use others' gaze direction to cue their own attention toward relevant stimuli in the environment within the first few months after birth (Reid & Striano, 2005). By the end of the first year, infants also direct others' attention toward objects and events, thus actively initiating episodes of joint attention with others (Tomasello, Carpenter, & Liszkowski, 2007). In addition to outlining joint attention development on the behavioral level (see Table 6.1 for an overview), we discuss the neural correlates of joint attention that are currently studied using neuroimaging and electrophysiological techniques. Furthermore, the early functions of joint attention during infancy are considered. It becomes evident that a biopsychosocial perspective, incorporating different data sources and levels of analysis, has

TABLE 6.1. Developmental Onsets of Important Joint Attention Behaviors

Age	Observed joint attention behavior
Neonate	• Detection of eye contact (Farroni, Csibra, Simion, & Johnson, 2002) • Rudimentary gaze cueing (Farroni, Massaccesi, Pividori, & Johnson, 2004)
3–4 months	• Gaze following to objects within the infant's immediate visual field (D'Entremont, Hains, & Muir, 1997) • Effects of others' eye gaze and head direction on infants' object processing (Hoehl, Wahl, & Pauen, 2014; Wahl, Michel, Pauen, & Hoehl, 2012)
6 months	• Following of another person's gaze direction up to the first object in the scan path (Butterworth & Jarrett, 1991)
8–9 months	• Following of a person's head turns even when the person's eyes are closed (Brooks & Meltzoff, 2002) • Expectation that eye gaze has a target, that is, it is not directed toward an empty location (Csibra & Volein, 2008)
12 months	• Gaze following behind barriers (Moll & Tomasello, 2004) • Infants follow a person's gaze to relatively precise locations within a room (Butterworth & Jarrett, 1991) and toward locations behind themselves (Deak, Flom, & Pick, 2000) • The status of the eyes gains importance for infants' gaze following (Meltzoff & Brooks, 2007; Tomasello, Hare, Lehmann, & Call, 2007) • Use of communicative gestures (Carpenter, Nagell, & Tomasello, 1998) • Declarative pointing in order to initiate joint attention (Liszkowski, Carpenter, Henning, Striano, & Tomasello, 2004)

deepened our understanding of joint attention development and its functions in infancy. Based on recent advances in our understanding of the mechanisms and neural correlates of joint attention across development, we point out open questions and conclude with suggestions for future directions in research.

Detecting Another Person's Attention Toward Oneself

A basic prerequisite for engaging in joint attention interactions is detecting that another person's attention is focused on oneself. Several behavioral cues can indicate this, such as eye contact, calling someone's name, and acting contingently to the other person's behavior. Infants are sensitive to all of these cues from very early on in development.

Newborn infants look longer at a picture of a woman with open eyes than at a picture of the same woman with closed eyes (Batki, Baron-Cohen, Wheelwright, Connellan, & Ahluwalia, 2000). This finding was taken as initial evidence that newborns possess an innate neural module that allows them to detect the presence of eyes in a stimulus. In a preferential looking experiment with pictures presented side by side, 2- to 5-day-old infants preferred to look at a woman who directed her eye gaze toward them, thus establishing eye contact, as compared with the same woman averting her eyes to the side (Farroni, Csibra, Simion, & Johnson, 2002). This shows that newborns detect whether or not eyes are present. In addition, it shows that newborns are sensitive to the presence of eye contact. Although this early sensitivity is likely based on subcortical brain mechanisms and thus not consciously controlled (Johnson, 2005), it may affect how infants perceive faces on the cortical level. Gliga and Csibra (2007) suggested that eyes, a very salient high-contrast visual stimulus, may attract newborns' attention to faces, thus feeding information to cortical regions devoted to the processing and discrimination of faces leading to increased functional specialization of these regions across early development.

Neurophysiological studies with slightly older infants support this view. Using event-related potentials (ERPs), Farroni et al. (2002) found that 4-month-olds respond with an increased amplitude of the occipital N290 component to faces with eye contact as compared to faces with side-averted gaze. This effect is not simply due to the greater symmetry in faces with eye contact, as it is only found when upright faces are presented but not when inverted faces are shown (Farroni, Johnson, & Csibra, 2004). The N290 is thought to be a developmental precursor of the adult N170, which is involved in structural face processing (Hoehl & Peykarjou, 2012). In 3-month-olds the N290 is increased for faces compared with matched visual noise stimuli (Halit, Csibra, Volein, & Johnson, 2004). It is also greater in amplitude for human as compared with ape faces (Halit, de Haan, & Johnson, 2003), and is sensitive to the orientation of human faces but not cars (Peykarjou & Hoehl, 2013). Thus, direct eye contact leads to increased cortical face processing by 4 months of age. This fits well with the behavioral observation that eye contact during familiarization supports later face recognition in 4-month-olds (Farroni, Massaccesi, Menon, & Johnson, 2007).

Eye contact also modulates infants' oscillatory brain activity. The electroencephalogram (EEG) contains information about how the power or amplitude of oscillatory activity at different frequencies varies across time, which can be assessed using wavelet analysis (Csibra & Johnson, 2007). For instance, high-frequency gamma-band activity (i.e., neuronal activity oscillating at a frequency above 20 hertz) has been related to perceptual binding, attentional processes, and the matching of sensory signals with memory contents (Saby & Marshall, 2012). In adults, induced gamma-band activity correlates with hemodynamic brain activity as measured by functional magnetic resonance imaging (fMRI; Fiebach, Gruber, & Supp, 2005). Therefore, infants' oscillatory brain activity has been related to neuroimaging findings in adults in order to explore whether regions of the "social brain" (Adolphs, 2009) are already involved in infants' processing of social signals. A more direct way to do this is to use functional near-infrared imaging (fNIRS), which also delivers a measure of the hemodynamic response but is less costly and easier to apply with infants than fMRI.

Four-month-olds respond with bursts of gamma-band EEG activity over right frontal channel sites when viewing static faces with eye contact as compared to the same faces with eye gaze averted to the side (Grossmann, Johnson, Farroni, & Csibra, 2007). Functional neuroimaging work with adults has shown that the right medial prefrontal cortex (PFC) is activated when adults perceive static faces with eye contact (Kampe, Frith, & Frith, 2003). Grossmann et al. (2007) therefore suggest that similar brain regions may be involved in eye contact detection in adults and young infants. The medial PFC is particularly interesting in this context as it is generally involved in the detection of communicative signals directed toward the self, independent of sensory modality: This brain region is also activated when adult participants hear someone else calling their name as compared with hearing another name (Kampe et al., 2003).

Further similarities between infants' and adults' brain activations were found using dynamic stimuli. Grossmann et al. (2008) observed increased frontal gamma activity in 4-month-olds when perceiving a person who raised his eyebrows and smiled while maintaining eye contact, but not when the person averted his gaze to the side. Thus, infants were sensitive to the self-relevance of communicative signals and did not simply respond to the physical change in the stimulus when the person raised his eyebrows and smiled. In the same study, fNIRS was applied to assess infants' hemodynamic responses to the same stimuli. Increased brain activation during eye contact as compared with averted gaze and baseline was observed in the right frontopolar cortex and right superior posterior temporal cortex. Correspondingly, dynamic gaze shifts toward the observer induced increased activation in posterior superior temporal sulcus in adults (Ethofer, Gschwind, & Vuilleumier, 2011). In addition, Schilbach et al. (2006) found that a ventral portion of the medial PFC is involved in adults' analysis of dynamic facial gestures as communicative in contrast to arbitrary face movements, whereas a more dorsal region of the medial PFC was sensitive to eye contact in the same study.

In adults, the medial PFC responds to multimodal social cues signaling that a person addresses the perceiver. In infants, multimodal social signals indicating communicative intent also elicit analogous brain responses, especially in the frontal cortex. For instance, newborns respond with increased frontal brain activity as measured with fNIRS to infant-directed speech as compared with adult-directed speech (Saito et al., 2007). In 5-month-olds, both seeing faces with eye contact as compared with averted gaze and hearing someone call their own name as compared with another name elicits hemodynamic responses in the frontal cortex (Grossmann, Parise, & Friederici, 2010).

Parise and Csibra (2013) assessed prefrontal gamma-band EEG activity and ERPs in response to infant-directed speech and eye contact in 5-month-old infants. In the first experiment both kinds of communicative signals were presented independently from each other. Infants showed increased prefrontal gamma activity for self-relevant signals in both modalities, that is, during eye contact and infant-directed speech. ERPs revealed increased amplitude of a positive peak around 300 milliseconds after stimulus onset over central channels for self-relevant as compared with non-self-relevant stimuli. In the second experiment of this study multimodal stimuli were presented. The same positive peak over central channels was sensitive to the presence or absence of self-relevance in these stimuli. Amplitude was smaller for averted gaze paired with adult-directed speech as compared with stimuli featuring eye contact or infant-directed speech either presented in combination or combined with nonostensive cues from the other modality. Interestingly, the effects of self-relevant ostensive signals from both modalities were nonadditive. The authors conclude that the presence of an ostensive communicative cue triggers obligatory brain processes, which are neither heightened nor diminished by congruent or incongruent cues from another modality. This finding speaks for qualitative instead of quantitative differences in processing ostensive versus nonostensive communicative signals indicating another person's attention toward the self. The functional significance of the positive ERP component and its specificity for ostensive signals remains to be tested in further research. Nonetheless, this study is informative as it demonstrates that infants are very sensitive to the presence of ostensive signals directed at them.

All of the studies reviewed thus far tested infants' sensitivity to being addressed by another person in a dyadic person–person context. As joint attention involves two persons sharing attention toward an external entity, an interesting question is whether infants are also sensitive to being addressed by another person in a triadic person–object–person interaction. In a study by

Striano and Stahl (2005) 3-, 6-, and 9-month-olds smiled and gazed more at an adult who broke a dyadic interaction to alternate gaze between the infant and an object (establishing a triadic interaction) as compared with the adult only looking away from the infant toward the object and never back at the infant. The experimenter spoke in a positive tone of voice and smiled equally in both conditions, so results suggest that infants were sensitive to the presence or absence of eye contact in a triadic interaction. In a second experiment, infants of the same age groups also detected more subtle manipulations in the adult's interactive behavior. Infants gazed and smiled at the experimenter significantly less when she broke eye contact for 1 second each time before turning toward an object compared with an uninterrupted triadic interaction. This suggests that infants are sensitive to the referential nature of another person's eye-gaze shifts by 3 months of age. The same effect was not observed in 6-week-old infants, suggesting that infants' sensitivity to eye contact in triadic interactions develops between 6 weeks and 3 months of age (Striano, Stahl, Cleveland, & Hoehl, 2007).

Thus far, we conclude that infants are remarkably sensitive to being addressed by an interactive partner, both in dyadic and triadic interactions. Similar brain activations, particularly in the frontal cortex, are found when infants perceive self-relevant communicative cues in different modalities (visual/auditory) and these activations are similar to brain responses observed in adults who are addressed by another person. Monitoring another person's attention in relation to the self is an essential aspect of engaging in joint attention interactions. It is therefore not surprising that this ability develops early in life and that certain brain regions are consistently involved in the related mechanisms across development. A second important skill is being able to follow someone's attention toward an external object or event. This is often accomplished by following others' gaze direction. The next section therefore focuses on infants' ability to follow others' gaze and the neural correlates of this behavior.

Shifting Attention in the Direction of Others' Gaze

Following others' direction of regard enables us to determine another person's attention focus. Gaze following is useful because it guides our own attention toward relevant objects and events in the environment and supports social learning and joint attention (see also the next section).

Very young infants' attention is cued in the direction of others' eye gaze. Farroni, Massaccesi, Pividori, and Johnson (2004) presented 2- to 5-day-old infants with schematic faces whose pupils moved from the middle to the left or right side of the eye. The centrally presented face then disappeared and an object was shown on the left or right side of the screen, its position being either congruous with the direction of the previous eye-gaze shift or not. Newborn infants were faster in making saccades toward the peripheral object when the eyes of the schematic face had moved in the congruous direction before. Hood, Willen, and Driver (1998) reported a similar gaze-cueing effect using realistic photographs in infants by 3 months of age.

Farroni, Mansfield, Lai, and Johnson (2003) carried out further experiments with 4-month-olds to test the specificity of this effect. Interestingly, gaze cueing was only observed when upright faces were presented. Thus, it is not simply the motion of the pupils alone that triggers the effect. Furthermore, a period of mutual gaze had to precede the motion of the eyes for gaze-cueing effects to occur and the pupil motion had to be visible. This suggests that even if gaze cueing in very young infants may rely on rather low-level or automatic mechanisms, some prerequisites have to be met that enable gaze cueing in the context of a social interaction including eye contact but not otherwise.

The effects reported thus far were observed in artificial experimental setups with a face appearing on the screen and disappearing before the target of the gaze shift was presented. This is usually done because young infants tend to maintain their gaze fixated on the centrally presented face when a peripheral target appears (Hood et al., 1998). The target is also presented very close to the face, such that rather small saccades are sufficient for infants to turn their focus on them. One important question is therefore how overt gaze following in more natural social interactions develops.

The first experimental demonstration of infant gaze following was published by Scaife and Bruner (1975). The authors found that infants followed an adult's line of regard indicated by eye gaze and head orientation by 2–4 months of age and that gaze following occurred more frequently with increasing age across the first year. D'Entremont, Hains, and Muir (1997) reported gaze following in infants from 3 months of age when the object was presented within the visual field of the infant. At 6 months infants follow others' line of regard, but they may end up looking at the first object appearing in their scan path (Butterworth & Jarrett, 1991). Their ability to detect the exact focus of others' attention becomes more precise by 12 months of age (Butterworth & Jarrett, 1991). At this age infants also follow others' gaze to locations outside of their current field of view. For instance, 12-month-olds turn around if they see someone looking at a location behind them (Deak, Flom, & Pick, 2000). At 8 and 12 months of age infants expect a person's eye gaze to have a target even if it is not visible to them: They look longer when an occluder is removed from the location a person had previously gazed at revealing an empty location as opposed to an object (Csibra & Volein, 2008). By 12 months they also locomote to look behind a barrier after observing an adult looking behind it (Moll & Tomasello, 2004).

Thus, infants' gaze following becomes more precise and more flexible across the first year. During this time changes also occur with respect to whose gaze infants preferably follow. A longitudinal study using eye tracking showed that a "stranger preference" in terms of following gaze shifts to objects occurs between 4 and 6 months of age (Gredebäck, Fikke, & Melinder, 2010). The authors found that infants more frequently followed their mother's than a stranger's gaze toward an object at 2 months of age. Older infants, however, increasingly followed a stranger's gaze direction. Consistent with this finding, infants at 7 and 9 months of age coordinate attention toward a toy more frequently with a stranger compared with their mother in a free-play situation (Striano & Bertin, 2005). It is currently unclear why infants become more interested in what strangers look at than their caregivers by 4–6 months of age. It is possible that they are more wary of strangers and therefore track more carefully what they are looking at.

Though infants readily and frequently follow others' line of regard by the end of the first year, it has been a matter of debate to what extent, if at all, infants at this age rely on information from the eyes instead of head orientation alone in these studies. For instance, Corkum and Moore (1995) reported that 12-month-olds follow someone's head turn to the side even if the person maintains eye contact with them. In a later experiment the authors found that only 18-month-olds, but not younger infants, followed an experimenter's isolated eye movements (Moore & Corkum, 1998). A more recent study showed that eye gaze influences 12-month-olds' attention allocation to the ceiling more than head orientation (Tomasello, Hare, Lehmann, & Call, 2007). Correspondingly, Meltzoff and Brooks (2007) reported that 10- to 11-month-olds follow someone's head turn to the side when the person's eyes are open, but refrain from doing so when his or her eyes are closed, indicating an understanding of "looking" as involving open eyes. However, younger infants in these experiments followed head turns even when the experimenter's eyes were closed (Meltzoff & Brooks, 2007). Thus, although the age at which the status of the eyes becomes relevant for infants' following of others' attention focus varies in different studies between 10 and 18 months, it is quite unequivocal that younger infants are more affected by head direction and hardly seem to take into account the eyes at all.

These findings from live gaze following studies seem to contradict the above-mentioned effects of eye-gaze cues on spatial attention allocation very early in development. Moore and Corkum (1998) have therefore argued that early attention cueing through eye gaze may not depend on awareness of the other person's attention focus and should be distinguished from more deliberate gaze following and joint attention in older infants. If these processes can be distinguished developmentally, different neural structures may be involved in reflexive gaze cueing and more controlled joint attention processes.

In adults the perception of averted eye gaze activates the intraparietal sulcus (IPS; Hoffman & Haxby, 2000). The IPS is also involved in visual-orienting tasks and is part of the frontoparietal spatial attention network (Corbetta, 1998). Fitting the notion that gaze cues recruit more general spatial attention mechanisms, reflexive gaze shifts induced by task-irrelevant eye-gaze cues have been associated with activation in this frontoparietal network, in particular the frontal eye field, IPS, and posterior parietal cortex (Cazzato, Macaluso, Crostella, & Aglioti, 2012). In infants the neural correlates of reflexive gaze shifts are less well researched. However, Grossmann et al. (2007) reported bursts of oscillatory gamma EEG activity over the right parietal regions in response to averted eye gaze in 4-month-olds, suggesting that similar attention mechanisms may be involved in young infants' gaze perception. Involvement of IPS during reflexive gaze cueing does not imply that it is insensitive to the social context of gaze shifts, though. In adults, this region, along with the superior temporal sulus, is also sensitive to whether a perceived gaze shift to the side is goal directed or not (Mosconi, Mack, McCarthy, & Pelphrey, 2005; Pelphrey, Singerman, Allison, & McCarthy, 2003).

Neural correlates of deliberate joint attention interactions have been investigated in adults using virtual characters who contingently responded to participants' gaze behavior (Schilbach et al., 2010). Consciously following another person's eye gaze recruits the anterior portion of the medial PFC (Schilbach et al., 2010), which is also implicated in the detection of communicative signals directed toward the self (Schilbach et al., 2006).

Using fNIRS and videos of virtual characters, Grossmann and Johnson (2010) observed activation in the left dorsal PFC when 5-month-old infants observed a character turn his head to look at an object following a period of mutual gaze as opposed to the character looking toward empty space or turning toward the object without establishing eye contact first. The same region was active when 5-month-olds saw a virtual character looking toward an object they had turned their own gaze toward before (Grossmann, Lloyd-Fox, & Johnson, 2013). These findings suggest that young infants recruit similar brain areas in the PFC in joint attention interactions as those observed in adults.

Overall, neuroimaging findings suggest that different brain regions underlie reflexive gaze cueing and deliberate gaze following and joint attention. Whereas gaze cueing relies on the frontoparietal attention network including IPS, conscious gaze following and joint attention induce activation in the medial PFC in adults. Since both cortical regions are implicated in eye-gaze processing and joint attention already from early on in infancy, their involvement in the developmental trajectory from early attention cueing to a later emerging understanding of "looking" as involving the eyes is not yet clear. Mundy, Card, and Fox (2000) suggested that infants' early gaze-cueing and gaze-following skills (i.e., their ability to respond to joint attention) rely on a posterior orienting attention system including the parietal cortex as postulated by Posner and Petersen (1990). According to Mundy et al. (2000), infants' somewhat later-developing ability to initiate joint attention (see section below) is associated with the later-maturing anterior attention regulation network, whose functions include the capacity to share attention across tasks or foci and the regulation of voluntary orienting (Posner & Petersen, 1990). Further research on the neural correlates of early gaze-cueing effects—as well as more studies on brain mechanisms involved in joint attention and the processing of eye gaze and head orientation in older infants—are warranted in order to specify the roles these brain regions and networks play in the development of different aspects of joint attention across infancy.

Another important question is whether infants are able to encode the relationship between a person and the target of his or her gaze. ERP research has shown that infants discriminate object-directed from object-averted gaze by 4 months of age (Hoehl, Reid, Mooney, & Striano, 2008; Senju, Johnson, & Csibra, 2006). However, infants associate a person with the particular target of his or her gaze only later in development. In a study by Woodward (2003) 7-, 9-, and 12-month-olds readily followed an actor's gaze toward one of two objects. Infants were habituated to the actor always directing her gaze at the same object. In the test trials the object locations were switched and the adult looked either at the same location now featuring the other object or turned toward the other location where the old object was now located. Only 12-month-olds, but not younger infants, looked longer in test trials in which the adult looked at the new object compared with the new location, suggesting that they detected that the target of the actor's gaze had changed. Younger infants only detected this change when the actor's gaze was accompanied by a grasp. However, as shown by Johnson, Ok, and Luo (2007), 9-month-olds are also able to encode the relationship between a looker and the particular target of her gaze when given multiple cues emphasizing that the model is looking at the object from several angles.

The finding by Johnson et al. (2007) demonstrates that infants' performance in live gaze-following tasks depends on the richness of social cues provided to them. Furthermore, infants' responding to social cues depends on whether they are directly addressed by the other person. As outlined in the previous section of this chapter, infants are sensitive to ostensive cues signaling communicative intent directed at them from early on in development. The presence of these cues increases their responding to joint attention bids as shown by Senju and Csibra (2008). In this study an actor was presented turning his gaze toward one of two objects on a table in front of him. Six-month-olds' gaze following toward the cued object was increased when the person had established eye contact before shifting attention toward the object. In another condition without eye contact a similar effect was found for infant-directed speech as compared with adult-directed speech.

Interestingly, the presence of certain ostensive social cues seems to induce "gaze" following even in the absence of an actual human person. Johnson, Slaughter, and Carey (1998) presented 12-month-olds with a soft, brown, amorphously shaped, asymmetrical object shifting its orientation toward one of two targets. Infants followed the object's orientation with their gaze if it had facial features and/or if it had acted contingently to their own behavior previously. Using eye tracking, Deligianni, Senju, Gergely, and Csibra (2011) also found that 8-month-olds follow the orientation of teapot-shaped objects after these had responded contingently to the infants' looking behavior, supporting the role of temporal contingency in inducing gaze following in infants.

Very early in development infants detect temporal contingencies between their own actions and events in the environment (Gergely, 2000). Gergely (2000) suggested that the preference of (imperfect) contingencies by 3 months of age may attune infants to increasingly explore the "social world" and to detect social agents. Around the same age infants smile more in a contingent interaction with their mother as compared with a noncontingent or imitative interaction (Striano, Henning, & Stahl, 2005). Contingent behavior may indicate the presence of a social agent with attentional and perceptual abilities and communicative intentions, leading infants to follow the orientation of a contingently behaving object even in the absence of facial features and eyes (Deligianni et al., 2011; Johnson et al., 1998).

In sum, eye-gaze cues bias infants' attention toward peripheral targets from birth on. This ability does not, however, imply a conscious understanding of eyes as being necessary for seeing. Infants at 8 and 12 months readily follow a communicative agent's orientation in the absence of eyes and they follow an adult's head orientation even when his or her eyes are closed until 10–11 months of age. Although these early gaze-cueing and "gaze"-following effects could rely on rather automatic mechanisms involving the frontoparietal attention network, they require the presence of an agent addressing the infant directly, either by making eye contact with the infant, speaking in infant-directed speech, or responding contingently to the infant's behavior. Thus, they do not occur irrespective of the social context and may already have a function in guiding infants' attention toward socially relevant information in the environment. In the following section we therefore focus on the early functions of gaze cueing and gaze following.

Early Functions of Gaze Following: Effects on Infants' Object Processing

A newborn infant encounters a tremendous amount of visual input and is faced with the task of making sense and structuring these novel perceptual experiences. One of the most frequently encountered visual stimuli for infants is the human face. Newborns prefer to look at faces compared with other similarly complex visual patterns (Johnson et al., 1991) and they are influenced in their attention allocation to stimuli in the environment by facial cues such as eye gaze (Farroni, Massaccesi, et al., 2004). These findings led to the suggestion that eye gaze may help infants to discern socially relevant visual input from early on in development, thus helping them to structure their visual environment (Hoehl et al., 2009; Reid & Striano, 2007). Thereby, the perceptual input is parsed into manageable components and social information is highlighted.

Supporting this view, a number of studies have demonstrated that social cues, especially eye gaze, affect the processing of unfamiliar objects in early infancy. Reid and Striano (2005) presented 4-month-olds with a central face shifting eye gaze to the left or right. Two objects were shown next to either side of the face. Then the face disappeared and both objects were presented again in a visual preference task either at the same location as previously or with switched locations. Infants looked significantly longer at objects that had *not* been cued by the adult's eye gaze before, irrespective of location. This suggests that the cued objects were more thoroughly encoded and therefore more familiar to the infants. Noncued objects presumably appeared more novel and therefore more interesting to the infants. Infants' ERPs revealed increased neural processing of noncued objects in the same age group, thus also suggesting facilitated processing of cued objects (Reid, Striano, Kaufman, & Johnson, 2004). In an eye-tracking study with 12-month-olds a similar effect was found, although restricted to the first of two test trials indicating that older infants are able to quickly catch up on processing the previously neglected noncued object resulting in only a brief visual preference effect (Theuring, Gredebäck, & Hauf, 2007).

A series of experiments has investigated this effect further using the same general paradigm with 4-month-old infants. One study found that the effect is modulated by familiarity of the face (Hoehl, Wahl, Michel, & Striano, 2012). In this ERP study only the caregiver's face, and not a stranger's, elicited increased neural responses for noncued as compared with cued objects in 4-month-olds. Consistent with the finding that very young infants more often follow their mother's gaze than a stranger's (Gredebäck et al., 2010), these results suggest that 4-month-olds' object processing is more affected by their caregiver's gaze cues as compared with an unfamiliar person's. An open question is whether this is due to the perceptual familiarity of the caregiver's face or the relationship the infant has already formed with this person.

Wahl, Michel, Pauen, and Hoehl (2012) reported longer looking times and increased ERP responses for noncued as compared with cued objects when the actor's gaze shift was accompanied by a congruous head turn. Importantly, no effect on the behavioral level and only a marginally significant effect on the neural level were found when a car turned toward the left or right side, thus cueing one of the objects with a similar motion as the head turn. This finding demonstrates that the effect of social cues on infants' processing of novel objects is not simply due to attention biases caused by movement cues in general. As in the above-reviewed gaze-cueing studies with infants at the same age, a social agent and ostensive cues signaling communicative intent (in this case, eye contact) seem to be required. In addition, just as the effects of eye-gaze cues on infants' spatial attention, the effects of social cues on object processing in early infancy do not rely on a conscious understanding of eyes as being necessary for seeing. Hoehl, Wahl, and Pauen (2014) found longer looking times and increased ERP responses for noncued versus cued objects both when isolated eye-gaze cues were used and when only the actor's head turned to the side with the eyes looking straight ahead toward the infant. Given the similarity of experimental setups and stimuli used in gaze-cueing studies and studies on object processing, the parallels regarding the results are not surprising. However, social cues affect infants' object processing also in more ecologically valid live social interaction paradigms.

In a series of studies, Cleveland and colleagues (Cleveland, Schug, & Striano, 2007; Cleveland & Striano, 2007) had an adult engage with infants of different age groups in a live triadic interaction involving a toy object. In a joint attention condition the adult engaged with the infants by establishing eye contact, smiling, and talking in infant-directed speech. Then she turned her head and gaze toward an object on a table in front of her and continued talking in a positive tone of voice. During familiarization the adult alternated gaze between the infant and the toy. In a nonjoint attention condition the adult alternated gaze between the object on the table and a spot at the ceiling but never looked at the infant while also talking in a positive voice. After this familiarization with the object, a visual preference task was conducted using the familiarized object and a novel object that the infants had not previously seen. Seven- and 9-month-olds showed a clear novelty preference only when they were familiarized with the "old" objects in a joint attention interaction. A nonsignificant tendency in the same direction was found in 5-month-olds but not in 4-month-olds. This suggests that the above-reviewed eye-tracking and ERP paradigms may be somewhat more sensitive in detecting effects of social cues on young infants' object processing than live studies. This may be due to the fact that live social interactions are much more complex. However, by 7 months of age infants show a clear advantage in encoding information about a novel object in a joint attention interaction as compared with a situation where an adult does not engage with them directly.

A promising methodological approach is combining live social interactions with neurophysiological measures that can inform us about cognitive processes above and beyond looking times. Several studies have used ERPs to measure the effects of live joint attention interactions on infants' object processing and learning. Striano et al. (2006) showed that 9-month-olds' attention toward a novel object is increased by an adult looking at the object together with the infant following a period of eye contact, thus establishing joint attention. When the adult only looked at the object without engaging with the participant first, infants' brain response indicating the amount of attention directed at the object (the negative central [Nc] component) was significantly smaller (see Parise, Reid, Stets, & Striano, 2008, for a similar effect in 5-month-olds). This suggests that

9-month-olds' processing of objects is affected by eye contact in a live joint attention interaction. This may account for better subsequent memory performance for objects encountered within a triadic joint attention interaction as demonstrated by Cleveland and Striano (2007). This notion is supported by the finding that joint attention during a learning episode affects 9-month-olds' subsequent ERP responses to objects in immediate and delayed recognition tasks (Kopp & Lindenberger, 2011). Furthermore, facilitating effects of joint attention on word learning were found in 18- to 21-month-old infants (Hirotani, Stets, Striano, & Friederici, 2009).

As demonstrated by the above-reviewed studies, ERPs are useful for studying effects of social interactions on information processing in infants. However, ERPs provide only limited information on brain processes that are not phase locked to the temporal onset of a stimulus. Therefore, induced oscillations are used in addition to ERPs to study object processing (Csibra, Davis, Spratling, & Johnson, 2000; Saby & Marshall, 2012; Southgate, Csibra, Kaufman, & Johnson, 2008). One frequency band that is especially relevant in the context of joint attention interactions is the alpha range. Desynchronization or suppression of oscillatory brain activity in the alpha frequency range (8–13 hertz in adults, 6–9 hertz in infants) has typically been interpreted as reflecting cortical excitation (Pfurtscheller, 2003). In contrast, high-amplitude alpha-band power—that is, synchronization—is considered to reflect an idling state (Pfurtscheller, Stancak, & Neuper, 1996; Scheeringa, Petersson, Kleinschmidt, Jensen, & Bastiaansen, 2012), or inhibition of activity in areas not involved in the present task (Neuper & Pfurtscheller, 2001).

In an EEG study on joint attention in adults, desynchronization of signal power in the alpha range was found when two participants looked at the same object simultaneously following a short period of eye contact compared with both participants looking at different objects (Lachat, Hugueville, Lemarechal, Conty, & George, 2012). On posterior electrodes this effect was interpreted as indicating higher arousal during joint attention resulting from mutual awareness of a common attention focus. The effect extended to central channels where it was interpreted as a mu response originating from the motor system. The mu rhythm is an alpha range response typically recorded over central electrodes, which is suppressed during performing an action as well as during observation of another person's actions in adults and in infants (Marshall & Meltzoff, 2011). It is therefore often interpreted as a neural correlate of the link between action perception and action production in the brain (Muthukumaraswamy & Johnson, 2004). Mu suppression during action observation is thought to reflect motor resonance, which supports the coordination of two persons' actions (Sebanz, Bekkering, & Knoblich, 2006) and imitation (Meltzoff & Decety, 2003). Lachat and colleagues (2012) reasoned that mu desynchronization during joint attention may reflect an attention "mirroring" process during which one's own and another person's attention focus are coordinated.

A similar alpha suppression effect as in adults was recently observed in 9-month-olds (Hoehl, Michel, Reid, Parise, & Striano, 2014). Analyses were conducted on infants' brain responses when looking at an object together with an adult during a live interaction. Infants responded with desynchronization of alpha-band activity only when the adult had engaged in eye contact with them prior to turning to the object, but not when the adult only looked at the object without engaging with the infant first. This result is in line with the previous finding of an increased Nc ERP response for objects perceived together with an adult following a period of eye contact (Striano et al., 2006). Amplitude of the Nc is thought to reflect the amount of attention directed at a visual stimulus and is related to autonomic arousal (Reynolds & Richards, 2005). In contrast to the Nc, however, event-related desynchronization of alpha-band activity is not considered an obligatory response to a stimulus (Klimesch, 2012). No alpha synchronization or desynchronization effect was observed in the no eye contact condition, whereas an Nc deflection was found in both conditions in the ERP analyses. Alpha desynchronization may thus more specifically tap into the neural processes underlying triadic social interaction and mutual awareness of a joint attention focus. Further studies are required, however, to examine the exact functional role of this response in encoding information during a joint attention interaction.

Initiating Joint Attention as a Rewarding Experience

Thus far this chapter has focused on infants' responding to joint attention bids from others. By the end of the first year infants are also able to initiate triadic joint attention interactions. Important indicators of this ability are pointing gestures that can be observed by 11 to 12 months of age (Carpenter, Nagell, & Tomasello, 1998).

An important distinction has been made between imperative pointing and declarative pointing (Liszkowski, Carpenter, Henning, Striano, & Tomasello, 2004; Tomasello, Carpenter, & Liszkowski, 2007). One example for imperative pointing is gesturing at an object as a request for an adult to hand the object to the infant. This requires a basic understanding that others are causal agents who can be "used" by the infant to achieve some desired goal. Declarative pointing is, in contrast to imperative pointing, not observed in nonhuman primates (Call & Tomasello, 1996). Declarative pointing is motivated by a desire to share attention toward an external object or event with another person. This requires the ability to understand others as social interactive partners with attentional and perceptual abilities and with whom experiences can be shared. It has been questioned, though, whether 12-month-olds' pointing stems from a motivation to share an experience with another person or merely from a desire to elicit an emotional reaction from the adult toward themselves (Moore & Corkum, 1994).

Liszkowski et al. (2004) therefore examined the motivations behind 12-month-olds' pointing gestures experimentally. Infants in this study interacted with an adult experimenter. During test trials an interesting event occurred somewhere in the room (a stuffed toy animal appeared from behind a curtain), prompting infants to point toward it. The adult reacted to infants' pointing either by sharing attention and interest by alternating gaze between the infant and the event while speaking in a positive tone of voice, or by attending only to the event, only to the infant, or by ignoring both the infant and the event. When the adult reacted to the infant's pointing by sharing attention, infants pointed in a greater proportion of test trials and tended to point for longer periods of time than in the other conditions, suggesting that they enjoyed the experience. When the adult attended only to the infant or to the event, infants pointed more frequently within each test trial, presumably in an attempt to engage the adult in a joint attention interaction involving attention toward both the infant and the event. Furthermore, when an adult misinterprets infants' pointing by attending to a different nearby referent, 12-month-olds repeat their pointing in order to redirect the adult's attention focus and establish joint attention even if the adult responded enthusiastically to the first wrong referent (Liszkowski, Carpenter, & Tomasello, 2007). In contrast, when the adult attended to the correct referent, but expressed indifference, infants pointed significantly less within and across trials. This pattern of results speaks against the notion that infants' pointing is primarily motivated by a desire to induce an emotional reaction toward themselves and supports the idea that infants point to share an experience with another person.

The idea that sharing attention with someone is inherently rewarding is supported by neuroimaging work with adults. Schilbach et al. (2010) had participants interact with virtual characters that responded contingently to the participants' gaze behavior. When participants perceived a virtual character following their own gaze toward a target after a period of eye contact, activations were observed in the striatum, which is part of the reward network in the brain.

It is currently unclear to what extent the neural reward system is involved in infants' initiation of joint attention. This is because electrophysiological (EEG) and neuroimaging (fNIRS) methods that are most commonly used with infant participants do not inform us about activations of subcortical structures, such as the brain structures involved in representing rewards (Schilbach et al., 2010). However, distinct neural correlates of responding to joint attention bids by others and actively initiating joint attention have been identified in infants using EEG. Mundy et al. (2000) found that a pattern of left parietal activation and right parietal deactivation at 14 months correlates with the ability to respond to joint attention at 14 and 18 months. In the same study, left frontal and central baseline EEG activity at 14 months predicted infants' initiating of joint attention in a live social interaction at 18 months of age. Since left frontal activation has been associated with approach behavior, sensitivity to rewards, and social orientation in infancy (Davidson & Fox, 1982; Fox, 1991), this observation fits with the notion that brain areas implicated in motivational processes and sensitivity to rewards are also involved in infants' initiating of joint attention.

Conclusions and Future Directions

In the present chapter we have reviewed joint attention development from a biopsychosocial perspective considering behavioral, electrophysiological, and brain-imaging research. We have distinguished separate aspects of joint attention beginning with the ability to detect when another person's attention is directed at the self through ostensive, communicative signals. Infants' early sensitivity to these signals is well documented. For instance, newborns prefer to look at a face with eye contact as compared to a face with averted gaze (Farroni et al., 2002). By 3 months of age infants are sensitive to interruptions of eye contact in triadic interactions involving another person and an object (Striano & Stahl, 2005). Furthermore, young infants are sensitive to infant-directed speech (Saito et al., 2007), being called by their name (Mandel, Jusczyk, & Pisoni, 1995), and they detect when an interactive partner acts contingently to their own behavior (Striano et al., 2005). Interestingly, the self-relevance of different communicative signals seems to be processed in the medial PFC, independent of sensory modality (i.e., visual or auditory), as suggested by neuroimaging work in adults (e.g., Kampe et al., 2003) and in infants (Grossmann et al., 2010; Parise & Csibra, 2013).

The ability to detect communicative signals directed toward the self may thus be the foundation upon which other joint attention skills, such as following and actively directing others' attention, are developed. In fact, the presence of self-relevant communicative signals prompts infants to follow an agent's eye gaze or body orientation with their own gaze. This enhancing effect on infants' gaze following was demonstrated for eye contact and infant-directed speech when a human model was shown (Senju & Csibra, 2008), as well as for contingent behavior with nonhuman agents lacking visual features and eyes (Deligianni et al., 2011; Johnson et al., 1998).

In addition, eye contact during a triadic live interaction affects infants' neural processing of novel objects (Hoehl, Michel, Reid, Parise, & Striano, 2014; Striano et al., 2006), as well as their later object recognition (Cleveland et al., 2007; Cleveland & Striano, 2007; Kopp & Lindenberger, 2011) and word learning (Hirotani et al., 2009). Although infants are sensitive to different kinds of communicative signals from early on, the effects of signals other than eye contact on infant learning have been less thoroughly studied to this point. Since similar brain responses are elicited when infants are addressed directly by another person through different modalities, it is conceivable that communicative cues like infant-directed speech, contingent behavior, and calling the infant's name affect infants' object processing and learning as well. Preliminary evidence that this may be the case comes from an ERP study that found that 5-month-olds respond with increased attention to objects when at the same time hearing their own name as compared with another name (Parise, Friederici, & Striano, 2010). One important direction of future research will thus be to determine whether learning about objects is similarly affected by different kinds of communicative signals. Furthermore, infants' and children's learning of other, more complex kinds of information depending on joint attention and communicative signals directed at the self will be an issue for further research. For instance, on the behavioral level it was shown that 18-month-old infants learn differently about the valence of an unfamiliar object when someone expresses an emotion toward the object in a communicative context in which they are directly addressed as compared with a noncommunicative context (Egyed, Király, & Gergely, 2013). In addition, 14-month-olds tend to imitate relatively inefficient arbitrary means actions more when these are demonstrated by a communicative model as compared with a model who does not address them directly (Gergely, Bekkering, & Király, 2002; Király, Csibra, & Gergely, 2013). It will be an interesting topic for future research to determine whether similar brain processes are involved in social learning of these kinds of information in joint attention interactions as opposed to incidental observations of another person's actions.

One avenue for future research will also be to investigate the roles of distinct neural substrates involved in aspects of joint attention: detecting self-relevant communicative signals that indicate another person's attention has been associated with activation of the medial PFC (Kampe et al., 2003). The ability to respond to joint attention by following others' attention focus should be further divided into relatively automatic or reflexive gaze cueing on the one hand, and deliberate gaze following depending on the status of another person's eyes on the other hand. Reflexive gaze cueing seems to rely on the frontoparietal spatial attention network including IPS in adults (Cazzato et al., 2012) and possibly also in infants (Grossmann et al., 2007), whereas deliberate gaze following in joint attention interactions induces activation in the medial PFC (Schilbach et al., 2010). In the same study activations in a structure belonging to the reward system in the brain, the striatum, were observed when participants perceived someone else following their own gaze (Schilbach et al., 2010). Although existing evidence suggests that infants experience initiating joint attention interactions as rewarding (Liszkowski et al., 2004; Mundy et al., 2000), research on the involvement of the reward and motivation network of the brain during joint attention interactions in infants is still lacking.

Finally, researchers may consider examining the role of joint attention in sensory modalities other than the visual domain. Joint attention interactions are rich multimodal experiences that may, for instance, involve listening to something or someone together. What are the effects of self-relevant communicative signals such as eye contact in these contexts? How is attending jointly to a sound, a taste, or a somatosensory sensation initiated? Is learning in the auditory or somatosensory domain affected by sharing attention to an auditory or tactile percept? All of these questions bear relevance for a deeper understanding of joint attention in infants' day-to-day social interactions and learning experiences but have yet received very little attention by researchers.

In recent years joint attention has become a hot topic in cognitive neuroscience and development research. As evidenced by the vast body of research reviewed in this chapter, we have learned much about the early development and functions, as well as the neural correlates of joint attention. Still, there are many open questions, especially when considering joint attention as a multimodal experience taking place in complex environments full of rich and multifaceted sensory experiences. In future studies researchers should continue to combine the advantages of ecologically valid live interactions with controlled experimental procedures and neurobehavioral measures as a challenging but promising approach to study the impact of joint attention on infants' social cognitive development and learning.

ACKNOWLEDGMENTS

The writing of this chapter was supported by Grant No. HO 4342/2-2 from the Deutsche Forschungsgemeinschaft.

REFERENCES

Adolphs, R. (2009). The social brain: Neural basis of social knowledge. *Annual Review of Psychology, 60,* 693–716.

Baldwin, D. A. (1995). Understanding the link of joint attention and language. In C. Moore & P. Dunham (Eds.), *Joint attention: Its origin and role in development* (pp. 131–158). Hillsdale, NJ: Erlbaum.

Baron-Cohen, S. (1994). How to build a baby that can read minds: Cognitive mechanisms in mindreading. *Current Psychology of Cognition, 13,* 513–552.

Barresi, J., & Moore, C. (1993). Sharing a perspective precedes the understanding of that perspective. *Behavioral and Brain Sciences, 16,* 513–514.

Batki, A., Baron-Cohen, S., Wheelwright, S., Connellan, J., & Ahluwalia, J. (2000). Is there an innate gaze module? Evidence from human neonates. *Infant Behavior and Development, 23,* 223–229.

Brooks, R., & Meltzoff, A. N. (2002). The importance of eyes: How infants interpret adult looking behavior. *Developmental Psychology, 38*(6), 958–966.

Brooks, R., & Meltzoff, A. N. (2005). The development of gaze following and its relation to language. *Developmental Science, 8*(6), 535–543.

Butterworth, G., & Jarrett, N. (1991). What minds have in common is space: Spatial mechanisms serving joint visual attention in infancy. *British Journal of Developmental Psychology, 9,* 55–72.

Call, J., & Tomasello, M. (1996). The effect of humans on the cognitive development of apes. In A. Russon (Ed.), *Reaching into thought: The minds of the great apes* (pp. 371–403). Cambridge, UK: Cambridge University Press.

Carpenter, M., Nagell, K., & Tomasello, M. (1998). Social cognition, joint attention, and communicative competence from 9 to 15 months of age. *Monographs of the Society for Research in Child Development, 63*(4), i–vi, 1–143.

Cazzato, V., Macaluso, E., Crostella, F., & Aglioti, S. M. (2012). Mapping reflexive shifts of attention in eye-centered and hand-centered coordinate systems. *Human Brain Mapping, 33*(1), 165–178.

Cleveland, A., Schug, M., & Striano, T. (2007). Joint attention and object learning in 5- and 7-month-old infants. *Infant and Child Development, 16*, 195–306.

Cleveland, A., & Striano, T. (2007). The effects of joint attention on object processing in 4- and 9-month-old infants. *Infant Behavior and Development, 30*(3), 499–504.

Corbetta, M. (1998). Frontoparietal cortical networks for directing attention and the eye to visual locations: Identical, independent, or overlapping neural systems? *Proceedings of the National Academy of Sciences of the United States of America, 95*(3), 831–838.

Corkum, V., & Moore, C. (1995). Development of joint visual attention in infants. In C. Moore & P. Dunham (Eds.), *Joint attention: Its origins and role in development* (pp. 61–83). Hillsdale, NJ: Erlbaum.

Csibra, G., Davis, G., Spratling, M. W., & Johnson, M. H. (2000). Gamma oscillations and object processing in the infant brain. *Science, 290*(5496), 1582–1585.

Csibra, G., & Gergely, G. (2011). Natural pedagogy as evolutionary adaptation. *Philosophical Transactions of the Royal Society London B: Biological Science, 366*(1567), 1149–1157.

Csibra, G., & Johnson, M. H. (2007). Investigating event-related oscillations in infancy. In M. de Haan (Ed.), *Infant EEG and event-related potentials* (pp. 289–304). Hove, UK: Psychology Press.

Csibra, G., & Volein, A. (2008). Infants can infer the presence of hidden objects from referential gaze information. *British Journal of Developmental Psychology, 26*, 1–11.

Davidson, R. J., & Fox, N. A. (1982). Asymmetrical brain activity discriminates between positive and negative affective stimuli in human infants. *Science, 218*(4578), 1235–1237.

Deak, G. O., Flom, R. A., & Pick, A. D. (2000). Effects of gesture and target on 12- and 18-month-olds' joint visual attention to objects in front of or behind them. *Developmental Psychology, 36*(4), 511–523.

Deligianni, F., Senju, A., Gergely, G., & Csibra, G. (2011). Automated gaze-contingent objects elicit orientation following in 8-month-old infants. *Developmental Psychology, 47*(6), 1499–1503.

D'Entremont, B., Hains, S. M., & Muir, D. W. (1997). A demonstration of gaze following in 3- to 6-month-olds. *Infant Behavior and Development, 20*(4), 569–572.

Egyed, K., Király, I., & Gergely, G. (2013). Communicating shared knowledge in infancy. *Psychological Science, 24*(7), 1348–1353.

Ethofer, T., Gschwind, M., & Vuilleumier, P. (2011). Processing social aspects of human gaze: A combined fMRI-DTI study. *Neuroimage, 55*(1), 411–419.

Farroni, T., Csibra, G., Simion, F., & Johnson, M. H. (2002). Eye contact detection in humans from birth. *Proceedings of the National Academy of Sciences USA, 99*(14), 9602–9605.

Farroni, T., Johnson, M. H., & Csibra, G. (2004). Mechanisms of eye gaze perception during infancy. *Journal of Cognitive Neuroscience, 16*(8), 1320–1326.

Farroni, T., Mansfield, E. M., Lai, C., & Johnson, M. H. (2003). Infants perceiving and acting on the eyes: Tests of an evolutionary hypothesis. *Journal of Experimental Child Psychology, 85*(3), 199–212.

Farroni, T., Massaccesi, S., Menon, E., & Johnson, M. H. (2007). Direct gaze modulates face recognition in young infants. *Cognition, 102*(3), 396–404.

Farroni, T., Massaccesi, S., Pividori, D., & Johnson, M. H. (2004). Gaze following in newborns. *Infancy, 5*(1), 39–60.

Fiebach, C. J., Gruber, T., & Supp, G. G. (2005). Neuronal mechanisms of repetition priming in occipitotemporal cortex: Spatiotemporal evidence from functional magnetic resonance imaging and electroencephalography. *Journal of Neuroscience, 25*(13), 3414–3422.

Fox, N. A. (1991). If it's not left, it's right. Electroencephalograph asymmetry and the development of emotion. *American Psychologist, 46*(8), 863–872.

Gergely, G. (2000). Reapproaching Mahler: New perspectives on normal autism, symbiosis, splitting and libidinal object constancy from cognitive developmental theory. *Journal of the American Psychoanalytic Association, 48*(4), 1197–1228.

Gergely, G., Bekkering, H., & Király, I. (2002). Rational imitation in preverbal infants. *Nature, 415*(6873), 755.

Gliga, T., & Csibra, G. (2007). Seeing the face through the eyes: A developmental perspective on face expertise. *Progress in Brain Research, 164*, 323–339.

Gredebäck, G., Fikke, L., & Melinder, A. (2010). The development of joint visual attention: A longitudinal study of gaze following during interactions with mothers and strangers. *Developmental Science, 13*(6), 839–848.

Grossmann, T., & Johnson, M. H. (2010). Selective prefrontal cortex responses to joint attention in early infancy. *Biology Letters, 6*(4), 540–543.

Grossmann, T., Johnson, M. H., Farroni, T., & Csibra, G. (2007). Social perception in the infant brain: Gamma oscillatory activity in response to eye gaze. *Social Cognitive and Affective Neuroscience, 2*(4), 284–291.

Grossmann, T., Johnson, M. H., Lloyd-Fox, S., Blasi, A., Deligianni, F., Elwell, C., et al., (2008). Early cortical specialization for face-to-face communication in human infants. *Proceedings of the Royal Society: Biological Sciences, 275*(1653), 2803–2811.

Grossmann, T., Lloyd-Fox, S., & Johnson, M. H. (2013). Brain responses reveal young infants' sensitivity to when a social partner follows their gaze. *Developmental Cognitive Neuroscience, 6*, 155–161.

Grossmann, T., Parise, E., & Friederici, A. D. (2010). The detection of communicative signals directed at the self in infant prefrontal cortex. *Frontiers in Human Neuroscience, 4*, 201.

Halit, H., Csibra, G., Volein, A., & Johnson, M. H. (2004). Face-sensitive cortical processing in early infancy. *Journal of Child Psychology and Psychiatry, 45*(7), 1228–1234.

Halit, H., de Haan, M., & Johnson, M. H. (2003). Cortical specialisation for face processing: Face-sensitive event-related potential components in 3- and 12-month-old infants. *Neuroimage, 19*(3), 1180–1193.

Hirotani, M., Stets, M., Striano, T., & Friederici, A. D. (2009). Joint attention helps infants learn new words: Event-related potential evidence. *Neuroreport, 20*(6), 600–605.

Hoehl, S., Michel, C., Reid, V. M., Parise, E., & Striano, T. (2014). Eye contact during live social interaction modulates infants' oscillatory brain activity. *Social Neuroscience, 9*(3), 300–308.

Hoehl, S., & Peykarjou, S. (2012). The early development of face processing: What makes faces special? *Neuroscience Bulletin, 28*(6), 765–788.

Hoehl, S., Reid, V., Mooney, J., & Striano, T. (2008). What are you looking at?: Infants' neural processing of an adult's object-directed eye gaze. *Developmental Science, 11*(1), 10–16.

Hoehl, S., Reid, V. M., Parise, E., Handl, A., Palumbo, L., & Striano, T. (2009). Looking at eye gaze processing and its neural correlates in infancy: Implications for social development and autism spectrum disorder. *Child Development, 80*(4), 968–985.

Hoehl, S., Wahl, S., Michel, C., & Striano, T. (2012). Effects of eye gaze cues provided by the caregiver compared to a stranger on infants' object processing. *Developmental Cognitive Neuroscience, 2*, 81–89.

Hoehl, S., Wahl, S., & Pauen, S. (2014). Disentangling the effects of an adult model's eye gaze and head orientation on young infants' processing of a previously attended object. *Infancy, 19*, 53–64.

Hoffman, E. A., & Haxby, J. V. (2000). Distinct representations of eye gaze and identity in the distributed human neural system for face perception. *Nature Neuroscience, 3*(1), 80–84.

Hood, B. M., Willen, J. D., & Driver, J. (1998). Adult's eyes trigger shifts of visual attention in human infants. *Psychological Science, 9*(2), 131–134.

Johnson, M. H. (2005). Subcortical face processing. *Nature Reviews Neuroscience, 6*(10), 766–774.

Johnson, M. H., Dziurawiec, S., Ellis, H., & Morton, J. (1991). Newborns' preferential tracking of face-like stimuli and its subsequent decline. *Cognition, 40*(1–2), 1–19.

Johnson, S. C., Ok, S. J., & Luo, Y. (2007). The attribution of attention: 9-month-olds' interpretation of gaze as goal-directed action. *Developmental Science, 10*(5), 530–537.

Johnson, S. C., Slaughter, V., & Carey, S. (1998). Whose gaze will infants follow?: The elicitation of gaze following in 12-month-olds. *Developmental Science, 1*(2), 233–238.

Kampe, K. K., Frith, C. D., & Frith, U. (2003). "Hey John": Signals conveying communicative intention toward the self activate brain regions associated with "mentalizing," regardless of modality. *Journal of Neuroscience, 23*(12), 5258–5263.

Király, I., Csibra, G., & Gergely, G. (2013). Beyond rational imitation: Learning arbitrary means actions from communicative demonstrations. *Journal of Experimental Child Psychology, 116*(2), 471–486.

Klimesch, W. (2012). Alpha-band oscillations, attention, and controlled access to stored information. *Trends in Cognitive Sciences, 16*(12), 606–617.

Kopp, F., & Lindenberger, U. (2011). Effects of joint attention on long-term memory in 9-month-old infants: An event-related potentials study. *Developmental Science, 14*(4), 660–672.

Kristen, S., Sodian, B., Thoermer, C., & Perst, H. (2011). Infants' joint attention skills predict toddlers' emerging mental state language. *Developmental Psychology, 47*(5), 1207–1219.

Lachat, F., Hugueville, L., Lemarechal, J. D., Conty, L., & George, N. (2012). Oscillatory brain correlates of live joint attention: A dual-EEG study. *Frontiers in Human Neuroscience, 6*, 156.

Liszkowski, U., Carpenter, M., Henning, A., Striano, T., & Tomasello, M. (2004). Twelve-month-olds point to share attention and interest. *Developmental Science, 7*(3), 297–307.

Liszkowski, U., Carpenter, M., & Tomasello, M. (2007). Reference and attitude in infant pointing. *Journal of Child Language, 34*(1), 1–20.

Mandel, D. R., Jusczyk, P. W., & Pisoni, D. B. (1995). Infants' recognition of the sound patterns of their own names. *Psychological Science, 6*(5), 314–317.

Marshall, P. J., & Meltzoff, A. N. (2011). Neural mirroring systems: Exploring the EEG mu rhythm in human infancy. *Developmental Cognitive Neuroscience, 1*(2), 110–123.

Meltzoff, A. N., & Brooks, R. (2007). Eyes wide shut: The importance of eyes in infant gaze-following and understanding other minds. In R. Flom & K. Lee (Eds.), *Gaze following: Its development and significance* (pp. 217–241). Mahwah, NJ: Erlbaum.

Meltzoff, A. N., & Decety, J. (2003). What imitation tells us about social cognition: A rapprochement between developmental psychology and cognitive neuroscience. *Philosophical Transactions of the Royal Society of London B: Biological Sciences, 358*(1431), 491–500.

Meltzoff, A. N., & Moore, M. K. (1977). Imitation of facial and manual gestures by human neonates. *Science, 198*(4312), 75–78.

Moll, H., & Tomasello, M. (2004). 12- and 18-month-old infants follow gaze to spaces behind barriers. *Developmental Science, 7*(1), F1–F9.

Moore, C., & Corkum, V. (1994). Social understanding at the end of the first year of life. *Developmental Review, 14*(4), 349–372.

Moore, C., & Corkum, V. (1998). Infant gaze following based on eye direction. *British Journal of Psychology, 16*, 495–503.

Mosconi, M. W., Mack, P. B., McCarthy, G., & Pelphrey, K. A. (2005). Taking an "intentional stance" on eye-gaze shifts: A functional neuroimaging study of social perception in children. *NeuroImage, 27*(1), 247–252.

Mundy, P., Card, J., & Fox, N. (2000). EEG correlates of the development of infant joint attention skills. *Developmental Psychobiology, 36*(4), 325–338.

Muthukumaraswamy, S. D., & Johnson, B. W. (2004). Changes in rolandic mu rhythm during observation of a precision grip. *Psychophysiology, 41*(1), 152–156.

Neuper, C., & Pfurtscheller, G. (2001). Event-related dynamics of cortical rhythms: Frequency-specific features and functional correlates. *International Journal of Psychophysiology, 43*(1), 41–58.

Parise, E., & Csibra, G. (2013). Neural responses to multimodal ostensive signals in 5-month-old infants. *PLoS ONE, 8*(8), e72360.

Parise, E., Friederici, A. D., & Striano, T. (2010). "Did you call me?" 5-month-old infants own name guides their attention. *PLOS ONE, 5*(12), e14208.

Parise, E., Reid, V. M., Stets, M., & Striano, T. (2008). Direct eye contact influences the neural processing of objects in 5-month-old infants. *Social Neuroscience, 3*(2), 141–150.

Pelphrey, K. A., Singerman, J. D., Allison, T., & McCarthy, G. (2003). Brain activation evoked by perception of gaze shifts: The influence of context. *Neuropsychologia, 41*(2), 156–170.

Peykarjou, S., & Hoehl, S. (2013). Three-month-olds' brain responses to upright and inverted faces and cars. *Developmental Neuropsychology, 38*(4), 272–280.

Pfurtscheller, G. (2003). Induced oscillations in the alpha band: Functional meaning. *Epilepsia, 44*(Suppl. 12), 2–8.

Pfurtscheller, G., Stancak, A., Jr., & Neuper, C. (1996). Event-related synchronization (ERS) in the alpha band—an electrophysiological correlate of cortical idling: A review. *International Journal of Psychophysiology, 24*(1–2), 39–46.

Posner, M. I., & Petersen, S. E. (1990). The attention system of the human brain. *Annual Reviews in Neuroscience, 13*, 25–42.

Reid, V. M., & Striano, T. (2005). Adult gaze influences infant attention and object processing: Implications for cognitive neuroscience. *European Journal of Neuroscience, 21*(6), 1763–1766.

Reid, V. M., & Striano, T. (2007). The directed attention model of infant social cognition. *European Journal of Developmental Psychology, 4*(1), 100–110.

Reid, V. M., Striano, T., Kaufman, J., & Johnson, M. H. (2004). Eye gaze cueing facilitates neural processing of objects in 4-month-old infants. *Neuroreport, 15*(16), 2553–2555.

Reynolds, G. D., & Richards, J. E. (2005). Familiarization, attention, and recognition memory in infancy: An event-related potential and cortical source localization study. *Developmental Psychology, 41*(4), 598–615.

Saby, J. N., & Marshall, P. J. (2012). The utility of EEG band power analysis in the study of infancy and early childhood. *Developmental Neuropsychology, 37*(3), 253–273.

Saito, Y., Aoyama, S., Kondo, T., Fukumoto, R., Konishi, N., Nakamura, K., et al. (2007). Frontal cerebral blood flow change associated with infant-directed speech. *Archives of Disease in Childhood: Fetal and Neonatal Edition, 92*(2), F113–F116.

Scaife, M., & Bruner, J. S. (1975). The capacity for joint visual attention in the infant. *Nature, 253*(5489), 265–266.

Scheeringa, R., Petersson, K. M., Kleinschmidt, A., Jensen, O., & Bastiaansen, M. C. (2012). EEG alpha power modulation of FMRI resting-state connectivity. *Brain Connect, 2*(5), 254–264.

Schilbach, L., Wilms, M., Eickhoff, S. B., Romanzetti, S., Tepest, R., Bente, G., et al. (2010). Minds made for sharing: Initiating joint attention recruits reward-related neurocircuitry. *Journal of Cognitive Neuroscience, 22*(12), 2702–2715.

Schilbach, L., Wohlschlaeger, A. M., Kraemer, N. C., Newen, A., Shah, N. J., Fink, G. R., et al. (2006). Being with virtual others: Neural correlates of social interaction. *Neuropsychologia, 44*(5), 718–730.

Sebanz, N., Bekkering, H., & Knoblich, G. (2006). Joint action: Bodies and minds moving together. *Trends in Cognitive Sciences, 10*(2), 70–76.

Senju, A., & Csibra, G. (2008). Gaze following in human infants depends on communicative signals. *Current Biology, 18*(9), 668–671.

Senju, A., Johnson, M. H., & Csibra, G. (2006). The development and neural basis of referential gaze perception. *Social Neuroscience, 1*(3–4), 220–234.

Southgate, V., Csibra, G., Kaufman, J., & Johnson, M. H. (2008). Distinct processing of objects and faces in the infant brain. *Journal of Cognitive Neuroscience, 20*(4), 741–749.

Striano, T., & Bertin, E. (2005). Coordinated affect with mothers and strangers: A longitudinal analysis of joint engagement between 5 and 9 months of age. *Cognition and Emotion, 19*(5), 781–790.

Striano, T., Henning, A., & Stahl, D. (2005). Sensitivity to social contingencies between 1 and 3 months of age. *Developmental Science, 8*(6), 509–518.

Striano, T., & Reid, V. M. (2006). Social cognition in the first year. *Trends in Cognitive Sciences, 10*(10), 471–476.

Striano, T., Reid, V. M., & Hoehl, S. (2006). Neural mechanisms of joint attention in infancy. *European Journal of Neuroscience, 23*(10), 2819–2823.

Striano, T., & Stahl, D. (2005). Sensitivity to triadic attention in early infancy. *Developmental Science, 8*(4), 333–343.

Striano, T., Stahl, D., Cleveland, A., & Hoehl, S. (2007). Sensitivity to triadic attention between 6 weeks and 3 months of age. *Infant Behavior and Development, 30*(3), 529–534.

Theuring, C., Gredebäck, G., & Hauf, P. (2007). Object processing during a joint gaze following task. *European Journal of Developmental Psychology, 4*(1), 65–79.

Tomasello, M., Carpenter, M., Call, J., Behne, T., & Moll, H. (2005). Understanding and sharing intentions: The origins of cultural cognition. *Behavioral and Brain Sciences, 28*(5), 675–691, discussion 691–735.

Tomasello, M., Carpenter, M., & Liszkowski, U. (2007). A new look at infant pointing. *Child Development, 78*(3), 705–722.

Tomasello, M., Hare, B., Lehmann, H., & Call, J. (2007). Reliance on head versus eyes in the gaze following of great apes and human infants: The cooperative eye hypothesis. *Journal of Human Evolution, 52*(3), 314–320.

Tronick, E., Als, H., Adamson, L., Wise, S., & Brazelton, T. B. (1978). The infant's response to entrapment between contradictory messages in face-to-face interaction. *Journal of the American Academy for Child Psychiatry, 17*(1), 1–13.

Wahl, S., Michel, C., Pauen, S., & Hoehl, S. (2012). Head and eye movements affect object processing in 4-month-old infants more than an artificial orientation cue. *British Journal of Psychology, 31*(2), 212–230.

Woodward, A. (2003). Infants' developing understanding of the link between looker and object. *Developmental Science, 6*(3), 297–311.

CHAPTER 7

The Development of Declarative Memory in Infancy and Implications for Social Learning

Patricia J. Bauer and Jacqueline S. Leventon

The ability to recall the past is fundamental to mental life. It allows us to remember discrete events and experiences, both the mundane (e.g., where the car is parked at the grocery store) and the significant (e.g., graduations, weddings, and births). The capacity also contributes to developments outside of memory, including those that support social interaction and learning from others. To state the obvious, for infants, memory is crucial to tasks as fundamental as recognizing the faces of one's caregivers and learning to interpret the vocalizations they make in the course of interactions (otherwise known as language). Perhaps less obvious is the role of memory in learning about the world from others. It is by watching others and remembering how they behave that infants learn—and remember—what to approach in the world around them and conversely, what to avoid. Memory is thus crucial not only for keeping track of the location of the car but also for understanding how to navigate a world inhabited by others of the same species.

Historically, assessing the emergence and early development of the foundational ability to recall the past posed significant challenges because of the response limitations of infants—they are unable to engage in the memory paradigm of choice, namely, verbal report. In part for this reason, until the middle 1980s, it was widely believed that the ability to recall the past was late to emerge. Development in the middle 1980s of a nonverbal test of recall, coupled with an expanding body of information about the development of the neural substrate responsible for recall, led to revision of the assumption of a mnemonically incompetent infant. In this chapter we review the neural foundations of memory and its development, and illustrate links between neural developments and changes in memory behavior throughout infancy. We then discuss the implications of changes in memory ability for learning from others in social situations. We begin with the important "social" task of ensuring shared reference regarding the particular type of memory under consideration, namely, declarative memory.

"Memory": A Singular Noun but a Plural Construct

To fully understand how memory develops in infancy—and thus how it might relate to social learning and memory—one must first determine what type of memory is being discussed. This determination is essential because, although the noun—*memory*—is singular, memory is not a unitary construct. There is a widely recognized distinction between two dissociable mnemonic constructs, namely, declarative (explicit) and nondeclarative (implicit) memory (e.g., Squire, Knowlton, & Musen, 1993). Declarative memory permits conscious recall of past events, whereas nondeclarative memory supports acquisition of motor skills, habits, classical conditioning, and perceptual priming. In contrast to declarative memories, these forms of behavior do not depend on conscious access or awareness and thus are not available to verbal report.

In the context of development, the distinction between memory systems is important because the different types of memory depend on different neural substrates with different developmental courses. The formation and maintenance of nondeclarative memories relies on a number of different neural circuits. For example, classical conditioning largely depends on the cerebellum, whereas habit learning relies on the integrity of the striatum. In general, the neural substrates that support nondeclarative forms of memory develop early and perhaps as a consequence, behavioral changes are not especially pronounced (see Lloyd & Newcombe, 2009). In contrast, as described in the next section, declarative memory depends on a network involving the cortex and structures in the medial temporal lobe. Some components of the system have a protracted developmental course, which has implications for declarative memory behavior.

The Neural Substrate Underlying Declarative Memory

The capacity for declarative memory of past events and experiences is multifaceted. There are multiple stages in the life of a memory, each of which is a potential source of developmental change. Moreover, the processes of encoding information present in the environment, consolidating and storing that information as a memory trace, and retrieving the trace when necessary involve a complex neural network that includes structures in the temporal lobe (including hippocampus and entorhinal, parahippocampal, and perirhinal cortices) and cortical areas (including prefrontal cortex and association areas; e.g., Dickerson & Eichenbaum, 2010; Eichenbaum & Cohen, 2001; Markowitsch, 2000; Milner, 2005; Zola & Squire, 2000). The structures themselves and the connectivity among them undergo substantial postnatal development. Each of these aspects of declarative memory are elaborated below.

The Life of a Memory: Trace Formation, Consolidation, and Retrieval

Memories begin their lives as experiences. Consider the rich experience of a mother holding a toy in front of an infant, shaking it to draw her or his attention, and gently cooing "What a nice toy." The perceptual information generated by this experience initially is registered in primary sensory areas, such as in the visual cortex (for the visual stimulus of the mother and the toy) and auditory cortex (for the auditory stimulus of the verbalization). Inputs from these areas are sent (projected) to unimodal association areas, where the information is integrated into modality-specific perceptions (i.e., information is not yet integrated across modalities). These association areas then project to polymodal association cortices in the prefrontal, posterior, and limbic areas where information from the various sensory modalities begins to be combined. In addition, the information from these various modalities is maintained over delays of seconds in these association areas (Petrides, 1995). As such, prefrontal areas are involved in processing and encoding initial perceptual experiences.

For information about the "nice toy" to be maintained over time, aspects of the experience must undergo a process of stabilization into a memory trace and integration of the trace into long-term memory. This process—known as *consolidation*—results from the associated actions of structures in the medial temporal lobe and cortical association areas (McGaugh, 2000). Information from the polymodal association areas travels to the perirhinal and parahippocampal cortices in the medial temporal lobe before being projected into the entorhinal cortex and the hippocampus proper, where the various components of an event are bound into a single representation—mother's behavior toward this particular toy. Simultaneously, association areas are active in integrating information about mother and the new toy with representations of her and toys already in long-term storage (e.g., McKenzie & Eichenbaum, 2011). Consolidated memory traces are ultimately stored in the neocortex.

Finally, recall or retrieval of a memory trace critically relies on the prefrontal cortex (Cabeza, McIntosh, Tulving, Nyberg, & Grady, 1997; Cabeza et al., 2004; Maguire, 2001). Damage to this area of the brain results in retrieval deficits that have been observed for the free recall of information relative to recognition, memory for temporal order relative to memory for individual items, memory for the specific features of events, and memory for the source of the presented information. Imaging data indicate that the prefrontal cortex is active when retrieving episodic memories from long-term stores (reviewed in Gilboa, 2004).

Developments in the Neural Substrate Underlying Declarative Memory

As reflected in the previous section, the process of creating, storing, and later retrieving declarative memories involves a number of neural "moving parts." Critically, aspects of the neural structures themselves, as well as the connections between and among them, undergo a protracted course of postnatal development. The development of the neural substrate underlying the formation and later recall of declarative memories has been the subject of numerous previous reviews (Bauer, 2006, 2007, 2009, 2014; Lukowski & Bauer, 2014; Nelson, 2000; Nelson, de Haan, & Thomas, 2006; Richmond & Nelson, 2008) and so we summarize it only briefly here. Components of the medial temporal lobe develop prenatally or during the early postnatal period. For example, Seress and Abraham (2008) indicate that hippocampal cells are generated during the first half of prenatal development and have migrated to their final destinations by birth. Synapses are apparent by about 15-weeks gestation. The number of hippocampal synapses and synaptic density increases until about 6 months of age, at which time adult levels are reached. At this same time, glucose utilization (an indicator of energy use) also reaches adult levels, likely in relation to the increased number of synapses (Chugani, 1994; Chugani & Phelps, 1986).

Other components of the neural circuitry are later to mature. For example, the development of the dentate gyrus of the hippocampus is protracted (Seress & Abraham, 2008). This area of the brain includes about 70% of the adult complement of cells at birth; the remaining cells are produced postnatally. Neurogenesis in this region has been confirmed in childhood and beyond (Tanapat, Hastings, & Gould, 2001). Morphologically the structure is adult-like around 12 to 15 months after birth. Increases in synaptic density are also protracted relative to what is observed in other regions of the hippocampus: synaptic density in this region increases starting around 8 to 12 months after birth and peaks around 18 to 20 months. Adult levels of synapses are reached during the early school years (Eckenhoff & Rakic, 1991).

The implications of the later-maturing dentate gyrus on formation and recall of declarative memories have yet to be identified. However, there is reason to believe that this late-developing structure may be a rate-limiting variable in the development of recall in infancy (Bauer, 2007, 2009; Nelson, 1995, 1997, 2000). As previously described, information integrated in polymodal association areas is projected to the entorhinal cortex for processing by the hippocampus proper. This projection into the hippocampus can occur either through a "long route" or through a "short route." The long route includes projections from the entorhinal cortex through the dentate gyrus into the hippocampus proper; in the short route, the dentate gyrus is bypassed completely. Processing via the short route seems to support some aspects of memory (Nelson, 1995, 1997), although rodent data suggest that adult-typical memories require transmission through the dentate gyrus (Czurkó, Czéh, Seress, Nadel, & Bures, 1997; Nadel & Willner, 1989).

The development of association areas is also protracted (Bachevalier, 2001). All six layers of the prefrontal cortex are not found until the seventh month of gestation. Synaptic density in this region increases until 8 months after birth and reaches its peak between 15 and 24 months. Maximum synaptic density may be apparent as early as 15 months after birth, and synapses appear adult-like in their morphology at 24 months (Huttenlocher, 1979). Throughout the infancy period, changes in blood flow and glucose utilization are also apparent, such that these measurements exceed adult levels by 8 to 12 months and 13 to 14 months, respectively (Chugani, Phelps, & Mazziotta, 1987).

Consequences of Developments in the Underlying Neural Substrate

As is apparent from this brief review, the neural network that supports memory trace formation and later recall includes various regions that develop at different times. As such, the substrate can function as an integrated unit only once the components have reached functional maturity. "Functional maturity" has been identified as occurring when the peak number of synapses has been realized, whereas "full maturity" occurs when the synapses have been pruned to adult levels (Goldman-Rakic, 1987). This analysis suggests that the ability to form memories that later can be recalled should become apparent or emerge near the end of the first year of life, with continued developments over the second year and beyond (see Barbas, 2000; Fuster, 2002, for discussion). This proposed time line is based on the apparent increases in synaptic density in the dentate gyrus between 8 and 20 months of age (Eckenhoff & Rakic, 1991) and in the prefrontal cortex between 8 and 24 months (Huttenlocher, 1979; Huttenlocher & Dabholkar, 1997). Developments in these areas continue throughout childhood (for the dentate gyrus, see Eckenhoff & Rakic, 1991) and beyond (for the prefrontal cortex, see Huttenlocher & Dabholkar, 1997). The fit between this time line and the available data is the subject of the next section.

Assessing Long-Term Declarative Memory in Infancy

As noted above, before the 1980s, it was widely believed that infants lacked the capacity to form declarative memories of past events. The perspective was consistent with the dominant theoretical perspective at the time. A central tenet of Jean Piaget's *genetic epistemology* (see Flavell, 1963, for an introduction to the perspective) was that for the first 18 to 24 months of life, infants lacked symbolic capacity and thus, the ability to mentally re-present (and thus recall) objects and events (e.g., Piaget, 1952). Instead, they were thought to live in a "here-and-now" world that included physically present entities, yet the entities had no past and no future.

The perspective on infants' mnemonic abilities began to change in the middle 1980s in part as a result of the development of a nonverbal analogue to verbal report, namely, elicited and deferred imitation (see Bauer, 2013; Lukowski & Bauer, 2014, for other sources of change in perspective). Elicited and deferred imitation entail use of objects to demonstrate an action or sequence of actions that either immediately (elicited imitation), after some delay (deferred imitation), or both, infants are invited to imitate. For example, an adult uses two nesting cups and a block to "make a rattle," by putting the block inside one cup, inverting it into the other cup, and shaking the cups to make a rattling sound. Piaget (1952) himself had identified deferred imitation as one of the hallmarks of the development of symbolic thought. Meltzoff (1985) and Bauer and colleagues (Bauer & Mandler, 1989; Bauer & Shore, 1987) brought the technique under experimental control. In a common version of the procedure (see Bauer, 2004), the infant is given the props for a sequence prior to any modeling or instruction. Using the above example, infants would be given the two cups and the block with the invitation to "Look at this stuff. What can you do with this stuff?" Infants' production of the target actions (a measure of item memory) and sequences of action (a measure of memory organization) during this uninstructed baseline is compared with their performance after production of the sequence by the adult (either immediately or after some delay). Differences in behavior are attributed to memory for the adult's actions. Over long delays (i.e., on the order of weeks or months), performance after exposure to the model is also compared with baseline performance on novel sequences, to control for developmental increases in problem solving.

Early research using imitation-based tasks demonstrated that infants as young as 9 months of age were able to defer imitation of an action for 24 hours (Meltzoff, 1988b). Bauer and Shore (1987) demonstrated that over a 6-week delay, infants 17 to 23 months of age remembered not only individual actions but temporally ordered sequences of action. These and other findings reviewed below strongly suggested that even infants are able to recall past events, and have led to acceptance of imitation-based tasks as a nonverbal measure of declarative memory, and more specifically, as a nonverbal analogue of verbal report. Because the significant similarities between imitation and verbal report paradigms have been discussed elsewhere (e.g., Bauer, 2002, 2004, 2007; Bauer, DeBoer, & Lukowski, 2007; Mandler, 1990; Meltzoff, 1990), we present only a brief review of three primary points. First, under some circumstances, once they acquire language, children are able to talk about events experienced in imitation tasks (e.g., Bauer, Wenner, & Kroupina, 2002; Cheatham & Bauer, 2005; see Bauer, 2007, for discussion of the constraints on this ability). For example, when presented with the cups and block she had used to make a rattle as a 20-month-old, a 3-year-old might remark "It's a rattle!" The ability to verbally label and discuss memories formed in the context of imitation suggests that the representations are declarative, mnemonic formats that are amenable to later verbal recall (nondeclarative memories are not linguistically accessible).

Second, adults with medial temporal lobe amnesia, in whom declarative memory processes are compromised, are also impaired on an adult version of the imitation task (McDonough, Mandler, McKee, & Squire, 1995). Adolescents who have experienced hippocampal damage early in life are also impaired (Adlam, Vargha-Khadem, Mishkin, & de Haan, 2005). The common pattern of impairment suggests that the tasks depend on the same neural substrate. Third, performance on imitation-based tasks at 20 months is related to scores on standardized tests of memory at age 6 years (Riggins, Cheatham, Stark, & Bauer, 2013), suggesting continuity in the processes over long periods of developmental time. As a result of these features, imitation-based tasks are well accepted as a nonverbal test of recall (e.g., Bauer, 2002; Nelson & Fivush, 2000; Rovee-Collier & Hayne, 2000; Schneider & Bjorklund, 1998; Squire et al., 1993). Below we summarize what has been learned about the development of declarative memory in infancy using imitation-based tasks, followed by discussion of the implications of changes in memory behavior for learning through social interaction. Because the strongest evidence of declarative memory comes from recall (rather than recognition), we focus the review on measures of recall.

Characteristics of Recall in Infancy

Use of the elicited imitation paradigm has indicated that the ability to recall information over the long term undergoes significant development during infancy. In particular, developments are apparent in terms of the duration of time over which infants recall and the robustness of their memories. Major developments in each of these areas are discussed below (see also Bauer, 2007, 2014).

Duration of Time over Which Memory Is Apparent

The length of time over which memory is apparent increases significantly over the first months of life. Importantly, because like any complex behavior, the length of time an experience is remembered is multiply determined, there is no "growth chart" function that specifies the length of time over which infants of a given age should remember. Nonetheless, across numerous studies there is evidence that with age, infants tolerate lengthier retention intervals. For example, at 6 months of age, infants remember the individual actions involved in events over a 24-hour delay (Barr, Dowden, & Hayne, 1996; Collie & Hayne, 1999). Thus 1 day after seeing the rattle modeled, they may put the block into one of the cups, or invert one cup into the other. This suggests that a fledgling capacity for long-term recall has emerged by at least the second half of the first year of life.

As infants near their first birthdays, they remember information over increasingly long delays. Nine-month-olds remember the individual target actions that comprise two-step event sequences for up to 1 month (Carver & Bauer, 1999, 2001). Ten- and 11-month-olds remember this information for up to 3 months (Carver & Bauer, 2001). By the time children are 13 to 14 months old, they remember individual target actions over delays ranging from 4 to 6 months (Bauer, Wenner, Dropik, & Wewerka, 2000; Meltzoff, 1995). Twenty-month-olds remember individual target actions for up to and potentially exceeding 12 months (see Bauer et al., 2000, for the longest duration that has been tested to date, to our knowledge).

Developments in the duration of time over which information is retained are also apparent in memory for temporal order information. Memory for order information is particularly challenging for infants as is indicated by protracted development of the ability and substantial amounts of within-group variability. Only approximately one-quarter of 6-month-olds remember actions in correct temporal order (Barr et al., 1996; though in Collie & Hayne, 1999, none of the infants recalled temporal order information). That is, 1 day after seeing the rattle modeled, only 25% of 6-month-olds will first put the block into one of the cups and then go on to invert the cup into another. Memory for temporal order at 9 months exceeds that which is apparent at 6 months, but is by no means robust. Approximately half of tested infants remember the temporal order of multistep event sequences after delays of 5 weeks; this finding has been replicated in three independent samples (Bauer, Wiebe, Carver, Waters, & Nelson, 2003; Bauer, Wiebe, Waters, & Bangston, 2001; Carver & Bauer, 1999). By 13 months of age the substantial individual variability in ordered recall has resolved: 78% of 13-month-olds exhibit ordered recall after 1 month (Bauer et al., 2000).

Another development in ordered recall is the ability to accurately reproduce arbitrarily ordered sequences. Arbitrarily ordered sequences are those for which there are no inherent constraints on the order in which the actions occur. In the morning routine, it does not matter whether one brushes one's teeth before or after taking a shower. In contrast, other sequences have inherent constraints such that in order to reach a particular end state or goal, actions must be performed in a particular order. With the goal of clean teeth in mind, one must apply toothpaste to the brush before—not after—brushing. Similarly, with the goal of making a rattle in mind, one must put the block inside the cup before—not after—shaking the cup.

In the first 2 years of life, temporal constraints on the order in which actions occur (commonly referred to as *enabling relations*) facilitate ordered recall at immediate imitation (e.g., Bauer & Mandler, 1992; Bauer & Thal, 1990) and after a delay (e.g., Bauer & Dow, 1994; Bauer & Hertsgaard, 1993; Bauer & Mandler, 1989). The effect is apparent even among 9-month-old infants (Carver & Bauer, 1999, 2001). In contrast, accurate ordered recall of sequences that are arbitrarily ordered is a later development. Consider the sequence of "making a picture" drawing on paper, attaching a decorative sticker to the paper, and tracing a shape. It is not until approximately 20 months of age that infants perform this type of sequence in other than chance temporal order (e.g., Bauer, Hertsgaard, Dropik, & Daly, 1998). Even at this age, infants show reliable recall of arbitrarily ordered sequences that are few but not many steps in length (three steps vs. five steps). Recall of arbitrarily ordered sequences is also influenced by the duration of time over which children are tested: recall is reliable immediately after the presentation of the sequences, but not after 2 weeks. Nevertheless, by the time infants are 28 months of age, they recall arbitrarily ordered sequences well even after a delay (Bauer et al., 1998).

The Robustness of Memory

Age-related developments in recall abilities are also apparent in terms of the robustness of memory. One index of robustness is the number of experiences required to support long-term recall (e.g., Bauer & Leventon, 2013). Younger infants generally require a greater number of exposures to to-be-remembered information to evidence long-term retention. For example, at 6 months of age, infants who witnessed a sequence demonstrated six times remembered it, whereas same-age infants who saw a sequence demonstrated only three times did not (Barr et al., 1996). By 9 months, however, infants require only two (Bauer et al., 2001) or three (Meltzoff, 1988b) exposures to remember individual actions over delays of 24 hours and more.

The number of experiences required to support ordered recall typically is greater than the number required to support recall of individual actions. For example, although 9-month-olds required only two exposures to remember the target actions of sequences for 1 week, they required three exposures to remember the actions in temporal order (Bauer et al., 2001). Similarly, over a 1-month delay, whereas a single experience of an event is sufficient to support 16-month-olds' recall of the individual target actions of sequences, only with the aid of verbal reminders do they also recall the temporal order of the sequences. Over the same delay, 20-month-olds remember both the actions and order of events experienced only one time (Bauer & Leventon, 2013). These findings speak to the gradual emergence of the ability to preserve memories of one-time experiences over long periods of time.

A second index of the robustness of memory is the extent to which the same cues must be present at encoding and retrieval in order for infants to recall. This question is often addressed by changing the props or other cues presented at encoding versus at the time of the test. An example is Hayne, MacDonald, and Barr (1997), in which a puppet sequence could be enacted with either a cow or a duck puppet. The sequence involved removing a mitten from the puppet's hand, shaking the mitten (which contained a bell), and then putting the mitten back on the puppet's hand. Eighteen- and 21-month-olds presented with the same puppet at encoding and at a 24-hour delayed recall test (cow–cow) remembered the sequence. In contrast, when the infants experienced one puppet at encoding and a different puppet at test (cow–duck), only the older infants showed evidence of recall (see also Hayne, Boniface, & Barr, 2000; Herbert & Hayne, 2000).

Other findings suggest that infants' memories are more robust, surviving changes in props, testing context, models, and medium of experience. In Bauer and Dow (1994), infants 16 and 20 months of age showed evidence of recall over a week delay when tested with perceptually distinct yet functionally similar props. For instance, at encoding, they saw the rattle made with round nesting cups and a block. One week later, they showed evidence of recall by making the rattle using square stacking cups and a rubber ball (see also Bauer & Lukowski, 2010; Lechuga, Marcos-Ruiz, & Bauer, 2001; Lukowski, Wiebe, & Bauer, 2009). Infants also evidence recall when changes are made to the context in which testing occurs so that they are dissimilar at encoding and test (e.g., Barnat, Klein, & Meltzoff, 1996; Hanna & Meltzoff, 1993; Klein & Meltzoff, 1999), when different individuals perform the modeled actions and conduct the recall test (e.g., Hanna & Meltzoff, 1993), and when event sequences are initially presented on television and recall memory later is assessed behaviorally using three-dimensional props (Meltzoff, 1988a; although, see Barr & Hayne, 1999).

One possible source of flexibility in recall may be forgetting of specific features of the original encoding context. In other words, flexibility may be born of forgetting. This possibility is contraindicated by findings that infants flexibly use their memory representations even in the face of accurate memory for the original events. In Bauer and Dow (1994), 16- and 20-month-old infants used novel, functionally equivalent props to produce event sequences, and also performed reliably in a forced-choice procedure in which they selected the original props from an array of distracters. Moreover, Bauer and Lukowski (2010) found that memory for the specific features of event sequences is positively correlated with later memory for them. Together, these findings indicate that although flexibility in memory may develop over time (e.g., Herbert & Hayne, 2000), there is substantial flexibility in memory at least by late in the first year of life. We now turn to discussion of possible reasons for the developmental changes just summarized, in terms of developments in the basic processes of memory.

Developments in the Basic Processes of Memory

Each of the phases in the life of a memory—trace formation (or encoding), consolidation and storage, and retrieval—is a possible source of the age-related changes in memory performance just described. Though the different processes are difficult to cleanly separate from one another (e.g., when encoding ends and consolidation begins is a challenging question to address), they clearly build on one another. Much like the enabling relations described earlier, the processes occur in a temporal order such that a memory must be encoded before it can be consolidated and stored, and it must be consolidated and stored before it can be retrieved. For this reason, we describe the processing in the nominal order in which they occur: encoding, consolidation and storage, and retrieval.

Encoding

As described previously, unimodal and polymodal association areas are responsible for the initial registration and short-term maintenance of information registered by sensory organs. The prefrontal cortex in particular undergoes significant postnatal development. As such, developments in this brain region may be related to changes in the rapidity and efficiency with which information is initially registered and passed on for additional processing. Consistent with this suggestion, in a longitudinal study, Bauer and colleagues (Bauer et al., 2006) found differences in the patterns of event-related potential (ERP) responses to familiar stimuli between 9 and 10 months of age that correlated with age-related improvements in recall after a 1-month delay. ERPs are scalp recordings of the electrical activity of postsynaptic potentials that propagate to the surface of the scalp via the volume-conducting properties of the brain. Because the recordings are time locked to the presentation of visual or auditory stimuli, they provide a snapshot of cognition in action. In Bauer et al. (2006) infants were exposed to event sequences at each of ages 9 and 10 months. At each age, to assess whether the infants had encoded the sequences, immediately after seeing the events modeled, infants were presented with photographs of props from familiar and novel sequences on a computer screen; their brain activity was recorded using ERPs. Beginning as early as 260 milliseconds after stimulus onset and continuing to 1,500 milliseconds, at 9 months, the infants showed larger neural responses (greater amplitude) to novel stimuli than to familiar stimuli. In contrast, at 10 months, the infants showed larger neural responses to familiar stimuli than to novel stimuli. These different patterns indicate age-related changes in the efficacy of encoding of the stimuli. The developmental change was associated with increased recall: infants remembered more of the events to which they had been exposed at 10 months, relative to events to which they had been exposed at 9 months.

Behavioral data also suggest that encoding improves with age. One way of assessing variability in encoding is to determine the rapidity with which infants learn event sequences to criterion, a procedure that ensures full encoding. Fifteen-month-olds are faster to learn to criterion relative to 12-month-olds; 18-month-olds are faster to learn to criterion relative to 15-month-olds (Howe & Courage, 1997). These findings, among others, indicate that older infants learn information more quickly relative to those who are younger. Indeed, across development, older children learn more rapidly than younger children (Howe & Brainerd, 1989).

Consolidation and Storage

As indicated earlier, medial temporal lobe structures are responsible for the stabilizing and integration of information for long-term retention. In adults, cellular changes related to synaptic connectivity and memory consolidation are apparent from hours to months after the occurrence of to-be-remembered events. Importantly, memory traces are vulnerable to disruption and forgetting throughout this consolidation period: lesions to the hippocampus during the period of consolidation result in deficits in memory, whereas lesions imposed after the consolidation period has ended do not (e.g., Kim & Fanselow, 1992; Takehara, Kawahara, & Kirino, 2003). Given that some of the neural structures responsible for successful consolidation undergo protracted development, achieving a consolidated memory trace may be more challenging for a less mature organism relative to an adult. As a result, the memories of infants and younger children may be especially susceptible to forgetting (e.g., Bauer, 2004, 2005, 2006).

The possible implications of consolidation and storage processes have been evaluated both behaviorally, using elicited imitation, and neurally, with ERPs. To assess mnemonic abilities in 9-month-old infants, Bauer and colleagues (2003) presented infants with two-step event sequences. As in Bauer et al. (2006), described above, to assess whether the infants had encoded the sequences, we administered an immediate recognition test using ERPs. One week later, how well memories had been consolidated and stored was assessed with a second ERP test. One month later, delayed recall was assessed behaviorally. After the monthlong delay, approximately half of the infants demonstrated ordered recall of one or more of the original sequences, whereas the other half of the infants did not. Although both groups of infants showed evidence of having encoded the sequences (based on the first ERP test—they had differential responses to familiar and novel stimuli), only the infants who recalled the sequences after the delay also showed evidence of successful consolidation and storage (based on the second ERP test). These findings indicate that individual differences in consolidation and storage processes are related to variability in long-term recall memory (see also Carver, Bauer, & Nelson, 2000, for similar findings).

The finding that variability in consolidation and storage processes contributes to long-term recall performance has also been established in infants tested during the second year of life. Bauer, Cheatham, Cary, and Van Abbema (2002) presented 16- and 20-month-old infants with multistep event sequences and tested their memory for them immediately after presentation to assess encoding and after a delay of 24 hours. The younger infants forgot a significant amount of the information they had learned before the delay, such that they performed 65% of the target actions and 57% of the pairs of actions they had learned the previous day. The 20-month-olds did not show significant forgetting over the same delay. In other research, infants 20 months of age evidence significant forgetting 48 hours after the experience of to-be-remembered events (Bauer, Van Abbema, & de Haan, 1999).

Just as in the first year, in the second year of life, the vulnerability of memory traces during the initial period of consolidation is related to the robustness of recall after 1 month. This is apparent from another of the experiments in Bauer, Cheatham, et al. (2002), this one involving 20-month-olds only. The infants were exposed to multistep events and then tested for memory for some of the events immediately, some of the events after 48 hours (a delay after which, based on Bauer et al., 1999, some forgetting was expected), and some of the events after 1 month. Although the infants exhibited high levels of initial encoding (as measured by immediate recall), they nevertheless exhibited significant forgetting after both 48 hours and 1 month. How well they remembered the events after 48 hours predicted 25% of the variance in recall 1 month later; variability in level of encoding did not predict significant variance (see also Pathman & Bauer, 2013). This effect is a conceptual replication of that observed with 9-month-olds in Bauer et al. (2003; see Bauer, 2005; Bauer, Güler, Starr, & Pathman, 2011; Howe & Courage, 1997, for additional evidence of a role for postencoding processes in long-term recall).

Retrieval

As described, memory retrieval is dependent on the prefrontal cortex, a brain structure that undergoes significant postnatal development. As such, changes in this structure are likely implicated in behavioral advances in recall. Though this logical possibility is often noted (e.g., Liston & Kagan, 2002), most studies of memory in infancy do not permit empirical test of it because few studies feature procedures that permit assessment of age-related differences in encoding and in consolidation and storage. Without these assessments, it is difficult to determine whether memories are inaccessible after a delay due to consolidation and storage failure or whether the memory remains but cannot be accessed using the provided cues (retrieval failure).

One of the studies that permits assessment of the contributions of consolidation and/or storage relative to retrieval processes is Bauer et al. (2000; see also

Bauer et al., 2003, described earlier). The study provided data on infants of multiple ages (13, 16, and 20 months) tested over a range of delays (1 to 12 months). Because immediate recall of half of the events was tested, measures of encoding are available. Because the infants were given what amounted to multiple test trials, without intervening study trials, there were multiple opportunities for retrieval. Third, immediately after the recall tests, relearning was tested. That is, after the second test trial the experimenter demonstrated each event once, and allowed the infants to imitate. Since Ebbinghaus (1885), relearning has been used to distinguish between an intact but inaccessible memory trace and a trace that has disintegrated. Specifically, if the number of trials required to relearn a stimulus was smaller than the number required to learn it initially, savings in relearning was said to have occurred. Savings presumably accrue because the products of relearning are integrated with an existing (though not necessarily accessible) memory trace. Conversely, the absence of savings is attributed to storage failure: there is no residual trace on which to build. In developmental studies, age-related differences in relearning would suggest that the residual memory traces available to infants of different ages are differentially intact.

To eliminate encoding processes as a potential source of developmental differences in long-term recall, in a reanalysis of the data from Bauer et al. (2000), subsets of 13- and 16-month-olds and subsets of 16- and 20-month-olds were matched for levels of encoding (as measured by immediate recall; Bauer, 2005). The amount of information the infants forgot over the delays then was examined. For both comparisons, even though they were matched for levels of encoding, younger infants exhibited more forgetting relative to older infants. The age effect was apparent on both test trials. Moreover, in both cases, for older infants, levels of performance after the single relearning trial were as high as those at initial learning. In contrast, for younger infants, performance after the relearning trial was lower than at initial learning. Together, the findings suggest that infants of different ages lose mnemonic information differentially over time. These data also suggest that difficulties with consolidation and storage, as opposed to retrieval processes, are a prime source of variability in long-term recall abilities across ages.

Summary

Developmental changes in the basic process of memory formation and later recall are largely consistent both with the characteristics of memory behavior outlined above, and with what is known about developmental changes in the neural substrate that supports declarative memory in general and recall in particular. First, changes in encoding-related processes are consistent with developmental changes in the prefrontal cortex. One consequence of more efficient encoding is that infants require fewer experiences of events in order to remember them over a delay. Second, changes in consolidation and storage processes are consistent with developmental changes in medial–temporal structures, and in the dentate gyrus of the hippocampus in particular. Consequences of more efficient and more effective consolidation and storage are that memories are retained over longer periods of time, and memory representations are better structured and organized (as reflected in improved memory for the temporal order in which events occurred). Third, changes in retrieval processes likely are linked with changes in the prefrontal cortex, rendering memory traces more accessible to retrieval even over long periods of time. In the next section, we explore the implications of these neural and behavioral developments for learning from others in social situations.

Using Memory in Social Contexts: The Case of Social Referencing

Infants learn a great many things over the first months and years of life. Many of their learning experiences come from their own exploration of the world—from banging, mouthing, and visually inspecting objects, for example. As described above, they also learn a great deal from others, simply by watching. Indeed, the fact that infants watch and then use what they observe to guide their own action is the basis for the imitation-based means of testing memory in infancy. The success of the task rests squarely on a skill known as *social referencing*, an ability that infants exploit well beyond the elicited and deferred imitation task.

Social referencing is a complex skill that is readily apparent by the end of the first year of life. Broadly defined, social referencing is the search for and use of another's emotional expression or reaction to inform an ambiguous situation and guide behavior. For example, when encountering a strange new object, such as a cow or duck puppet (Hayne et al., 1997), a 12-month-old may look to her or his caregiver (or the experimenter) to inform approach or avoidance of the object. Positive emotional information (typically present in imitation-based tasks), may lead to approach behavior; negative emotional information often supports avoidance. The skills involved in social referencing depend critically on advances in memory development. That is, the capacity to encode and remember emotional information toward a specific referent allows the infant to call on this experience and respond appropriately in future occurrences.

Social referencing has been primarily examined in three behavioral paradigms: visual cliff, stranger, and novel object. In the visual cliff paradigm, the infant is placed on the "safe" side of a covered, but transparent cliff (thus, *visual cliff*). When infants reach the drop off, they typically reference their caregivers to guide behavior (e.g., Sorce, Emde, Campos, & Klinnert, 1985). In the stranger paradigm, social referencing behavior is elicited when a novel person (stranger) approaches the infant (e.g., Feinman, 1982). And in the novel object paradigm, one or more novel objects are presented to the infant, prompting social referencing behavior (e.g., Hornik, Reisenhoover, & Gunner, 1987). Across these three paradigms, a key feature is that an ambiguous situation prompts social referencing and regulated behavior based on the emotional expression from the referee.

Component Structure of Social Referencing

Social referencing can be separated into three components: seeking information (joint attention), association of information with referent, and regulation of behavior (Feinman, 1982). As will become clear, memory processes play a critical role, especially at the final stage of social referencing: regulation of behavior.

Joint Attention

Joint attention is the shared gaze between two or more individuals toward an object of visual reference. In short, the simple act of looking at an object to which another is also looking is an act of joint attention. Joint attention emerges throughout the first year of life and is supported by the developments in automatic and intentional attention networks (Mundy & Newell, 2007). Information seeking associated with social referencing (i.e., in ambiguous situations) has been observed in infants as young as 7 months (Striano & Rochat, 2000). Joint attention is tied to the present moment, involving a combination of attention and working memory processes. Though it is certainly in operation during encoding, because joint attention is not directly tied to long-term memory processes, we do not discuss it further.

Association of Information with Referent

The association of emotional information with its referent comprises linking the new information with a specific element of the emotional event. It involves joint attention if the infant first needs to solicit the attention of the caregiver to provide information about the event. However, considerable evidence indicates that infants can link emotional information with specific referents without explicitly seeking information, in an incidental learning paradigm. For example, 12-month-olds who received a negative message (e.g., disgust) about a novel object interacted less with that object among a group of neutral distractors (and less than infants who received a positive message about the object; Hornik et al., 1987). Further, interaction with the neutral distractors did not differ between infants in the "disgust" and "joy" conditions. Such findings demonstrate that infants link the emotional information with a specific referent as opposed to the event and context as a whole. Encoding and subsequent memory for the specific features of an event (as in Bauer & Dow, 1994; Bauer & Lukowski, 2010, discussed above), may support association of emotional information with its referent. That is, similar processes may be engaged when encoding the specific features of an event and when associating emotional information with a specific referent in the event.

Regulation of Behavior

Perhaps the most obvious connection between memory and social referencing is to the third component, namely, regulation of behavior. Although many investigations of social referencing examine behavior immediately after the provision of emotional information, some feature delays ranging from minutes to days to weeks. In studies featuring delays, social referencing has been examined in behavior, visual attention (looking time studies), and neural attention (ERP studies). As described earlier, 12-month-olds interacted less with an object of negative reference (disgust) than with neutral distractors, or when the object was positively referenced (joy; Hornik et al., 1987). Notably, the effect was still present after an 8-minute delay, when the caregiver was no longer providing the emotional information. Thus, the emotional information in association with its referent must have been encoded into long-term memory since there was nothing inherent in the objects or context to inform behavior at the delay. Further, there is evidence for retention of both negative (disgust) and positive (joy) emotional information in 14-month-olds following a delay of 1 hour (Hertenstein & Campos, 2004). Infants participated in either the negative or positive conditions, and emotional messages were provided by an experimenter, unsolicited by the infant. Fourteen-month-olds interacted less with the object of negative reference and more with the object of positive reference than a neutral comparison object after a 1-hour delay. Eleven-month-olds showed the same effects after a 3-minute delay but not after a 1-hour delay. Thus, similar to the developmental trajectories observed in the literature on recall of event sequences reviewed earlier, older infants seemingly retain (and use) emotion information over longer delays, relative to younger infants.

It is important to note that social referencing *behavior* as a measure of retention of learned emotional information is a strict measure of memory, and may underestimate infants' memory and social referencing capacities since it relies on an explicit, overt behavior. Less action-based methodological approaches can inform infants' acquisition and retention of emotional information, such as looking time and ERP designs, which inform visual and neural behavior, respectively. In one such study, 12-month-olds demonstrated memory for emotional information and regulation of visual attention after a 24-hour delay (Flom & Johnson, 2011). First, infants were habituated to an experimenter expressing disgust toward one of two objects, and joy toward the other. After delays of 5 minutes, 24 hours, and 1 month, infants' preference between the objects was examined in a visual paired-comparison design. Infants looked significantly longer toward the positively referenced object at the 5-minute and 24-hour delays, and showed no preference at the 1-month delay. Because the nature of the paradigm pits the responses toward each object against each other, it does not permit conclusions on whether the preference indicates memory for one or both of the emotional pairings (as each would predict the same behavior: less time at the negative object vs. more time at the positive object). However, at least one of the pairings must have been retained in order for infants to demonstrate a preference (or avoidance). Thus, memory for an emotional event is retained for at least 1 day.

ERP paradigms have the power to clarify the patterns of attention, since neural responses are measured to discrete stimuli (as opposed to a mixed response between two stimuli, as in Flom & Johnson, 2011). Further, ERP paradigms may be more sensitive than looking time designs in that they do not depend on an explicit visual behavior. ERP components that represent attentional responses are robust and have indicated sensitivity to emotional information in infants as young as 3 months of age (e.g., Hoehl & Striano, 2008). To date, two studies have capitalized on ERP methodologies to examine the response to novel objects associated with emotional information. In each study, the emotional information was paired with objects in a traditional behavioral social referencing paradigm, and ERPs were collected at a different point in time. Because the emotional information was no longer present during the collection of ERPs, the responses are a robust test of memory for the emotional event.

Following a behavioral social referencing paradigm in which one of each of three objects was associated with a negative (disgust), positive (joy), or neutral message, 12-month-olds' ERPs showed a larger response to the negative object after a 20-minute delay (Carver & Vaccaro, 2007). That is, 12-month-olds showed enhanced neural attention toward the negative object in contrast to the positive and neutral objects. Further research clarifies the difference in attention among the three objects. Similar to the traditional behavioral paradigm of examining the change in behavior to emotionally referenced objects, Leventon and Bauer (2013) examined the change in neural response to emotionally referenced objects. ERPs were collected before and after one of each of three objects were paired with a negative (fear), positive (joy), or neutral message. The post-emotion responses alone were similar to the previous study, indicating larger responses to the negatively referenced object (after a 5-minute delay). Yet the change in response clarifies the finding: Neural responses decreased to the neutral object specifically, and were sustained to the negative and positive object. Further, infants who attended more to the objects during the emotional events showed an increased neural response to the negative object and a decreased response to the positive object. The findings indicate that neural attention is regulated in accordance with learned emotional information (both negative and positive), and that retention is maintained for at least 20 minutes.

In summary, limited—but consistent—evidence in behavior, visual attention, and neural response indicates that infants encode and remember emotional information associated with specific referents over delays that necessitate long-term memory processes. Together, joint attention and memory skills support social referencing behavior. Further, social referencing is dependent on the development of a complex network of neural responses involved in memory, emotion processing, joint attention, and regulation of behavior. It is to this network that we now turn.

Neural Substrate Supporting Social Referencing

As reviewed earlier, medial–temporal lobe areas including the hippocampal formation as well as association areas in the prefrontal cortex are necessary to form and retrieve long-term memories. It is not until late in the first year of life that these areas reach functional maturity, and further development is protracted across childhood and into early adulthood. Emotion processing is tied to an equally broad network, with subcortical structures such as the amygdala implicated in emotional reactivity, and prefrontal areas such as the orbitofrontal cortex and anterior cingulate involved in emotional regulation (Davidson, Jackson, & Kalin, 2000). Attentional biases to fearful faces in infants as young as 3 months of age suggest early functionality of the amygdala (e.g., Hoehl & Striano, 2008). Regulation of emotion emerges later in infancy and continues into the school-age years and adolescence (Posner & Rothbart, 1998). Joint attention involves a distributed network of posterior (automatic) and anterior (intentional) attention processes (Mundy & Newell, 2007). The functional maturity of all of these networks working in concert supports the sophisticated skill we call social referencing.

Memory and Emotion: Contextual Factors

As the work summarized in this chapter makes clear, infants form and retain memories of specific past events, and they pair information about emotional valence with specific referents, even over a delay. Interestingly, the retention intervals in social referencing paradigms fall short of what infants of the same age demonstrate in elicited and deferred imitation paradigms. In 12-month-olds, the maximum delay over which social referencing behavior has been observed is 24 hours, yet by this age, infants demonstrate memory for the actions of event sequences over a 3-month delay. What might explain the difference? One possible explanation is the context of remembering in the two paradigms. In both imitation-based and social referencing tasks, infants must encode information about objects. Yet in the case of social referencing, infants must use information from the wider social context of the event as well. Specifically, in order for infants to change their behavior or attention (outcome measures of social referencing paradigms), in addition to information about objects, they must also encode information about the emotion of another person, remember the emotional information, apply it to the current event, and then modify their behavior accordingly. Infants may remember the emotional information, but if they fail to apply it to the current event or modify their behavior, their memory would not be detected.

The different contexts of remembering in imitation-based and social referencing paradigms may help to explain more than differences in retention intervals. They may also contribute to differences in the impact of environmental variation on behavior. Social referencing is impacted by context as early as the first stage of information seeking. Most notably, it is in *ambiguous* situations where social referencing behaviors are best elicited (e.g., Gunnar & Stone, 1984; Sorce et al., 1985). Thus, the information seeking in social referencing is more likely in the specific context where it is unclear if the infant should approach or avoid. The setting in which social referencing is tested may also impact expression of the behavior. For example, Walden and Baxter (1989) examined social referencing behavior in a familiar child care setting versus an unfamiliar laboratory setting. They found that infants regulated their behavior to both positive and negative information in both settings. Interestingly, infants referenced their caregivers sooner and more frequently in the familiar setting relative to the unfamiliar setting. In contrast, in imitation-based tasks in which emotion is not used to suggest approach or avoidance, changes in context have little—if any—impact on behavior. That is, infants evidence memory in imitation-based tasks whether tested in the laboratory, their homes, or their day care centers (Hanna & Meltzoff, 1993). As noted earlier, they evidence memory even when the context changes between the time of encoding and the time of test (Hanna & Meltzoff, 1993). Thus, whereas contextual variation seemly impacts the seeking, associating, and regulatory use of emotion information, it does not impact the underlying ability that supports the inferential chain, namely, memory.

Summary and Directions for Future Research

The capacity to form, retain, and later retrieve memory representations of the experiences of our daily lives is one that most adults take for granted. Yet the ability is far from simple. It involves a number of neural structures that function as a network to transform ongoing perceptual experiences into enduring memory traces. The structures themselves and the network in which they participate undergo protracted courses of development. As they develop over the first months of life, changes in memory-related behavior are apparent. As early as the second half of the first year, infants show evidence of recall of past events and experiences. Yet their memories are temporally restricted, lasting only hours, and they are not especially robust, seemingly requiring multiple trials to establish an enduring trace. By the end of the second year of life, memory is both temporally extended and robust. The timing of changes in memory behavior corresponds with the timing of developmental changes in the neural substrate known to support recall.

The changes also have consequences for the uses to which memory is put. One especially salient example is that of social referencing. As outlined here, the ability to use the cues that others emit during social interactions requires that the information be associated with the referent and that the association be used to regulate behavior. To be maximally effective, the information must be retained over time, to regulate behavior not only in the moment but over the long term.

Research on developmental changes in infant memory enjoyed a heyday in the latter part of the 20th century, heralded in large part by the methodological innovation of imitation-based paradigms that permitted tests of recall in preverbal infants. Researchers employed elicited and deferred imitation in tests of memory in the first and second years of life and found unqualified evidence that even at these young ages, infants remember past events. The work brought into stark relief the need for modification of the dominant theoretical perspective that infants lived exclusively in a "here-and-now" world without a past or a future. Yet as discussed in Bauer and Leventon (2013), the fact that infants remember past events does not require the conclusion that their memories are functionally equivalent to those of older children and adults. On the contrary, there are substantial changes in memory both within the infancy period (as reviewed above) and well beyond. Especially salient changes beyond infancy, in childhood, are apparent in the specificity of memory (e.g., memory for the source of experience; e.g., Drummey & Newcombe, 2002), in its accessibility (i.e., older children are less dependent on external cues and reminders; e.g., Pillemer, Picariello, & Pruett, 1994), and in its deliberate and strategic use (as reviewed in Bjorklund, Dukes, & Brown, 2009). How the early memory abilities described here relate to these later abilities is only beginning to be explored (see Riggins et al., 2013) and certainly merits additional empirical attention.

Future research also will be required to more fully understand relations between the different processes involved in memory trace construction, maintenance, and subsequent retrieval. Behavioral research (e.g., Bauer et al., 2011; Pathman & Bauer, 2013) and investigations using ERP (e.g., Bauer et al., 2003, 2006) indicate that not all—or even the majority—of variance in long-term recall is explained by measures of encoding into memory or by age-related differences in retrieval success. Instead, measures of the integrity of memory traces in the period in between—the period associated with the consolidation of memory traces—account for substantial variance. They continue to explain significant unique variance well into the preschool years (Bauer, Larkina, & Doydum, 2012). A full account of the development of the ability to recall the past seemingly will require more complete explication of the relative variance explained by each phase in the life of a memory.

Another potentially highly productive avenue for future research is direct examination of relations between developmental changes in long-term memory and changes in social referencing. As noted above, social referencing intimately relies on memory, in order that information associated with a specific referent be retained and later used to regulate behavior. Though the association between these behavioral domains is obvious on the face of it, there have not been direct empirical tests of the degree of shared variance across these tasks. The amount of shared variance may or may not be large. As discussed above, the "injection"of emotion into the memory context—as in the case of social referencing—seemingly alters the infants' sensitivity to the larger context of the learning experience. Given that both memory and social referencing are amenable to investigation by behavioral measures and ERP tests, the possibilities for co-investigation seem especially rich.

Finally, in the case of both memory for events and social referencing, we emphasized the implications for behavior of developmental changes in the neural substrates supporting the abilities. The adult literatures are rich with insights into relations between neural structure and function and behavior in both the cognitive and affective domains. By comparison, the developmental literature is in its infancy, and the literature on structure–function–behavior relations in the period of infancy could appropriately be described as "embryonic." Yet even in infancy, approaches are being developed to allow investigators to peer into the brain as it engages in cognition and emotion processing tasks. In addition to ERPs, as described here, the literature features reports of use of magnetoencephalography (MEG; e.g., Roberts et al., 2014), near-infrared spectroscopy (NIRS; e.g., Aslin & Mehler, 2005), and functional magnetic resonance imaging (fMRI; e.g., Dehaene-Lambertz, Dehaene, & Hertz-Pannier, 2002). These techniques permit assessment of the time course and neural generators of behavior and hold great promise for elucidation of structure–function–behavior relations in infancy. For example, MEG may can be used to better localize responses in the brain, while also providing impressive temporal resolution. Because it does not require that the subject remain perfectly still, it is especially attractive for developmental research. NIRS also shows substantial promise as a tool for developmental cognitive neuroscience. Like fMRI, it detects changes in blood flow concentration associated with neural activity. Like MEG, it can be used with squirmy research participants, such as infants (though the fact that it can be used to scan cortical tissue only represents a limitation). These and future such techniques still on the drawing board promise substantial advance in our understanding of memory in infancy (and beyond) and its implications for social learning.

ACKNOWLEDGMENTS

Support for the authors' research summarized in this chapter was provided by Grant Nos. HD28425 and HD42483 from the National Institute of Child Health and Human Development to Patricia J. Bauer. We thank the infants and parents who took part in our research, as well as those who have contributed to the larger literature described herein.

REFERENCES

Adlam, A.-L. R., Vargha-Khadem, F., Mishkin, M., & de Haan, M. (2005). Deferred imitation of action sequences in developmental amnesia. *Journal of Cognitive Neuroscience, 17*, 240–248.

Aslin, R. N., & Mehler, J. (2005). Near-infrared spectroscopy for functional studies of brain activity in human infants: Promise, prespects, and challenges. *Journal of Biomedical Optics, 10*, 1–12.

Bachevalier, J. (2001). Neural bases of memory development: Insights from neuropsychological studies in primates. In C. A. Nelson & M. Luciana (Eds.), *Handbook of developmental cognitive neuroscience* (pp. 365–379). Cambridge, MA: MIT Press.

Barbas, H. (2000). Connections underlying the synthesis of cognition, memory, and emotion in primate prefrontal cortices. *Brain Research Bulletin, 52*, 319–330.

Barnat, S. B., Klein, P. J., & Meltzoff, A. N. (1996). Deferred imitation across changes in context and object: Memory and generalization in 14-month-old children. *Infant Behavior and Development, 19*, 241–251.

Barr, R., Dowden, A., & Hayne, H. (1996). Developmental changes in deferred imitation by 6- to 24-month-old infants. *Infant Behavior and Development, 19*, 159–170.

Barr, R., & Hayne, H. (1999). Developmental changes in imitation from television during infancy. *Child Development, 70*, 1067–1081.

Bauer, P. J. (2002). Long-term recall memory: Behavioral and neuro-developmental changes in the first 2 years of life. *Current Directions in Psychological Science, 11*, 137–141.

Bauer, P. J. (2004). New developments in the study of infant memory. In D. M. Teti (Ed.), *Blackwell handbook of research methods in developmental science* (pp. 467–488). Oxford, UK: Blackwell.

Bauer, P. J. (2005). Developments in declarative memory: Decreasing susceptibility to storage failure over the second year of life. *Psychological Science, 16*, 41–47.

Bauer, P. J. (2006). Constructing a past in infancy: A neuro-developmental account. *Trends in Cognitive Sciences, 10*, 175–181.

Bauer, P. J. (2007). *Remembering the times of our lives: Memory in infancy and beyond.* Mahwah, NJ: Erlbaum.

Bauer, P. J. (2009). The cognitive neuroscience of the development of memory. In M. L. Courage & N. Cowan (Eds.), *The development of memory in infancy and childhood* (2nd ed., pp. 115–144). New York: Psychology Press.

Bauer, P. J. (2013). Memory. In P. D. Zelazo (Ed.), *Oxford handbook of developmental psychology: Vol. 1. Body and mind* (pp. 505–541). New York: Oxford University Press.

Bauer, P. J. (2014). The development of forgetting: Childhood amnesia. In P. J. Bauer & R. Fivush (Eds.), *The Wiley-Blackwell handbook on the development of children's memory* (pp. 519–544). West Sussex, UK: Wiley-Blackwell.

Bauer, P. J., Cheatham, C. L., Cary, M. S., & Van Abbema, D. L. (2002). Short-term forgetting: Charting its course and its implications for long-term remembering. In S. P. Shohov (Ed.), *Advances in psychology research* (Vol. 9, pp. 53–74). Huntington, NY: Nova Science.

Bauer, P. J., DeBoer, T., & Lukowski, A. F. (2007). In the language of multiple memory systems: Defining and describing developments in long-term declarative memory. In L. M. Oakes & P. J. Bauer (Eds.), *Short- and long-term memory in infancy and early childhood: Taking the first steps towards remembering* (pp. 240–270). New York: Oxford University Press.

Bauer, P. J., & Dow, G. A. (1994). Episodic memory in 16- and 20-month-old children: Specifics are generalized, but not forgotten. *Developmental Psychology, 30,* 403–417.

Bauer, P. J., Güler, O. E., Starr, R. M., & Pathman, J. (2011). Equal learning does not result in equal remembering: The importance of post-encoding processes. *Infancy, 16,* 557–586.

Bauer, P. J., & Hertsgaard, L. A. (1993). Increasing steps in recall of events: Factors facilitating immediate and long-term memory in 13.5- and 16.5-month-old children. *Child Development, 64,* 1204–1223.

Bauer, P. J., Hertsgaard, L. A., Dropik, P., & Daly, B. P. (1998). When even arbitrary order becomes important: Developments in reliable temporal sequencing of arbitrarily ordered events. *Memory, 6,* 165–198.

Bauer, P. J., Larkina, M., & Doydum, A. O. (2012). Explaining variance in long-term recall in 3- and 4-year-old children: The importance of post-encoding processes. *Journal of Experimental Child Psychology, 113,* 195–210.

Bauer, P. J., & Leventon, J. (2013). Memory for one-time experiences in the second year of life: Implications for the status of episodic memory. *Infancy, 18,* 755–781.

Bauer, P. J., & Lukowski, A. F. (2010). The memory is in the details: Relations between memory for the specific features of events and long-term recall during infancy. *Journal of Experimental Child Psychology, 107,* 1–14.

Bauer, P. J., & Mandler, J. M. (1989). One thing follows another: Effects of temporal structure on one- to two-year-olds' recall of events. *Developmental Psychology, 25,* 197–206.

Bauer, P. J., & Mandler, J. M. (1992). Putting the horse before the cart: The use of temporal order in recall of events by one-year-old children. *Developmental Psychology, 28,* 441–452.

Bauer, P. J., & Shore, C. M. (1987). Making a memorable event: Effects of familiarity and organization on young children's recall of action sequences. *Cognitive Development, 2,* 327–338.

Bauer, P. J., & Thal, D. J. (1990). Scripts or scraps: Reconsidering the development of sequential understanding. *Journal of Experimental Child Psychology, 50,* 287–304.

Bauer, P. J., Van Abbema, D. L., & de Haan, M. (1999). In for the short haul: Immediate and short-term remembering and forgetting by 20-month-old children. *Infant Behavior and Development, 22,* 321–343.

Bauer, P. J., Wenner, J. A., Dropik, P. L., & Wewerka, S. S. (2000). Parameters of remembering and forgetting in the transition from infancy to early childhood. *Monographs of the Society for Research in Child Development, 65*(4).

Bauer, P. J., Wenner, J. A., & Kroupina, M. G. (2002). Making the past present: Later verbal accessibility of early memories. *Journal of Cognition and Development, 3,* 21–47.

Bauer, P. J., Wiebe, S. A., Carver, L. J., Lukowski, A. F., Haight, J. C., Waters, J. M., et al. (2006). Electrophysiological indices of encoding and behavioral indices of recall: Examining relations and developmental change late in the first year of life. *Developmental Neuropsychology, 29,* 293–320.

Bauer, P. J., Wiebe, S. A., Carver, L. J., Waters, J. M., & Nelson, C. A. (2003). Developments in long-term explicit memory late in the first year of life: Behavioral and electrophysiological indices. *Psychological Science, 14,* 629–635.

Bauer, P. J., Wiebe, S. A., Waters, J. M., & Bangston, S. K. (2001). Reexposure breeds recall: Effects of experience on 9-month-olds' ordered recall. *Journal of Experimental Child Psychology, 80,* 174–200.

Bjorklund, D. F., Dukes, C., & Brown, R. D. (2009). The development of memory strategies. In M. Courage & N. Cowan (Eds.), *The development of memory in childhood* (pp. 145–175). Hove East Sussex, UK: Psychology Press.

Cabeza, R., McIntosh, A. R., Tulving, E., Nyberg, L., & Grady, C. L. (1997). Age-related differences in effective neural connectivity during encoding and recall. *NeuroReport, 8,* 3479–3483.

Cabeza, R., Prince, S. E., Daselaar, S. M., Greenberg, D. L., Budde, M., Dolcos, F., et al. (2004). Brain activity during episodic retrieval of autobiographical and laboratory events: An fMRI study using a novel photo paradigm. *Journal of Cognitive Neuroscience, 16,* 1583–1594.

Carver, L. J., & Bauer, P. J. (1999). When the event is more than the sum of its parts: Nine-month-olds' long-term ordered recall. *Memory, 7,* 147–174.

Carver, L. J., & Bauer, P. J. (2001). The dawning of a past: The emergence of long-term explicit memory in infancy. *Journal of Experimental Psychology: General, 130,* 726–745.

Carver, L. J., Bauer, P. J., & Nelson, C. A. (2000). Associations between infant brain activity and recall memory. *Developmental Science, 3,* 234–246.

Carver, L. J., & Vaccaro, B. G. (2007). 12-month-old infants allocate increased neural resources to stimuli associated with negative adult emotion. *Developmental Psychology, 43*(1), 54–69.

Cheatham, C. L., & Bauer, P. J. (2005). Construction of a more coherent story: Prior verbal recall predicts later verbal accessibility of early memories. *Memory, 13,* 516–532.

Chugani, H. T. (1994). Development of regional blood glucose metabolism in relation to behavior and plasticity. In G. Dawson & K. Fischer (Eds.), *Human behavior and the developing brain* (pp. 153–175). New York: Guilford Press.

Chugani, H. T., Phelps, M., & Mazziotta, J. (1987). Positron emission tomography study of human brain functional development. *Annals of Neurology, 22,* 487–497.

Chugani, H. T., & Phelps, M. E. (1986). Maturational changes in cerebral function determined by 18FDG positron emission tomography. *Science, 231,* 840–843.

Collie, R., & Hayne, H. (1999). Deferred imitation by 6- and 9-month-old infants: More evidence of declarative memory. *Developmental Psychobiology, 35,* 83–90.

Czurkó, A., Czéh, B., Seress, L., Nadel, L., & Bures, J. (1997). Severe spatial navigation deficit in the Morris water maze after single high dose of neonatal X-ray irradiation in the rat. *Proceedings of the National Academy of Sciences, 94,* 2766–2771.

Davidson, R. J., Jackson, D. C., & Kalin, N. H. (2000). Emotion, plasticity, context, and regulation: Perspectives from affective neuroscience. *Psychological Bulletin, 126*(6), 890–909.

Dehaene-Lambertz, G., Dehaene, S., & Hertz-Pannier, L. (2002). Functional neuroimaging of speech perception in infancy. *Science, 298,* 2013–2015.

Dickerson, B. C., & Eichenbaum, H. (2010). The episodic memory system: Neurocircuitry and disorders. *Neuropsychopharmacology, 35,* 86–104.

Drummey, A. B., & Newcombe, N. S. (2002). Developmental changes in source memory. *Developmental Science, 5,* 502–513.

Ebbinghaus, H. (1885). *On memory* (H. A. Ruger & C. E. Bussenius, Trans.). New York: Teachers' College Press.

Eckenhoff, M., & Rakic, P. (1991). A quantitative analysis of synaptogenesis in the molecular layer of the dentate gyrus in the rhesus monkey. *Developmental Brain Research, 64,* 129–135.

Eichenbaum, H., & Cohen, N. J. (2001). *From conditioning to conscious recollection: Memory systems of the brain.* New York: Oxford University Press.

Feinman, S. (1982). Social referencing in infancy. *Merrill-Palmer Quarterly, 28,* 445–470.

Flavell, J. (1963). *The developmental psychology of Jean Piaget.* Princeton: Van Nostrand.

Flom, R., & Johnson, S. (2011). The effects of adults' affective expression and direction of visual gaze on 12-month-olds' visual preferences for an object following a 5-minute, 1-day, or 1-month delay. *British Journal of Developmental Psychology, 29,* 64–85.

Fuster, J. M. (2002). Frontal lobe and cognitive development. *Journal of Neurocytology, 31,* 373–385.

Gilboa, A. (2004). Autobiographical and episodic memory—one and the same?: Evidence from prefrontal activation in neuroimaging studies. *Neuropsychologia, 42,* 1336–1349.

Goldman-Rakic, P. S. (1987). Circuitry of primate prefrontal cortex and regulation of behavior by representational memory. In F. Plum (Ed.), *Handbook of physiology: The nervous system, higher functions of the brain* (Vol. 5, pp. 373–417). Bethesda, MD: American Physiological Society.

Gunnar, M. R., & Stone, C. (1984). The effects of positive maternal affect on infant responses to pleasant, ambiguous, and fear-provoking toys. *Child Development, 55*(4), 1231–1236.

Hanna, E., & Meltzoff, A. N. (1993). Peer imitation by toddlers in laboratory, home, and day-care contexts: Implications for social learning and memory. *Developmental Psychology, 29,* 702–710.

Hayne, H., Boniface, J., & Barr, R. (2000). The development of declarative memory in human infants: Age-related changes in deferred imitation. *Behavioral Neuroscience, 114,* 77–83.

Hayne, H., MacDonald, S., & Barr, R. (1997). Developmental changes in the specificity of memory over the second year of life. *Infant Behavior and Development, 20,* 233–245.

Herbert, J., & Hayne, H. (2000). Memory retrieval by 18–30-month-olds: Age-related changes in representational flexibility. *Developmental Psychology, 36,* 473–484.

Hertenstein, M. J., & Campos, J. J. (2004). Retention effects of an adult's emotional displays on infant behavior. *Child Development, 75*(2), 595–613.

Hoehl, S., & Striano, T. (2008). Neural processing of eye gaze and threat-related emotional facial expressions in infancy. *Child Development, 79*(6), 1752–1760.

Hornik, R., Risenhoover, N., & Gunnar, M. (1987). The effects of maternal positive, neutral, and negative affective communications on infant responses to new toys. *Child Development, 58,* 937–944.

Howe, M. L., & Brainerd, C. J. (1989). Development of children's long-term retention. *Developmental Review, 9,* 301–340.

Howe, M. L., & Courage, M. L. (1997). Independent paths in the development of infant learning and forgetting. *Journal of Experimental Child Psychology, 67,* 131–163.

Huttenlocher, P. R. (1979). Synaptic density in human frontal cortex: Developmental changes and effects of aging. *Brain Research, 163,* 195–205.

Huttenlocher, P. R., & Dabholkar, A. S. (1997). Regional differences in synaptogenesis in human cerebral cortex. *Journal of Comparative Neurology, 387,* 167–178.

Kim, J. J., & Fanselow, M. S. (1992). Modality-specific retrograde amnesia of fear. *Science, 256,* 675–677.

Klein, P. J., & Meltzoff, A. N. (1999). Long-term memory, forgetting, and deferred imitation in 12-month-old infants. *Developmental Science, 2,* 102–113.

Lechuga, M. T., Marcos-Ruiz, R., & Bauer, P. J. (2001). Episodic recall of specifics and generalisation coexist in 25-month-old children. *Memory, 9,* 117–132.

Leventon, J. S., & Bauer, P. J. (2013). The sustained effect of emotional signals on neural processing in 12-month-olds. *Developmental Science, 16*(4), 485–498.

Liston, C., & Kagan, J. (2002). Memory enhancement in early childhood. *Nature, 419,* 896.

Lloyd, M. E., & Newcombe, N. S. (2009). Implicit memory in childhood: Reassessing developmental invariance. In M. L. Courage & N. Cowan (Eds.), *The development of memory in infancy and childhood* (pp. 93–113). New York: Taylor & Francis.

Lukowski, A. F., & Bauer, P. J. (2014). Long-term memory in infancy and early childhood. In P. J. Bauer & R. Fivush (Eds.), *The Wiley-Blackwell handbook on the development of children's memory* (pp. 230–254). West Sussex, UK: Wiley-Blackwell.

Lukowski, A. F., Wiebe, S. A., & Bauer, P. J. (2009). Going beyond the specifics: Generalization of single actions, but not temporal order, at nine months. *Infant Behavior and Development, 32*, 331–335.

Maguire, E. A. (2001). Neuroimaging studies of autobiographical event memory. *Philosophical Transactions Royal Society of London, 356*, 1441–1451.

Mandler, J. M. (1990). Recall of events by preverbal children. In A. Diamond (Ed.), *The development and neural bases of higher cognitive functions* (pp. 485–516). New York: New York Academy of Science.

Markowitsch, H. J. (2000). Neuroanatomy of memory. In E. Tulving & F. I. M. Craik (Eds.), *The Oxford handbook of memory* (pp. 465–484). New York: Oxford University Press.

McDonough, L., Mandler, J. M., McKee, R. D., & Squire, L. R. (1995). The deferred imitation task as a nonverbal measure of declarative memory. *Proceedings of the National Academy of Sciences, 92*, 7580–7584.

McGaugh, J. L. (2000). Memory: A century of consolidation. *Science, 287*, 248–251.

McKenzie, S., & Eichenbaum, H. (2011). Consolidation and reconsolidation: Two lives of memories? *Neuron, 28*, 224–233.

Meltzoff, A. N. (1985). Immediate and deferred imitation in fourteen- and twenty-four-month-old infants. *Child Development, 56*, 62–72.

Meltzoff, A. N. (1988a). Imitation of televised models by infants. *Child Development, 59*, 1221–1229.

Meltzoff, A. N. (1988b). Infant imitation and memory: Nine-month-olds in immediate and deferred tests. *Child Development, 59*, 217–225.

Meltzoff, A. N. (1990). The implications of cross-modal matching and imitation for the development of representation and memory in infants. In A. Diamond (Ed.), *The development and neural bases of higher cognitive functions* (pp. 1–31). New York: New York Academy of Science.

Meltzoff, A. N. (1995). What infant memory tells us about infantile amnesia: Long-term recall and deferred imitation. *Journal of Experimental Child Psychology, 59*, 497–515.

Milner, B. (2005). The medial temporal-lobe amnesic syndrome. *Psychiatric Clinics of North America, 28*, 599–611.

Mundy, P., & Newell, L. (2007) Attention, joint attention and social cognition. *Current Directions in Psychological Science, 16*, 269–274.

Nadel, L., & Willner, J. (1989). Some implications of postnatal maturation of the hippocampus. In V. Chan-Palay & C. Köhler (Eds.), *The hippocampus: New vistas* (pp. 17–31). New York: Liss.

Nelson, C. A. (1995). The ontogeny of human memory: A cognitive neuroscience perspective. *Developmental Psychology, 31*, 723–738.

Nelson, C. A. (1997). The neurobiological basis of early memory development. In N. Cowan (Ed.), *The development of memory in childhood* (pp. 41–82). Hove East Sussex, UK: Psychology Press.

Nelson, C. A. (2000). Neural plasticity and human development: The role of early experience in sculpting memory systems. *Developmental Science, 3*, 115–136.

Nelson, C. A., de Haan, M., & Thomas, K. (2006). Neural bases of cognitive development. In W. Damon & R. M. Lerner (Series Eds.), D. Kuhn & R. Siegler (Eds.), *Handbook of child psychology: Vol. 2. Cognition, perception, and language* (6th ed., pp. 3–57). Hoboken, NJ: Wiley.

Nelson, K., & Fivush, R. (2000). Socialization of memory. In E. Tulving & F. I. M. Craik (Eds.), *The Oxford handbook of memory* (pp. 283–295). New York: Oxford University Press.

Pathman, T., & Bauer, P. J. (2013). Beyond initial encoding: Measures of the post-encoding status of memory traces predict long-term recall in infancy. *Journal of Experimental Child Psychology, 114,* 321–338.

Petrides, M. (1995). Impairments on nonspatial self-ordered and externally ordered working memory tasks after lesions of the mid-dorsal part of the lateral frontal cortex in monkeys. *Journal of Neuroscience, 15,* 359–375.

Piaget, J. (1952). *The origins of intelligence in children.* New York: International Universities Press.

Pillemer, D. B., Picariello, M. L., & Pruett, J. C. (1994). Very long-term memories of a salient preschool event. *Applied Cognitive Psychology, 8,* 95–106.

Posner, M. I., & Rothbart, M. K. (1998). Attention, self-regulation, and consciousness. *Philosophical Transactions of the Royal Society of London B, 353,* 1915–1927.

Richmond, J., & Nelson, C. A. (2008). Mechanisms of change: A cognitive neuroscience approach to declarative memory development. In C. A. Nelson & M. Luciana (Eds.), *Handbook of developmental cognitive neuroscience* (2nd ed., pp. 541–552). Cambridge, MA: MIT Press.

Riggins, T., Cheatham, C., Stark, E., & Bauer, P. J. (2013). Elicited imitation performance at 20 months predicts memory abilities in school age children. *Journal of Cognition and Development, 14,* 593–606.

Roberts, T. P., Paulson, D. N., Hirschkoff, G., Pratt, K., Mascarenas, A., Miller, P., et al. (2014). Artemis 123: Development of whole-head infant MEG system. *Frontiers in Human Neuroscience, 8,* 99.

Rovee-Collier, C., & Hayne, H. (2000). Memory in infancy and early childhood. In E. Tulving & F. I. M. Craik (Eds.), *The Oxford handbook of memory* (pp. 267–282). New York: Oxford University Press.

Schneider, W., & Bjorklund, D. F. (1998). Memory. In W. Damon & R. M. Lerner (Series Eds.), D. Kuhn & R. Siegler (Eds.), *Handbook of child psychology: Vol. 2. Cognition, perception, and language* (6th ed., pp. 467–521). Hoboken, NJ: Wiley.

Seress, L., & Abraham, H. (2008). Pre- and postnatal morphological development of the human hippocampal formation. In C. A. Nelson & M. Luciana (Eds.), *Handbook of developmental cognitive neuroscience* (2nd ed., pp. 187–212). Cambridge, MA: MIT Press.

Sorce, J. F., Emde, R. N., Campos, J., & Klinnert, M. D. (1985). Maternal emotional signalings: Its effect on the visual cliff behavior of 1-year-olds. *Developmental Psychology, 21*(1), 195–200.

Squire, L. R., Knowlton, B., & Musen, G. (1993). The structure and organization of memory. *Annual Review of Psychology, 44,* 453–495.

Striano, T., & Rochat, P. (2000). Emergence of selective social referencing in infancy. *Infancy, 1*(2), 253–264.

Takehara, K., Kawahara, S., & Kirino, Y. (2003). Time-dependent reorganization of the brain components underlying memory retention in trace eyeblink conditioning. *Journal of Neuroscience, 23,* 9897–9905.

Tanapat, P., Hastings, N. B., & Gould, E. (2001). Adult neurogenesis in the hippocampal formation. In C. A. Nelson & M. Luciana (Eds)., *Handbook of developmental cognitive neuroscience* (pp. 93–105). Cambridge, MA: MIT Press.

Walden, T. A., & Baxter, A. (1989). The effects of context and age on social referencing. *Child Development, 60*(6), 1511–1518.

Zola, S. M., & Squire, L. R. (2000). The medial temporal lobe and the hippocampus. In E. Tulving & F. I. M. Craik (Eds.), *The Oxford handbook of memory* (pp. 485–500). New York: Oxford University Press.

CHAPTER 8

Infant Word Learning
in Biopsychosocial Perspective

Catherine S. Tamis-LeMonda and Marc H. Bornstein

In his book *Word and Object*, the philosopher Willard Quine (1960) proposed a hypothetical scenario in which an English speaker hears someone of an unfamiliar language exclaim "Gavagai!" just as a rabbit hops past. The English speaker might reasonably infer that gavagai means rabbit, yet countless other possibilities exist: gavagai might refer to the rabbit's color, a part of the rabbit, the rabbit's movement or direction, the ground beneath the rabbit, and so forth. Researchers of language development often cite Quine's scenario to illustrate the enormous challenge that infants face in learning language. How do infants crack the language code? How do they transition from communicative novices to relatively competent users of conventional words and sentences in a brief span of 2 to 3 years?

This question has inspired vigorous theoretical debate and countless empirical studies on the human capacities and social proclivities that underlie the remarkable skill of language. Research on this topic is inspired by the distinct theoretical traditions that characterize the study of learning and development more broadly. For example, theories of language learning vary in the mechanisms of acquisition they emphasize. Some researchers have interpreted language learning to result from innate core capacities of infants, following the tradition of Chomsky's (1965) writings on the language acquisition device. Others highlight powerful learning processes, such as attention and statistical learning that enable infants to extract meaning from visual and auditory streams (Baldwin, Markham, Bill, Desjardins, & Irwin, 1996; Saffran, Aslin, & Newport, 1996; Smith & Yu, 2008). Relatedly, theories of language learning also differ

152

in the extent to which they align with Piaget's (1952) characterization of infants as "little scientists" or alternatively with the view that infants are serendipitous beneficiaries of *supportive social interactions* (Vygotsky, 1978; Bruner, 1984).

As is true of the scientific endeavor more broadly, these varying theoretical traditions are imbued in researchers' questions, procedures, and measures. For example, the little scientist metaphor is reflected in laboratory-based observations of infant responses to computer-generated stimuli; such studies characterize infants as "probability detectors" who are sensitive to statistical regularities in sensory input. In contrast, research on the social context of language development is typically based on naturalistic observations of infants' interactions with others, and describes the ways that social input scaffolds infant language learning.

However, neither of these perspectives offers a complete answer to how infants transition to the world of language. Word learning is a dynamic, emergent system that is multiply determined, complex, and self-organizing (Thelen, 1993). Accordingly, we present a unified, multilevel biopsychosocial perspective of infant word learning that characterizes infants as "little scientists in social worlds." We describe the biological and social capacities of infants that facilitate word learning, while simultaneously demonstrating how social input from parents and other caregivers supports the word-learning task by capitalizing on infant capacities.

The Infant's Contribution

Infant biology contributes to the language-learning process at several levels. Structural features of the infant *brain* function to support an early emerging left-hemisphere advantage for the channeling of speech. Infants' *sensory and motor capacities* enable them to perceive and engage with the objects and people of their world, including hearing and producing the sounds of the language(s) around them. Infants' abilities to *detect environmental contingencies* and *statistical regularities* allow them to make sense out of the otherwise chaotic overload of sensory input that surrounds them.

The Infant Brain

The *mature* human brain has specialized regions in the left cerebral hemisphere for the understanding and production of language (Dronkers, Plaisant, Iba-Zizen, & Cabanis, 2007). *Wernicke's area* is commonly acknowledged to be involved in understanding spoken and written language (Démonet et al., 1992); lesions to this area result in "Wernicke's aphasia," a condition that entails impairments in language comprehension, word-finding deficits, and substitution errors even while speech retains natural-sounding rhythms and relatively normal syntax (Harpaz, Levkovitz, & Lavidor, 2009). By contrast, *Broca's area* is linked to speech production (Cabeza & Nyberg, 2000; Cantalupo & Hopkins, 2001), and "Broca's aphasia" is associated with deficits in language production such that individuals typically understand what is being said to them, but experience problems with fluency, articulation, repetition, and the production of complex grammatical structures both orally and in writing (Amici, Gorno-Tempini, Ogar, Dronkers, & Miller, 2006; Benson & Ardila, 1996; Goodglass, 1993).

However, the functional specialization of the mature brain does not yet exist in the infant brain. Infants who experience damage to Wernicke's and Broca's areas do not display the language aphasias seen in adults with corresponding brain damage, because other areas of the young, developing brain take over the language functions that would otherwise fall under the purview of these areas (Johnson, 1998). How then, does the human *infant brain*, a mass of gray and white matter, develop into a *mature* brain characterized by anatomical and functional specialization for language processing? What particular organization of the infant brain provides the springboard for language learning in the human species?

There is growing evidence that early *structural asymmetry* of the brain creates a left-hemisphere advantage for the channeling of speech. Indeed, humans possess the most asymmetrical brain of mammals, even those of primate lineage (Glasel et al., 2011), and interhemispheric structural asymmetry is evident in the first weeks of postnatal life. Brain asymmetry means that certain regions of the brain—located in the left hemisphere—are especially suited (compared with other regions) for processing rapid, temporal transitions, such as those that characterize speech (Boemio, Fromm, Braun, & Poeppel, 2005; Zatorre & Belin, 2001). When 2-month-olds listen to the speech of either the mother or a stranger, the left planum temporale is activated. In contrast, when they listen to music, which is not characterized by the same rapid sound transitions as speech, there is symmetrical brain activation in the two hemispheres (Dehaene-Lambertz et al., 2010).

There is also evidence that the left temporal and frontal areas of the brain govern infant sensitivity to speech sounds that occur with high probability; newborns respond differently to repetitive syllabic sequences (like /gamama/) compared with nonrepetitive ones (like /gamada/; Gervain, Macagno, Cogoi, Peña, & Mehler, 2008). And, infants between 3 and 7 months show preferential activation in left-hemispheric locations that are similar to those described in the adult brain when listening to voices (Blasi et al., 2011; Grossmann, Oberecker, Koch, & Friederici, 2010). Event-related potential (ERP) studies confirm that the bias toward left-hemisphere processing for language is present in infancy (Cheour-Luhtanen et al., 1995; Kuhl, 1998; Molfese, Burger-Judisch, & Hans, 1991). A few months later—12 to 18 months of age—infants begin to understand words and demonstrate brain activation in the left frontal temporal areas when exposed to familiar words; this activation occurs about 400 milliseconds after word onset (Travis et al., 2011), which aligns with activation patterns documented in adults. The relatively late timing of the activation reflects higher-order cognitive processes rather than lower-level perceptual ones, indicating that infants are processing the familiar words.

Perception

Infants' *capacities to perceive and engage with the objects and people of their world* are the human building blocks to word learning. Infants are able to see, smell, touch, and taste "apples" and to hear the word *apple* spoken. By the close of the first year, before beginning formal production, infants' skills in vision and audition rival adult levels (Bornstein, Arterberry, & Lamb, 2013). In fact, the auditory system is well developed before birth: fetuses exposed to select passages read to them by their mothers suck more on a pacifier postnatally to hear those passages than do infants who had not been so exposed (DeCasper & Spence, 1986).

Moreover, infants are able to *connect* experiences across sensory modalities, thereby experiencing different perceptual inputs as a whole. For example, infants attend more to visual displays of objects that they have touched in the dark than to those they have not touched (Rose, 1994). They look more to video displays of events that match versus do not match the sounds they are hearing, such as watching a hopping animal whose movements coincide with the sounds of impact (Spelke, 1976, 1979), or attending to a face whose expression matches the emotional tone of the voice (Kahana-Kalman & Walker-Andrews, 2001). These cross-modal connections are fundamental to word learning, because learning words requires infants to link meanings across multiple sense modalites.

Finally, infants display perceptual biases that increase the odds that they will selectively attend to certain types of visual and auditory inputs over others. For example, infants prefer faces (particularly dynamic faces) over other complex stimuli (Johnson & Morton, 1991). Moreover, these preferences exist in newborns, who have not yet had experiences interacting with others. In a study conducted over three decades ago, newborn infants (averaging 9 minutes of age) displayed head and eye movements that indicated their preference to track a moving schematic face to moving scrambled faces and blank head outlines (Goren, Sarty, & Wu, 1975). The preference for faces is thought to be subserved by primitive, possibly subcortical circuits of the brain that function to bias the newborn's visual attention (Johnson & Morton, 1991), much like the hemispheric biases for language processing described earlier. These attentional biases, and subsequent experiences with faces, lead to the eventual emergence of specialized circuits for face processing as found in adults (de Haan, Johnson, & Halit, 2003).

Although there has been controversy around the age(s) at which infant face preference is reliably observed, early biases in visual attention mean that the word-learning infant will be especially motivated to look at people who are moving, talking, and motioning about something interesting in the world. In turn, infants benefit from the social information available in others' affective expressions, direction of gaze, mouth movements, and the gestures that accompany their spoken language, as we elaborate on later in this chapter. It is therefore unsurprising that infants attend more to live tutors than they do to video or audio presentations of the same speech information, and that they learn from their observations of live tutors only (Kuhl, Tsao, & Liu, 2003).

Contingency Detection

The ability to connect information across sensory modalities, as described above, depends on the *detection of environmental contingencies*. Infants will only connect the sight, touch, smell, and taste of apple with the spoken word *apple* if the word and its referent are temporally bound. Tight temporal connection among stimuli is critical for infant learning because the likelihood that two events will come to be associated depends on their co-occurrence within a brief time window. Information encountered after a time window has closed is not associated with the initial event (Rovee-Collier, 1995).

Contingency detection may be present from birth (Gewirtz & Palàez-Nogueras, 1992) or, at minimum, well before the emergence of language. Two-month-olds modified the amplitudes of sucking a pacifier when auditory input was contingent on sucking, suggesting that they were aware of the consequences of their actions (Rochat & Striano, 1999). They also derive pleasure from the experience of contingency; one group of 2-month-olds heard music in response to their pulling an arm string, and a control group heard the same music played randomly with no connection to their string pulling (Lewis, Alessandri, & Sullivan, 1990). The infants in the contingent music condition showed more interest and smiling than did infants in the control condition.

Contingency detection is especially salient during social interactions (Rovee-Collier, 1987; Stern, 1985; Tarabulsy, Tessier, & Kappas, 1996), as evidenced by infants' distress when social contingencies are disrupted. The classic illustration of infants' reactions to social contingency disruption is seen in the "still-face paradigm" (SFP), where mothers are instructed to maintain unresponsive and expressionless faces, speak in a flat tone, and minimize body movement and contact with their infants who sit across from them (e.g., Cohn & Tronick, 1983; Tronick, Brazelton, & Als, 1978). Three-month-old infants who interacted with their mothers in an SFP condition displayed higher levels of distress and gaze aversion and lower positive affect (e.g., smiling) than did infants engaged in normal interactions (Cohn & Tronick, 1987). Others have also shown infants to be especially sensitive to the lack of contingency in normal social interactions with their parents as evidenced by their vivid (and unhappy) response when mothers become still-faced (Goldstein, Schwade, & Bornstein, 2009; Tronick, Brazelton, & Als, 1978) or when synchronous interactions with mothers are replaced via video with noncontingent actions (Bigelow, MacLean, & MacDonald, 1996). In neither case are adults attempting to elicit negative affect; they are merely not responding as they normally would. The finding that even young infants react negatively to noncontingent maternal behavior attests to the importance of contingency rules by which infants and mothers normally interact (Moore et al., 2009).

Moreover, infants' negative behavioral responses in the SFP are accompanied by physiological reactions mediated by the parasympathetic nervous system, including increased heart rate and decreased vagal tone (Moore & Calkins, 2004). Infants with high physiological reactions in the SFP maintain those reactions longer (i.e., even after their mothers reengaged them) than infants who were less physiologically aroused.

Infants' adverse reactions to the SFP, as well as general abilities to discriminate between adult behaviors that occur contingently and behaviors that take place randomly, have been documented across numerous studies with infants of different ages (e.g., Bigelow, 1998; Bigelow & Rochat, 2006; Bloom, 1988; Bloom, Russell, & Wassenberg, 1987; Field, 1987; Murray & Trevarthen, 1985; Rochat, 2001; Watson, 1985), leading to the suggestion that infants are born with a "contingency detection module" that analyzes temporal conditional probabilities and enables infants to detect contingent relations in the environment (Gergely, 2003; Gergely & Watson, 1996, 1999). Alternatively, the contingent structure of social interactions might be something that is a bottom-up process that is built up out of everyday experiences. Infants normally develop in a responsive, social environment (described below) and may therefore be quick to pick up on recurring temporal structures in social interactions. Natural environmental contingencies, therefore, support infants' ability to perceive contingent regularities in others' behavior (Baldwin, Baird, Saylor, & Clark, 2001; Feldman, 2003).

Statistical Learning

Before learning the meaning of words, infants must be able to discover which elements of the continuous speech stream constitute "words." To do this, they must figure out which sounds belong together as a unit, and which are unrelated. This process is referred to as phonotactic learning or statistical learning more generally. Word learning would not proceed if infants were unable to solve this segmenting problem. Analyses of speech sounds show that people tend to run words together when talking without pausing between words or otherwise indicating word boundaries. This is true even when adults talk directly to infants. Consequently, the number of ways to divide or segment a sentence into possible words is very large, and infants must solve this daunting word expedition problem.

For example, in English, the sounds /n/ and /k/ can occur together in a syllable, but only at the end (*sink*) and only in that order (*sikn*, *nkis*, and *knis* are not possible words in English). Although there are similarities in these rules across languages, there are also clear differences. For example, in Dutch, /kn/ is a possible word onset—the Dutch word for *knee* (*knie*) is pronounced like the English, except that the Dutch pronounce the initial /k/. Infants must be able to spontaneously group together syllables that have this kind of statistical consistency to find words in the streams of auditory input (Estes, 2009; Lany & Saffran, 2011).

Research indicates that infants are able to detect these statistical regularities as early as 8 months of age. In a seminal study of statistical learning (Saffran, Aslin, & Newport, 1996), 8-month-old infants were familiarized with 2 minutes of a synthesized continuous speech stream of strings of syllables—such as *bidakupadotigolabubidaku*—that contained no pauses or other cues (e.g., intonational patterns) to word boundaries. The transitional probabilities between pairs of syllables were manipulated to be 1.0 (always occurring adjacent to each other, thereby signaling a "word") or .33 (rarely occurring together, thereby signaling word boundaries). After the 2-minute exposure, infants were tested with familiar "words" (e.g., syllable pairs that always co-occurred such as *bida*) versus "nonwords" (syllables heard during the 2-minute learning phase, but in different orders). Infants dishabituated to the novel syllable pairings, indicating that they had extracted the serial order information from the auditory input.

By 8 months of age, infants' statistical learning skills enable them to segment "words" in artificial and natural languages (Pelucchi, Hay, & Saffran, 2009). Moreover, infants are able to detect neighboring sounds in both their primary language(s) and foreign language(s), and are able to draw on this ability to detect the breaking points in continuous streams of visual events (Roseberry, Richie, Hirsh-Pasek, Golinkoff, & Shipley, 2011). In one study, American (English speaking) and Dutch babies were presented with lists of words that were allowable in Dutch but not English (such as *knoest*), or allowable in English but not Dutch (such as *stewed*, whose final *d* is not permitted in Dutch). Infants preferred to listen to lists consistent with their own language's phonotactics (Jusczyk, Friederici, Wessels, Svenkerud, & Jusczyk, 1993).

Statistical learning is vital to language acquisition because it accounts not only for how infants parse speech streams but also how they come to construct word-to-world mappings, for example, by recognizing that the likelihood of hearing the word *apple* in the presence of an apple is greater than hearing the word *orange*, *knife*, *plate*, and so forth. Learning how to map words to objects and events requires infants to track co-occurrences across two streams of events (words and referents) simultaneously (Smith & Yu, 2008). To test infants' capacities in word-referent mapping, 12- and 14-month-old infants were presented with slides that contained two objects and two words, thereby creating ambiguity within trials as to which word referred to which object. However, across trials, the investigators manipulated the probabilities of word and object pairings, and found that infants deciphered which words mapped to which objects reliably based on the likelihoods of word–object co-occurence. Both groups of infants looked reliably longer to the target (i.e., word–object pairings that occurred with high likelihood) than to the distracter (words that did not co-occur with objects), indicating that they were able to accumulate and use information across trials to figure out word meanings (Smith & Yu, 2008).

Summary

Infants' enter the world poised to learn language. The asymmetrical structure of the infant *brain* leads to a left-hemispheric advantage for the processing of rapid, temporal transitions such as those that characterize speech. This biological bias interacts with environmental inputs (i.e., exposure to language) in the early emergence of an efficient cortical network for language processing. Infants' *sensory capacities* enable them to perceive and integrate information across sensory modalities, and early perceptual biases toward animate, dynamic faces provide fertile ground for engaging in social interactions that support word learning. Infants are *sensitive to environmental contingencies*, including the contingency structures of social interactions, enabling them to learn about and anticipate regularities in the temporal structures of social interactions. Finally, studies of *statistical learning* suggest that infants are "probability detectors" who continuously update the likelihoods that speech sounds (phonemes) will co-occur as "words," and that words co-occur with and thus refer to objects and events in the world.

Experiential Correlates

As reviewed above, biological building blocks for learning words include left-hemisphere biases for processing speech; capacities to perceive and connect auditory, visual, and other inputs; and abilities to detect environmental contingencies and statistical regularities in sensory input. However, biological explanations are limited in their explanatory scope because language unfolds in a social context and primary caregivers provide the ingredients for infant word learning. Moreover, the process of learning language in the real world is quite different from and messier than the process of learning artificial words or syllable configurations in controlled laboratory settings. In laboratory settings, infants have little to do but attend to the visual and auditory information presented to them. In naturalistic settings, in contrast, there is an abundance of information available. Infants are faced with competing demands as to where to look, what to listen to, and with whom to engage. The words they hear from other people can refer to countless objects and events around them. Yet, somehow, infants are able to sift through the clutter to disambiguate meaning. They are able to do so because social interactions contain valuable cues that scaffold word learning.

The importance of social interactions for infant word learning is illustrated by research contrasting learning under live versus artificial conditions. In one study, 9-month-old English-speaking infants who were presented with televised or audio recordings of Mandarin speakers did not learn the phonetic contrasts of Mandarin, whereas infants exposed to live social interactions showed impressive learning. Learning was assessed both by infant head turns to changes to Mandarin contrasts (Kuhl et al., 2003) as well as ERPs (Kuhl, 2007). Similarly, toddlers (ages 15 months to 2 years) were more successful at learning object labels from live tutors than from television (Krcmar, Grela, & Lin, 2007), and only children over 3 years of age learned verbs from television (Roseberry, Hirsh Pasek, Parish-Morris, & Golinkoff, 2009). In another study, the importance of live interactions for word learning was demonstrated by manipulating adult presence during word presentations. Infants who were focused on exploring a novel toy heard an adult say, "A toma! It's a toma." For some infants, the speaker was in view and talking to the infant. For other infants, the speaker was hidden behind a screen and had previously been seen talking on the telephone. Infants in the former condition learned that the object was a "toma." By contrast, infants in the latter condition did not learn the word (Baldwin et al., 1996).

Collectively, the above results are striking because based on simple associative views of word learning (or phonetic learning as in Kuhl's research), hearing a new word and attending to a new toy should be sufficient for word learning, but this is not the case. Simple co-occurrence of a word and infants' attention to an object are not sufficient for word learning if social aspects of the situation do not support linking the word and object. Indeed, the "social brain 'gates' the computational mechanisms involved in human language learning" (Kuhl, 2007, p. 110).

What then might explain the essentialism of social interaction for word learning? In the sections below, we highlight features of parent input to infants that support the task of learning new words. Specifically, we describe the properties of *child-directed speech and action*, which function to elicit infant attention; the temporal features of parental *contingent responsiveness*, which aids infants' linking of words to objects in the world; the *didactic content* of parental speech, which promotes infant word growth; the *physical cues* parents use to mark the referents of speech; and the ways that parents *developmentally scaffold word learning* by providing language to infants that is attuned to infants' changing skills.

Child-Directed Speech and Action

Parents package the language they direct to infants to facilitate word learning. Mothers and fathers (as well as infant caregivers and even adults who are not parents) adjust their speech in many ways when addressing infants. This special dialect is variously called baby talk, motherese, parentese, or more neutrally child-directed speech. The characteristics of child-directed speech cross multiple levels from prosody (higher pitch, greater range of frequencies, more varied and exaggerated intonation) to simplicity (shorter utterances, slower tempo, longer pauses between phrases, fewer embedded clauses, fewer auxiliaries) to redundancy (more repetition over shorter amounts of time, more immediate repetition) to vocabulary (special forms like *mama*) to content (restriction of topics to the infant's world; e.g., Snow, 1977; see Ma, Golinkoff, Houston, & Hirsh-Pasek, 2011, for a review).

Adults in many cultures tend to use a different register of speech when addressing infants and young children compared with their normal speech to other adults. This special register is characterized by a slower rate, a higher pitch, exaggerated prosodic contours, and longer vowels and pauses. In one study, the fundamental frequency as well as utterance duration and pause duration of French, Italian, German, Japanese, British English, and American English mothers' and fathers' naturalistic speech to preverbal infants was analyzed (Fernald, Taeschner, Dunn, Papousek, de Boysson-Bardies, et al., 1989). Regardless of language, mothers and fathers alike used higher mean, minimum, and maximum pitch (fundamental frequency) and a greater variability in pitch. They also used shorter utterances and longer pauses in child-directed speech than in adult-directed speech.

Further, when mothers talk with infants and young children, they almost always focus on the here and now, referring to objects and people that are present (e.g., Snow et al., 1976). In addition, words that adults use when addressing infants tend to be concrete (Phillips, 1973), phonologically simple (Ferguson, 1964), and contain a remarkably high rate of simple labels, descriptors, and questions (Tamis-LeMonda, Baumwell, & Cristofaro, 2012).

Sometimes, mothers even highlight specific words for infants by speaking to them in a louder voice. One investigator measured the relative loudness of labels and nonlabels in mothers' speech while mothers showed toys to their 1-year-olds. Labels had nearly a .50 probability of being the loudest word (Messer, 1981). Thus, relative loudness (like pitch) could cue infants to map new words onto referent objects. Others have pointed to links between the prosody of maternal speech and infants' object focus. For example, mothers' speech to infants consistently positions words at points of perceptual prominence in the speech stream—notably on exaggerated fundamental frequency peaks in utterance-initial or -final position—whereas in speech to adults the use of a prosodic emphasis is more variable (Golinkoff & Alioto, 1995; Seidl & Johnson, 2006).

Finally, parents tailor the grammatical complexity of their language in line with infant language skill. Child-directed speech contains shorter and simpler sentences as reflected in shorter mean length of utterance, fewer subordinate clauses (Longhurst & Stepanich 1975; Phillips, 1973), and a higher redundancy as reflected in type-token ratios (Phillips, 1973).

Although most work on child-directed speech is based on mothers, findings generalize to father–infant communicative interactions. In one study, mother–child and father–child dyads were video recorded on separate occasions while playing with their 2-year-olds. Fathers and mothers alike modified their language complexity to align with the language complexity of their toddlers' language. Both mothers and fathers used fewer words, and less grammatically complex and less diverse language with less linguistically competent infants than did parents of more linguistically advanced infants (Tamis-LeMonda, Baumwell, & Cristofaro, 2012).

Child-directed speech may be intuitive and nonconscious, and cross-cultural developmental research has confirmed its presence in many cultural communities around the globe (Kitamura, Thanavishuth, Burnham, & Luvsaneeyanawin, 2002). Studies of a number of European, U.S., and Asian linguistic communities have documented similar features of adult speech directed to young children (e.g., Blount & Padgug, 1976; Ferguson, 1964; Grieser & Kuhl, 1988; Kelkar, 1964), although there is also evidence for a lack of child-directed speech in certain communities (e.g., Ochs, 1982; Ochs & Schieffelin, 1984; Schieffelin, 1979; Pye, 1986). Notably, the signing of caregivers to infants involves slow and highly repetitive and exaggerated movements (Masataka, 1992), suggesting that child-directed speech is not restricted to the hearing population. When communicating with their infants, even deaf mothers modify their sign language in very much the way hearing mothers use child-directed speech (Erting, Thumann-Prezioso, & Benedict, 2000). Children as young as 4 years of age also engage in the same systematic language adjustments when speaking to an infant (Weppelman, Bostow, Schiffer, Elbert-Perez, & Newman, 2003).

In addition to speech modifications, adults modify their *actions* when interacting with infants versus with other adults. When communicating with infants, adults exaggerate their movements, which is referred to as "motionese" or infant-directed action (Brand, Baldwin, & Ashburn, 2002; Brand, Shallcross, Sabatos, & Massie, 2007; Koterba & Iverson, 2009). When middle-class, European American mothers of infants were asked to demonstrate how to use novel objects (e.g., a neon green "twisty" that could form different shapes and be taken apart and put back together) to either their babies or another adult they had a close relationship with (e.g., partner, friend, or mother), their demonstrations were qualititively different depending on the message recipient. Mothers' demonstrations to their infants were closer, more interactive, enthusiastic, repetitive, simpler, and included a greater range of motion compared with their demonstrations to adults (Brand et al., 2002).

Why might child-directed speech and action facilitate infant word learning? It could be that the prosodic patterning of child-directed speech elicits attention, modulates arousal, communicates affect, and supports infants' segmenting of the speech stream (Fernald, 2004; Soderstrom, Blossom, Foygel, & Morgan, 2008). First, with regard to eliciting attention, infants are more responsive to mothers' child-directed speech than their adult-directed speech. Infants also prefer child-directed speech than adult-directed speech spoken by strangers (Fernald et al., 1989). This amplified attention to child-directed speech might assist word learning because infants who pay more attention generally also show advanced language and communication skills (Arterberry, Midgett, Putnick, & Bornstein, 2007; Colombo et al., 2008).

Second, the sound and rhythm of child-directed speech might regulate infant arousal and communicate affect to the infant. Certain similar intonation contours in mothers' speech recur with regularity in particular interactions among American English, German, and Mandarin Chinese speakers (Papoušek & Papoušek, 2002). Mothers use rising pitch contours to engage infant attention and elicit infant response, falling contours to soothe a distressed infant, and bell-shaped contours to maintain infant attention. The prosodic patterns of child-directed speech may provide infants with supportive cues about the intentions of the speaker.

Finally, the prosodic modifications of child-directed speech facilitate the infant's speech processing and language comprehension. Exaggerated prosody helps infants segment the speech stream and provides acoustic cues to the grammatical structure of linguistic messages (Soderstrom, 2007; Soderstrom et al., 2008). For example, infants discriminate speech sounds embedded in multisyllabic sequences better in streams of child-directed speech than in streams of adult-directed speech, and children who show delayed onset of speech had mothers who did not use exaggerated pitch in their speech (D'Odorico & Jacob, 2006). Within the first few months of life, infants neurologically process child-directed speech differently from other auditory stimuli. Electroencephalogram (EEG) activity resulting from hearing child-directed speech is greatest in the temporal regions (Naoi et al., 2012).

Similar to the attention-eliciting functions seen in child-directed speech, "motionese" is likely to maintain infants' attention and highlight the structure and meaning of action. Infants sustained longer looking times when their primary caregivers moved a novel object (e.g., a toothbrush case) with either high amplitude or high repetition or both—the two parameters on which infant-directed action differ from adult-directed action (Brand et al., 2002)— than when they moved the object with both low amplitude and low repetition (Koterba & Iverson, 2009).

Responsiveness

Another key feature of parenting that facilitates word learning is responsiveness (Tamis-LeMonda, Kuchirko, & Tafuro, 2013; Tamis-LeMonda, Kuchirko, & Song, 2014). The behaviors that naturally flow from infants' interest in the people around them—namely, looks, vocalizations, facial expressions, and arm, leg, and torso movements—are catalysts for parental engagement. Parents and other infant caregivers follow infants' exploratory and communicative behaviors with prompt, contingent, and appropriate in-kind behaviors (e.g., looking to, pointing to, and labeling a "giraffe" in reply to an infant point to a giraffe). These behaviors, which we refer to as "parental responsiveness," are basic to the social feedback loop of "infant act–parent react effect on child" (Bornstein, Tamis-LeMonda, Hahn, & Haynes, 2008). Thus, responsiveness reflects a central element of recurring and meaningful sequences in everyday exchanges between child and parent that generalizes across contexts (e.g., laboratory and home; Lohaus, Keller, Ball, Elben, & Völker, 2001).

Infants benefit from parental responsiveness well before they produce conventional words. For example, real-time changes are observed in the sophistication of infants' babbling following maternal responsiveness. In one study, mothers and their infants were randomly assigned to one of two social-interaction conditions. In the contingent feedback condition, mothers were instructed to verbally respond to their infants' babbling. In the noncontingent feedback condition, infants received verbal input from their mothers that was temporally dissociated from infant babbling (Goldstein & Schwade, 2008). Infants who experienced contingent social feedback modified their babbling to mirror the phonological structure of their mothers' input, whereas infants exposed to the noncontingent feedback condition did not.

At the end of the first year and through the second year of life, infants are entering the world of language: they are increasingly able to understand and produce words and simple phrases, and benefit from verbal input that is temporally and conceptually connected to their actions on the world (Tamis-LeMonda, Cristofaro, Rodriguez, & Bornstein, 2006). At this time, mothers' responsiveness to infants' vocalizations, bids to mother, exploration and play with objects, and emotional displays predict the sizes of infants' vocabularies (Tamis-LeMonda, Bornstein, Kahana-Kalman, Baumwell, & Cyphers, 1998), the diversity of infants' communications (Beckwith & Cohen, 1989), and the timing of language milestones (Nicely, Tamis-LeMonda, & Bornstein, 1999; Tamis-LeMonda et al., 1998; Tamis-LeMonda, Bornstein, & Baumwell, 2001). For example, in two longitudinal studies, mothers' responsiveness predicted the ages at which children achieved milestones such as first words, vocabulary spurt, and combinatorial speech (Tamis-LeMonda et al., 1998, 2001). To assess the onsets of infant language skills, mothers were prospectively interviewed about their infants' receptive and productive vocabularies and skills at using language in simple sentences every 2 weeks from when infants were 9 months through 21 months of age. Additionally, mothers' contingent responsiveness to infants' communicative and exploratory behaviors was coded from video-recorded interactions of naturalistic play actions at home. Infants of high-responsive mothers (90th percentile) at 9 and 13 months achieved language milestones 4 to 6 months earlier than did infants of low-responsive mothers (10th percentile).

Although the above studies are correlational, and therefore limit researchers' ability to draw causal inferences, there is strong evidence that the facilitative role of responsiveness for child learning and development is not merely an epiphenomenon of genetic heritability or unobservable characteristics of children and/or parents. Parental responsiveness predicts the language skills of adopted children (Stams, Juffer, & van IJzendoorn, 2002) and infant learning under laboratory manipulations (Goldstein, King, & West, 2003). Moreover, interventions that target responsiveness in parents effectively enhance children's language and cognitive skills (e.g., Landry, Smith, Swank, & Guttentag, 2008; Mendelsohn et al., 2005, 2007).

What mechanisms might explain associations between parental responsiveness and infant word learning? Responsive behaviors on the part of parents are temporally connected to (i.e., *contiguous*) and conceptually dependent on (i.e., *contingent*) infant actions. These features of responsiveness promote word learning by capitalizing on infants' abilities to detect environmental contingencies and extract statistical regularities in word-to-world mappings.

To what extent do parents display behaviors that are temporally and conceptually connected to their infants' preceding actions? That is, under natural circumstances, without any prompting, are parents more likely to engage in visual (gaze), verbal (language), and physical (e.g., gestures, object touch) behaviors within 2 to 5 seconds of infant exploratory or communicative actions than to engage in those same behaviors in the absence of infant action? Research on the parental talk to infants indicates that contiguity and contingency are hallmarks of social interactions.

To illustrate, mothers were observed interacting with their 14-month-olds during play and book sharing and video recordings were coded for the temporal onsets and offsets of various infant and mother exploratory and communicative behaviors (e.g., looking and touching objects, infant vocalizations and maternal talk; Tamis-LeMonda, Kuchirko, et al., 2013). Sequential analysis was applied to these sequences of infant–mother interactions. This statistical approach relies on Bayesian analyses, in which the observed distribution of behaviors is used to estimate the likelihoods or conditional probabilities of *behavior* Y *given behavior* X (e.g., mother talking to the infant after the infant explores an object, vocalizes, or gestures). These conditional probabilities present a reasonable test of the dependent relation between infant and parent behaviors because they control for base-rate behaviors of the "given" or preceding behavior, and statistics that are generated from the conditional probabilities also consider the base-rate occurrence of parent behaviors.

Mothers were more likely to use language in response to their 14-month-old infants' object exploration (i.e., within 3 seconds of infant action) than in the presence of infant off-task behaviors. Thus, as soon as infants looked to, manipulated, and picked up objects of interest to them, their mothers provided verbal input that was connected to their infants' object-directed actions. The tight temporal connection between infant object engagement and parent verbal input heightens the odds that infants will hear words for the objects/events that are most visually salient to them. When an infant picks up an object for exploration, the infant's visual field is dominated by that single object, as shown in studies that use head-mounted eye trackers to document the visual world from the infant's perspective (Bornstein & Arterberry, 2010; Spencer et al., 2009). The predominant focus on a single object can be explained by the biological reality that children have short arms that function to keep objects close to their eyes when they hold them (Spencer et al., 2009). In turn, infants are more likely to learn words for objects that are visually salient than they are to learn words for objects that do not dominate their visual fields (Yu & Smith, 2012).

Responsiveness to infants' *vocalizations*, in particular, promotes infants' admission into the turn-taking feature of communication. Adults conversing with each other regularly match timing factors in their speech. Turn taking is fundamental to the structure of adult dialogue: It is impolite to interrupt, so instead people wait their turn to speak. From an extremely early age, infants produce a variety of sounds, and their caregivers respond differently to different infant vocalizations depending on how they interpret them (Hsu & Fogel, 2003; Markova & Legerstee, 2006; Papoušek, 2007). For infants, turn taking is an important first lesson in pragmatics (do not talk when someone else is talking). Mothers promote turn taking by responding with a vocalization immediately following infant vocalization, and they often prolong pauses after their own vocalizations to increase the likelihood that infant vocalizations will become part of a conversational chain. Turn taking may be a socializing aspect of mother–infant conversation. Paralleling the sequential analytic findings on mother response to infant object exploration, the likelihoods of mothers talking following infant vocalizations increased relative to when infants were not communicating (Tamis-LeMonda, Tafuro, Kuchirko, Song, & Kahana-Kalman, 2013).

Parental responsiveness also functions to increase the predictability of interactions, thereby promoting more optimal developmental environments for children (Chapple, 1970; Cohn & Elmore, 1988; Dunham & Dunham, 1995; Tarabulsy et al., 1996; Van Egeren, Barratt, & Roach, 2001). Social contingencies generate expectancies of predictable partner reactions in relation to one's own behaviors, and vice versa. The ability to detect contingencies is one of the quintessential features of adaptation (Canfield & Haith, 1991), and learning contingencies between one's own behavior and environmental events is a key adaptation in childhood (Millar & Weir, 1992).

Finally, parental responsiveness indirectly promotes word learning by supporting infants' skills at emotion regulation. In a study of infants' physiological arousal in the SFP (Moore & Calkins, 2004), 3-month-old infants who experienced high levels of synchrony in their play interactions with mothers (reflected in mothers' coordination of moment-to-moment affective states with those of their infants) were better able to suppress their vagal tone responses in the SFP than were infants who experienced low levels of synchrony in their play interactions. The regulation of emotional arousal is important to learning words, because both word production and emotions recruit cognitive resources, and language learning is disadvantaged when emotion arousal is high (Bloom, 1993; Cole, Armstrong, & Pemberton, 2010). In one in-depth, longitudinal study of infants at the early period of word learning, the more time infants spent in neutral affect during play (compared with time spent in extreme forms of emotional arousal), the younger they were in achieving the language skills of first words, the vocabulary spurt, and the transition to multiword speech (Bloom & Capatides, 1987). Thus, to the extent that parental responsiveness supports infants' abilities to regulate their emotional arousal, infants who experience high levels of parental responsiveness are in essence "ready to learn."

The Informational Content of Social Input

Beyond these temporal features of parental input, the "content" or information available to infants during social interactions influences word learning. Two aspects of informational content that support infants' word learning are *didactic* features and *embodied* features (Bornstein, 2002; Tamis-LeMonda, Kuchirko, & Song, 2014).

Didactic language is verbal input that refers to objects, activities, or events in the environment by describing, labeling, or asking about the unique qualities of the referent or event (e.g., "That's a spoon" and "What color is the spoon?"; "The rabbit's hopping" and "Where is he going?"). When parents respond to their infants' exploratory or communicative initiatives, the likelihood of their using didactic language is increased. In one study, mothers' verbal responses were coded as *referential* (i.e., didactic forms of language in which mothers refer to or ask about objects/events: e.g., "Yellow cup") or *regulatory* (i.e., statements that direct infants' actions: e.g., "Do it"). Mothers' referential language increased following infant vocalizations, gestures, and/or object exploration, whereas regulatory language decreased in the presence of these actions (Tamis-LeMonda, Kuchirko, et al., 2013a; Tamis-LeMonda, Tafuro, et al., 2013). Mothers' referential but not regulatory language was associated with infants' productive vocabulary. Others show that the diversity of parental language to infants (i.e., the use of *different* word types and different communicative functions) is associated with children's vocabulary size, rate of vocabulary growth, and communicative diversity in early language development (e.g., Hart & Risley, 1995; Hoff, 2003, 2006; Huttenlocher, Haight, Bryk, Seltzer, & Lyons, 1991; Tamis-LeMonda et al., 2012).

Embodied input refers to the multimodal coordination of parents' language with physical cues to meaning, for example, by looking to, touching, or pointing to objects they simultaneously name and describe following infant object engagement (Tamis-LeMonda, Kuchirko, et al., 2013; Tamis-LeMonda, Tafuro, et al., 2013). Parents regularly provide their infants with a range of nonverbal supports to communication and language learning. Gesture is one such support (Goldin-Meadow, 2006a, 2006b, 2009). For example, a mother might point and at the same time ask the question "What is that?" or "Is that a ball?" or say "Look! A ball." When responding to infants' exploratory or communicative actions mothers are more likely to coordinate gestural and manual cues of reference (points to objects, touching/manipulating objects) with didactic language than with regulatory language (Tamis-LeMonda, Kuchirko, & Song, 2014). Language that is accompanied by physical cues such as gesture is found to support infant word learning (e.g., Matatyaho & Gogate, 2008; Rowe & Goldin-Meadow, 2009; Tamis-LeMonda, Baumwell, et al., 2012).

Why might didactic language and embodied input promote word learning? Didactic language is rich in lexical diversity (i.e., the number of different words offered to infants) and facilitates infants' vocabulary growth more than does language low in lexical diversity (e.g., simple affirmations, such as "Yes!" and "Okay!"; Song, Spier, & Tamis-LeMonda, 2014). As infants are exposed to more words, and come to learn those words, the resultant growth in their vocabularies facilitates the processing of new information. In one study of bilingual infants, a composite measure of vocabulary was associated with processing speed in each language (i.e., based on Spanish and English; Marchman, Fernald, & Hurtado, 2010). A recent study confirms the association among child-directed talk, vocabulary growth, and processing speed in a study of infants from low-income, Spanish-speaking families. Infants who experienced more child-directed speech became more efficient at processing familiar words in real time and had larger expressive vocabularies by 24 months (Weisleder & Fernald, 2013).

The enhanced processing of new information by infants who hear more language and who have larger vocabularies may be explained by inhibitory processes. If an infant encounters a new word (e.g., *cat*) that contains partially overlapping meaning with a word that is already known (e.g., *dog*), learning the new word is facilitated when the semantic representation of the familiar word is sufficiently specified (Friedrich & Friederici, 2010) or richly instantiated (Dapretto & Bjork, 2000). In this example, the incoming information (new word *cat*) activates several possible semantic representations, making it necessary for the infant to suppress activity patterns associated with inaccurate representations (Friedrich & Friederici, 2010). Richer semantic networks facilitate this process.

In terms of embodied input, multimodal information capitalizes on infants' capacity to use nonspeech contextual information to learn words (Yu, Ballard, & Aslin, 2005). The synchronization of actions and words creates a unitary experience for infants who perceive such stimuli as "belonging together" (Rader & Zukow-Goldring, 2010). Moreover, physical actions, such as points, are likely to result in joint attention, which in turn facilitates word learning (Tomasello & Farrar, 1986). When mothers teach infants a name for a novel toy, they also have a strong tendency to move the toy in synchrony with their verbal label, which may help infants make the association (Gogate, Bahrick, & Watson, 2000). In this regard, gestures make parents' intentions salient and "narrow the search space" (Zukow-Goldring, 2006).

Developmental Scaffolding

There exists powerful evidence for the developmental attunement of parents' responses to infants (Bornstein, 2013). That is, parents continually modify *what they respond to* and *how they respond* in line with the changing skills of their infants. In one study, mothers *labeled and described* objects in response to their 1-year-olds' vocalizations, but asked questions of their older toddlers more skilled at language (Bornstein et al., 2008). Mothers also shifted from responding to basic object exploration at 9 months to responding to advanced forms of object play at later ages. Mothers are more likely to respond when their 2-year-olds produce new words than when their toddlers produce words that have been in their vocabularies for some time (Masur, 1997). Between the infant ages of 14 and 24 months, mothers increased their didactic responses to infant vocalizations, but decreased their responses to infant gestures (Tamis-LeMonda, Tafuro, et al., 2013). Finally, mothers of 13-month-old crawling infants show different patterns of responding to their infants' social bids than do mothers of 13-month-old walking infants, mainly because the two groups of infants bid in different ways. Crawling infants predominantly bid from stationary positions (e.g., while sitting), whereas walking infants bid by carrying objects over to their mothers half the time (Karasik, Tamis-LeMonda, & Adolph, 2011). Mothers in turn use noun phrases (e.g., "Red ball") in response to stationary bids, but predicate phrases (e.g., "Roll it to me") in response to moving bids (Karasik, Tamis-LeMonda, & Adolph, 2013). Collectively, these studies indicate that parents are attuned to and respond in new ways to emerging skills in infants.

Why is developmental attunement important? As infants develop their language skills, they attend to and require different cues to learn new words. During the earliest period of word learning, infants have an immature principle of reference and primarily learn words for objects that are salient to them and coincide with their attentional focus. At this time, infants require more frequent word repetitions and multiple cues to learn words than do infants who are more advanced in their lexicons and understanding of reference (Hollich et al., 2000). Novice word learners predominantly learn words that align with objects that are salient and coincide with their perspective, whereas more expert word learners are able to learn words for objects that are signaled from other peoples' perspectives. In this regard, caregivers' developmental attunement to infants' changing language skills scaffolds word learning by providing infants with the supports needed to understand communicative intentions at particular times in the developmental trajectory. As an example, repetitious contingent labeling of a "ball" will yield greater value to an infant who does not yet know the word than it will to the one who does. In contrast, infants with more advanced lexicons are able to participate in simple conversations and will benefit from being asked simple referential questions (e.g., "What is that?").

Social Interaction and the Developing Brain

The sections above highlight the features of social interaction that support infant word learning at a behavioral level. Notably, research in developmental neuroscience is beginning to identify connections between social interactions and language learning at the level of the brain, and suggests that infant exposure to language influences the brain's neural circuitry even before infants speak their first words (Kuhl, 2010).

As infants are exposed to language and in turn grow in their language skills, their responses to speech are increasingly lateralized in the left hemisphere, their concentrations of gray matter and white matter change (Deniz Can, Richards, & Kuhl, 2013), and there are discernable changes in temporal patterns of brain activation when exposed to words (Travis et al., 2011). Moreover, research on bilingual infants indicates greater brain tissue density in the areas of the brain related to language, memory, and attention, with the highest levels of tissue density among those who were exposed to a second language prior to age 5 (Mechelli, Price, Friston, & Ashburner, 2005).

In a longitudinal study of Spanish–English bilingual children, associations among early brain measures of phonetic discrimination in both languages (based on ERPs), degree of exposure to each language in the home, and children's later bilingual word-production skills were assessed. Infants' amount of exposure to each of their native languages in the home predicted their phonetic discrimination abilities, and both language exposure and early neural discrimination skills predicted later word production in both languages (Garcia-Sierra et al., 2011). Moreover, the degree of social engagement infants demonstrated during language-learning sessions predicted the degree of learning indexed by ERPs as well as behavioral measures of word and phoneme learning (Conboy & Kuhl, 2011). Research with adults also offers valuable insights into the ways that exposure to language influences brain activity. In one study, Japanese adults with limited English exposure were trained on the phonemes of /r/ and /l/, speech sounds that are typically not detected by adult Japanese speakers (Zhang, Kuhl, Imada, Iverson, Pruitt, et al., 2009). Participants were exposed to the English phonemes with a software program that mimicked the exaggerated features of infant-directed speech as described above. At the end of the 12-session training, adults showed behavioral improvements in their ability to distinguish between the English phonemes. Notably, functional neuroimaging of brain activity indicated that learning induced increases to neural sensitivity and efficiency. Moreover, individual differences in adults' phoneme discrimination scores were associated with pre–post changes to neural sensitivity.

Moreover, the ability of bilingual adults to perceive foreign speech sounds is associated with the volume of Heschl's gyrus (HG), a brain structure that contains the auditory cortex. In one study, Spanish–Catalan bilingual adults who had been exposed to two languages since childhood were compared with a group of Spanish monolinguals. The two groups were demographically matched on education, socioeconomic status, and musical experience. Bilinguals had larger gray matter volumes in HG than did monolinguals. These differences indicate that learning a second language leads to an increased size of the auditory cortex rather than being explained by demographic measures or selection biases in the samples (Ressel, Pallier, Ventura-Campos, Díaz, Roessler, et al., 2012).

Collectively, this new wave of studies with infants and adults indicates a bottom-up process of developmental influence, whereby social interactions and exposure to language results in changes to neural response and brain structure. Findings such as these underscore the importance of taking a biopsychosocial approach to the study of early language development.

Cultural Context

The capacities of infants and features of parenting reviewed above have been observed in infants and parents around the world. Moreover, although parents from different cultural communities might differ in *how often* they engage in child-directed speech and action, responsiveness, didactic talk, and so forth, there is evidence that these features of parenting uniformly support children's word learning.

Nonetheless, the social contexts in which word learning unfold are culturally embedded. For example, parents' views, socialization goals, and the larger sociocultural context shape *how much and how* parents talk and respond to their infants, *what* they talk about and respond to, and *why* they talk (Bornstein, 2015; Bornstein & Lansford, 2010). Parents from different cultural communities differ in the extent to which they make communicative accommodations when interacting with their infants and likewise differ in the types of infant signals they find to be salient (Ochs & Schieffelin, 1984; Tamis-LeMonda & Song, 2013).

For example, middle-income mothers from Japan and the United States differ in their frequencies of responding to their 3-month-olds' gazes, smiles, and vocalizations (Bornstein, Cote, Haynes, Suwalsky, & Bakeman, 2012; Fogel, Toda, & Kawai, 1988). In another study, U.S. mothers responded to infant object play (e.g., stacking blocks) more than social play (e.g., feeding a doll), whereas Japanese mothers responded more to social play than to object play (Tamis-LeMonda, Bornstein, Cyphers, Toda, & Ogino, 1992). A comparison of maternal responsiveness across six cultural communities indicated that mothers from Berlin and Los Angeles were more likely to respond to infant nondistress vocalizations and gaze than were mothers from Bejiing, Delhi, and the Nso of Cameroon (Kärtner et al., 2008), whereas Nso mothers responded more often to infant touch than did mothers from other cultures. In a study of New York City mothers, Mexican immigrant mothers were more likely to respond to their 14-month-olds' gestures with referential language than were Dominican and African American mothers (Tamis-LeMonda, Song, et al., 2012), aligning with the cultural emphasis on learning through observation and physical cues. Again, however, in the context of these differences, mothers from all cultural communities displayed contiguity, contingency, and embodiment in their responses, suggesting universality in many core features of parenting.

Parents from different cultural communities also display different *types* of responses to their infants' behaviors. Mothers from France, Japan, and the United States differ in their extradyadic (directing infant attention to the environment) and dyadic (directing attention to mother) responses to their 5-month-olds. U.S. mothers were more extradyadic in their responsiveness than were French and Japanese mothers, whereas Japanese mothers were more dyadic in their responsiveness than were other mothers (Bornstein et al., 1992). These patterns of responding may reflect different cultural emphases on individual exploration (extradyadic) versus social connection (dyadic). For example, mothers of infants in many cultures use affect-laden speech, but as children achieve more sophisticated levels of motor exploration and cognitive comprehension mothers increasingly orient, comment, and prepare children for the world outside the dyad by infusing their speech to children with increasing amounts of information (Bornstein et al., 1992).

These cultural and individual differences in the amounts and types of specific parental behaviors, however, do not change their *associations* to infant learning, because averages are statistically independent of correlations. In fact, across families from different cultural communities and socioeconomic strata, parent lexical diversity, responsiveness, multimodal input, and so forth has been shown to promote children's language learning and development (e.g., Bornstein & TamisLeMonda, 1989, 1997; Bornstein, Tamis-LeMonda, & Haynes, 1999; Rodriguez & Tamis-LeMonda, 2011; Tamis-LeMonda et al., 2001;

Tamis-LeMonda, Shannon, & Cabrera, 2004; Weisleder & Fernald, 2013). For example, the responsiveness of Italian and Canadian mothers was associated with children's verbal skills and, although specific associations emerged in each culture, each association turned on presumed linear relations between maternal responsiveness and child language outcomes (Hsu & Lavelli, 2005).

Conclusions

The development of language is one of the most heralded achievements of infancy. It is thus unsurprising that scholars have long questioned the capacities in infants and the characteristics of social input that enable infants to "crack the language code." We advanced a biopsychosocial perspective of language development that unites an account of word learning in which infants' biological, perceptual, and computational capacities enable them to make meaning out of sensory input with a sociocultural account in which infants benefit from interactions with attuned and dynamic social partners (Bornstein, 2013; Kuhl, 2007; Tamis-LeMonda, Kuchirko, & Tafuro, 2013).

Infants enter the world of language armed with biological building blocks that pave the way for learning words, including a left-hemispheric bias for processing speech, capacities to perceive and integrate sensory information across modalities, and general learning abilities to detect social contingencies and statistical regularities in environmental input. For their part, parents facilitate infant word learning by offering input that builds on infants' natural capacities and proclivities. *Child-directed speech and action* elicit infant attention and facilitate segmenting actions and sounds into meaningful units. The features of parental *responsiveness*—contiguity and contingency—increase the likelihood that the words infants hear will be temporally and conceptually aligned with the objects and events that are most salient and of greater interest to them. The *didactic content* of parental input promotes growth in vocabulary and in turn faster processing of new information. The embodied, *multimodal* feature of parent input provides infants with physical cues, such as gestures and touch, which function to mark the referents of the words that are spoken. Finally, *developmental attunements* in social interactions reflect the reciprocal and dynamic process of word learning: parents scaffold infant learning and development by "upping the ante" as infants gain new skills.

Collectively, the studies reviewed in this chapter highlight the value of an integrative approach to early word learning in which the synergistic connections among brain processes, infant social proclivities and capacities, and caregiver supportive interactions are considered. Nonetheless, research is only at the frontier of integrating science across these multiple levels. New techniques for studying brain structures and processes, including EEG/ERPs, magnetoencephalography (MEG), functional magnetic resonance imaging (fMRI), and near-infrared spectroscopy (NIRS), have yielded exciting information on the neural underpinnings to early language learning. However, this work has yet to consider how variations in the quality of infant–parent social interactions might play out in infant neural response. Future research should capitalize on the new tools available in neuroscience *and* behavioral coding to address the question of *why* it is that infants best learn language in the presence of supportive social partners. Although developmentalists have made great strides in identifying the key features of social interactions that facilitate infant word learning, and have offered rich theoretical interpretation of why these features of input might matter (e.g., Tamis-LeMonda et al., 2014), much remains to be learned about how variations in social input play out at the level of brain response.

ACKNOWLEDGMENTS

We acknowledge funding from National Science Foundation BCS Grant No. 021859 and IRADS Grant No. 0721383 and the Intramural Research Program of the National Institute of Child Health and Human Development, National Institutes of Health. We are grateful to the hundreds of mothers and children who have participated in our research over the years. This chapter summarizes selected aspects of Catherine S. Tamis-LeMonda's research, and portions of the text have appeared in previous scientific publications cited in the references.

REFERENCES

Amici, S., Gorno-Tempini, M. L., Ogar, J. M., Dronkers, N. F., & Miller, B. L. (2006). An overview on primary progressive aphasia and its variants. *Behavioural Neurology, 17*(2), 77–87.

Arterberry, M. E., Midgett, C., Putnick, D. L., & Bornstein, M. H. (2007). Early attention and literacy experiences predict adaptive communication. *First Language, 27*(2), 175–189.

Baldwin, D. A., Baird, J. A., Saylor, M. M., & Clark, M. A. (2001). Infants parse dynamic action. *Child Development, 72*(3), 708–717.

Baldwin, D. A., Markham, E. M., Bill, B., Desjardins, R. N., & Irwin, J. M. (1996). Infants' reliance on a social criterion for establishing word–object relations. *Child Development, 67*, 3135–3153.

Beckwith, L., & Cohen, S. E. (1989). Maternal responsiveness with preterm infants and later competency. *New Directions for Child and Adolescent Development, 43*, 75–87.

Benson, D. F., & Ardila, A. (1996). *Aphasia: A clinical perspective.* New York: Oxford University Press.

Bigelow, A. E. (1998). Infants' sensitivity to familiar imperfect contingencies in social interaction. *Infant Behavior and Development, 21*(1), 149–162.

Bigelow, A. E., MacLean, B. K., & MacDonald, D. (1996). Infants' response to live and replay interactions with self and mother. *Merrill-Palmer Quarterly, 42*, 596–611.

Bigelow, A. E., & Rochat, P. (2006). Two-month-old infants' sensitivity to social contingency in mother–infant and stranger–infant interaction. *Infancy, 9*(3), 313–325.

Blasi, A., Mercure, E., Lloyd-Fox, S., Thomson, A., Brammer, M., Sauter, D., et al. (2011). Early specialization for voice and emotion processing in the infant brain. *Current Biology, 14*(21), 1220–1224.

Bloom, K. (1988). Quality of adult vocalizations affects the quality of infant vocalizations. *Journal of Child Language, 15*(3), 469–480.

Bloom, K., Russell, A., & Wassenberg, K. (1987). Turn taking affects the quality of infant vocalizations. *Journal of Child Language, 14*(2), 211–227.

Bloom, L. (1993). *Language development from two to three.* New York: Cambridge University Press.

Bloom, L., & Capatides, J. B. (1987). Expression of affect and the emergence of language. *Child Development, 58*(6), 1513–1522.

Blount, B. G., & Padgug, E. J. (1976). Mother and father speech: Distribution of parental speech features in English and Spanish. *Papers and Reports on Child Language Development, 12*, 47–59.

Boemio, A., Fromm, S., Braun, A., & Poeppel, D. (2005). Hierarchical and asymmetric temporal sensitivity in human auditory cortices. *Nature Neuroscience, 8*(3), 389–395.

Bornstein, M. H. (2002). Parenting infants. In M. H. Bornstein (Ed.), *Handbook of parenting: Vol. 1. Children and parenting* (2nd ed., pp. 3–43). Mahwah, NJ: Erlbaum.

Bornstein, M. H. (2013). Mother–infant attunement: A multilevel approach via body, brain, and behavior. In M. Legerstee, D. W. Haley, & M. H. Bornstein (Eds.), *The infant mind: Origins of the social brain* (pp. 266–298). New York: Guilford Press.

Bornstein, M. H. (2015). Children's parents. In M. H. Bornstein & T. Leventhal (Eds.), *Handbook of child psychology and developmental science: Vol. 4. Ecological settings and processes in developmental systems* (7th ed., pp. 55–132). Hoboken, NJ: Wiley.

Bornstein, M. H., & Arterberry, M. E. (2010). The development of object categorization in young children: Hierarchical inclusiveness, age, perceptual attribute, and group versus individual analyses. *Developmental Psychology, 46*(2), 350–365.

Bornstein, M. H., Arterberry, M. E., & Lamb, M. E. (2013). *Development in infancy: A contemporary introduction* (5th ed.). New York: Psychology Press.

Bornstein, M. H., Cote, L. R., Haynes, O. M., Suwalsky, J. T., & Bakeman, R. (2012). Modalities of infant–mother interaction in Japanese, Japanese American immigrant, and European American dyads. *Child Development, 83*(6), 2073–2088.

Bornstein, M. H., & Lansford, J. E. (2010). Parenting. In M. H. Bornstein (Ed.), *The handbook of cultural developmental science: Part 1. Domains of development across cultures* (pp. 259–277). New York: Psychology Press.

Bornstein, M. H., & Tamis-LeMonda, C. S. (1989). Maternal responsiveness and cognitive development in children. In M. H. Bornstein (Ed.), *Maternal responsiveness: Characteristics and consequences* (pp. 49–61). San Francisco: Jossey-Bass.

Bornstein, M. H., & Tamis-LeMonda, C. S. (1997). Maternal responsiveness and infant mental abilities: Specific predictive relations. *Infant Behavior and Development, 20*(3), 283–296.

Bornstein, M. H., Tamis-LeMonda, C. S., Hahn, C., & Haynes, O. M. (2008). Maternal responsiveness to young children at three ages: Longitudinal analysis of a multidimensional, modular, and specific parenting construct. *Developmental Psychology, 44*(3), 867–874.

Bornstein, M. H., Tamis-LeMonda, C. S., & Haynes, O. M. (1999). First words in the second year: Continuity, stability, and models of concurrent and predictive correspondence in vocabulary and verbal responsiveness across age and context. *Infant Behavior and Development, 22*(1), 65–85.

Bornstein, M. H., Tamis-LeMonda, C. S., Tal, J., Ludemann, P., Toda, S., Rahn, C. W., et al. (1992). Maternal responsiveness to infants in three societies: The United States, France, and Japan. *Child Development, 63*(4), 808–821.

Brand, R. J., Baldwin, D. A., & Ashburn, L. A. (2002). Evidence for "motionese": Modifications in mothers' infant-directed action. *Developmental Science, 5*(1), 72–83.

Brand, R. J., Shallcross, W. L., Sabatos, M. G., & Massie, K. P. (2007). Fine-grained analysis of motionese: Eye gaze, object exchanges, and action units in infant- versus adult-directed action. *Infancy, 11*(2), 203–214.

Bruner, J. S. (1984). Pragmatics of language and language of pragmatics. *Social Research: An International Quarterly, 51*(4), 969–984.

Cabeza, R., & Nyberg, L. (2000). Neural basis of learning and memory: Functional neuroimaging evidence. *Current Opinion in Neurology, 13*(4), 415–421.

Canfield, R. L., & Haith, M. M. (1991). Young infants' visual expectations for symmetric and asymmetric stimulus sequences. *Developmental Psychology, 27*(2), 198–208.

Cantalupo, C., & Hopkins. W. D. (2011). Asymmetric Broca's area in great apes: A region of the ape brain is uncannily similar to one linked with speech in humans. *Nature, 414*(6863), 505.

Chapple, E. D. (1970). *Culture and biological man: Explorations in behavioral anthropology.* New York: Holt, Rinehart & Winston.

Cheour-Luhtanen, M., Alho, K., Kujala, T., Sainio, K., Reinikainen, K., Renlund, M., et al. (1995). Mismatch negativity indicates vowel discrimination in newborns. *Hearing Research, 82*(1), 53–58.

Chomsky, N. (1965). *Aspects of the theory of syntax* (No. 11). Cambridge, MA: MIT Press.

Cohn, J. F., & Elmore, M. (1988). Effect of contingent changes in mothers' affective expression on the organization of behavior in 3-month-old infants. *Infant Behavior and Development, 11*(4), 493–505.

Cohn, J. F., & Tronick, E. Z. (1983). Three-month-old infants' reaction to simulated maternal depression. *Child Development, 54*(1), 185–193.

Cohn, J. F., & Tronick, E. Z. (1987). Mother–infant face-to-face interaction: The sequence of dyadic states at 3, 6, and 9 months. *Developmental Psychology, 23*(1), 68.

Cole, P. M., Armstrong, L. M., & Pemberton, C. K. (2010). The role of language in the development of emotion regulation. In S. D. Calkins & M. A. Bell (Eds.), *Child development at the intersection of emotion and cognition* (pp. 59–77). Washington, DC: American Psychological Association.

Colombo, J., Shaddy, D. J., Blaga, O. M., Anderson, C. J., Kannass, K. N., & Richman, W. A. (2008). Early attentional predictors of vocabulary in childhood. In J.

Colombo, P. McCardle, & L. Freund (Eds.), *Infant pathways to language: Methods, models, and research directions* (pp. 143–168). New York: Psychology Press.

Conboy, B. T., & Kuhl, P. K. (2011). Impact of second-language experience in infancy: Brain measures of first- and second-language speech perception. *Developmental Science, 14*, 242–248.

Dapretto, M., & Bjork, E. L. (2000). The development of word retrieval abilities in the second year and its relation to early vocabulary growth. *Child Development, 71*(3), 635–648.

de Haan, M., Johnson, M. H., & Halit, H. (2003). Development of face-sensitive event-related potentials during infancy: A review. *International Journal of Psychophysiology, 51*(1), 45–58.

DeCasper, A. J., & Spence, M. J. (1986). Prenatal maternal speech influences newborns' perception of speech sounds. *Infant Behavior and Development, 9*(2), 133–150.

Dehaene-Lambertz, G., Montavont, A., Jobert, A., Allirol, L., Dubois, J., Hertz-Pannier, L., et al. (2010). Language or music, mother or Mozart?: Structural and environmental influences on infants' language networks. *Brain and Language, 114*(2), 53–65.

Démonet, J.-F., Chollet, F., Ramsay, S., Cardebat, D., Nespoulous, J. L., Wise, R., et al. (1992). The anatomy of phonological and semantic processing in normal subjects. *Brain, 115*(6), 1753–1768.

Deniz Can, D., Richards, T., & Kuhl, P. K. (2013). Early gray-matter and white-matter concentration in infancy predict later language skills: A whole brain voxel-based morphometry study. *Brain and Language, 124*(1), 34–44.

D'Odorico, L., & Jacob, V. (2006). Prosodic and lexical aspects of maternal linguistic input to late-talking toddlers. *International Journal of Language and Communication Disorders, 41*(3), 293–311.

Dronkers, N. F., Plaisant, O., Iba-Zizen, M. T., & Cabanis, E. A. (2007). Paul Broca's historic cases: High resolution MR imaging of the brains of Leborgne and Lelong. *Brain, 130*(5), 1432–1441.

Dunham, P. J., & Dunham, F. (1995). Optimal social structures and adaptive infant development. In C. Moore & P. J. Dunham (Eds.), *Joint attention: Its origins and role in development.* Hillsdale, NJ: Erlbaum.

Erting, C. J., Thumann-Prezioso, C., & Benedict, B. S. (2000). Bilingualism in a deaf family: Fingerspelling in early childhood. In P. E. Spencer, C. J. Erting, & M. Marschark (Eds.), *The deaf child in the family and at school: Essays in honor of Kathryn P. Meadow-Orlans* (pp. 41–54). Mahwah, NJ: Erlbaum.

Estes, K. G. (2009). From tracking statistics to learning words: Statistical learning and lexical acquisition. *Language and Linguistics Compass, 3*(6), 1379–1389.

Feldman, R. (2003). Infant–mother and infant–father synchrony: The coregulation of positive arousal. *Infant Mental Health Journal, 24*(1), 1–23.

Ferguson, C. A. (1964). Baby talk in six languages. *American Anthropologist, 66*(6-2), 103–114.

Fernald, A. (2004). Hearing, listening, and understanding: Auditory development in infancy. In G. Bremner & A. Fogel (Eds.), *Blackwell handbook of infant development* (pp. 35–70). London: Blackwell.

Fernald, A., Taeschner, T., Dunn, J., Papousek, M., de Boysson-Bardies, B., & Fukui, I.

(1989). A cross-language study of prosodic modifications in mothers' and fathers' speech to preverbal infants. *Journal of Child Language, 16*(3), 477–501.

Field, T. (1987). Affective and interactive disturbances in infants. In J. D. Osofsky (Ed.), *Handbook of infant development* (2nd ed., pp. 972–1005). New York: Wiley-Interscience.

Fogel, A., Toda, S., & Kawai, M. (1988). Mother–infant face-to-face interaction in Japan and the United States: A laboratory comparison using 3-month-old infants. *Developmental Psychology, 24*(3), 398–406.

Friedrich, M., & Friederici, A. D. (2010). Maturing brain mechanisms and developing behavioral language skills. *Brain and Language, 114*(2), 66–71.

Garcia-Sierra, A., Rivera-Gaxiola, M., Percaccio, C. R., Conboy, B. T., Romo, H., Klarman, L., et al. (2011). Bilingual language learning: An ERP study relating early brain responses to speech, language input, and later word production. *Journal of Phonetics, 39,* 546–557.

Gergely, G. (2003). What should a robot learn from an infant?: Mechanisms of action interpretation and observational learning in infancy. *Connection Science, 15*(4), 191–209.

Gergely, G., & Watson, J. S. (1996). The social biofeedback theory of parental affect-mirroring: The development of emotional self-awareness and self-control in infancy. *International Journal of Psycho-Analysis, 77,* 1181–1212.

Gergely, G., & Watson, J. S. (1999). Early socio-emotional development: Contingency perception and the social–biofeedback model. In P. Rochat (Ed.), *Early social cognition: Understanding others in the first months of life* (pp. 101–136). Hillsdale, NJ: Erlbaum.

Gervain, J., Macagno, F., Cogoi, S., Peña, M., & Mehler, J. (2008). The neonate brain detects speech structure. *Proceedings of the National Academy of Sciences, 105*(37), 14222–14227.

Gewirtz, J. L., & Peláez-Nogueras, M. (1992). B. F. Skinner's legacy in human infant behavior and development. *American Psychologist, 47*(11), 1411–1422.

Glasel, H., Leroy, F., Dubois, J., Hertz-Pannier, L., Mangin, J. F., & Dehaene-Lambertz, G. (2011). A robust cerebral asymmetry in the infant brain: The rightward superior temporal sulcus. *Neuroimage, 58*(3), 716–723.

Gogate, L., Bahrick, L., & Watson, J. (2000). A study of multimodal motherese: The role of temporal synchrony between verbal labels and gestures. *Child Development, 71*(4), 878–894.

Goldin-Meadow, S. (2006a). Nonverbal communication: The hand's role in talking and thinking. In D. Kuhn, R. S. Siegler, W. Damon, & R. M. Lerner (Eds.), *Handbook of child psychology: Vol. 2. Cognition, perception, and language* (6th ed., pp. 336–369). Hoboken, NJ: Wiley.

Goldin-Meadow, S. (2006b). Talking and thinking with our hands. *Current Directions in Psychological Science, 15*(1), 34–39.

Goldin-Meadow, S. (2009). How gesture promotes learning throughout childhood. *Child Development Perspectives, 3*(2), 106–111.

Goldstein, M. H., King, A. P., & West, M. (2003). Social interaction shapes babbling: Testing parallels between birdsong and speech. *Proceedings of the National Academy of Sciences, 100*(13), 8030–8035.

Goldstein, M. H., & Schwade, J. A. (2008). Social feedback to infants' babbling facilitates rapid phonological learning. *Psychological Science, 19*(5), 515–523.

Goldstein, M. H., Schwade, J. A., & Bornstein, M. H. (2009). The value of vocalizing: Five-month-old infants associate their own noncry vocalizations with responses from caregivers. *Child Development, 80*(3), 636–644.

Golinkoff, R. M., & Alioto, A. (1995). Infant-directed speech facilitates lexical learning in adults hearing Chinese: Implications for language acquisition. *Journal of Child Language, 22*(3), 703–726.

Goodglass, H. (1993). *Understanding aphasia.* San Diego, CA: Academic Press.

Goren, C. C., Sarty, M., & Wu, P. Y. (1975). Visual following and pattern discrimination of face-like stimuli by newborn infants. *Pediatrics, 56*(4), 544–549.

Grieser, D. L., & Kuhl, P. K. (1988). Maternal speech to infants in a tonal language: Support for universal prosodic features in motherese. *Developmental Psychology, 24*(1), 14–20.

Grossmann, T., Oberecker, R., Koch, S. P., & Friederici, A. D. (2010). The developmental origins of voice processing in the human brain. *Neuron, 65*(6), 852–858.

Hart, B., & Risley, T. R. (1995). *Meaningful differences in the everyday experience of young American children.* Baltimore: Brookes.

Harpaz, Y., Leckovitz, Y., & Lavidor. M. (2009). Lexical ambiguity resolution in Wernicke's area and its right homologue. *Cortex, 45*(9), 1097–1103.

Hoff, E. (2003). Causes and consequences of SES-related differences in parent-to-child speech. In M. H. Bornstein (Ed.), *Socioeconomic status, parenting, and child development* (pp. 147–160). Mahwah, NJ: Erlbaum.

Hoff, E. (2006). How social contexts support and shape language development. *Developmental Review, 26*(1), 55–88.

Hollich, G. J., Hirsh-Pasek, K., Golinkoff, R. M., Brand, R. J., Brown, E., Chung, H. L., et al. (2000). Breaking the language barrier: An emergentist coalition model for the origins of word learning. *Monographs of the Society for Research in Child Development, 65*(3, Serial No. 262).

Hsu, H. C., & Fogel, A. (2003). Social regulatory effects on infant nondistress vocalization on maternal behavior. *Developmental Psychology, 39*(6), 976–991.

Hsu, H. C., & Lavelli, M. (2005). Perceived and observed parenting behavior in American and Italian first-time mothers across the first 3 months. *Infant Behavior and Development, 28*(4), 503–518.

Huttenlocher, J., Haight, W., Bryk, A., Seltzer, M., & Lyons, T. (1991). Early vocabulary growth: Relation to language input and gender. *Developmental Psychology, 27*(2), 236–248.

Johnson, M. H. (1998). The neural basis of cognitive development. In W. Damon (Ed.) & D. Kuhn & R. S. Siegler (Vol. Eds.), *Handbook of child psychology: Vol. 2. Cognition, perception, and language* (5th ed., pp. 1–49). New York: Wiley.

Johnson, M. H., & Morton, J. (1991). *Biology and cognitive development: The case of face recognition.* Oxford: Blackwell.

Jusczyk, P. W., Friederici, A. D., Wessels, J. M., Svenkerud, V. Y., & Jusczyk, A. M. (1993). Infants' sensitivity to the sound patterns of native language words. *Journal of Memory and Language, 32*(3), 402–420.

Kahana-Kalman, R., & Walker-Andrews, A. S. (2001). The role of person familiarity in young infants' perception of emotional expressions. *Child Development, 72*(2), 352–369.

Karasik, L., Tamis-LeMonda, C. S., & Adolph, K. E. (2013). Crawling and walking infants elicit different verbal responses from mothers. *Developmental Science, 17*(3), 388–395.

Karasik, L. B., Tamis-LeMonda, C. S., & Adolph, K. E. (2011). Transition from crawling to walking and interactions with objects and people. *Child Development, 82*(4), 1199–1209.

Kärtner, J., Keller, H., Lamm, B., Abels, M., Yovsi, R. D., Chaudhary, N., et al. (2008). Similarities and differences in contingency experiences of 3-month-olds across sociocultural contexts. *Infant Behavior and Development, 31*(3), 488–500.

Kelkar, A. R. (1964). Marathi baby talk. *Word: Journal of the International Linguistic Association, 20*(1), 40–54.

Kitamura, C., Thanavishuth, C., Burnham, D., & Luksaneeyanawin, S. (2002). Universality and specificity in infant-directed speech: Pitch modifications as a function of infant age and sex in a tonal and non-tonal language. *Infant Behavior and Development, 24*(4), 372–392.

Koterba, E. A., & Iverson, J. M. (2009). Investigating motionese: The effect of infant-directed action on infants' attention and object exploration. *Infant Behavior and Development, 32*(4), 437–444.

Krcmar, M., Grela, B., & Lin, K. (2007). Can toddlers learn vocabulary from television?: An experimental approach. *Media Psychology, 10*(1), 41–63.

Kuhl, P. K. (1998). The development of speech and language. In T. J. Carew, R. Menzel, & C. J. Shatz (Eds.), *Mechanistic relationships between development and learning* (pp. 53–73). New York: Wiley.

Kuhl, P. K. (2007). Is speech learning "gated" by the social brain? *Developmental Science, 10*(1), 110–120.

Kuhl, P. K. (2010). Brain mechanisms in early language acquisition. *Neuron, 67*, 713–727.

Kuhl, P. K., Tsao, F. M., & Liu, H. M. (2003). Foreign-language experience in infancy: Effects of short-term exposure and social interaction on phonetic learning. *Proceedings of the National Academy of Sciences, 100*(15), 9096–9101.

Landry, S. H., Smith, K. E., Swank, P. R., & Guttentag, C. (2008). A responsive parenting intervention: The optimal timing across early childhood for impacting maternal behaviors and child outcomes. *Developmental Psychology, 44*(5), 1335–1353.

Lany, J., & Saffran, J. R. (2011). Interactions between statistical and semantic information in infant language development. *Developmental Science, 14*(5), 1207–1219.

Lewis, M., Alessandri, S. M., & Sullivan, M. W. (1990). Violation of expectancy, loss of control, and anger expressions in young infants. *Developmental Psychology, 26*(5), 745–751.

Lohaus, A., Keller, H., Ball, J., Elben, C., & Völker, S. (2001). Maternal sensitivity: Components and relations to warmth and contingency. *Parenting: Science and Practice, 1*(4), 267–284.

Longhurst, T. M., & Stepanich, L. (1975). Mothers' speech addressed to one-, two-, and three-year-old normal children. *Child Study Journal, 5*, 3–11.

Ma, W., Golinkoff, R. M., Houston, D., & Hirsh-Pasek, K. (2011). Word learning in infant- and adult-directed speech. *Language Learning and Development, 7*(3), 209–225.

Marchman, V. A., Fernald, A., & Hurtado, N. (2010). How vocabulary size in two languages relates to efficiency in spoken word recognition by young Spanish–English bilinguals. *Journal of Child Language, 37*(4), 817.

Markova, G., & Legerstee, M. (2006). Contingency, imitation, and affect sharing: Foundations of infants' social awareness. *Developmental Psychology, 42*(1), 132–141.

Masataka, N. (1992). Motherese in a signed language. *Infant Behavior and Development, 15*(4), 453–460.

Masur, E. F. (1997). Maternal labeling of novel and familiar objects: Implications for children's development of lexical constraints. *Journal of Child Language, 24*(2), 427–439.

Matatyaho, D. J., & Gogate, L. J. (2008). Type of maternal object motion during synchronous naming predicts preverbal infants' learning of word–object relations. *Infancy, 13*(2), 172–184.

Mechelli, A., Price, C. J., Friston, K. J., & Ashburner, J. (2005). Voxel-based morphometry of the human brain: Methods and applications. *Current Medical Imaging Reviews, 1*(2), 105–113.

Mendelsohn, A. L., Dreyer, B. P., Flynn, V., Tomopoulos, S., Rovira, I., Tineo, W., et al. (2005). Use of videotaped interactions during pediatric well-child care to promote child development: A randomized, controlled trial. *Journal of Developmental and Behavioral Pediatrics, 26*(1), 34–41.

Mendelsohn, A. L., Valdez, P. T., Flynn, V., Foley, G. M., Berkule, S. B., Tomopoulos, S., et al. (2007). Use of videotaped interactions during pediatric well-child care: Impact at 33 months on parenting and on child development. *Journal of Developmental and Behavioral Pediatrics, 28*(3), 206–212.

Messer, D. (1981). The identification of names in maternal speech to infants. *Journal of Psycholinguistic Research, 10*(1), 69–77.

Millar, W. S., & Weir, C. G. (1992). Relations between habituation and contingency learning in 5 -to 12-month old infants. *Current Psychology of Cognition, 12*(3), 209–222.

Molfese, D. L., Burger-Judisch, L. M., & Hans, L. L. (1991). Consonant discrimination by newborn infants: Electrophysiological differences. *Developmental Neuropsychology, 7*(2), 177–195.

Moore, G. A., & Calkins, S. D. (2004). Infants' vagal regulation in the still-face paradigm is related to dyadic coordination of mother–infant interaction. *Developmental Psychology, 40*(6), 1068–1080.

Moore, G. A., Hill-Soderlund, A. L., Propper, C. B., Calkins, S. D., Mills-Koonce, W. R., & Cox, M. J. (2009). Mother–infant vagal regulation in the face-to-face still-face paradigm is moderated by maternal sensitivity. *Child Development, 80*(1), 209–223.

Murray, L., & Trevarthen, C. (1985). Emotional regulation of interactions between two-month-olds and their mothers. In T. M. Field & N. A. Fox (Eds.), *Social perception in infants* (pp. 177–197). Norwood, NJ. Ablex.

Naoi, N., Minagawa-Kawai, Y., Kobayashi, A., Takeuchi, K., Nakamura, K., Yama-mato, J., et al. (2012). Cerebral responses to infant-directed speech and the effect of talker familiarity. *Neuroimage, 59*(2), 1735–1744.

Nicely, P., Tamis-LeMonda, C. S., & Bornstein, M. H. (1999). Mothers' attuned responses to infant affect expressivity promote earlier achievement of language milestones. *Infant Behavior and Development, 22*(4), 557–568.

Ochs, E. (1982). Talking to children in Western Samoa. *Language in Society, 11*(01), 77–104.

Ochs, E., & Schieffelin, B. B. (1984). Language acquisition and socialization: Three developmental stories and their implications. In R. Shweder & R. LeVine (Eds.), *Culture theory: Essays on mind, self, and emotion* (pp. 276–320). Cambridge, UK: Cambridge University Press.

Papoušek, H. (2007). Communication in early infancy: An area of intersubjective learn-ing. *Infant Behavior and Development, 30*(2), 258–266.

Papoušek, H., & Papoušek, M. (2002). Intuitive parenting. In M. H. Bornstein (Ed.), *Handbook of parenting: Vol 2. Biology and ecology of parenting* (2nd ed., pp. 183–203). Mahwah, NJ: Erlbaum.

Pelucchi, B., Hay, J. F., & Saffran, J. R. (2009). Learning in reverse: Eight-month-old infants track backwards transitional probabilities. *Cognition, 113*(2), 244–247.

Phillips, J. R. (1973). Syntax and vocabulary of mothers' speech to young children: Age and sex comparisons. *Child Development, 44*(1), 182–185.

Piaget, J. (1952). *The origins of intelligence in children.* New York: International Uni-versity Press.

Pye, C. (1986). Quiché Mayan speech to children. *Journal of Child Language, 13*(1), 85–100.

Quine, W. V. (1960). *Word and object.* Cambridge, MA: MIT Press.

Rader, N. D. V., & Zukow-Goldring, P. (2010). How the hands control attention during early word learning. *Gesture, 10*(2–3), 202–221.

Ressel, V., Pallier, C., Ventura-Campos, N., Díaz, B., Roessler, A., Ávila, C., et al. (2012). An effect of bilingualism on the auditory cortex. *The Journal of Neurosci-ence, 32*(47), 16597–16601.

Rochat, P. (2001). *The infant's world.* Cambridge, MA: Harvard University Press.

Rochat, P., & Striano, T. (1999). Social–cognitive development in the first year. In P. Rochat (Ed.), *Early social cognition: Understanding others in the first months of life* (pp. 3–34). Mahwah, NJ: Erlbaum

Rodriguez, E., & Tamis-LeMonda, C. S. (2011). Trajectories of the home learning envi-ronment across the first five years: Associations with children's language and lit-eracy skills at prekindergarten. *Child Development, 82*(4), 1058–1075.

Rose, S. A. (1994). From hand to eye: Findings and issues in infant cross-modal transfer. In D. J. Lewkowicz & R. Lickliter (Eds.), *The development of intersensory percep-tion: Comparative perspectives* (pp. 265–284). Hillsdale, NJ: Erlbaum.

Roseberry, S., Hirsh-Pasek, K., Parish-Morris, J., & Golinkoff, R. M. (2009). Live action: Can young children learn verbs from video? *Child Development, 80*(5), 1360–1375.

Roseberry, S., Richie, R., Hirsh-Pasek, K., Golinkoff, R. M., & Shipley, T. F. (2011).

Babies catch a break: 7- to 9-month-olds track statistical probabilities in continuous dynamic events. *Psychological Science, 22*(11), 1422–1424.

Rovee-Collier, C. (1987). Learning and memory in infancy. In J. D. Osofsky (Ed.), *Handbook of infant development* (2nd ed. pp. 98–148). New York: Wiley.

Rovee-Collier, C. (1995). Time windows in cognitive development. *Developmental Psychology, 31*(2), 147–169.

Rowe, M., & Goldin-Meadow, S. (2009). Differences in early gesture explain SES disparities in child vocabulary size at school entry. *Science, 323*(5916), 951–953.

Saffran, J. R., Aslin, R. N., & Newport, E. L. (1996). Statistical learning by 8-month-old infants. *Science, 274*(5294), 1926–1928.

Schieffelin, B. B. (1979). Getting it together: An ethnographic approach to the study of the development of communicative competence. In E. Ochs & B. B. Schieffelin (Eds.), *Developmental pragmatics* (pp. 93–108). New York: Academic Press.

Seidl, A., & Johnson, E. K. (2006). Infant word segmentation revisited: Edge alignment facilitates target extraction. *Developmental Science, 9*(6), 565–573.

Smith, L., & Yu, C. (2008). Infants rapidly learn word–referent mappings via cross-situational statistics. *Cognition, 106*(3), 1558–1568.

Snow, C. E. (1977). Mothers' speech research: From input to interactions. In C. E. Snow & C. A. Ferguson (Eds.), *Talking to children: Language input and acquisition* (pp. 31–49). London: Cambridge University Press.

Snow, C. E., Arlman-Rupp, A., Hassing, Y., Jobse, J., Joosten, J., & Vorster, J. (1976). Mothers' speech in three social classes. *Journal of Psycholinguistic Research, 5*(1), 1–20.

Soderstrom, M. (2007). Beyond babytalk: Re-evaluating the nature and content of speech input to preverbal infants. *Developmental Review, 27*(4), 501–532.

Soderstrom, M., Blossom, M., Foygel, I., & Morgan, J. L. (2008). Acoustical cues and grammatical units in speech to two preverbal infants. *Journal of Child Language, 35*(4), 869–902.

Song, L., Spier, E. T., & Tamis-LeMonda, C. S. (2014). Reciprocal influences between maternal language and children's language and cognitive development in low-income families. *Journal of Child Language, 41*(2), 305–326.

Spelke, E. (1976). Infants' intermodal perception of events. *Cognitive Psychology, 8*(4), 553–560.

Spelke, E. S. (1979). Perceiving bimodally specified events in infancy. *Developmental Psychology, 15*(6), 626–636.

Spencer, J. P., Blumberg, M. S., McMurray, B., Robinson, S. R., Samuelson, L. K., & Tomblin, J. B. (2009). Short arms and talking eggs: Why we should no longer abide the nativist–empiricist debate. *Child Development Perspectives, 3*(2), 79–87.

Stams, G. J. J., Juffer, F., & van IJzendoorn, M. H. (2002). Maternal sensitivity, infant attachment, and temperament in early childhood predict adjustment in middle childhood: The case of adopted children and their biologically unrelated parents. *Developmental Psychology, 38*(5), 806–821.

Stern, D. N. (1985). *The interpersonal world of the infant.* New York: Basic Books.

Tamis-LeMonda, C. S., Baumwell, L., & Cristofaro, T. (2012). Parent–child conversations during play. *First Language, 32*(4), 413–438.

Tamis-LeMonda, C. S., Bornstein, M. H., & Baumwell, L. (2001). Maternal responsiveness and children's achievement of language milestones. *Child Development, 72*(3), 748–767.

Tamis-LeMonda, C. S., Bornstein, M. H., Cyphers, L., Toda, S., & Ogino, M. (1992). Language and play at one year: A comparison of toddlers and mothers in the United States and Japan. *International Journal of Behavioral Development, 15*(1), 19–42.

Tamis-LeMonda, C. S., Bornstein, M. H., Kahana-Kalman, R., Baumwell, L., & Cyphers, L. (1998). Predicting variation in the timing of linguistic milestones in the second year: An events-history approach. *Journal of Child Language, 25*(3), 675–700.

Tamis-LeMonda, C. S., Cristofaro, T. N., Rodriguez, E. T., & Bornstein, M. H. (2006). Early language development: Social influences in the first years of life. In L. Balter & C. S. Tamis-LeMonda (Eds.), *Child psychology: A handbook of contemporary issues* (2nd ed., pp. 79–108). New York: Psychology Press.

Tamis-LeMonda, C. S., Kuchirko, Y., & Song, L. (2014). Why is infant language learning facilitated by parents' contingent speech? *Current Directions in Psychological Science, 23*(2), 121–126.

Tamis-LeMonda, C. S., Kuchirko, Y., & Tafuro, L. (2013). From action to interaction: Mothers' contingent responsiveness to infant exploration across cultural communities. *IEEE Transactions on Autonomous Mental Development, 5*(3), 202–209.

Tamis-LeMonda, C. S., Shannon, J. D., & Cabrera, N. (2004). Mothers and fathers at play with their 2- and 3-year-olds. *Child Development, 75*(6), 1806–1820.

Tamis-LeMonda, C. S., & Song, L. (2013). Parent–infant communicative interactions in cultural context. In R. M. Lerner, E. Easterbrooks, & J. Mistry (Eds.), *Handbook of psychology* (2nd ed., pp. 143–170). Hoboken, NJ: Wiley.

Tamis-LeMonda, C. S., Song, L., Leavell Smith, A., Kahana Kalman, R., & Yoshikawa, H. (2012). Ethnic differences in mother–infant language and gestural communications are associated with specific skills in infants. *Developmental Science, 15*(3), 384–397.

Tamis-LeMonda, C. S., Tafuro, L., Kuchirko, Y., Song, L., & Kahana-Kalman, R. (2013). *Mothers' responsiveness and child development: A focus on mother–infant interactions in low-income, ethnically diverse families.* Paper presented at the Society for Research on Child Development, Seattle, WA.

Tarabulsy, G. M., Tessier, R., & Kappas, A. (1996). Contingency detection and the contingent organization of behavior in interactions: Implications for socioemotional development in infancy. *Psychological Bulletin, 120*(1), 25–41.

Thelen, E. (1993). Self-organization in developmental processes: Can systems approaches work? In M. Gunnar & E. Thelen (Eds.), *Systems in development: The Minnesota Symposia on Child Psychology* (Vol. 22, pp. 77–117). Hillsdale, NJ: Erlbaum.

Tomasello, M., & Farrar, M. J. (1986). Joint attention and early language. *Child Development, 57*(6), 1454–1463.

Travis, K. E., Leonard, M. K., Brown, T. T., Hagler, D. J., Curran, M., Dale, A. M., et al. (2011). Spatiotemporal neural dynamics of word understanding in 12- to 18-month-old infants. *Cerebral Cortex, 21*(8), 1832–1839.

Tronick, E. Z., Als, H., Adamson, L., Wise, S., & Brazelton, T. B. (1978). The infant's response to entrapment between contradictory messages in face-to-face interaction. *Journal of the American Academy of Child Psychiatry, 17*(1), 1–13.

Tronick, E., Brazelton, T. B., & Als, H. (1978). The structure of face-to-face interaction and its developmental functions. *Sign Language Studies, 18*, 1–16.

Van Egeren, L. A., Barratt, M. S., & Roach, M. A. (2001). Mother–infant responsiveness: Timing, mutual regulation, and interactional context. *Developmental Psychology, 37*(5), 684–697.

Vygotsky, L. (1978). *Mind in society: The development of higher psychological processes.* Cambridge, MA: Harvard University Press.

Watson, J. S. (1985). Contingency perception in early social development. In T. M. Field & N. A. Fox (Eds.), *Social perception in infants* (pp. 157–176). Norwood, NJ: Ablex.

Weisleder, A., & Fernald, A. (2013). Talking to children matters: Early language experience strengthens processing and builds vocabulary. *Psychological Science, 24*(11), 2143–2152.

Weppelman, T. L., Bostow, A., Schiffer, R., Elbert-Perez, E., & Newman, R. S. (2003). Children's use of the prosodic characteristics of infant-directed speech. *Language and Communication, 23*(1), 63–80.

Yu, C., Ballard, D. H., & Aslin, R. N. (2005). The role of embodied intention in early lexical acquisition. *Cognitive Science, 29*(6), 961–1005.

Yu, C., & Smith, L. B. (2012). Embodied attention and word learning by toddlers. *Cognition, 125*(2), 244–262.

Zatorre, R. J., & Belin, P. (2001). Spectral and temporal processing in human auditory cortex. *Cerebral Cortex, 11*(10), 946–953.

Zhang, Y., Kuhl, P., Imada, T., Iverson, P., Pruitt, J., Stevens, E. B., et al. (2009). Neural signatures of phonetic learning in adulthood: A magnetoencephalography study. *NeuroImage, 46*(1), 226–240.

Zukow-Goldring, P. (2006). Assisted imitation: Affordances, effectivities, and the mirror system in early language development. In M. A. Arbib (Ed.), *From action to language* (pp. 469–500). Cambridge, UK: Cambridge University Press.

PART III

SOCIAL AND EMOTIONAL PROCESSES

CHAPTER 9

Introduction to Part III

Reweaving the Strands—Biology, Behavior, Context

Ross A. Thompson

The study of behavioral development is dauntingly (or compellingly) complex because of its multifaceted origins. At any moment, behavior derives from a richly interwoven network of neurobiological, physiological, cognitive, socio-emotional, cultural, and contextual processes. These processes evolve developmentally and are mutually influential as individuals grow and mature. For those who study behavioral development, this complexity affords exciting but challenging opportunities for thinking integratively across levels of functioning and levels of context.

When people are faced with complex systems, however, the natural inclination is to simplify them. This has certainly been true of developmental science, in which debates over the preeminence of nature or nurture—and within them, the predominance of genes, conditioning, culture, maturation, or socialization—have colored its history and theory. Despite recurrent claims that the nature–nurture debate is scientifically obsolete, moreover, each generation of scientists has reinstantiated it. Maybe this is because the tension between nature and nurture has deep origins in Western and Eastern cultures. From ancient Platonic beliefs and Confucian thought to Enlightenment philosophy to the present, the dichotomy between intrinsic (especially biological) tendencies and social (especially parental) influences on human development has appeared inescapable.

Conceptualizing human development in this manner, of course, has consequences. In the early 1970s, President Nixon's ambivalence about Head Start derived, in part, from arguments within the scholarly community concerning the genetics of intelligence, which were interpreted as undermining the efficacy of early intervention for disadvantaged children. Several decades later, a National Research Council committee was commissioned to write a report on early childhood development (subsequently titled *From Neurons to Neighborhoods*; Committee on Integrating the Science of Early Childhood Development, National Research Council, 2000), owing, in part, to public concern about whether parenting influences were important in light of scientific arguments that genetics, not parenting, guides behavioral development within the normal range.

There are several reasons, however, why the present moment offers a unique opportunity to move beyond the nature–nurture polarity (Thompson, 2015). First, developmental neuroscience has provided scientists and the public with a model of a biologically dynamic, experience-driven developmental system that deeply integrates the influences of nature and nurture. The understanding that experience shapes a plastic brain, while scientifically familiar (see Hunt, 1961), is a new contribution to public understanding and provides a powerful conceptual framework to guide the thinking of parents, policymakers, and future scientists. Second, technological advances are providing a much more incisive understanding of the biological processes at work in behavioral development and how they interact with experiential catalysts. While technology cannot alone do the interpretive work needed for integrating biology with behavior, it has provided new ways of understanding their interaction. Third, we are on the vanguard of significant new advances in developmental science that will help to consolidate new understandings of the developmental dynamic of nature and nurture. Epigenetics is, in particular, showing how even gene expression (and possibly also structure; see Charney, 2012) is also a biologically dynamic, experience-driven developmental process.

The contributors to Part III, and to this volume, illustrate how much progress we have made. In this brief introduction, my goal is to consider the implications of the biopsychosocial models that are emerging from current developmental science for our understanding of socioemotional development. In doing so, I also consider the broader sociocultural context of these models, especially their implications for policy and practice, because of their significance for the understanding of human development that practitioners and policymakers enlist into their decisions concerning children. I profile two areas in which biopsychosocial models are proving to be especially provocative of new thinking: stress reactivity and emotion regulation. I close with some interpretive cautions, caveats, and concluding thoughts.

Developing Stress Reactivity

The understanding that experience shapes developing biological and behavioral systems has long been familiar to developmental science. More recently, the view that biological systems are designed to incorporate experience (whether positive or negative) into their organization and development has been articulated in the findings of developmental neuroscience and, in recent years, behavioral epigenetics. Such a view is based on the recognition that organisms must adapt, behaviorally and biologically, to the environmental conditions into which they are born. This adaptation is crucial to survival and growth, but it requires early sensitivity to cues signaling these environmental conditions and the reorganization of developing systems accordingly.

The development of language is a well-known example. Because newborns cannot anticipate living in Paris, London, Tokyo, Kiev, Beijing, or elsewhere, their brains must be prepared to learn any language, and this is consistent with research evidence that 6-month-olds can discriminate among a great variety of human speech phonemes (Werker, 2003). But this perceptual capacity is lost by age 1 as the child overhears the language(s) spoken at home and language-relevant brain regions reorganize to more efficiently learn one or two specific languages, paving the way for the vocabulary explosion of the second year (Kuhl, 2007; Kuhl et al., 2008). In this respect, the development of biological and behavioral systems relevant to language acquisition is experientially guided to foster efficient language acquisition.

What we observe of early language learning may be part of a broader developmental process that guides other developing biological and behavioral systems. According to the *predictive adaptive response model* and similar formulations, very young organisms are sensitive to cues of the environmental conditions relevant to their survival and, beginning prenatally, their development adapts accordingly (Gluckman & Hanson, 2005). Biological and behavioral adaptations like these can render the child more capable of functioning in these environmental conditions and enhance chances of long-term survival and growth if those conditions endure. If those conditions change significantly, however, deleterious developmental outcomes may ensue. An important cue concerning environmental conditions, for example, pertains to food sufficiency. When mothers are undernourished, fetal malnutrition is associated with decreased energy metabolism and slower growth rate that may prepare for a postnatal life of food insufficiency (Barker, 2002; Nathanielsz, 1999). But studies also show that when fetal malnutrition is followed by food prosperity and consequent weight gain, it is a significant predictor of coronary heart disease and other correlates of adult metabolic syndrome (Gluckman & Hanson, 2005). In these circumstances, children grew up in conditions of plenty for which they were biologically unprepared.

There are other environmental cues relevant to survival and growth, such as those signaling the relative safety, adversity, or reliability of living conditions. According to life history theory (Stearns, 1992), the quality of parental care provides cues concerning these conditions to which developing organisms must adapt to function more effectively in those settings. Life history theory has provided a framework for understanding, for example, the association of early maternal care and attachment security with later outcomes such as risk taking, pubertal timing, and reproductive strategy (e.g., Belsky, Steinberg, Houts, Halpern-Felsher, & NICHD Early Child Care Research Network, 2010; Chisholm, 1996). In this view, the support or harshness of early caregiving experience signals broader environmental safety or adversity, and the adaptations that result are both biological and behavioral in nature, deriving from common experiential catalysts, to ensure survival and reproductive success.

It would be expected that the quality of parental care would be the primary avenue for conveying environmental cues concerning safety or danger to a young organism. And, as the fetal malnutrition research illustrates, it would not be surprising to find that sensitivity to these cues begins before birth. Elevated and extended prenatal exposure to maternal cortisol owing to the mother's stress, for example, is associated with a larger neonatal cortisol response and slower recovery (Davis, Glynn, Waffarn, & Sandman, 2011). In one prospective longitudinal study, maternal depression during pregnancy was associated with heightened cortisol levels when infants were observed at 3 months in a moderately challenging procedure (Oberlander et al., 2008). In another longitudinal study, early gestational exposure to maternal cortisol was associated with emotional difficulties and larger volume in the right amygdala in girls at age 7 (Buss et al., 2012). These findings are consistent with substantial animal research documenting heightened stress reactivity in the offspring of experimentally stressed pregnant females (Weinstock, 2008). Prenatal stress exposure contributes to changes in developing neurobiological systems that help to account for children's greater reactivity to challenge and threat, consistent with the view that these prenatal conditions foster biological adaptations to a postnatal life of adversity and challenge.

These "fetal programming" effects anticipate the effects of direct experiences of stress after children are born. There is growing evidence that early adversity and stress alter developing biological systems as well as behavior. In a longitudinal study of children living in poverty, for example, environmental characteristics like poor housing quality, economic strain, and poor parenting were associated with disrupted activity of the hypothalamic–pituitary–adrenocortical (HPA) axis, a major component of biological stress reactivity, in children from 7 months to age 4 (Blair et al., 2011). Another study of poor children found that toddlers living in families characterized by violence between parents and mothers' "emotional unavailability" to the child also exhibited disruptions in normal HPA activity (Sturge-Apple, Davies, Cicchetti, & Manning, 2012). In older children, dysregulated HPA activity was associated with lower family socioeconomic status, and older children showing this pattern of HPA disruption were more likely to have mothers with symptoms of depression (Lupien, King, Meaney, & McEwen, 2000). Children exposed to chronic stress, which is associated with poverty, family conflict, and/or parenting problems, exhibit atypical patterns of biological stress responding that are adaptations to the aversive environmental conditions in which they live.

Contrary to the concept of "toxic stress," however, there are at least two kinds of HPA dysregulation that have been identified in children in these circumstances (Bruce, Gunnar, Pears, & Fisher, 2013). In one, children become hyperreactive to stress in the form of higher basal or acute HPA levels that may reflect adaptations to chronic threat or danger. In another, children become hyporesponsive in the form of suppressed HPA reactivity or lower basal levels that may develop in response to the deprivation or withdrawal of social support. These different patterns are important, especially in their association with different aspects of parental nurturance—protection from threat and nurturant care—that likely constitute significant cues to young organisms about the safety or danger of the world in which they live. They also illustrate the associations between contextual challenge, relational experience, and the organization of biological systems in young children.

Children in conditions of chronic stress also exhibit behavioral problems, such as heightened vigilance, emotional reactivity, and self-regulatory difficulties that may be manifested in poorer coping, cognitive and attention problems, poorer emotion regulation, and difficulty in social functioning (Blair & Raver, 2012; Evans & Kim, 2013). These behavioral problems are associated with dysregulation of the HPA system and its effects on the limbic and cortical systems that regulate HPA activity, including prefrontal areas and limbic structures, especially the amygdala, hypothalamus, and hippocampus (Ulrich-Lai & Herman, 2009). Thus, consistent with a biopsychosocial model, the behavioral characteristics of children in chronic stress have complex and multifaceted biological bases. Moreover, chronic stress is associated with other biological challenges that further contribute to these behavioral consequences. Stress is associated with sharp increases in autonomic activity, including elevated blood pressure, sleep disruptions, and other correlates (El-Sheikh & Erath, 2011). Stress also undermines immune response to infectious challenges, increasing cytokine response and generally embedding "proinflammatory tendencies" into biological functioning (Miller, Chen, & Parker, 2011). Considered together, the biological and behavioral correlates of chronic stress, especially experienced in childhood, are consistent with the portrayal of allostatic load: the progressive dysregulation of biological systems attributable to the long-term effects of chronic stress activation (Danese & McEwen, 2012).

Biopsychosocial research on the effects of chronic stress in the early years is consistent with the model of a biologically dynamic, experience-driven developmental system, in which biological and behavioral systems adapt to cues concerning the environmental conditions in which children must live. If early experiences of family conflict, limited resources, and poor parenting signal the continuing probability of aversive conditions, then it makes sense that biological systems reorganize to contribute to the allocation of mental resources to threat vigilance, foster quick and strong reactions to perceptions of danger, enable rapid mobilization of energy, and related characteristics. There are, of course, important trade-offs to such an orientation. Mental resources devoted to vigilance cannot as readily be devoted to learning, problem solving, and other long-term investments in general behavioral competence. A social orientation to threat detection also makes it more difficult to develop constructive relationships. Moreover, a behavioral pattern adapted to conditions of adversity based on family experience may be poorly suited to other settings—such as at school and with peers—that require a different and more constructive repertoire of behavioral skills. These biological adaptations are also taxing. Consistent with the concept of allostatic load, considerable research documents the long-term physical and mental health vulnerabilities of individuals who grow up or live in conditions of chronic stress (Danese & McEwen, 2012).

Fortunately, studies of early stress reactivity also document the social buffering of stress for children. Stated simply, when caregivers can provide social and emotional support to children experiencing threat or challenge, children's reactivity is diminished and over time HPA functioning can become normalized (Hostinar, Sullivan, & Gunnar, 2014). This conclusion, which has been demonstrated in studies with children and animals, further illustrates the biopsychosocial connections among context, psychological functioning, and biological organization. It also provides the basis for considering the kinds of interventions that might benefit children experiencing chronic stress, especially because their parents are likely to be stressed by the same conditions that create difficulty for children, or parents themselves are sources of stress. In either case, it is important either to help parents provide a more safe, secure caregiving environment for their offspring (in the form of two-generation interventions), or to enlist other adults who can do so, to better buffer stress for children (Thompson & Haskins, 2014).

There are a number of illustrations of interventions for young children in adversity that have been guided by an appreciation of the interaction of context, relationships, and biological functioning. Intervention studies of young children in foster care by Phil Fisher and Mary Dozier show, for example, that when foster parents were provided support to reduce their own stress and guidance in developing warm, responsive relationships with foster children that encouraged the child's self-regulation, children showed progressively more typical patterns of HPA reactivity over the course of the intervention (Dozier, Peloso, Lewis, Laurenceau, & Levine, 2008; Dozier et al., 2006; Fisher, Stoolmiller, Gunnar, & Burraston, 2007; Fisher, Van Ryzin, & Gunnar, 2011). In each study, moreover, foster children showed increasing evidence of developing supportive attachments to their foster parents. Another research team showed that after 3½ years of participation in a conditional cash-transfer antipoverty program in Mexico, preschool children showed more typical levels of basal HPA functioning, and children of the most depressed mothers showed the greatest benefit (Fernald & Gunnar, 2009). In another example, an intervention program for at-risk 4-year-olds was shown to be effective in normalizing cortisol reactivity and this led, in turn, to reductions in children's aggression by the follow-up assessment (O'Neal et al., 2010). Each of these studies illustrates the coordinated changes in behavior and biology in children deriving from biologically informed interventions to alter the social context of their lives to increase support and the buffering of stress.

There are limits, of course, to the social buffering of children's stress reactivity. The interventions described in these studies occurred over periods of months or years, underscoring that such benefits do not come easily or quickly. Moreover, other studies have shown that for young children in extremely aversive circumstances, even years of supportive adoptive care were ineffective in fostering HPA axis recovery (Gunnar, Morison, Chisholm, & Schuder, 2001). But in addition to providing further illustration of experience-driven developmental changes in biological functioning, these studies also highlight the importance of their relational context. In most of these interventions, researchers focused on improving caregiver responsiveness and warmth, often by removing sources of stress on the adult's experience, so they could provide more reliable support to children under stress. This suggests the importance of relational support in the family environment to the stability and normalization of biological and behavioral stress reactivity, and of the significance of two-generation interventions to accomplish this in children at risk (Thompson, 2014).

The research on early stress reactivity is important for several other reasons. First, in documenting how early adversity "gets under the skin" to affect the developing organization of multiple biological systems, these studies cast a fresh light on the challenges of children who live in poverty, dysfunctional families, or other aversive conditions. Academic underachievement, behavioral problems, and the self-regulatory difficulties characteristic of children in chronic stress derives, in part, from the "biological programming" of early experience (Farah et al., 2006; Hackman & Farah, 2008). Understanding the biopsychosocial origins of these behavioral problems provides a corrective to simple characterizations of these children as difficult, uncooperative, or unmotivated, and suggests that providing social support as a stress buffer may be important to promoting early cognitive and social competence. Second, these studies highlight the value of biologically informed interventions to provide assistance, focused especially on relational support as a buffer on stress and self-regulatory assistance to foster behavioral competence. These interventions can occur in the family or in out-of-home care and early education settings. Concerning the latter, research-informed interventions to strengthen the self-regulatory skills in children at risk in their preschool programs have been shown to be effective in strengthening social and cognitive competencies (e.g., Raver et al., 2009, 2011). Third, research on stress reactivity underscores the importance of early intervention in light of the relative plasticity of developing biological and behavioral systems in the early years (Thompson & Haskins, 2014). Studies of the experiential shaping of the HPA system and other biological processes add weight to a focus on the early years for the identification of children at psychosocial risk and intervention to assist them.

Developing Emotion Regulation

Understanding the development of emotion regulation and the origins of individual differences in self-regulatory capability is also important for scientific and practical reasons. Emotion regulation is associated with social competence, academic achievement, and personal well-being (Calkins & Leerkes, 2011; Thompson, 2015), and distinguishing children with developmentally appropriate skills from those who struggle with emotional self-control has been a long-standing focus of research and intervention. This is especially true in developmental psychopathology in which poor emotion self-regulation is a typical correlate of children with internalizing or externalizing disorders, who are maltreated or living in troubled families, or face other challenges (see, e.g., Kring & Sloan, 2010). Parents are also concerned with fostering competent emotion regulation in offspring. Because parents typically overestimate how much young children can manage their feelings, conflict between these expectations and children's actual self-regulatory abilities can be a family challenge (Newton & Thompson, 2010).

As a biopsychosocial process, therefore, the development of emotion regulation integrates influences from socialization and culture with neurobiological maturation and with children's understanding of emotion management. In interaction over time, these processes contribute to the development of self-regulatory competence through the maturation of prefrontal brain regions, the growth of executive functions, better understanding of cultural expectations for emotional control, more sophisticated representations of emotion regulation strategies, and the support and coaching of parents and other adults (Thompson, 2011, 2015). Emotion regulation is, however, a biologically dynamic, experience-driven developmental process. Although it is typical to think of children becoming progressively more competent at emotional self-regulation as they mature, some developmental transitions—such as during adolescence—can conditionally undermine self-regulatory competence. According to some views, vulnerability to emotion-instigated risk taking increases during adolescence because of rapidly developing subcortical brain areas and hormonal changes accompanying puberty that enhance sensitivity to social reward, while prefrontal cortical areas that underlie self-regulation remain relatively immature (Casey & Caudle, 2013). These biological changes pose challenges to effective emotion self-regulation in certain circumstancees, especially in the context of peer experiences that enhance these vulnerabilities.

The development of emotion regulation is biologically dynamic and experience driven in other ways. Following traditional models of emotion, the development of emotion regulation is often portrayed as the imposition of cognitive controls (such as executive functions) or cortical controls (such as prefrontal cortical regulation) to inhibit emotional activation. This view is useful but incomplete because of the mutual influences of many brain areas relevant to emotion activation and control. Contemporary research on the neurobiology of emotion indicates that responses to emotional stimuli activate complex neural networks that are widely distributed throughout the brain, integrating areas typically regarded as important to emotion activation (including the amygdala, hypothalamus, brain stem, and striatum) with those viewed as crucial to emotion regulation (including the lateral and medial prefrontal cortex and anterior cingulate). There is increasing evidence from neuroimaging studies that these multilevel emotion-relevant areas are *coactive* in response to emotion stimuli rather than functioning primarily in activation–inhibition associations (Kober et al., 2008; Ochsner et al., 2009; Ulrich-Lai & Herman, 2009). Stated differently, emotion regulation can function in a conventional "top-down" fashion (such as how prefrontal processes regulate amygdala function) or in a "bottom-up" fashion (such as how conditioned fear arising from limbic processes alters higher-level threat detection).

The mutual, bidirectional influences between higher and lower brain systems makes emotion regulation a more dynamic process than a simplified inhibitory model because of the multiple sources of regulatory influence throughout the system. This is true of both typical and atypical functioning. Affective psychopathology is associated, for example, with disrupted interactions between cortical and limbic systems that normally function to modulate emotional arousal. This has been found in studies of depression and anxiety in children and adults, with changes in the functioning and coordination of limbic and cortical emotion-related areas coinciding with treatment efficacy (Johnstone, van Reekum, Urry, Kalin, & Davidson, 2007; Lewis et al., 2008; Nitschke et al., 2009). Thus, risk for affective psychopathology can arise from various levels of the neurobiology of emotion and their interaction, with different potential avenues for therapeutic intervention (Ochsner et al., 2009).

These neurobiological systems are also shaped by the quality of early experience and thus reflect developmental history (Calkins & Hill, 2007). This conclusion is consistent with the research reviewed earlier on the development of stress reactivity and the social buffering of stress that highlighted the potential for the development of dysregulated patterns of emotional reactivity in conditions of inadequate care. Neurobiological systems governing self-regulation, such as parasympathetic regulation, are also developmentally influenced by the quality of early experience, particularly the nurturance and support of caregivers (Propper & Moore, 2006). In many respects, it would be surprising not to find this to be true. Responding appropriately to emotional stimuli requires adapting the organization of biological and behavioral emotion systems to cues concerning environmental threat or security conveyed by the quality of parental care. In aversive circumstances, emotions systems affording sensitivity to threat and quick and strong reactivity are more likely to benefit the organism than those promoting emotion modulation and complex secondary appraisals of events.

Early experiential influences on developing systems of emotion and self-regulation can have far-reaching consequences, moreover, if they contribute to biases in emotion appraisals encoded in the functioning of neurobiological systems involved in emotional arousal. Fear conditioning is one example of how early experience can enhance perceptual sensitivity to cues of danger at lower levels of the neuroaxis that bias higher-level emotion appraisals (Ochsner et al., 2009; Surguladze et al., 2003). Early emotional biases can have enduring influences on emotion responding in part through their influence on higher cognitive processes (e.g., anxious rumination; Calkins & Hill, 2007). In one study, 2-year-olds who were behaviorally identified as emotionally inhibited or uninhibited were later studied as adults, and functional magnetic resonance imaging (fMRI) analyses revealed heightened amygdala activation in the inhibited group when viewing novel (vs. familiar) faces, but no differences in the uninhibited group (Schwartz, Wright, Shin, Kagan, & Rauch, 2003). Early experience is important for the developing organization of emotion-relevant neurobiological systems and their interaction.

In concert with these neurobiological changes, early experiences also influence the development of behavioral strategies of emotion self-regulation. From a functionalist perspective, children (and adults) manage their emotions to accomplish goals, and these goals are both developmentally changing and socioculturally shaped (Thompson, 2011, 2015). Children increasingly understand, for example, that some ways of responding emotionally may be more appropriate when parents are present than with peers because of the responses they can expect from each partner (Thompson & Waters, 2010). In other contexts, emotion regulation strategies are adapted to the specific, sometimes powerful, emotional demands of everyday experience. Young children who are behaviorally inhibited and prone to anxiety disorders show hypervigilance in situations associated with fearful events, attentionally orienting to anxiety-provoking stimuli, with a tendency to construe benign situations as disproportionately threatening (Fox, Henderson, Marshall, Nichols, & Ghera, 2005). These appraisal and preappraisal processes develop to accomplish the immediate goal of avoiding anxiety-provoking events despite their broader dysfunctional consequences for behavioral competence. Children in families characterized by frequent marital conflict engage in strategies to preserve a sense of security in their parents' relationship but which also render them more vulnerable to emotional problems. These strategies include trying to mediate, comfort, or pacify parents; aggressing against one or both parents; and maintaining perceptual vigilance to cues of impending conflict, with each strategy potentially costing further enmeshment in parental conflict (Davies & Woitach, 2008). Children who are maltreated maintain heightened vigilance for signs of adult anger that may foreshadow further abuse, and have difficulty attentionally disengaging from such cues even though it heightens their own emotional vulnerability (Pollak, 2008). This enables them to anticipate a potentially abusive encounter with an adult (and the possibility of avoidance or escape) even though this vigilance is emotionally demanding and socially costly when generalized to other partners. In these contexts, children's emotion regulation strategies purchase immediate coping and potential relief from emotional challenges at the cost of longer-term behavioral competence and emotional well-being. Their strategies enable them to function more adaptively in the contexts in which these strategies develop, but they may not function comparably in other contexts. Emotion regulation is, for them, a double-edged sword.

An important task for biopsychosocial analysis is to better understand how these contextual demands on emotion regulation contribute to linked biological, behavioral, and representational processes relevant to how children manage their emotions in these situations. How do the neurobiological systems mediating hypervigilance to danger or heightened reactivity to threat influence children's representations of emotion and their management? How do their strategies for emotion regulation differ when escape or avoidance is possible compared with when it is not? For children whose HPA reactivity is hyporesponsive in the context of neglect or withdrawal of support, how do they represent emotional experience and its regulation? In what ways can the availability of extrafamilial social support function as a psychosocial and/or neurobiological buffer for such children (Thompson & Goodwin, in press)? These and other research questions arise from efforts to link biological, psychological, and contextual processes relevant to developing emotion regulation for at-risk children.

These questions underscore that simple characterizations of children in these circumstances as "emotionally dysregulated" is only the beginning of an incisive analysis of their management of emotion. Emotion regulation is effective only in relation to the contexts in which emotion is managed and the goals of the individual. For children in difficult contexts, the inherent trade-offs that are involved in purchasing immediate coping at the cost of longer-term behavioral competence makes it easier to see why children in these contexts respond as they do, and why their longer-term adjustment is threatened as a result. The problem is not that they are deficient in coping skills, but that they are striving to cope with emotionally impossible demands with limited options. This recognition focuses attention to the kinds of assistance that might be possible to provide children with greater options for coping with difficult circumstances, including the availability of social support from individuals within and outside the family (Thompson & Haskins, 2014).

Cautions, Caveats, and Conclusions

The contributors to this section, and to this volume, underscore the considerable scientific potential of biopsychosocial models of socioemotional development—and of development more generally. In addition to the opportunity to truly bridge the nature–nurture polarity, such models provide a forum in which to better understand the mutual influences of biology, behavior, and context. As researchers are increasingly understanding development as a biologically dynamic, experience-driven process, such models are increasingly warranted. Yet we have a long way to go toward realizing the scientific potential of this approach, and several obstacles to overcome along the way.

One obstacle concerns the limited state of our current understanding of the biology of human behavior. The astonishing advances in neuroscience, molecular genetics, and developmental biology have both dramatically expanded current understanding and overturned conclusions that were conventional knowledge just a couple of decades ago. They invite humility in our current understanding of these biological foundations. In a scientific context in which different imaging studies indicate somewhat different psychological correlates of specified brain areas, where molecular genetics analyses struggle to replicate previously reported associations between specific alleles and behavioral characteristics, and the "missing heritability" problem looms large (Plomin, 2013; Turkheimer, 2011), it is clear that researchers seeking to develop informative biopsychosocial models must seek clearer understanding of the biological side of this interaction.

This leads to a second obstacle: the challenge of connecting biology to behavior. Until our understanding of the behavioral correlates of the activation of specific brain regions or gene alleles is better specified, applications of neuroscience or molecular genetics to behavioral development risk misapplication and overgeneralization. This is especially true when the behavior we seek to explain biologically is nonspecific. One example is the current debate about the influence of developmental neurobiology on adolescent risk taking (Thompson, 2012). As Casey and Caudle (2013) have noted, some brain-based explanations of adolescent risk taking have been overgeneralized to apply, it seems, to stereotyped portrayals of the rebellious, delinquent teenager. This is a problem because the stereotype is not reality: only a small proportion of adolescents exhibit serious problems with drug use, criminality, and other risky behaviors (Steinberg, 2008). Thus, understanding how the neurobiological changes associated with adolescence are behaviorally influential requires a more specific characterization of the behavioral vulnerability to be biologically explained (in this case, context-dependent challenges involving heightened reward, especially with peers). Biopsychosocial models need specific, research-based conceptualizations of behavior and biology to forge an informative integration.

One reason it is challenging to connect biology with behavior is that we are informed and haunted by our history. Alongside the nature–nurture dichotomy, psychologists have long adopted a materialist orientation to psychological phenomena, preferring biologically based explanations that appear tangible and perceptible over phenomenological explanations that, while also measurable, seem more subjective and even ethereal (see Barrett, 2009). Consequently, identifying the biological substrate of behavior is a more intuitively acceptable approach to understanding biopsychosocial processes than studying the psychological bases of biology, such as the experiential foundations of synaptogenesis or the emotional processes contributing to behavioral epigenetics. It will require time and effort to move beyond the materialist orientation of our history to fully appreciate the mutual influences of biology and behavior throughout development and in psychological functioning.

A final, but formidable, obstacle to be overcome concerns the technological innovations that simultaneously inform developmental science but can also misinform it. In a remarkable collection of articles about physiological measures of emotion from a developmental perspective (Dennis, Buss, & Hastings, 2012), contributors illuminated the uses of biological methods, recording technology, and statistical modeling and the interpretive pitfalls that can accompany their use. The timing of measurement in relation to the time course of emotion, the interpretation of biological activity in psychologically relevant terms, developmental changes in biological systems, and the use of statistical methods (and sample sizes) appropriate to the amount of data generated are some of the challenges these authors profiled. These challenges should not, of course, deter developmental researchers from enlisting these methods into their studies, but they should instill thoughtful care and caution in their implementation and interpretation.

In a similar manner, these cautions and caveats concerning the future of research on biopsychosocial models of development derive from excitement concerning their scientific potential and the expectation that it will continue. We have a long way to go, but much progress has been made in reweaving the strands, and there is reason for excitement about the future.

REFERENCES

Barker, D. J. (2002). Fetal programming of coronary heart disease. *Trends in Endocrinology and Metabolism, 13,* 364–368.

Barrett, L. F. (2009). The future of psychology: Connecting mind to brain. *Perspectives on Psychological Science, 4,* 326–339.

Belsky, J., Steinberg, L., Houts, R. M., Halpern-Felsher, B. L., & the NICHD Early Child Care Research Network. (2010). Development of reproductive strategy in females: Early maternal harshness → earlier menarche → increased sexual risk taking. *Developmental Psychology, 46,* 120–128.

Blair, C., & Raver, C. C. (2012). Child development in the context of adversity: Experiential canalization of brain and behavior. *American Psychologist, 67,* 309–318.

Blair, C., Raver, C. C., Granger, D., Mills-Koonce, R., Hibel, L., & the Family Life Project Key Investigators. (2011). Allostasis and allostatic load in the context of poverty in early childhood. *Development and Psychopathology, 23,* 845–857.

Bruce, J., Gunnar, M. R., Pears, K. C., & Fisher, P. A. (2013). Early adverse care, stress neurobiology, and prevention science: Lessons learned. *Prevention Science, 14,* 247–256.

Buss, C., Davis, E. P., Shahbaba, B., Pruessner, J. C., Head, K., & Sandman, C. A. (2012). Maternal cortisol over the course of pregnancy and subsequent child amygdala and hippocampus volumes and affective problems. *Proceedings of the National Academy of Sciences, 109,* E1312–E1319.

Calkins, S. D., & Hill, A. (2007). Caregiver influences on emerging emotion regulation: Biological and environmental transactions in early development. In J. Gross (Ed.), *Handbook of emotion regulation* (pp. 229–248). New York: Guilford Press.

Calkins, S. D., & Leerkes, E. M. (2011). Early attachment processes and the development of emotional self-regulation. In K. D. Vohs & R. F. Baumeister (Eds.), *Handbook of self-regulation* (pp. 355–373). New York: Guilford Press.

Casey, B. J., & Caudle, K. (2013). The teenage brain: Self control. *Current Directions in Psychological Science, 22,* 82–87.

Charney, E. (2012). Behavior genetics and postgenomics. *Behavioral and Brain Sciences, 35,* 331–410.

Chisholm, J. S. (1996). The evolutionary ecology of attachment organization. *Human Nature, 1,* 1–37.

Committee on Integrating the Science of Early Childhood Development, National Research Council. (2000). *From neurons to neighborhoods: The science of early childhood development.* Washington, DC: National Academy Press.

Danese, A., & McEwen, B. (2012). Childhood experiences, allostasis, allostatic load, and age-related disease. *Physiology and Behavior, 106,* 29–39.

Davies, P. T., & Woitach, M. J. (2008). Children's emotional security in the interparental relationship. *Current Directions in Psychological Science, 17,* 269–274.

Davis, E. P., Glynn, L. M., Waffarn, F., & Sandman, C. A. (2011). Prenatal maternal stress programs infant stress regulation. *Journal of Child Psychology and Psychiatry, 52,* 119–129.

Dennis, T. A., Buss, K. A., & Hastings, P. D. (Eds.). (2012). Physiological measures of emotion from a developmental perspective: State of the science. *Monographs of the Society for Research in Child Development, 77*(Serial No. 303).

Dozier, M., Peloso, E., Lewis, E., Laurenceau, J.-P., & Levine, S. (2008). Effects of an attachment-based intervention on the cortisol production of infants and toddlers in foster care. *Development and Psychopathology, 20,* 845–859.

Dozier, M., Peloso, E., Lindheim, O., Gordon, M. K., Manni, M., Sepulveda, S., et al. (2006). Developing evidence-based interventions for foster children: An example of a randomized clinical trial with infants and toddlers. *Journal of Social Issues, 62,* 767–785.

El-Sheikh, M., & Erath, S. A. (2011). Family conflict, autonomic nervous system functioning, and child adaptation: State of the science and future directions. *Development and Psychopathology, 23*, 703–721.

Evans, G. W., & Kim, P. (2013). Childhood poverty, chronic stress, self-regulation, and coping. *Child Development Perspectives, 7*, 43–48.

Farah, M. J., Shera, D. M., Savage, J. H., Betancourt, L., Giannetta, J. M., Brodsky, N. L., et al. (2006). Childhood poverty: Specific associations with neurocognitive development. *Brain Research, 1110*, 166–174.

Fernald, L. C. H., & Gunnar, M. R. (2009). Poverty-alleviation program participation and salivary cortisol in very low-income children. *Social Science and Medicine, 68*, 2180–2189.

Fisher, P. A., Stoolmiller, M., Gunnar, M. R., & Burraston, B. O. (2007). Effects of a therapeutic intervention for foster preschoolers on diurnal cortisol activity. *Psychoneuroendocrinology, 32*, 892–905

Fisher, P. A., Van Ryzin, M. J., & Gunnar, M. R. (2011). Mitigating HPA axis dysregulation associated with placement changes in foster care. *Psychoneuroendocrinology, 36*, 531–539.

Fox, N. A., Henderson, H. A., Marshall, P. J., Nichols, K. E., & Ghera, M. M. (2005). Behavioral inhibition: Linking biology and behavior within a developmental framework. *Annual Review of Psychology, 56*, 235–262.

Gluckman, P., & Hanson, M. (2005). *The fetal matrix.* Cambridge, UK: Cambridge University Press.

Gunnar, M. R., Morison, S. J., Chisholm, K., & Schuder, M. (2001). Salivary cortisol levels in children adopted from Romanian orphanages. *Development and Psychopathology, 13*, 611–628.

Hackman, D. A., & Farah, M. J. (2008). Socioeconomic status and the developing brain. *Trends in Cognitive Sciences, 13*, 65–73.

Hostinar, C. E., Sullivan, R. M., & Gunnar, M. R. (2014). Psychobiological mechanisms underlying the social buffering of the hypothalamic–pituitary–adrenocortical axis: A review of animal models and human studies across development. *Psychological Bulletin, 140*, 256–282.

Hunt, J. M. (1961). *Intelligence and experience.* New York: Ronald Press.

Johnstone, T., van Reekum, C. M., Urry, H. L., Kalin, N. H., & Davidson, R. J. (2007). Failure to regulate: Counterproductive recruitment of top-down prefrontal-subcortical circuitry in major depression. *Journal of Neuroscience, 27*, 8877–8884.

Kober, H., Barrett, L. F., Joseph, J., Bliss-Moreau, E., Lindquist, K., & Wager, T. D. (2008). Functional grouping and cortical–subcortical interactions in emotion: A meta-analysis of neuroimaging studies. *NeuroImage, 42*, 998–1031.

Kring, A., & Sloan, D. (Eds.). (2010). *Emotion regulation and psychopathology.* New York: Guilford Press.

Kuhl, P. K. (2007). Is speech learning "gated" by the social brain? *Developmental Science, 10*, 110–120.

Kuhl, P. K., Conboy, B. T., Coffey-Corina, S., Padden, D., Rivera-Gaxiola, M., & Nelson, T. (2008). Phonetic learning as a pathway to language: New data and native language magnet theory expanded (NLM-e). *Philosophical Transactions of the Royal Society B: Biological Sciences, 363*, 979–1000.

Lewis, M. D., Granic, I., Lamm, C., Zelazo, P. D., Stieben, J., Todd, R. M., et al. (2008). Changes in the neural bases of emotion regulation associated with clinical improvement in children with behavior problems. *Development and Psychopathology, 20,* 913–939.

Lupien, S. J., King, S., Meaney, M. J., & McEwen, B. S. (2000). Child's stress hormone levels correlate with mother's socioeconomic status and depressive state. *Biological Psychiatry, 48,* 976–980.

Miller, G. E., Chen, E., & Parker, K. J. (2011). Psychological stress in childhood and susceptibility to the chronic diseases of aging: Moving toward a model of behavioral and biological mechanisms. *Psychological Bulletin, 137,* 959–997.

Nathanielsz, P. W. (1999). *Life in the womb: The origin of health and disease.* Ithaca, NY: Promethean Press.

Newton, E. K., & Thompson, R. A. (2010). Parents' views of early social and emotional development: More and less than meets the eye. *Zero to Three, 31,* 10–15.

Nitschke, J. B., Sarinopoulos, I., Oathes, D. J., Johnstone, T., Whalen, P. J., Davidson, R. J., et al. (2009). Anticipatory activation in the amygdala and anterior cingulate in generalized anxiety disorder and prediction of treatment response. *American Journal of Psychiatry, 166,* 302–310.

Oberlander, T. F., Weinberg, J., Papsdorf, M., Grunau, R., Misri, S., & Devlin, A. M. (2008). Prenatal exposure to maternal depression, neonatal methylation of human glucocorticoid receptor gene (*NR3C1*) and infant cortisol stress responses. *Epigenetics, 3,* 97–106.

Ochsner, K. N., Ray, R. R., Hughes, B., McRae, K., Cooper, J. C., Weber, J., et al. (2009). Bottom-up and top-down processes in emotion generation: Common and distinct neural mechanisms. *Psychological Science, 20,* 1322–1331.

O'Neal, C. R., Brotman, L. M., Huang, K.-Y., Gouley, K. K., Kamboukos, D., Calzada, E. J., et al. (2010). Understanding relations among early family environment, cortisol response, and child aggression via a prevention experiment. *Child Development, 81,* 290–305.

Plomin, R. (2013). Child development and molecular genetics: 14 years later. *Child Development, 84,* 104–120.

Pollak, S. D. (2008). Mechanisms linking early experience and the emergence of emotions: Illustrations from the study of maltreated children. *Current Directions in Psychological Science, 17,* 370–375.

Propper, C., & Moore, G. A. (2006). The influence of parenting on infant emotionality: A multi-level psychobiological perspective. *Developmental Review, 26,* 427–460.

Raver, C. C., Jones, S. M., Li-Grining, C., Zhai, F., Bub, K., & Pressler, E. (2011). CSRP's impact on low-income preschoolers' preacademic skills: Self-regulation as a mediating mechanism. *Child Development, 82,* 362–378.

Raver, C. C., Jones, S. M., Li-Grining, C., Zhai, F., Metzger, M. M., & Solomon, B. (2009). Targeting children's behavior problems in preschool classrooms: A cluster-randomized controlled trial. *Journal of Consulting and Clinical Psychology, 77,* 302–316.

Schwartz, C., Wright, C., Shin, L., Kagan, J., & Rauch, S. (2003). Inhibited and uninhibited infants "grown up": Adult amygdalar response to novelty. *Science, 300,* 1952–1953.

Stearns, S. C. (1992). *The evolution of life histories.* Oxford, UK: Oxford University Press.

Steinberg, L. (2008). *Adolescence* (8th ed.). New York: McGraw-Hill.

Sturge-Apple, M. L., Davies, P. T., Cicchetti, D., & Manning, L. G. (2012). Interparental violence, maternal emotional unavailability and children's cortisol functioning in family contexts. *Developmental Psychology, 48,* 237–249.

Surguladze, S. A., Brammer, M. J., Young, A. W., Andrew, C., Travis, M. J., Williams, S. C. R., et al. (2003). A preferential increase in the extrastriate response to signals of danger. *NeuroImage, 19,* 1317–1328.

Thompson, R. A. (2011). Emotion and emotion regulation: Two sides of the developing coin. *Emotion Review, 3,* 53–61.

Thompson, R. A. (2012). Bridging developmental neuroscience and the law: Child–caregiver relationships. *Hastings Law Journal, 63,* 1443–1468.

Thompson, R. A. (2014). Stress and child development. *The Future of Children, 24,* 41–59.

Thompson, R. A. (2015). Relationships, regulation, and early development. In R. M. Lerner (Ed.), *Handbook of child psychology and developmental science: Vol. 3. Social and emotional development* (7th ed., pp. 201–246). New York: Wiley.

Thompson, R. A., & Goodvin, R. (in press). Social support and developmental psychopathology. In D. Cicchetti (Ed.), *Developmental psychopathology* (3rd ed.). New York: Wiley.

Thompson, R. A., & Haskins, R. (2014, Spring). Early stress gets under the skin: Promising initiatives to help children facing chronic adversity. *The Future of Children Policy Brief,* 1–7.

Thompson, R. A., & Waters, S. F. (2010). The development of emotion regulation: Parent and peer influences. In R. Sanchez-Aragon (Ed.), *Regulación Emocional: Una Travesia de la Cultura a la Formacion de las Relaciones Personales [Emotion regulation: A crossing from culture to the development of personal relationships]* (pp. 125–157). Mexico: Universidad Nacional Autonoma de Mexico [National Autonomous University of Mexico].

Turkheimer, E. (2011). Still missing. *Research in Human Development, 8,* 227–241.

Ulrich-Lai, Y. M., & Herman, J. P. (2009). Neural regulation of endocrine and autonomic stress responses. *Nature Reviews Neuroscience, 10,* 397–409.

Weinstock, M. (2008). Long-term behavioural consequences of prenatal stress. *Neuroscience and Biobehavioral Reviews, 32,* 1073–1086.

Werker, J. F. (2003). Baby steps to learning language. *Journal of Pediatrics, 143,* 62–69.

CHAPTER 10

A Psychobiological Perspective on Emotional Development within the Family Context

Esther M. Leerkes and Stephanie H. Parade

In this chapter, we examine the mechanisms by which the family environment and infants' biological reactivity and regulation are related to infants' emotional development. Although emotional development during infancy involves the acquisition of a number of fundamental skills, we focus on studies that predict emotion and behavioral regulation because deficits in these areas have long-term implications for subsequent social relations, academic performance, and mental health (Calkins, 2009). We recognize that the family context begins to exert an effect on infants' biological development and subsequent well-being during the prenatal period (e.g., Luecken et al., 2013), but inclusion of this rapidly growing literature is beyond the scope of this chapter. Thus we focus on the postnatal family context, specifically maternal and paternal caregiving behavior, and expressed affect and interparental relationship dynamics. Two biological systems are addressed: the hypothalamic–pituitary–adrenocortical (HPA) system and the parasympathetic branch of the autonomic nervous system (PNS) with an emphasis on infant vagal regulation. We lay out three pathways: (1) sensitive parental behavior, regulated parental affect, and harmonious couple dynamics promote adaptive physiological arousal and regulation, which in turn support children's adaptive emotional development; (2) the family context interacts with infants' physiological reactivity and regulation to predict subsequent emotional development; and (3) infant characteristics, including physiological arousal and regulation, and the family context influence each other and

206

subsequent child outcomes via a series of transactions. Recommendations for future research are noted throughout the review.

Overview of Relevant Biological Systems and Links with Emotional Development

Constitutionally based individual differences in reactivity to the environment and the ability to regulate that reactivity, referred to as temperament, is widely accepted to set children on distinct developmental trajectories that influence later socioemotional outcomes, and this perspective has existed, in at least rudimentary form, for over a century (Rothbart, 2011). For example, infants who are easily distressed and struggle to regulate their distress effectively are predisposed to later psychopathology (Crockenberg, Leerkes, & Barrig Jo, 2008). Efforts to understand the biological mechanisms that underlie these individual differences and to understand how they work in conjunction with the environment to predict subsequent outcomes have proliferated in recent decades with attention to neural activation in specific brain regions and hormonal and autonomic responses to stressful and nonstressful stimuli (Fox, Henderson, Pérez-Edgar, & White, 2008). Two biological systems that have received a good deal of attention in the literature to date are the HPA system and the PNS. Focus on these systems is well justified in the study of infant emotional development because both (1) are demonstrated to "come online" in early development, (2) are of integral importance to the regulation of state and mood, (3) are well-grounded in parallel animal research, and (4) have reasonably good methods in place to measure their functioning in infancy and beyond.

The HPA System

The HPA axis is a neuroendocrine system believed to underlie links between family context and children's emotional and behavioral health. When exposed to stress the HPA axis is activated and a hormonal cascade is set into motion. Corticotropin-releasing hormone (CRH) is secreted from the hypothalamus-stimulating production of adrenocorticotropic hormone (ACTH) in the anterior pituitary. These processes result in the release of glucocorticoids from the adrenal cortex that contribute to negative feedback by binding to glucocorticoid receptors that inhibit production of additional CRH and ATCH. This negative feedback loop represents HPA system effort to maintain homeostasis. In humans, cortisol is the primary glucocorticoid released and is a commonly assessed measure of HPA activity (see Gunnar & Cheatham, 2003, for a review). A temporary increase in cortisol production in response to acute stress is adaptive, and the cortisol stress response is detectable at birth (Jansen, Beijers, Riksen-Walraven, & de Weerth, 2010; Gunnar & Cheatham, 2003). Although cortisol production typically increases in response to stress, basal levels of cortisol are necessary for the developing brain, and cortisol plays a pivotal role in metabolic and immune functioning (Sapolsky, Romero, & Munck, 2000). A typical diurnal pattern of basal cortisol production that peaks upon awakening then declines across the day is evident by 12 months (Larson, White, Cochran, Donzella, & Gunnar, 1998; Watamura, Donzella, Kertes, & Gunnar, 2004).

Although cortisol production in response to stress is adaptive in the moment, accumulating evidence suggests that chronic activation of the HPA axis in infancy and early childhood contributes to dysregulated HPA functioning (Gunnar & Vazquez, 2001, 2006; McEwen, 2012). Dysregulated HPA functioning as a consequence of stress exposure may be reflected through either hyper- or hypoactivity of the HPA axis, the direction of which is hypothesized to depend on the chronicity, timing, and severity of stress exposure (Bruce, Gunnar, Pears, & Fisher, 2013; Miller, Chen, & Zhou, 2007; Tarullo & Gunnar, 2006). *Hypercortisolism*, excessive activation of the HPA axis, may manifest itself as an initial response to chronic stress as the neuroendocrine system repeatedly mobilizes itself to prepare for threat. This increasing sensitivity of the HPA axis is reflected in an exaggerated cortisol stress response. However, over time repeated stress exposure may result in a down regulation of the HPA axis as the system attempts to maintain homeostasis and adapt to contextual stressors. Consequently, *hypocortisolism* is reflected in a blunted diurnal rhythm (attenuated basal cortisol upon awakening), as well as a blunted cortisol stress response.

Both hypo- and hyperactivity of the HPA axis have the potential to exert influence on infant emotion regulation and behavior problems. Hypercortisolism may spill over to increased stress sensitivity in affective and behavioral domains of functioning, placing infants at risk for difficulties with emotional and behavioral regulation (Repetti, Taylor, & Seeman, 2002). Supporting this perspective, infant cortisol in response to stress at 6 months was positively associated with maternal ratings of infant negative affect in later infancy and early childhood (Huot, Brennan, Stowe, Plotsky, & Walker, 2004). Recent meta-analyses suggest that higher basal cortisol is linked with higher externalizing problems among preschoolers (Alink et al., 2008) and a diagnosis of depression in childhood and adolescence (Lopez-Duran, Kovacs, & George, 2009). In contrast, hypocortisolism may contribute to attenuated behavioral and emotional responsiveness to stress, and subsequently place infants at risk for difficulties responding to and processing emotion (Susman, 2006). Consistent with this possibility, an attenuated profile of both basal cortisol and cortisol stress reactivity was associated with higher internalizing symptoms (Badanes, Watemura, & Hankin, 2011), and attenuated basal cortisol was linked to lower effortful control (Zalewski, Lengua, Kiff, & Fisher, 2012) and more adjustment problems (Lengua, Zalewski, Fisher, & Moran, 2013) among preschoolers. Moreover, emerging evidence suggests that exposure to atypical patterns of HPA activity in infancy and early childhood has lasting effects on brain architecture and neurocircuitry involved in learning, memory, and social information processing (Shonkoff et al., 2012). Consequently, the HPA axis is a relevant biological system for emotional development in infancy.

The PNS

The autonomic nervous system is responsible for controlling a number of organs and their function in response to the environment and consists of two distinct branches. The sympathetic branch is linked with reactivity to the environment that promotes a fight-or-flight response. Although there is some exciting evidence linking the caregiving context to infants' sympathetic functioning and infants' sympathetic functioning to well-being (e.g., Hill-Soderlund et al., 2008), there is a richer body of work in relation to infants' autonomic functioning in the parasympathetic branch as indexed by the vagal system, hence we focus on the latter. The parasympathetic branch of the autonomic nervous system influences the manner in which individuals regulate their state, emotions, and behavior (Porges, 2003). Of particular interest, the vagus nerve sends input to the heart that causes changes in cardiac activity that allows the body to transition between sustaining metabolic processes and generating responses to the environment (Porges, 2007). This parasympathetic influence on heart rate can be readily measured in infants by measuring the variability in heart rate that occurs at the frequency of spontaneous breathing known as respiratory sinus arrhythmia (RSA). In the absence of a stressor, high vagal tone is considered adaptive because it maintains homeostasis (i.e., a steady low heart rate) and allows for a greater response or larger reduction when environmental stressors occur. Thus, high resting vagal tone is generally viewed as a physiological marker of socioemotional adjustment and competent emotion regulation (Porges, 2007). Consistent with this view, prior research indicates that infants with high resting vagal tone demonstrate greater attention to and appropriate reactions to changes in the environment, better behavioral and physiological regulation when presented with stressors, and fewer behavior problems over time (see Propper & Holochwost, 2013, for a review).

Vagal withdrawal that reflects vagal *regulation* of the heart when an organism is challenged is indexed by decreases in RSA during situations where coping or emotional and behavioral regulation are required (Porges, 2003, 2007). Vagal regulation is often described as the functioning of the "vagal brake" because a decrease, or withdrawal, in vagal input to the heart has the effect of stimulating increases in heart rate. During demanding tasks, such a response reflects physiological processes that allow the infant to shift focus from internal homeostatic demands to other demands that require internal processing such as the generation of coping strategies to control affective arousal. Thus, vagal withdrawal is thought to be a physiological strategy that supports active coping (Porges,

1991). Consistent with this view, infants' greater vagal withdrawal during challenge is associated with the use of more adaptive regulatory behaviors, greater soothability, fewer behavior problems, and greater sociability both concurrently and over time (see Calkins, 2011; Propper & Holochwost, 2013, for reviews).

In sum, evidence supports the view that individual differences in HPA and PNS functioning in infancy and early childhood predict children's subsequent emotional well-being. Next we turn to the role of the family context in promoting adaptive HPA and PNS functioning during infancy. We begin with the role of caregiving.

Links between Caregiving and the Infant's Biological Arousal and Regulation

Sensitive caregiving (i.e., consistent prompt responses to infant signals that are appropriate to the signal, context, and infant's developmental level) is positively associated with indicators of infants' emotional well-being including secure attachment, adaptive emotion regulation, and fewer behavior problems (Crockenberg & Leerkes, 2011). It has been argued that sensitive caregiving is linked with these outcomes because it promotes trust in the caregiver that needs will be met, models and reinforces effective self-regulation and social behavior, and instills a sense of competence each of which promote adaptive development (Leerkes, Blankson, & O'Brien, 2009). However, different mechanisms are likely at play for caregiving behavior to influence infants' biological reactivity and regulation. In fact, drawing on his work with rodents, Hofer (1995) argued that specific elements embedded in sensitive caregiving such as touch, body heat, the nutrients in milk, and maternal scents operate as "hidden regulators" that affect infant physiology and behavior in the moment and over time. For example, experimental evidence demonstrates that rats that experience maternal separation or poor caregiving have higher heart rates, greater HPA reactivity to mild stressors, and less adaptive behavior during stressful tasks compared with rats experiencing normal maternal care (Hofer, 1995; Meaney & Szyf, 2005; Sánchez, Ladd, & Plotsky, 2001). This impressive body of work has greatly influenced efforts to understand links between caregiving and stress reactivity and regulation among humans.

Caregiving and Infant HPA Functioning

Consistent with the animal literature, the human infant HPA system is regulated by social interaction (Gunnar & Donzella, 2002; Levine, 2005). At birth, healthy infants exhibit a strong cortisol stress response but over time infants have been observed to enter into a "hyporesponsive period" in which the cortisol stress response dampens, presumably to protect the developing brain

(Gunnar & Quevedo, 2007). Sensitive caregiving, characterized by consistent and appropriate responses to infant distress, is theorized to maintain the hyporesponsive period by promoting a sense of safety and security for the infant and thus buffering the HPA axis from stress (Gunnar, 1998; Gunnar & Donzella, 2002). In contrast, unresponsive parental care, deprived rearing environments, and maltreatment contribute to activation of the HPA system and a shortened hyporesponsive period that results in atypical patterns of cortisol production for the developmental stage (Dozier, Peloso, Lewis, Laurenceau, & Levine, 2008; Tarullo & Gunnar, 2006).

Consistent with this view, sensitive maternal behavior (sometimes inferred from a secure or organized mother–infant attachment) is associated with more adaptive HPA functioning including quicker cortisol recovery from a range of stressors including bathing, physical or emotional separation from the mother, and tasks designed to elicit frustration and fear, reflecting regulation, during infancy (see Gunnar & Vazquez, 2006; Repetti, Robles & Reynolds, 2011, for reviews). Recent evidence suggests a comparable concurrent effect for sensitive *paternal* behavior independent of maternal behavior (Mills-Koonce et al., 2011). Moreover, evidence from recent randomized control trials for maltreated infants and infants in foster care support causal interpretations by demonstrating that infants randomly assigned interventions designed to enhance parenting quality demonstrated more adaptive HPA functioning than infants in control conditions (Cicchetti, Rogosch, Toth, & Sturge-Apple, 2011; Dozier et al., 2008).

Recently, scholars have identified links between specific parenting practices highly related to the hidden regulators identified by Hofer (1995) and infants' cortisol reactivity and regulation. For example, cosleeping predicted lower cortisol reactivity following bathing at 5 weeks of age (Tollenaar, Beijers, Jansem, Riksen-Walraven, & de Weerth, 2011) and during the Strange Situation at 12 months (Beijers, Riksen-Walraven, & de Weerth, 2013), independent of a host of controls including maternal sensitivity for both and infant attachment status for the latter. Likewise, longer breast-feeding duration predicted more rapid cortisol recovery following the Strange Situation at 12 months (Beijers et al., 2013). However, a protective effect of cosleeping and breast-feeding on stress reactivity has not been observed during more severe stressors such as vaccinations (de Weerth & Buitelaar, 2007; Davis & Granger, 2009; Larson et al., 1998; Tollenaar et al., 2011). Finally, infants in a modified still-face procedure, in which mothers were allowed to touch them, demonstrated lower cortisol reactivity and higher subsequent recovery than infants in the traditional still-face procedure without maternal touch (Feldman, Singer, & Zagoory, 2010). Thus, it appears that engagement in proximal parenting behaviors in early infancy is related to more optimal HPA responding to mild stressors.

Although large-scale prospective investigations of the long-term effects of early caregiving on subsequent HPA functioning are scant, the available evidence is generally consistent with key hypotheses derived from the animal literature about the importance of early caregiving for later stress regulation. That is, the association between sensitive caregiving during infancy and adaptive HPA functioning is still apparent in later childhood and adolescence (Murray, Halligan, Goodyer, & Herbert, 2010; Schmid et al., 2013), demonstrating lasting effects of early care on stress regulation. Moreover, maternal sensitivity assessed during infancy but not at age 5 was related to adaptive HPA functioning among 13-year-olds (Murray et al., 2010), demonstrating the unique importance of early relative to later caregiving experiences.

Caregiving and Infant PNS Functioning

The animal literature has also influenced theorizing about how human caregiving may influence the development of the PNS. Drawing on Hofer's (1995) work, Feldman (2007) posits that synchronous social interaction between the caregiver and infant contribute to coordinated biological rhythms between the caregiver and infant that essentially promote physiological homeostasis reflected in high resting vagal tone. In turn, a characteristic pattern of high resting vagal tone may allow for greater vagal suppression when presented with a stressor (Propper & Holochwost, 2013). In contrast, negative or asynchronous interactions with a caregiver may contribute to a characteristically low vagal tone as necessitated by the consistent need to self-regulate, which may hamper the ability to suppress further when presented with a stressor. Over time, chronic exposure to stress within the caregiving context could contribute to physiological burnout resulting in underregulation over time (Hill-Soderlund et al., 2008).

Recently, Porges and Furman (2011) noted that vagal fibers continue to myelinate through adolescence with the most rapid period occurring early in life, and a greater number of myelinated vagal fibers should be linked with more adaptive vagal regulation. Although they focus on the likelihood that greater myelination of the vagus nerve promotes more adaptive social interaction, it may also be the case that features of the infants' environment, including sensitive caregiving, promote greater myelination of vagal fibers in early infancy, which in turn promotes more adaptive vagal regulation. For example, stimulating social interactions with caregivers may provide important opportunities to both up regulate and down regulate vagal tone, which may contribute to activity-dependent myelination (Fields, 2005) of the vagus nerve. Although the exact mechanism remains uncertain, a good deal of evidence supports the view that early caregiving is linked with more adaptive vagal functioning among infants.

First, synchronous mother–infant interactions are linked with coordinated infant–mother heart rhythms (parallel accelerations or decelerations of heart rate within 1 second of each other; Feldman, Magori-Cohen, Galili, Singer, & Louzoun, 2011), higher basal vagal tone (Porter, 2003), and a normative response pattern during the still-face paradigm (i.e., greater vagal withdrawal during the still-face episode than the normal face-to-face play periods; Moore & Calkins, 2004). Second, sensitive maternal behavior has been associated with better vagal regulation, whereas negative, harsh, or controlling maternal behavior has been associated with less adaptive vagal regulation in response to stressors (Calkins, 2011; Conradt & Ablow, 2010; Moore et al., 2009). Less normative vagal regulation (i.e., higher vagal suppression during mild stressors and across contexts when other children display recovery) has also been demonstrated among infants with an insecure or disorganized attachment with mothers, which may be a product of a history of less sensitive maternal caregiving (Hill-Soderland et al., 2008; Frigerio et al., 2009; Oosterman, De Schipper, Fisher, Dozier, & Schuengel, 2010). Although links between mother behavior and infant vagal regulation have typically been assessed concurrently, some longitudinal evidence exists. Notably, maternal sensitivity at 5 months predicted infants' increased vagal regulation during moderately frustrating tasks from 5 to 10 months (Perry, 2013). Evidence from a randomized controlled intervention trial demonstrating that improved parenting was related to improved vagal regulation among young children from pre- to posttreatment provides compelling evidence that sensitive maternal behavior contributes to more effective vagal regulation over time (Graziano, Bagner, Sheinkopf, Vohr, & Lester, 2012).

Additionally, a good deal of evidence supports the notion that caregiver touch is related to better vagal functioning both in the moment and over time. For example, neonates demonstrated greater vagal regulation during a heel-stick procedure when held by their mothers (Gormally et al., 2001), and 6-month-old infants demonstrated more rapid vagal recovery (i.e., an increase in vagal tone) following the modified still face accompanied by touch compared with infants in the no-touch condition (Feldman et al., 2010). With regard to longitudinal effects, frequent skin-to-skin contact promoted more rapid vagal regulation (i.e., an increase in resting vagal tone over time) in a sample of preterm infants (Feldman & Eidelman, 2003), and frequent maternal stroking over the first 2 months of life buffered infants from the negative effects of maternal depression on vagal regulation in response to a stressor at 7 months (Sharp et al., 2012). Despite the compelling data related to touch, it is important to note than when multiple modes of interaction were examined simultaneously, mother–infant synchronous gaze and affective communication were more predictive of coordinated heart rhythms than was touch (Feldman et al., 2011), demonstrating the importance of caregiving modes other than touch among humans.

Caregiver Affect and the Infant's Biological Arousal and Regulation

In addition to caregiving behavior, there is reason to believe that caregivers' affect may play a role in shaping infants' biological arousal and regulation, although much less research has been conducted on this possibility to date.

That is, infants who are exposed to frequent parental anger, sadness, anxiety, or depression may be at increased risk for regulatory difficulties via three pathways. First, it has primarily been argued that parental negative affect or affect dysregulation undermines sensitive caregiving because it promotes the parent's focus on his or her own needs rather than the needs of his or her infant (Leerkes, 2010). In turn, compromised caregiving is linked with infants' poorer physiological and behavioral regulation as reviewed above, suggesting an indirect effect of parental affect on infant emotional adjustment via caregiving behavior. In fact, positive associations between dysregulated parental affect (i.e., elevated symptoms of depression and anxiety) and infant physiological dysregulation have been demonstrated, but the possibility that these effects were mediated by caregiving behavior was not tested (e.g., Laurent, Ablow, & Measelle, 2011; Laurent et al., 2013; Schuetze, Eiden, & Danielewicz, 2009). It is also possible that caregiver affect influences infant stress physiology directly. For example, maternal depression was associated with increased cortisol reactivity and reduced recovery in response to a mild stressor independent of insensitive maternal behavior in two studies (Azar, Paquette, Zoccolillo, Baltzer, & Tremblay, 2007; Feldman et al., 2009), suggesting that alternate mechanisms by which maternal affect influences infant physiology may exist, a point we return to below. Finally, parental negative affect and insensitive caregiving may have joint (i.e., interactive) effects on infant arousal and regulation. For example, in one study, young children demonstrated increased cortisol reactivity to a stressor only when their parents had a history of depression *and* engaged in hostile parenting behavior (Dougherty, Klein, Rose, & Laptook, 2011), suggesting that maternal negative affect is particularly likely to exacerbate infant reactivity in the context of insensitive caregiving.

In our own work, we have focused on mothers' parenting-related affect, specifically their affect, arousal, and regulation in response to infant crying. Using this approach, we demonstrated a direct effect of maternal anxiety in response to crying on infant attachment resistance and an indirect effect of maternal anger in response to crying on infant attachment avoidance through mothers' negative and punitive responses to infant distress (Leerkes, Parade, & Gudmundson, 2011). Preliminary results of our ongoing study of 259 mother–infant dyads also demonstrate the importance of mothers' own physiological arousal and regulation while interacting with their infants in relation to subsequent infant adjustment. That is, infants whose mothers demonstrated physiological dysregulation during a series of emotionally arousing caregiving tasks when they were 6 months old (i.e., high arousal as evidenced by skin conductance increases and poor regulation as evidenced by low vagal withdrawal relative to a resting baseline), were more likely to be classified as disorganized in the Strange Situation and to have elevated behavior problems at 13 months compared with infants whose mothers were aroused but well regulated during the caregiving tasks. Moreover, this effect of maternal dysregulation was not mediated by observed maternal sensitivity and was independent of trait-like indicators of mothers' general emotional well-being including depressive symptoms. These results underscore the importance of examining aspects of parenting beyond direct caregiving behavior when trying to understand the effect of family context on infants' emotional development and suggest that greater attention to caregivers' affect during parent–infant interaction is warranted.

Though these early results are exciting, an important unanswered question is how might direct effects of maternal affect or emotional well-being on infant physiology and well-being occur? Recent work linking parental depression to infants' HPA functioning rules out the possibility that such effects are solely accounted for by the prenatal environment or genetics. That is, in one study, patterns of elevated prenatal and/or *postnatal* maternal depressive symptoms were linked with infants' poorer cortisol recovery poststressor (Laurent et al., 2011), demonstrating that effects of postnatal depression are not fully explained by prenatal depression. In the other study, adoptive mothers' and fathers' heightened depressive symptoms predicted infants' lower daily cortisol, reflecting a blunted pattern and internalizing problems after controlling for the birth mothers' depressive symptoms, suggesting an effect of caregiver affect and behavior over and above genetic risk for regulatory problems (Laurent et al., 2013). Thus, we raise two possibilities as to how parental affect may be directly linked with infants' physiological arousal and regulation. First, if mothers behaviorally express their negative affect in the infants' presence it may cause the infant to become dysregulated via emotion contagion, and chronic exposure to parental negative affect may contribute to persistent activation of infants' stress response systems and less effective regulation over time (i.e., "burnout"; Moore, 2009). Second, in the context of proximal caregiving, the physiological components of mothers' affective dysregulation (e.g., rapid breathing, irregular heart rate, bodily tension) may contribute to infants' physiological dysregulation via synchronization leading to less optimal infant regulation over time (Feldman, 2007). Thus, parental negative affect may simultaneously increase infant arousal maximizing the infant's need for external assistance with regulation, while undermining the caregiver's ability to provide the needed support.

Summary and Future Directions

Across both biological systems, there is clear evidence that caregiving is linked with infants' physiological arousal and regulation in the moment and over time, which in turn predicts infants' longer-term emotional well-being. However, a number of questions remain, and we believe work in this area would be advanced by the more precise measurement of caregiving, alternative research designs, and more attention to caregiving by fathers. First, multiple modes of caregiving behavior such as gaze, touch, and vocalizations should be rated over time to determine which modes of caregiving are particularly relevant to certain regulatory outcomes (Calkins, 2011). Second, specific dimensions of sensitivity should be measured separately to determine if maternal sensitivity to distress is more predictive of infants' physiological regulation than is sensitivity to nondistress as has been demonstrated for behavioral regulation (Leerkes et al., 2009). Third, additional work on specific parenting practices—such as breast-feeding, cosleeping, and other nighttime routines—is needed. Results of such work may point to other biologically mediated pathways by which parenting promotes physiological regulation. For example, it may be the case that sensitive bedtime routines promote better sleep, which in turn predicts adaptive physiological regulation, or that the effects of breast-feeding on biological regulation are a function of nutrition and not proximal care.

Two design features also warrant greater consideration. First, most of the existing work in this area is correlational. Additional small-scale experimental research, in which specific features of caregiving are manipulated (e.g., touch, no touch; gaze at vs. gaze away from infant; proximal vs. distal conditions) during known stressors, and infants' HPA and PNS responses recorded would offer valuable insight as to which features of caregiving are most relevant to infant reactivity and regulation in the moment. Second, most of this research is based on concurrent observations of caregiver and infant behavior during tasks in which the caregiver is the stressor (e.g., still-face procedure), which poses interpretive challenges related to the direction of effects and generalizability of findings to contexts in which the caregiver is not involved. Thus, additional work is needed in which infants' physiological arousal and regulation are assessed across a range of stressors, some of which do not involve the caregiver.

Finally, it is clear that additional research on the links between paternal caregiving and affect and infants' biological reactivity and regulation is needed. Compelling arguments as to why fathering may be particularly salient for regulatory processes have been made (e.g., the likelihood of rough-and-tumble play eliciting opportunities to regulate), but remain relatively untested with few exceptions (Laurent et al., 2013; Mills-Koonce et al., 2011). The extent to which maternal and paternal caregiving and affect are linked with infants' biological regulation independent of (i.e., the relative predictive validity) or in conjunction with each other (i.e., interaction effects) remains unknown. Likewise, the extent to which factors such as the relative frequency with which mothers and fathers interact with their infants, the nature of the caregiving tasks in which they engage (e.g., comforting, play, bedtime), and the quality of the attachment between the infant and each caregiver moderate these associations require attention. One area of research that has considered the role of both fathers and mothers, to some extent, is work linking couple dynamics to infants' biological regulation.

Links between Interparental Dynamics
and the Infant's Biological Arousal and Regulation

The quality of the romantic relationship between parents represents a salient context for the development of infant emotion regulation. Theories of emotional security suggest that interparental conflict and dysfunction triggers emotional and physiological responses within the child that have the potential to undermine children's sense of safety and security and consequently, long-term adaptation (Cummings & Davies, 2010). Additionally, discord in the interparental dyad has the potential to drain parents' socioemotional resources and spill over to caregiver affect and parental behavior, contributing to difficulty with children's emotional and behavioral regulation. Supporting this perspective, destructive interparental conflict characterized by verbal and nonverbal hostility elicits infant distress, and depressive interparental conflict characterized by avoidance and withdrawal elicits infant frustration (Du Rocher Schudlich, White, Fleischhauer, & Fitzgerald, 2011). Furthermore, interparental aggression and conflict are negatively associated with maternal sensitivity (Finger, Hans, Bernstein, & Cox, 2009), which is linked with biological regulation as described above.

Despite knowledge that infants are more likely to be exposed to dysfunctional interparental dyadic functioning in the form of interparental conflict and violence than are older children (Fantuzzo, Boruch, Beriama, & Atkins, 1997), the majority of research considering links between interparental relationship dynamics and child adjustment has focused on older children. Recent work, however, has demonstrated that marital conflict in the first year is linked with less adaptive emotion regulation at 6 months (Crockenberg, Leerkes, & Lekka, 2007; Parade & Leerkes, 2011; Porter, Wouden-Miller, Silva, & Porter, 2003). Exposure to interparental violence may be particularly salient to infant emotional health as evidenced by associations with heightened trauma symptoms (Dejonghe, Bogat, Levendosky, von Eye, & Davidson, 2005) and externalizing problems in toddlerhood (DeJonghe, von Eye, Bogat, & Levendosky, 2011).

Interparental Dynamics and Infant HPA Functioning

As described above, conflict in the interparental dyad induces an emotional and physiological stress response (Cummings & Davies, 2010). In particular, interparental violence and aggression threatens the infant's sense of safety and well-being and results in activation of the HPA system (Davies, Sturge-Apple, Cicchetti, & Cummings, 2007). Over time, infants reared in highly conflictual homes may exhibit patterns of hyper- or hypocortisolism, contributing to regulatory difficulties. Supporting this view, interparental violence, aggression, and impaired dyadic functioning are linked with higher basal cortisol in toddlerhood, later childhood, and adolescence (Davies, Sturge-Apple, Cicchetti, Manning, & Zale, 2009; Pendry & Adam, 2007; Saltzman, Holden, & Hola-han, 2005), and in toddlerhood these links are mediated by toddlers' anger in response to interparental conflict (Davies et al., 2009).

Interparental conflict and aggression is also linked with context-specific infant cortisol reactivity. Recent research utilizing a simulated interparental conflict task in the laboratory demonstrated that interparental violence was linked with lower levels of cortisol reactivity to the conflict simulation at age 2 (a blunted pattern), but was not associated with cortisol reactivity to the Strange Situation (Sturge-Apple, Davies, Cicchetti, & Manning, 2012). Likewise, care-giver emotional unavailability was linked with lower cortisol reactivity to the Strange Situation but not to the conflict simulation. In contrast, intimate part-ner violence was linked with higher cortisol stress reactivity to a frustration- and fear-evoking laboratory battery at 2 years, but only among infants whose mothers were less sensitive at 7 months (Hibel, Granger, Blair, Cox, & The Family Life Project Key Investigators, 2011). The mixed pattern of findings may be the result of differences in the intensity of conflict (i.e., verbal conflict vs. violence) or untested moderators, such as child characteristics. Consistent with the latter, interparental aggression was linked with heightened cortisol reactiv-ity in response to the interparental conflict simulation among toddlers with an inhibited temperament, and was marginally associated with decreased cortisol reactivity among toddlers with a bold temperament (Davies, Sturge-Apple, & Cicchetti, 2011). This suggests that young children who are easily frightened are particularly susceptible to heightened arousal when confronted with inter-parental conflict, placing them at greater risk for subsequent problems than uninhibited children when reared in a high-conflict family.

Interparental Dynamics and Infant Vagal Functioning

Similar to the influence of interparental conflict on infant HPA functioning, exposure to interparental conflict activates the PNS, and over time repeated exposure to conflict is believed to contribute to blunted vagal tone and vagal withdrawal (El-Sheikh & Hinnant, 2011). Supporting the perspective that inter-parental conflict leads to blunting of PNS activity, interparental conflict was linked with lower basal vagal tone and lower vagal tone when interacting with the mother during the still-face procedure at 6 months (Moore, 2010; Porter et al., 2003). In contrast, interparental aggression was linked with higher basal vagal tone at age 2 (Davies et al., 2009). Differences in the valence of effect in these studies suggest that other factors, such as infant age and gender, may moderate links between interparental functioning and PNS activity in infants. Consistent with the latter possibility, conflict avoidance in the interparental dyad was linked with higher basal vagal tone among female infants but with lower basal vagal tone among male infants at 5 months (Graham, Ablow, &

Measelle, 2010). As Graham et al. (2010) suggest, parents may express their negative interparental dynamics differently when they are in the presence of girls than when they are in the presence of boys, leading to different patterns of PNS functioning. An alternate possibility is that male and female infants may be attending to and interpreting negative interparental behaviors differently.

Summary and Future Directions

Taken together, research examining the role of interparental dyadic functioning in the development of infant biological stress response systems is best described as emerging. In particular, work focused on interparental dyadic functioning and the PNS in infancy is scant. Collectively, the majority of work in this area has focused on older infants and toddlers; few studies have focused on interparental functioning and infant biological systems in the first months of life. Furthermore, this literature has largely considered behavioral aspects of interparental dyadic functioning, most notably conflict and interparental aggression or violence. It remains to be seen if less overt aspects of the interparental dyad such as relationship satisfaction and feelings of love and intimacy exert influence on the infant HPA axis and PNS. It is likely that these aspects of interparental functioning contribute to infant biological systems through processes of biobehavioral synchrony (Feldman, 2007) and spill over to parental affect and behavior (Stroud, Durbin, Wilson, & Mendelsohn, 2011). In future research, considering the role of interparental dyadic functioning in the prenatal period versus the postnatal period will be critically important given emerging literature suggesting that interparental violence in pregnancy has the potential to prenatally "program" aspects of the HPA system (Radtke et al., 2011).

Moving Beyond Parent-Driven Main-Effects Models

Up to this point, we have described the associations between family context and infant outcomes as a unidirectional effect from parent or family to child, but in fact, contemporary models of development are more complicated and take into account child characteristics in two distinct ways. First, infant characteristics, including their biologically based reactivity and regulation, and family context may interact to predict infant adjustment over time. Second, infants' biologically based reactivity and regulation may influence caregiving over time.

Child × Environment Effects

An additional pathway that has received empirical support is joint or interactive effects between family context and infants' emotion-related psychobiology or genotypes on emotional development. Theories of differential susceptibility and diathesis–stress/dual risk suggest that some infants are more likely to be influenced by environmental factors than are others due to individual infant characteristics, including physiological reactivity and regulation that make them more sensitive to environmental effects, or due to the accumulation of personal and contextual risks (see Belsky, Bakermans-Kranenburg, & van IJzendoorn, 2007, for a review of commonalities and differences in these two perspectives). Consistent with this view, there is evidence that the effects of caregiving on infants' physiological arousal and regulation vary by infant genotype. In one study, secure infants with genotypes believed to incur risk for heightened stress reactivity demonstrated less arousal and better recovery in response to a stressor as indexed by salivary alpha amylase than insecure infants with the same genotpyes (Frigerio et al., 2009). Likewise, an intervention to enhance sensitive caregiving and reduce externalizing symptoms contributed to infants' lower morning cortisol compared with infants who were not randomized to the intervention, but only among infants with the DRD4-7 repeat allele, which is linked with less efficient reuptake of dopamine (Bakermans-Kranenburg, van IJzendoorn, Mesman, Alink, & Juffer, 2008). Both studies suggest that sensitive caregiving is particularly likely to promote adaptive patterns of stress reactivity among infants at genetic risk for poor outcomes. A similar effect was demonstrated for vagal regulation in a compelling longitudinal study (Propper et al., 2008). Specifically, infants with the risk allele for the D2 dopamine receptor gene demonstrated initially compromised vagal regulation at 3 and 6 months regardless of maternal sensitivity, but by 12 months of age, infants with the risk allele and highly sensitive mothers demonstrated vagal regulation comparable to infants without the risk allele and significantly better than infants with the risk allele and insensitive mothers. This pattern suggests the long-term effect of sensitive caregiving on emotional outcomes via biological arousal and regulation would likely only be apparent for infants with these genetic risk factors (i.e., moderated mediation).

Other studies have demonstrated joint effects of infant physiology and parenting behavior on behavior problems. In one such study, baseline vagal tone and attachment classification interacted to predict behavior problems at 17 months such that attachment-based differences in behavior problems were apparent only among infants with high baseline vagal tone (Conradt, Measelle, & Ablow, 2013). High vagal tone infants classified as secure (reflecting a likely history of sensitive caregiving) appeared to benefit from positive caregiving as demonstrated by lower behavior problems, whereas high vagal tone infants classified as disorganized appeared to be negatively influenced by insensitive caregiving as demonstrated by heightened behavior problems. In another study, children with low vagal regulation in response to frustration at age 2 were only more likely to engage in a high level of disruptive behavior from age 2 to 5 if they experienced low maternal control as toddlers (Degnan, Calkins, Keane, &

Hill-Soderlund, 2008). This pattern suggests that children with early regulatory deficits are particularly dependent on their caregivers for external regulation.

Few studies have examined interactions between interparental dynamics and infants' biologically based arousal and regulation in relation to adjustment over time. Given the considerable body of literature demonstrating that higher vagal tone and withdrawal buffers older children from the deleterious effects of marital conflict (see El-Sheikh & Whitson, 2006), we expect a comparable effect in infancy. In the only infancy study we could identify, a high-quality caregiving environment that included good marital adjustment was linked with a decline in aggressive behavior across early childhood only among toddlers with moderate to high baseline vagal tone but not among toddlers with low baseline vagal tone (Eisenberg et al., 2012).

Child and Transactional Effects

Infant characteristics such as temperament are well known to predict parenting behavior and other aspects of the family context (Crockenberg & Leerkes, 2003). There is some evidence that individual differences in infants' HPA and PNS functioning operate in such a fashion. For example, neonates with higher resting vagal tone were subsequently observed to have more synchronous interactions with both their mothers and fathers, suggesting that the biological capacity for self-regulation contributed to more adaptive dyadic interactions or elicited more effective and attuned parenting over time (Feldman & Eidelman, 2007). Likewise, in a sample of preterm infants, mothers whose infants had better vagal regulation at 4 months were less likely to demonstrate a pattern of declining maternal positive affect and involvement across the first 2 years compared with mothers whose infants demonstrated poorer vagal regulation, perhaps because these infants were easier to care for or provided mothers with more positive reinforcement (Poehlmann et al., 2011). Over time, the preterm infants with higher vagal regulation demonstrated greater increases in positive affect and social competence, and a greater decrease in irritability and dysregulation. Although not directly tested, this pattern raises the intriguing possibility of transactive effects (Sameroff, 2009) whereby infant physiology and caregiving are related to each other concurrently and over time, and may contribute to change in each other over time. That is, infants with a greater biological capacity for self-regulation may elicit more sensitive caregiving, which in turn supports their emotional development over time. To date, we are aware of only two studies in which such reciprocal relations have been tested using a cross-lagged model, but neither tested moderating effects. In one, maternal sensitivity at age 2 predicted children's higher vagal regulation at age 4, which in turn predicted higher maternal sensitivity at age 5 (Perry, Mackler, Calkins, & Keane, 2014). In the other, children's low baseline vagal tone at age 2 predicted more negative maternal behavior at age 4, but maternal negative parenting at age 2 did not predict children's baseline vagal tone at age 4 (Kennedy, Rubin, Hastings, & Maisel, 2004). This pattern is consistent with the view that infant physiological reactivity and regulation influences subsequent parenting, and that parenting is more influential on the regulatory than the temperamental aspect of vagal functioning over time (Calkins, 2009).

Summary and Future Directions

As a set, the studies that test moderation demonstrate that the effects of family context on infants' emotional well-being over time are somewhat dependent on infants' biological reactivity and regulation. Additional work testing interactions between family context and infant biological reactivity and regulation is needed generally, but particularly in regard to parental affect and interparental dynamics, as interactions with caregiving quality has been examined somewhat more frequently to date. Work of this type is particularly important from an intervention perspective because it identifies those children who are at proportionately greater risk when in less optimal caregiving contexts.

Efforts to understand child-driven and transactive effects are rare in this area of research. Ultimately, additional careful longitudinal studies in which the caregiving context and infants' biological reactivity and regulation are assessed from early infancy on is needed to better understand the concurrent and cross-time links between caregiving and infants' physiological arousal and regulation, and the extent to which both are related to children's later emotional well-being. Given the time and expense inherent in this type of longitudinal work, exploiting data from popular paradigms such as the still-face procedure is an appealing avenue to examine short-term transactional effects between caregivers and infants (e.g., concurrent and cross-phase association between mother and infant physiology and behavior). If evidence of biological child effects on caregiving accrues, it paints a relatively bleak picture for infants with initially compromised physiological regulation. That is, infants who may be in greatest need of external assistance with self-regulation are somewhat less likely to get it, and the consequences of less sensitive care may be greater for them than for other infants, further underscoring the need for effective intervention with these families.

Conclusion

In sum, a good deal of evidence supports the view that infants who experience insensitive caregiving, negative parental affect, and/or interparental conflict demonstrate less adaptive patterns of physiological arousal and regulation, which are in turn linked with more behavior problems. Further, infants whose early physiological regulation is compromised appear to be at greatest risk for maladjustment when reared in suboptimal caregiving contexts, and their own characteristics somewhat increase the likelihood of encountering less positive caregiving contexts. The breadth of work in this area to date is impressive, but the value of this line of inquiry would be enhanced by further consideration of two important shortcomings.

First, there is a tendency for research groups to focus on a single or narrow set of psychobiological measures likely driven by the expense of and expertise needed for specialized equipment and procedures. This has resulted in few studies that measure and integrate findings from multiple biological systems. Research that integrates psychobiological measures from a range of physiological systems has the potential to contrast various mechanisms by which multiple systems affect emotional development including (1) a possible benefit of synchrony among systems, (2) dual risk across systems, (3) compensatory effects of one system on the effects of another system, and (4) causal pathways via spillover from one system to another. It seems likely that the family environment contributes to infants' emotional development through complex, yet coordinated, biological responses.

Second, although there are some exceptions, the studies conducted to date generally focus on caregiving involving one parent and one child when in fact a substantial number of infants have siblings and multiple caregivers, as well as multiple caregiving contexts with vastly different characteristics. Thus, efforts should be made to better understand the effects of the broader family system, home context, and other consistent daily contexts on trajectories of infant biobehavioral health. For example, it seems plausible that the presence of an older sibling with elevated externalizing symptoms may certainly influence day-to-day stress exposure for an infant, and depending on the quality of caregiving and the infant's initial levels of reactivity and regulation, this experience may lead to very different patterns of physiological reactivity and regulation over time. Likewise, family stress resulting from conditions of poverty, variations in home chaos, including instability in family composition, and other characteristics of the family environment beyond quality of direct care may give rise to different patterns of growth and change in reactivity and regulation over time. Although some of these effects may be mediated by caregiving quality, alternative pathways seem probable. Finally, the majority of U.S. infants experience some type of child care. Differences in the onset, duration, quality, and stability of child care experiences may have important implications for the development of physiological reactivity and regulation. Attention to these issues and the minor methodological issues noted throughout the review will further increase the value of this line of inquiry for both basic and applied science in early emotional development.

REFERENCES

Alink, L. A., van IJzendoorn, M. H., Bakermans-Kranenburg, M. J., Mesman, J., Juffer, F., & Koot, H. M. (2008). Cortisol and externalizing behavior in children and adolescents: Mixed meta-analytic evidence for the inverse relation of basal cortisol and cortisol reactivity with externalizing behavior. *Developmental Psychobiology, 50,* 427–450.

Azar, R., Paquette, D., Zoccolillo, M., Baltzer, F., & Tremblay, R. E. (2007). The association of major depression, conduct disorder, and maternal overcontrol with a failure to show a cortisol buffered response in 4-month-old infants of teenage mothers. *Biological Psychiatry, 62,* 573–579.

Badanes, L. S., Watamura, S., & Hankin, B. L. (2011). Hypocortisolism as a potential marker of allostatic load in children: Associations with family risk and internalizing disorders. *Development and Psychopathology, 23,* 881–896.

Bakermans-Kranenburg, M. J., van IJzendoorn, M. H., Mesman, J., Alink, L. A., & Juffer, F. (2008). Effects of an attachment-based intervention on daily cortisol moderated by dopamine receptor D4: A randomized control trial on 1- to 3-year-olds screened for externalizing behavior. *Development and Psychopathology, 20,* 805–820.

Beijers, R., Riksen-Walraven, J., & de Weerth, C. (2013). Cortisol regulation in 12-month-old human infants: Associations with the infants' early history of breastfeeding and co-sleeping. *Stress: The International Journal on the Biology of Stress, 16,* 267–277.

Belsky, J., Bakermans-Kranenburg, M. J., & van IJzendoorn, M. H. (2007). For better and for worse: Differential susceptibility to environmental influences. *Current Directions in Psychological Science, 16,* 300–304.

Bruce, J., Gunnar, M. R., Pears, K. C., & Fisher, P. A. (2013). Early adverse care, stress neurobiology, and prevention science: Lessons learned. *Prevention Science, 14,* 247–256.

Calkins, S. D. (2009). Regulatory competence and early disruptive behavior problems: The role of physiological regulation. In S. L. Olson & A. J. Sameroff (Eds.), *Biopsychosocial regulatory processes in the development of childhood behavioral problems* (pp. 86–115). New York: Cambridge University Press.

Calkins, S. D. (2011). Caregiving as coregulation: Psychobiological processes and child functioning. In A. Booth, S. M. McHale, & N. S. Landale (Eds.), *Biosocial foundations of family processes* (pp. 49–59). New York: Springer Science and Business Media.

Cicchetti, D., Rogosch, F. A., Toth, S. L., & Sturge-Apple, M. L. (2011). Normalizing the development of cortisol regulation in maltreated infants through preventive interventions. *Development and Psychopathology, 23,* 789–800.

Conradt, E., & Ablow, J. (2010). Infant physiological response to the still-face paradigm: Contributions of maternal sensitivity and infants' early regulatory behavior. *Infant Behavior and Development, 33,* 251–265.

Conradt, E., Measelle, J., & Ablow, J. C. (2013). Poverty, problem behavior, and promise: Differential susceptibility among infants reared in poverty. *Psychological Science, 24,* 235–242.

Crockenberg, S., & Leerkes, E. (2003). Infant negative emotionality, caregiving, and family relationships. In A. C. Crouter & A. Booth (Eds.), *Children's influence on family dynamics: The neglected side of family relationships* (pp. 57–78). Mahwah, NJ: Erlbaum.

Crockenberg, S. C., & Leerkes, E. M. (2011). Parenting infants. In D. W. Davis & M. C. Logsdon (Eds.), *Maternal sensitivity: A scientific foundation for practice* (pp. 125–143). Hauppauge, NY: Nova Science.

Crockenberg, S. C., Leerkes, E. M., & Barrig Jo, P. S. (2008). Predicting aggressive behavior in the third year from infant reactivity and regulation as moderated by maternal behavior. *Development and Psychopathology, 20,* 37–54.

Crockenberg, S. C., Leerkes, E. M., & Lekka, S. (2007). Pathways from marital aggression to infant emotion regulation: The development of withdrawal in infancy [Special section: Emergent family systems]. *Infant Behavior and Development, 30,* 97–113.

Cummings, E., & Davies, P. T. (2010). *Marital conflict and children: An emotional security perspective.* New York: Guilford Press.

Davies, P. T., Sturge-Apple, M. L., & Cicchetti, D. (2011). Interparental aggression and children's adrenocortical reactivity: Testing an evolutionary model of allostatic load. *Development and Psychopathology, 23,* 801–814.

Davies, P. T., Sturge-Apple, M. L., Cicchetti, D., & Cummings, E. (2007). The role of child adrenocortical functioning in pathways between interparental conflict and child maladjustment. *Developmental Psychology, 43,* 918–930.

Davies, P. T., Sturge-Apple, M. L., Cicchetti, D., Manning, L. G., & Zale, E. (2009). Children's patterns of emotional reactivity to conflict as explanatory mechanisms in links between interpartner aggression and child physiological functioning. *Journal of Child Psychology and Psychiatry, 50,* 1384–1391.

Davis, E., & Granger, D. A. (2009). Developmental differences in infant salivary alpha-amylase and cortisol responses to stress. *Psychoneuroendocrinology, 34,* 795–804.

de Weerth, C., & Buitelaar, J. K. (2007). Childbirth complications affect young infants' behavior. *European Child and Adolescent Psychiatry, 16,* 379–388.

Degnan, K. A., Calkins, S. D., Keane, S. P., & Hill-Soderlund, A. L. (2008). Profiles of disruptive behavior across early childhood: Contributions of frustration reactivity, physiological regulation, and maternal behavior. *Child Development, 79,* 1357–1376.

DeJonghe, E. S., Bogat, G., Levendosky, A. A., von Eye, A., & Davidson, W. (2005). Infant exposure to domestic violence predicts heightened sensitivity to adult verbal conflict. *Infant Mental Health Journal, 26,* 268–281.

DeJonghe, E. S., von Eye, A., Bogat, G., & Levendosky, A. A. (2011). Does witnessing intimate partner violence contribute to toddlers' internalizing and externalizing behaviors? *Applied Developmental Science, 15,* 129–139.

Dougherty, L. R., Klein, D. N., Rose, S., & Laptook, R. S. (2011). Hypothalamic–pituitary–adrenal axis reactivity in the preschool-age offspring of depressed parents: Moderation by early parenting. *Psychological Science, 22,* 650–658.

Dozier, M., Peloso, E., Lewis, E., Laurenceau, J., & Levine, S. (2008). Effects of an attachment-based intervention of the cortisol production of infants and toddlers in foster care. *Development and Psychopathology, 20,* 845–859.

Du Rocher Schudlich, T. D., White, C. R., Fleischhauer, E. A., & Fitzgerald, K. A. (2011). Observed infant reactions during live interparental conflict. *Journal of Marriage and Family, 73*, 221–235.

Eisenberg, N., Sulik, M. J., Spinrad, T. L., Edwards, A., Eggum, N. D., Liew, J., et al. (2012). Differential susceptibility and the early development of aggression: Interactive effects of respiratory sinus arrhythmia and environmental quality. *Developmental Psychology, 48*, 755–768.

El-Sheikh, M., & Hinnant, J. (2011). Marital conflict, respiratory sinus arrhythmia, and allostatic load: Interrelations and associations with the development of children's externalizing behavior. *Development and Psychopathology, 23*, 815–829.

El-Sheikh, M., & Whitson, S. A. (2006). Longitudinal relations between marital conflict and child adjustment: Vagal regulation as a protective factor. *Journal of Family Psychology, 20*, 30–39.

Fantuzzo, J., Boruch, R., Beriama, A., & Atkins, M. (1997). Domestic violence and children: Prevalence and risk in five major U.S. cities. *Journal of the American Academy of Child and Adolescent Psychiatry, 36*, 116–122.

Feldman, R. (2007). Parent–infant synchrony and the construction of shared timing: Physiological precursors, developmental outcomes, and risk conditions. *Journal of Child Psychology and Psychiatry, 48*, 329–354.

Feldman, R., & Eidelman, A. I. (2003). Skin-to-skin contact (kangaroo care) accelerates autonomic and neurobehavioural maturation in preterm infants. *Developmental Medicine and Child Neurology, 45*, 274–281.

Feldman, R., & Eidelman, A. I. (2007). Maternal postpartum behavior and the emergence of infant–mother and infant–father synchrony in preterm and full-term infants: The role of neonatal vagal tone. *Developmental Psychobiology, 49*, 290–302.

Feldman, R., Granat, A., Pariente, C., Kanety, H., Kuint, J., & Gilboa-Schechtman, E. (2009). Maternal depression and anxiety across the postpartum year and infant social engagement, fear regulation, and stress reactivity. *Journal of the American Academy of Child and Adolescent Psychiatry, 48*, 919–927.

Feldman, R., Magori-Cohen, R., Galili, G., Singer, M., & Louzoun, Y. (2011). Mother and infant coordinate heart rhythms through episodes of interaction synchrony. *Infant Behavior and Development, 34*, 569–577.

Feldman, R., Singer, M., & Zagoory, O. (2010). Touch attenuates infants' physiological reactivity to stress. *Developmental Science, 13*, 271–278.

Fields, R. D. (2005) Myelination: An overlooked mechanism of synaptic plasticity? *Neuroscientist, 11*, 528–531.

Finger, B., Hans, S. L., Bernstein, V. J., & Cox, S. M. (2009). Parent relationship quality and infant–mother attachment. *Attachment and Human Development, 11*, 285–306.

Fox, N. A., Henderson, H. A., Pérez-Edgar, K., & White, L. K. (2008). The biology of temperament: An integrative approach. In C. A. Nelson, & M. Luciana (Eds.), *Handbook of developmental cognitive neuroscience* (2nd ed.,pp. 839–853). Cambridge, MA: MIT Press.

Frigerio, A., Ceppi, E., Rusconi, M., Giorda, R., Raggi, M., & Fearon, P. (2009). The role played by the interaction between genetic factors and attachment in the stress response in infancy. *Journal of Child Psychology and Psychiatry, 50,* 1513–1522.

Gormally, S., Barr, R. G., Wertheim, L., Alkawaf, R., Calinoiu, N., & Young, S. N. (2001). Contact and nutrient caregiving effects on newborn infant pain responses. *Developmental Medicine and Child Neurology, 43,* 28–38.

Graham, A. M., Ablow, J. C., & Measelle, J. R. (2010). Interparental relationship dynamics and cardiac vagal functioning in infancy. *Infant Behavior and Development, 33,* 530–544.

Graziano, P. A., Bagner, D. M., Sheinkopf, S. J., Vohr, B. R., & Lester, B. M. (2012). Evidence-based intervention for young children born premature: Preliminary evidence for associated changes in physiological regulation. *Infant Behavior and Development, 35,* 417–428.

Gunnar, M., & Quevedo, K. (2007). The neurobiology of stress and development. *Annual Review of Psychology, 58,* 145–173.

Gunnar, M. R. (1998). Quality of early care and buffering of neuroendocrine stress reactions: Potential effects on the developing human brain. *Preventive Medicine: An International Journal Devoted to Practice and Theory, 27,* 208–211.

Gunnar, M. R., & Cheatham, C. L. (2003). Brain and behavior interface: Stress and the developing brain. *Infant Mental Health Journal, 24,* 195–211.

Gunnar, M. R., & Donzella, B. (2002). Social regulation of the cortisol levels in early human development. *Psychoneuroendocrinology, 27,* 199–220.

Gunnar, M. R., & Vazquez, D. (2006). Stress neurobiology and developmental psychopathology. In D. Cicchetti & D. J. Cohen (Eds.), *Developmental psychopathology: Vol 2. Developmental neuroscience* (2nd ed., pp. 533–577). Hoboken, NJ: Wiley.

Gunnar, M. R., & Vazquez, D. M. (2001). Low cortisol and a flattening of expected daytime rhythm: Potential indices of risk in human development. *Development and Psychopathology, 13,* 515–538.

Hibel, L. C., Granger, D. A., Blair, C., Cox, M. J., & The Family Life Project Key Investigators. (2011). Maternal sensitivity buffers the adrenocortical implications of intimate partner violence exposure during early childhood. *Development and Psychopathology, 23,* 689–701.

Hill-Soderlund, A. L., Mills-Koonce, W., Propper, C., Calkins, S. D., Granger, D. A., Moore, G. A., et al. (2008). Parasympathetic and sympathetic responses to the Strange Situation in infants and mothers from avoidant and securely attached dyads. *Developmental Psychobiology, 50,* 361–376.

Hofer, M. A. (1995). Hidden regulators: Implications for a new understanding of attachment, separation, and loss. In S. Goldberg, R. Muir, & J. Kerr (Eds.), *Attachment theory: Social, developmental, and clinical perspectives* (pp. 203–230). Hillsdale, NJ: Analytic Press.

Huot, R. L., Brennan, P. A., Stowe, Z. N., Plotsky, P. M., & Walker, E. F. (2004). Negative affect in offspring of depressed mothers is predicted by infant cortisol levels at 6 months and maternal depression during pregnancy, but not postpartum. In R. Yehuda & B. McEwen (Eds.), *Biobehavioral stress response: Protective and damaging effects* (pp. 234–236). New York: New York Academy of Sciences.

Jansen, J., Beijers, R., Riksen-Walraven, M., & de Weerth, C. (2010). Does maternal care-giving behavior modulate the cortisol response to an acute stressor in 5-week-old human infants? *Stress: The International Journal on the Biology of Stress, 13*, 491–497.

Kennedy, A. E., Rubin, K. H., Hastings, P. D., & Maisel, B. (2004). Longitudinal relations between child vagal tone and parenting behavior: 2 to 4 years. *Developmental Psychobiology, 45*, 10–21.

Larson, M. C., White, B., Cochran, A., Donzella, B., & Gunnar, M. (1998). Dampening of the cortisol response to handling at 3 months in human infants and its relation to sleep, circadian cortisol activity, and behavioral distress. *Developmental Psychobiology, 33*, 327–337.

Laurent, H. K., Ablow, J. C., & Measelle, J. (2011). Risky shifts: How the timing and course of mothers' depressive symptoms across the perinatal period shape their own and infants' stress response profiles. *Development and Psychopathology, 23*, 521–538.

Laurent, H. K., Leve, L. D., Neiderhiser, J. M., Natsuaki, M. N., Shaw, D. S., Harold, G. T., et al. (2013). Effects of prenatal and postnatal parent depressive symptoms on adopted child HPA regulation: Independent and moderated influences. *Developmental Psychology, 49*, 876–886.

Leerkes, E. M. (2010). Predictors of maternal sensitivity to infant distress. *Parenting: Science and Practice, 10*, 219–239.

Leerkes, E. M., Blankson, A., & O'Brien, M. (2009). Differential effects of maternal sensitivity to infant distress and nondistress on social-emotional functioning. *Child Development, 80*, 762–775.

Leerkes, E. M., Parade, S. H., & Gudmundson, J. A. (2011). Mothers' emotional reactions to crying pose risk for subsequent attachment insecurity. *Journal of Family Psychology, 25*, 635–643.

Lengua, L. J., Zalewski, M., Fisher, P. A., & Moran, L. (2013). Does HPA-axis dysregulation account for the effects of income on effortful control and adjustment in preschool children? *Infant and Child Development, 22*, 439–458.

Levine, S. (2005). Developmental determinants of sensitivity and resistance to stress. *Psychoneuroendocrinology, 30*, 939–946.

Lopez-Duran, N. L., Kovacs, M., & George, C. J. (2009). Hypothalamic–pituitary–adrenal axis dysregulation in depressed children and adolescents: A meta-analysis. *Psychoneuroendocrinology, 34*, 1272–1283.

Luecken, L. J., Lin, B., Coburn, S. S., MacKinnon, D. P., Gonzales, N. A., & Crnic, K. A. (2013). Prenatal stress, partner support, and infant cortisol reactivity in low-income Mexican American families. *Psychoneuroendocrinology, 38*, 3092–3101.

McEwen, B. S. (2012). Brain on stress: How the social environment gets under the skin. *Proceedings of the National Academy of Sciences USA, 109*(Suppl. 2), 17180–17185.

Meaney, M. J., & Szyf, M. (2005). Maternal care as a model for experience-dependent chromatin plasticity? *Trends in Neurosciences, 28*, 456–463.

Miller, G. E., Chen, E., & Zhou, E. S. (2007). If it goes up, must it come down?: Chronic stress and the hypothalamic–pituitary–adrenocortical axis in humans. *Psychological Bulletin, 133*, 25–45.

Mills-Koonce, W., Garrett-Peters, P., Barnett, M., Granger, D. A., Blair, C., & Cox, M. J. (2011). Father contributions to cortisol responses in infancy and toddlerhood. *Developmental Psychology, 47,* 388–395.

Moore, G. A. (2009). Infants' and mothers' vagal reactivity in response to anger. *Journal of Child Psychology and Psychiatry, 50,* 1392–1400.

Moore, G. A. (2010). Parent conflict predicts infants' vagal regulation in social interaction. *Development and Psychopathology, 22,* 23–33.

Moore, G. A., & Calkins, S. D. (2004). Infants' vagal regulation in the still-face paradigm is related to dyadic coordination of mother–infant interaction. *Developmental Psychology, 40,* 1068–1080.

Moore, G. A., Hill-Soderlund, A. L., Propper, C. B., Calkins, S. D., Mills-Koonce, W., & Cox, M. J. (2009). Mother–infant vagal regulation in the face-to-face still-face paradigm is moderated by maternal sensitivity. *Child Development, 80,* 209–223.

Murray, L., Halligan, S. L., Goodyer, I., & Herbert, J. (2010). Disturbances in early parenting of depressed mothers and cortisol secretion in offspring: A preliminary study. *Journal of Affective Disorders, 122,* 218–223.

Oosterman, M., De Schipper, J., Fisher, P., Dozier, M., & Schuengel, C. (2010). Autonomic reactivity in relation to attachment and early adversity among foster children. *Development and Psychopathology, 22,* 109–118.

Parade, S. H., & Leerkes, E. M. (2011). Marital aggression predicts infant orienting toward mother at six months. *Infant Behavior and Development, 34,* 235–238.

Pendry, P., & Adam, E. K. (2007). Associations between parents' marital functioning, maternal parenting quality, maternal emotion and child cortisol levels. *International Journal of Behavioral Development, 31,* 218–231.

Perry, N. B. (2013). *Maternal sensitivity and physiological processes as predictors of infant emotion regulation.* Unpublished doctoral dissertation, The University of North Carolina at Greensboro, Greensboro, NC.

Perry, N. B., Mackler, J. S., Calkins, S. D., & Keane, S. P. (2014). A transactional analysis of the relation between maternal sensitivity and child vagal regulation. *Developmental Psychology, 50*(3), 784–793.

Poehlmann, J., Schwichtenberg, A., Bolt, D. M., Hane, A., Burnson, C., & Winters, J. (2011). Infant physiological regulation and maternal risks as predictors of dyadic interaction trajectories in families with a preterm infant. *Developmental Psychology, 47,* 91–105.

Porges, S. W. (1991). Vagal tone: An autonomic mediator of affect. In J. Garber & K. A. Dodge (Eds.), *The development of emotional regulation and dysregulation.* Cambridge, UK: Cambridge University Press.

Porges, S. W. (2003). The polyvagal theory: Phylogenetic contributions to social behavior. *Physiology and Behavior, 79,* 503–513.

Porges, S. W. (2007). The polyvagal perspective. *Biological Psychology, 74,* 116–143.

Porges, S. W., & Furman, S. A. (2011). The early development of the autonomic nervous system provides a neural platform for social behaviour: A polyvagal perspective. *Infant and Child Development, 20,* 106–118.

Porter, C. L. (2003). Coregulation in mother–infant dyads: Links to infants' cardiac vagal tone. *Psychological Reports, 92,* 307–319.

Porter, C. L., Wouden-Miller, M., Silva, S., & Porter, A. (2003). Marital harmony and conflict: Linked to infants' emotional regulation and cardiac vagal tone. *Infancy, 4*, 297–307.

Propper, C., Moore, G., Mills-Koonce, W., Halpern, C., Hill-Soderlund, A. L., Calkins, S. D., et al. (2008). Gene–environment contributions to the development of infant vagal reactivity: The interaction of dopamine and maternal sensitivity. *Child Development, 79*, 1377–1394.

Propper, C. B., & Holochwost, S. J. (2013). The influence of proximal risk on the early development of the autonomic nervous system. *Developmental Review, 33*, 151–167.

Radtke, K. M., Ruf, M., Gunter, H. M., Dohrmann, K., Schauer, M., Meyer, A., et al. (2011). Transgenerational impact of intimate partner violence on methylation in the promoter of the glucocorticoid receptor. *Translational Psychiatry, 19*(1), e21.

Repetti, R. L., Robles, T. F., & Reynolds, B. (2011). Allostatic processes in the family. *Development and Psychopathology, 23*, 921–938.

Repetti, R. L., Taylor, S. E., & Seeman, T. E. (2002). Risky families: Family social environments and the mental and physical health of offspring. *Psychological Bulletin, 128*, 330–366.

Rothbart, M. K. (2011). *Becoming who we are: Temperament and personality in development.* New York: Guilford Press.

Saltzman, K. M., Holden, G. W., & Holahan, C. J. (2005). The psychobiology of children exposed to marital violence. *Journal of Clinical Child and Adolescent Psychology, 34*, 129–139.

Sameroff, A. (2009). *The transactional model of development: How children and contexts shape each other.* Washington, DC: American Psychological Association.

Sánchez, M., Ladd, C. O., & Plotsky, P. M. (2001). Early adverse experience as a developmental risk factor for later psychopathology: Evidence from rodent and primate models. *Development and Psychopathology, 13*, 419–449.

Sapolsky, R. M., Romero, L. M., & Munck, A. U. (2000). How do glucocorticosteroids influence stress responses?: Integrating permissive, suppressive, stimulatory and preparative actions. *Endocrine Reviews, 21*, 55–89.

Schmid, B., Buchmann, A. F., Trautmann-Villalba, P., Blomeyer, D., Zimmermann, U. S., Schmidt, M. H., et al. (2013). Maternal stimulation in infancy predicts hypothalamic–pituitary–adrenal axis reactivity in young men. *Journal of Neural Transmission, 120*, 1247–1257.

Schuetze, P., Eiden, R. D., & Danielewicz, S. (2009). The association between prenatal cocaine exposure and physiological regulation at 13 months of age. *Journal of Child Psychology and Psychiatry, 50*, 1401–1409.

Sharp, H., Pickles, A., Meaney, M., Marshall, K., Tibu, F., & Hill, J. (2012). Frequency of infant stroking reported by mothers moderates the effect of prenatal depression on infant behavioural and physiological outcomes. *PLoS ONE, 7*(10), e45446.

Shonkoff, J. P., Garner, A. S., Siegel, B. S., Dobbins, M. I., Earls, M. F., Garner, A. S., et al. (2012). The lifelong effects of early childhood adversity and toxic stress. *Pediatrics, 129*, e232–e246.

Stroud, C. B., Durbin, C., Wilson, S., & Mendelsohn, K. A. (2011). Spillover to triadic and dyadic systems in families with young children. *Journal of Family Psychology, 25*, 919–930.

Sturge-Apple, M. L., Davies, P. T., Cicchetti, D., & Manning, L. G. (2012). Interparental violence, maternal emotional unavailability and children's cortisol functioning in family contexts. *Developmental Psychology, 48*, 237.

Susman, E. J. (2006). Psychobiology of persistent antisocial behavior: Stress, early vulnerabilities and the attenuation hypothesis. *Neuroscience and Biobehavioral Reviews, 30*, 376–389.

Tarullo, A. R., & Gunnar, M. R. (2006). Child maltreatment and the developing HPA axis. *Hormones and Behavior, 50*, 632–639.

Tollenaar, M. S., Beijers, R. R., Jansen, J. J., Riksen-Walraven, J. A., & de Weerth, C. C. (2011). Maternal prenatal stress and cortisol reactivity to stressors in human infants. *Stress: The International Journal on the Biology of Stress, 14*, 53–65.

Watamura, S. E., Donzella, B., Kertes, D. A., & Gunnar, M. R. (2004). Developmental changes in baseline cortisol activity in early childhood: Relations with napping and effortful control. *Developmental Psychobiology, 45*, 125–133.

Zalewski, M., Lengua, L. J., Kiff, C. J., & Fisher, P. A. (2012). Understanding the relation of low income to HPA-axis functioning in preschool children: Cumulative family risk and parenting as pathways to disruptions in cortisol. *Child Psychiatry and Human Development, 43*, 924–942.

CHAPTER 11

A Biopsychosocial Framework
for Infant Temperament
and Socioemotional Development

Kristin A. Buss, Santiago Morales, Sunghye Cho, and Lauren Philbrook

Temperament theory provides a framework for understanding how socio-emotional development unfolds and research in this field has examined trajectories of individual variation across behavioral, biological, and social levels of analysis. In this chapter, we do not attempt a comprehensive review of the literature or concern ourselves with definitional or theoretical discussion of temperament, as these issues have been extensively covered in previous papers (Goldsmith et al., 1987; Shiner et al., 2012; Zentner & Shiner, 2012). Instead, we focus on a few aspects of temperament that highlight research using a biopsychosocial framework: fearful temperament/behavioral inhibition, exuberance, and the role that regulatory processes (e.g., effortful control, attention) play in predicting outcomes.

While definitions and theoretical models/approaches of temperament vary—especially an emphasis on particular definitional aspects—there are several core assumptions that most approaches share (Shiner et al., 2012) and guide this review. Zentner and Bates (2008) have offered a broad definition of infant and child temperament, as distinct from personality, by outlining a set of inclusion criteria. Temperament refers to (1) individual differences, within the normal range of behavior, across domains such as affect and attention (consistent with Rothbart's definition of reactivity and regulation), which can be measured in latency, duration, frequency and intensity; (2) its appearance early in the first few years of life with most aspects showing some initial variability in infancy; (3) being linked to a biological mechanism; and (4) stability across development and predicted variation in related outcomes. Borrowing from the conceptualization of temperament by Goldsmith and colleagues, temperament is viewed as the behavioral, biological, perceptual, and motor substrates (i.e., the raw material) of developing individual differences, where behavioral substrates combine with biological substrates to shape socioemotional behavior (Goldsmith, Lemery, Aksan, & Buss, 2000).

Although a comprehensive review of this literature is outside the scope of this chapter, we briefly summarize the most consistent set of findings linking early temperament traits with adjustment across childhood; we mainly focus on fearful temperament because it has received the most comprehensive treatment in the literature with respect to biopsychosocial models of development. We provide a brief review of the literature linking temperament to social and emotional outcomes, such as internalizing and externalizing symptoms. In this review, we focus on individual differences in both reactive and regulatory processes that predict maladaptive outcomes. We then turn to discussion of putative biomarkers—underlying physiological and neural mechanisms—that have been the focus of temperament research over the past decade. The second half of this chapter addresses one facet of the "social" component of the biopsychosocial model we propose, namely, parents and the parenting context. Variation in temperament influences social interaction and robust evidence exists demonstrating that parents' behavior influences, both directly and indirectly, developmental trajectories for particular children. Finally, we conclude the chapter by proposing a framework for future research on infant temperament.

Temperament and Socioemotional Adjustment

One of the key reasons that infant temperament research is so prolific is because temperamental variation in infancy emerges as a consistent and robust predictor of socioemotional adjustment across childhood. This section reviews some of the key literature linking early variations in temperament to adjustment—specifically, internalizing and externalizing problems.

Starting with the domain of fearful temperament, the pioneering work of Kagan on behavioral inhibition, which characterizes an extreme type of fearful temperament, is one of the best examples of a biopsychosocial temperament model. Behavioral inhibition is an extreme temperament type characterized in infancy by heightened motor and emotional reactivity to novelty (Kagan & Snidman, 1991), whereas behavior in toddlers is characterized by avoidance of unfamiliar adults and wariness of novel objects and situations (García Coll, Kagan, & Reznick, 1984; Kagan, Reznick, & Gibbons, 1989). Moreover, this inhibition in toddlers can be predicted from a pattern of high reactivity/distress to stimuli at 4 months (Kagan & Snidman, 1991). Research has revealed moderate stability throughout childhood with one-third to one-half of children remaining inhibited over time (Rubin, Burgess, & Hastings, 2002; Fox, Henderson, Marshall, Nichols, & Ghera, 2005; Kagan et al., 1989), especially for the subset of children who are most extreme in inhibition (Asendorpf, 1991). In early childhood, behaviorally inhibited children display social reticence and do not engage in, and often avoid, interaction with same-age peers (Rubin et al., 2002). One of the possible results of this cascade of events over early childhood is the emergence of social anxiety disorder. Indeed, there are now multiple studies that suggest that fearful temperament is the best early predictor of social anxiety symptoms in childhood and adolescence (Pérez-Edgar & Fox, 2005; Chronis-Tuscano et al., 2009). However, not all temperamentally fearful children develop anxiety problems, thus, the field is focused on uncovering the biological and social processes that account for this link.

Our own work has focused on elucidating which temperamentally fearful children are at greatest risk for social anxiety and social withdrawal more broadly. Although behavioral inhibition has emerged as the best early predictor of the development of social anxiety disorder, we know that not all inhibited children develop anxiety symptoms and some even become less inhibited over time (Degnan, Henderson, Fox, & Rubin, 2008; Fox, Henderson, Rubin, Calkins, & Schmidt, 2001). We hypothesized that this is due, in part, to heterogeneity in the identification of fearful children (Buss, 2011). The dominant approach to defining and measuring fearful temperament focuses predominantly on how much fear is observed in a novel laboratory setting and then averaging across situations to identify children at risk. An alternative approach focuses on assessing the pattern of fearful behavior across contexts and identifying patterns that are atypical, or dysregulated. Specifically, dysregulation was measured by taking into account the eliciting context of a toddler's behavior such that extreme fear in situations deemed to be low in threat would constitute a maladaptive response (Buss, 2011; Buss et al., 2013). This pattern of dysregulated fear can be reliably differentiated from behavioral inhibition (Buss, 2011) at age 2, predicts social wariness in preschool at age 5 (Buss, 2011), and social anxiety disorder symptoms at age 6 (Buss et al., 2013) over and above the risks associated with behavioral inhibition.

Other dimensions of temperament have also been implicated both in direct-effects models and in interaction with other temperament dimensions to predict externalizing behavior problems. Most notably, the temperamental dimension of exuberance has been implicated in the development of externalizing problems (Calkins, Fox, & Marshall, 1996; He et al., 2010; Stifter, Putnam, & Jahromi, 2008). Exuberance is characterized by high approach, high activity, boldness, and positivity in the face of novelty that can be identified in toddlers (Fox et al., 2001). Like behavioral inhibition, early predictors of this temperament have been identified in early infancy by a pattern of high-motor, high-positive behaviors (in contrast to the negativity associated with later behavioral inhibition). It has been suggested that exuberance is linked to externalizing via the specific characteristic of high-approach behavior, which increases the opportunity for experiencing frustration (Stifter et al., 2008; Polak-Toste & Gunnar, 2006). However, not all exuberant toddlers have adjustment difficulties and may be rated as higher in sociability (e.g., Hane, Fox, Henderson, & Marshall, 2008), and emerging work suggests that the positivity that is characteristic of exuberance may be protective of externalizing (Fox et al., 2001).

In our own work, we have found that a combination of low effortful control, high approach and low positivity at 24 months predicted observed, self- and adult-reported externalizing behaviors (Buss, Kiel, Morales, & Robinson, 2014). Turning to these interactive effects, some researchers have articulated self-regulation as a link between aspects of exuberant temperament and externalizing. Specifically, exuberance is associated with undercontrolled behavior including, most notably, low effortful control (Degnan et al., 2011; Calkins & Keane, 2009; Eisenberg et al., 2001; Janson & Mathiesen, 2008; Olson, Sameroff, Kerr, Lopez, & Wellman, 2005). Low effortful control—difficulty in inhibiting a dominant response in order to initiate a subdominant response (Rothbart, Ellis, & Posner, 2011)—in toddlers and preschoolers has consistently been implicated in the development of externalizing behavior problems (e.g., Eisenberg, Smith, Sadovsky, & Spinrad, 2004; Kochanska & Knaack, 2003; Rubin, Burgess, Dwyer, & Hastings, 2003). Thus, much of the research linking low self-regulation and externalizing has found evidence for interactive effects with other aspects of temperament (e.g., exuberance, impulsivity) (Murray & Kochanska, 2002).

Other regulatory processes such as attention have been explored in relation to temperament and socioemotional outcomes. One line of research has focused on attentional biases toward threat, fearful temperament, and anxiety development. Although the bulk of this work has been in adults, there is emerging developmental work. From this literature we know that anxious individuals have a heightened attention bias toward threat (Bar-Haim, Lamy, Pergamin, Bakermans-Kranenburg, & van IJzendoorn, 2007). Parallel results have been found in children who were classified as behaviorally inhibited in infancy (e.g., Pérez-Edgar et al., 2010). Moreover, there is evidence that attention biases toward threat moderate the relation between infant temperament and later anxiety—where those children and adolescents with a history of high fearfulness and attention bias toward threat displayed the most social withdrawal (Pérez-Edgar et al., 2010, 2011; Morales, Pérez-Edgar, & Buss, 2014). No studies have examined attention bias during infancy and its relation to fear behavior. However, Pérez-Edgar and colleagues (2010) examined individual differences in sustained attention and fearful temperament. At 9 months, infants were characterized as high and low in sustained attention to a video while distractors were presented—low sustained attention was thought to reflect vigilance. Infants with low sustained attention showed increasing levels of fearfulness throughout childhood, and attention and fearfulness interacted to predict social difficulties during adolescence. These results highlight how individual differences in attention during early development may shape how children process and respond to their environment throughout development. As children develop, these attentional biases interact with other self-regulatory processes (e.g., effortful control). For instance, Lonigan and Vasey (2009) found that fearful children only displayed a bias toward threat if they were also low on effortful control. Fearful children high on effortful control did not display such bias (Lonigan & Vasey, 2009). However, this literature does not address whether these biases reflect lack of attentional control (i.e., self-regulation) or merely reflect extreme fearful and anxious behavior. In sum, there is substantial literature demonstrating that early temperamental variation, encompassing both reactive and regulatory processes, in infancy predicts adjustment and maladjustment across childhood and into adolescence. In the following sections of this chapter, we review literature on biological and social environmental factors that influence how and when temperament predicts these social and emotional outcomes.

Biological Markers of Temperament

Because individual differences in socioemotional behavior (especially psychopathology) are increasingly recognized as neurodevelopmental in nature (Cicchetti & Gunnar, 2008; Mathew, Coplan, & Gorman, 2001), developmentalists have examined biological mechanisms (i.e., biomarkers) that inform developmental process. Consistent with the biopsychosocial model of temperament, research has implicated multiple components in the neural circuitry of temperament, such as the amygdala, cingulate cortex, prefrontal cortex, and autonomic nervous and neuroendocrine systems. For instance, Kagan hypothesized that hyperresponsivity of the amygdala and sympathetic nervous system (SNS) was central to the development of inhibited behavior (Kagan, 1994; Kagan, Reznick, & Snidman, 1988). Hyperreactivity across physiological systems is common among children with extreme temperament (e.g., fearful behavior). Rothbart's model of temperament has also specified neurobiological and physiological, as well as genetic, markers of self-regulation (Rothbart, Derryberry, & Posner, 1994). In this section, we provide a review of evidence for biological substrates of temperament in infancy. Several physiological correlates have been found for temperamental types and temperament dimensions, but the bulk of this physiological work has focused on the temperament dimension of fear (most often studied as behavioral inhibition) so we focus mainly on this work.

Autonomic Nervous System Markers of Temperament

The temperament literature is replete with studies linking temperament dimensions to reactivity of various autonomic indices, but we focus here on cardiac reactivity. Since the first studies on behavioral inhibition, differential patterns of cardiac activity have been found. Children characterized as behaviorally inhibited during infancy show higher and less variable heart rate (e.g., Kagan, Reznick, Clarke, Snidman, & García Coll, 1984), and infant negative affect more broadly (e.g., fear, anger, and sadness) has been associated with increases in heart rate reactivity during emotional challenges (Buss, Goldsmith, & Davidson, 2005).

It is important to note that heart rate variability is influenced by both the SNS and the parasympathetic nervous system (PNS). Most studies have used measures that reflect activity from only one system, most often the PNS. Respiratory sinus arrhythmia (RSA) is a PNS measure, which indexes activity from the vagus nerve by measuring the variations of the heart according to the respiratory cycle. The vagus nerve allows rapid acceleration and decceleration of the heart, providing a physiological mechanism for the individual to engage or disengage with the environment as needed to regulate emotion and behavior (Porges, 2007). As with heart rate variability, studies have found that high reactivity and negative affectivity are associated with lower RSA (Calkins, 1997; Huffman et al., 1998; Stifter & Fox, 1990), whereas positive affect and regulation tend to be associated with high RSA (Calkins, 1997; Beauchaine, 2001). Our group has found that context-specific fear—specifically high fear in low-threat situations—was related to higher SNS activity (i.e., faster preejection period [PEP]; Buss, Davidson, Kalin, & Hill Goldsmith, 2004). Similarly, other studies using SNS measures have found that behaviorally inhibited children have higher sympathetic activity as measured by heart rate period (e.g., Kagan et al., 1988). However, not all studies have found the expected associations between temperament and cardiac measures. For example, Marshall and Stevenson-Hinde (1998) did not find differences in any cardiac measures between fearful and nonfearful children.

Neuroendocrine Markers of Temperament

Another physiological marker that has been implicated in infant temperament literature is cortisol, which reflects activity from the hypothalamic–pituitary–adrenocortical (HPA) axis, activated under stress (McEwen & Seeman, 1999). Cortisol reactivity is believed to be highest when environmental challenges overwhelm the individual's coping resources (e.g., unpredictable or uncontrollable situations) and threaten the social self (Gunnar, Talge, & Herrera, 2009). As with cardiac physiology, some findings show that temperamentally fearful children have higher cortisol levels compared with nonfearful children (e.g., Kagan, Reznick, & Snidman, 1987), and notably under certain parenting environments (Nachmias, Gunnar, Mangelsdorf, Parritz, & Buss, 1996). However, these differences have not been consistently found (e.g., Schmidt, Fox, Schulkin, & Gold, 1999). When looking at potential moderators of this association, Nachmias and colleagues (1996) have identified mother–infant attachment as an important environmental context. In addition, our group has found that eliciting context is important to consider. For instance, only high fear in low-threat contexts was predictive of higher cortisol activity (Buss et al., 2004). Finally, cortisol is also often studied as a facet of allostatic load—the wear and tear of the body due to chronic physiological responses (Lupien et al., 2006). Although not typically studied in infancy, we examined allostatic load indexed by a composite of cortisol, RSA, sleep quality, and birth weight at 24 months and found that it predicted externalizing problems in preschool and kindergarten (Buss, Davis, & Kiel, 2011). In addition, 24-month fear predicted more anxiety symptoms when coupled with increased allostatic load under high levels of environmental stress.

Neural Markers of Temperament

While much of the earlier biological evidence was focused on the measures reviewed above, there has been a dramatic increase in research on neural markers of temperament, though the literature with functional magnetic resonance imaging (fMRI) methodology in young children is still scarce and no study, to our knowledge, has explored temperament using this methodology in infants or even young children. Despite the dearth of studies employing this methodology, the literature closely parallels the literature with nonhuman primates, which has also implicated the amygdala with fearful temperament and anxiety (e.g., Fox et al., 2012; Kalin, Shelton, & Davidson, 2004; Oler et al., 2010). Recent fMRI work with children selected during infancy as highly reactive has provided evidence for the hypothesis that the high levels of inhibition observed during childhood might be due to hyperactivity in the amygdala (Pérez-Edgar et al., 2007; Schwartz et al., 2011; Schwartz, Wright, Shin, Kagan, & Rauch, 2003). For example, Schwartz and colleagues (2011) found that highly reactive infants at 4 months of age showed increased amygdala reactivity to the presentation of faces when they were 18 years old. This was especially true for men (Schwartz et al., 2011).

In contrast, several studies have evaluated the relation between temperament and electrocortical measures in infants and young children. The most common of these measures has been hemispheric asymmetries in frontal electroencephalogram (EEG) activity, which has been used as an index of cortical activation believed to be related to unilateral limbic activity (Davidson, 2004). This asymmetric activity has been linked to withdrawal and approach behavior in infants, children, and adults with greater left activity related to approach and greater right activity related to withdrawal behavior. Studies find that infants with right-frontal asymmetry were characterized as more fearful compared to children with left asymmetry (Fox, Calkins, & Bell, 1994). In addition, right-frontal asymmetry has been found to predict moderate stability of behavioral inhibition and the association between inhibition and later outcomes, such as social reticence and internalizing (e.g., Fox et al., 2001). Other studies have found a direct relation between EEG asymmetry and socioemotional outcomes (e.g., Smith & Bell, 2010). For instance, Smith and Bell (2010) found that stable left EEG asymmetry at 10 and 24 months was associated with mother-rated externalizing behaviors, whereas stable right EEG asymmetry was predictive of internalizing behaviors.

As with other physiological measures there has been recent interest in the role of context. Diaz and Bell found that task-specific right EEG asymmetry was related to fear behaviors during that task after controlling for baseline EEG, even when fear behaviors were not correlated across tasks (Diaz & Bell, 2012). It is important to note that this study evaluated a sample not selected for high fear or negative affect, illustrating that the relation between EEG asymmetry and fear behaviors is not limited to infants who display extreme fear. These findings parallel our work, in which we found that right-frontal EEG asymmetry was related to withdrawal-related emotions (i.e., fear and sadness) during the laboratory task as well as higher basal and reactive cortisol levels in 6-month-olds (Buss et al., 2003).

Another electrocortical measure that has also been used to study temperament is the event-related potential (ERP). ERPs are electrophysiological responses, measured from the ongoing EEG signal, that are time locked to a particular event (e.g., cognitive, motor, or sensory). ERPs have been widely used to index constructs like attention and inhibitory control given their superior temporal resolution. In the temperament literature, ERPs have been used to examine how limbic activity (e.g., amygdala) shapes the way information in encoded and processed in the frontal cortex (e.g., anterior cingulated cortex), and have uncovered ERP biomarkers for emotion regulation processes that are characteristic of certain temperament types. Children characterized as inhibited during infancy show differences in ERP components that are consistent with hypotheses and imaging data showing differences in amygdala activity: mismatched negativity (Bar-Haim, Marshall, Fox, Schorr, & Gordon-Salant, 2003), error-related negativity (McDermott et al., 2009; Brooker & Buss, 2014), and brain stem auditory-evoked potentials (Woodward et al., 2001).

However, most of this work has been conducted later in childhood or in longitudinal studies with children characterized during infancy. One exception is a study by Marshall, Reeb, and Fox (2009) in which they compared ERP components among 9-month-old infants of different temperaments characterized at 4 months of age. They found that infants rated as high in negative reactivity— those who would later become behaviorally inhibited—displayed a heightened positive slow wave to novel tones compared with standard tones in an oddball paradigm. This effect was interpreted as increased attentional engagement to the novel tones, consistent with hypotheses about increased vigilance for fearful/anxious individuals (Marshall et al., 2009). In contrast, the positively reactive infants—those who become exuberant children—displayed an increased

P3 response to novel complex sounds, illustrating that temperamentally differ-ent infants show differences in electrophysiological indices that reflect an early response toward novelty (Marshall et al., 2009). Parallel findings have been found with other ERP components believed to indicate error monitoring and modification of subsequent behavior like the error-related negativity (McDer-mott et al., 2009) and the N2 (Henderson, 2010). In our own work, we found a different pattern of error-related negativity at 4.5 years for children charac-terized at age 2 as highly fearful versus nonfearful toddlers (Brooker & Buss, 2014).

Other studies have not found main effects of temperament but have found that some ERP components moderate the relation between infant temperament and socioemotional outcomes (Henderson, 2010; Reeb-Sutherland et al., 2009). For instance, the P3—in response to an auditory oddball task—moderated the relation between infant fearfulness and anxiety during adolescence, where ado-lescents with a history of high fearfulness and a larger P3 response, believed to index attention toward novelty, were at increased risk for anxiety (Reeb-Sutherland et al., 2009).

In summary, as mentioned at the outset of this section, disorders with roots in temperamental variation, such as anxiety, are regarded as neurodevelopmen-tal in nature (Insel et al., 2010). Across the studies reviewed in this section, a consistent pattern of findings emerges informing this work and biopsychosocial models of temperament. Multiple systems are implicated as markers of reactive and regulatory aspects of temperament, and dysregulation of these physiologi-cal systems is common among children at temperamental risk.

Temperament in Context: The Influence of Parenting

In infancy, social experiences are largely dominated by interactions with parents. Some temperament theories have explicitly established that the infant–caregiver relationship shapes individual differences in emotion expression because emo-tions are a central feature of infant–caregiver interactions (e.g., Thomas, Chess, & Birch, 1968). Interactions with caregivers serve as social regulatory processes that may influence the expression of temperament. Characteristics of the care-giving environment are linked to the developmental trajectories of the expres-sion of infants' constitutionally based temperament. Traditionally, temperament and parental socialization influences were viewed as largely independent enti-ties that may either fit optimally ("goodness of fit") or poorly. Based on recent evidence, however, there is a growing recognition that the association between child temperament and parenting behaviors exerts reciprocal influences (e.g., Sameroff, 2009) and are mutually shaped. Available evidence suggests that dif-ferent facets of children's temperament—encompassing emotional, behavioral, and physiological regulation—may elicit specific types of parenting behaviors from parents. Parental behaviors in turn have been shown to moderate or mediate the developmental trajectory of the expression of children's temperamental traits. In this section, we review various aspects of parenting and parent characteristics that have been studied with temperament in infancy and how they interact to predict social and emotional adjustment.

Parent Sensitivity and Parent–Infant Attachment

Formulations of parenting in infancy have mainly focused on parent sensitivity, defined as awareness and accurate interpretation of infant needs or interactional bids, followed by contingent and appropriate responses to them (Ainsworth, Blehar, Waters, & Wall, 1978). Infant trust in the parent to respond to his or her needs facilitates the development of secure base behavior and secure attachment (Ainsworth & Bell, 1970). Attachment security is associated with a host of positive developmental outcomes for children, including better emotion regulation skills and greater social competence (Sroufe, 2005). As children develop, sensitive parenting helps to facilitate the beginnings of a mutually responsive parent–child relationship characterized by each partner's feelings of responsibility to the other and responsiveness to the other's bids and needs (Maccoby, 1983, 1992; Maccoby & Martin, 1983). This mutually responsive orientation (Kochanska, 1997b) is theorized to facilitate parents' later socialization of the child and the development of more advanced social and emotional skills.

Recent work suggests that infants with varying temperamental traits are differentially responsive to equivalent forms of parenting (i.e., differential susceptibility; Belsky & Pluess, 2009). This susceptibility predicts children's socioemotional outcomes in a for-better or -worse manner. For example, prior work has found that child anger proneness moderates the association between maternal responsiveness at 7 months and receptive cooperation at 15 months (Kochanska, Aksan, & Carlson, 2005). Higher anger proneness was associated with more cooperation in the context of high maternal responsiveness, but low cooperation in the context of low maternal responsiveness.

Particular attention has been devoted to studying interactions between parenting quality and fearful child temperament. Generally, this research suggests that a parent–child relationship characterized by high levels of parental sensitivity may be particularly beneficial for fearful children. Higher inhibition in combination with an insecure attachment to the parent has been associated with a cortisol increase to novel stimuli and to the Strange Situation in 18-month-olds (Nachmias et al., 1996), and higher child fearfulness and attachment insecurity predicted greater cortisol reactivity to an inoculation in toddlers (Gunnar, Brodersen, Nachmias, Buss, & Rigatuso, 1996). Fearful children may be more likely to interpret situations as threatening, and without the external regulation of a sensitive parent, they may be more stressed by new or uncomfortable events (Nachmias et al., 1996). Children who are inhibited and have an insecure relationship with their parent have been shown to be at increased risk for developing anxiety in later childhood (Muris, van Brakel, Arntz, & Schouten, 2011; Shamir-Essakow, Ungerer, & Rapee, 2005).

Despite evidence suggesting that sensitive parenting may benefit fearful children, a number of studies have yielded equivocal findings about the effects of high levels of sensitive parenting for these children. It has been suggested that extremely high levels of parental sensitivity, characterized by consistent and prompt responsiveness to infant distress, serve to maintain infants' inhibited and anxious patterns of behaviors (Arcus, 2001; Mount, Crockenberg, Jó, & Wagar, 2010). Highly sensitive parenting behaviors that involve consistent and prompt attempts to shield children from possible threat or alleviate distress with excessive external regulatory support have been conceptualized as "overprotective" or "overindulgent" styles of parenting (Mount et al., 2010; see Buss & Kiel, 2013, for a detailed discussion). These behaviors are theorized to convey a heightened sense of vulnerability and deprive children of opportunities to independently develop age-appropriate soothing, regulatory, and social skills (Rapee, 1997). Although the specific risk conferred by overprotective parenting in anxiety development remains to be better understood, research has indicated that this type of sensitive but overprotective parenting behavior moderates (Rubin et al., 2002) and mediates (Kiel & Buss, 2011, 2014) the longitudinal association between temperamental fearfulness and social wariness later in development.

Parent-Focused versus Child-Focused Parenting

The degree to which parents are able to focus on their child's needs rather than their own has been associated with greater parental sensitivity. In a recent study by Leerkes and colleagues, mother-oriented cry processing was marked by anxious or angry feelings and prioritization of mothers' well-being, and infant-oriented responses were characterized by accurate detection of level of infant distress and prioritization of the infant's well-being (Leerkes, Weaver, & O'Brien, 2012). Mothers who endorsed higher levels of infant-oriented and lower levels of mother-oriented cry processing prenatally were found to be more sensitive to their 6-month-old infants than other mothers during distress-eliciting situations (Leerkes et al., 2012). Thus, mothers' ability to focus on their infant's needs rather than their own seems to be particularly relevant to their ability to sensitively respond to their infants when they are distressed. Parent sensitivity within different domains may be associated with specific behavior problems in later childhood, as for example, sensitivity to infant distress in situations that evoke fear may be associated with children's fearful or anxious behavior (Leerkes et al., 2012).

In early childhood, temperament has been shown to influence the degree to which mothers endorse parent- versus child-focused goals. Mothers of inhibited children have been found to be more likely than mothers of children who are not inhibited to endorse parent-centered strategies, such as higher levels of power assertion, in dealing with their children (Rubin & Mills, 1990). These mothers have also reported feeling more guilty and embarrassed about their children's behavior. Work from our own longitudinal studies has indicated that the relation between mothers' protective behavior and children's fearful temperament is strengthened when mothers accurately predict fearful behavior and endorse more parent-centered goals for handling their child's shyness (Kiel & Buss, 2012). The mother's anticipation of the distress coupled with a focus on her own goals (e.g., embarrassment by her child's fearfulness) leads her to attempt to find a "quick fix" that rapidly reduces the child's distress. Therefore, the child's temperament may influence the degree to which the parent endorses parent- versus child-focused goals, which may in turn influence parenting strategies. Consistent with this hypothesis, we found that mothers who were more embarrassed by their 2-year-old's shy behavior were more likely to behave intrusively with them, such as by carrying or pushing their children toward novel stimuli (Kiel & Buss, 2013).

Parental Control: Interactions with Temperament and Context

The effectiveness of parental control or discipline methods varies with child temperament (Bell, 1968) and interacts with temperament to predict a variety of outcomes. For example, gentle discipline, in the form of guidance de-emphasizing parental power over the child, has been identified as the most critical factor predicting aspects of moral development for behaviorally inhibited preschoolers (Kochanska, 1997a). Parents' use of power assertion is intended to help draw the child's attention to the importance of the message the parent is trying to deliver (Hoffman, 1982), and inhibited children are likely attentive to a potential wrongdoing because of their anxiety so do not require additional assertions of parental control to internalize the parent's directive (Kochanska, 1997a). In contrast, for exuberant children secure attachment and maternal responsiveness have been found to be the strongest predictors of conscience (Kochanska, 1997a). This pattern of findings for exuberant children may be explained by individual differences in effortful control. For instance, children with poorer effortful control may have more difficulty attending to and internalizing parental socialization messages (Kochanska, 1993).Exuberant temperament has also been shown to moderate the influence of parenting on the development of self-regulation. Exuberant toddlers whose mothers used more commands and prohibitive statements, but were positive in their directives, had higher levels of effortful control 2.5 years later (Cipriano & Stifter, 2010). By contrast, mothers' use of more redirections and reasoning characterized by a neutral or negative tone was associated with poorer effortful control for exuberant children. This research further suggests that a warm and positive relationship is particularly critical for fearless or exuberant children, and that power assertion and reasoning may be less effective discipline strategies.

Variability in parental control has also been shown to predict a range of internalizing behaviors for temperamentally fearful children. In addition, studies have shown that parental control may be associated with a developmental trajectory characterized by externalizing behaviors for a constellation of temperamental traits including irritability, frustration, and anger proneness. These divergent patterns may be explained by the notion that parenting behaviors may serve to "amplify" aspects of negative emotionality (Bates & Pettit, 2007), such that specific parenting dimensions such as overcontrol may exacerbate children's temperamental fearful or frustration reactivity.

For inhibited toddlers, there is evidence that parents' appraisal of children's fearfulness or regulatory competence may influence or elicit controlling behaviors (Belsky, Rha, & Park, 2000; Rubin, Nelson, Hastings, & Asendorpf, 1999). These parenting behaviors include overprotective or intrusive behaviors that may either restrict children's autonomy to independently explore, approach, or withdraw from potentially threatening situations. As we reviewed above, these behaviors are viewed as sensitive, but accumulating evidence suggests these behaviors can have unintended consequences for fearful children. For example, Kiel and Buss (2011) found that mothers of inhibited toddlers were more likely to respond to their toddlers in a protective manner in novel laboratory tasks as the accuracy of mothers' prediction of toddler fearful behaviors increased. This finding indicated that when mothers anticipate their toddlers to respond fearfully to novel situations, they exert control to prevent children's experience of fear or distress. Overprotective parenting behaviors in turn predicted children's social withdrawal behaviors during kindergarten age, suggesting that parental control may reinforce and thereby maintain children's fearful disposition. Thus, findings indicate that the transactional processes linking parental appraisal of children's fearfulness and regulatory capacity elicit parents' controlling behaviors that may shape a trajectory of internalizing behaviors by reinforcing children's fearful, avoidant, and dependent behaviors (Dadds & Roth, 2001; Kiel & Buss, 2011).

In contrast, parental control for toddlers with temperamental traits broadly characterized as difficult has been linked to an externalizing trajectory. Degnan and colleagues found that toddlers' high level of frustration interacted with high level of maternal control to predict high levels of disruptive behaviors at age 5 years (Degnan, Calkins, Keane, & Hill-Soderlund, 2008). Likewise, van Aken and colleagues reported that maternal negative control during structured play predicted an increase in toddler externalizing behaviors for boys who were rated as having a difficult temperament (van Aken, Junger, Verhoeven, van Aken, & Dekovic, 2007). Available evidence suggests that the adverse effects of parental control on children with difficult temperament may be similar to the "coercive interaction style" that has been described for older children with behavioral problems (Patterson, 1982), whereby parental perception of infants' difficult temperament evokes proactive control behaviors that involve physical restraint (Lee & Bates, 1985) and power assertion (Kochanska & Kim, 2012). Parental attempts to restrict children's control may reinforce and escalate infants' resistance to control behaviors. For example, Kochanska and Kim (2012) reported that toddlers' anger proneness likewise predicted an increase in parents' power-assertive behaviors, which in turn predicted a range of externalizing behavior outcomes at school age.

In addition to fit with a child's temperament, adaptive parenting must also be appropriate to context (Grusec & Davidov, 2010). In the context of novel stimuli, child temperament may influence which parenting strategies are most effective. Exuberant children, who are more fearless and quicker to approach novelty, may require more parental control than inhibited or fearful children, who may require parental encouragement to engage with a new environment. Parental control in these contexts is important for exuberant children because it helps them to learn self-regulation by showing restraint in unfamiliar and potentially unsafe circumstances (Cipriano & Stifter, 2010). On the other hand, parental encouragement of child exploration is appropriate for fearful children because it helps them to regulate their fear and learn about their environment (Fox et al., 2005). As noted earlier, work from our longitudinal study has indicated that it may not be appropriate for parents to provide protection and comfort in low-threat novel contexts, as a recent study demonstrated that higher levels of maternal protection in low-threat situations were longitudinally associated with greater social withdrawal behavior in toddlers (Kiel & Buss, 2012).

In this section, we reviewed several, albeit a fraction, of the studies that demonstrate the role that the parenting context has on the expression of temperament and socioemotional development across development. However, we now turn to research that integrates physiology, behavior, and parenting that is needed in order to fully test the theoretical biopsychosocial models of development.

Physiology, Parenting, and Temperament

We review a handful of studies that highlight the interactions among these temperament, biological, and parenting factors, as well as work examining adjustment outcomes across development. Studies of this nature also demonstrate how using several indicators provide a more nuanced description of the way in which maternal characteristics can influence infants' temperament.

As reviewed above, EEG frontal asymmetry has been related to withdrawal and approach behavior in early development. Although some of this work suggests that EEG asymmetry is a marker for trait-like individual differences, work has also found that EEG asymmetry can be influenced by environmental factors such as maternal caregiving practices (e.g., Hane & Fox, 2006; Hane, Henderson, Reeb-Sutherland, & Fox, 2010). Consistent with rodent models developed by Meaney and Champagne (Champagne & Mashoodh, 2009; Meaney, 2010), Hane and colleagues (2010) characterized mothers' caregiving behavior as high quality or low quality during usual caregiving situations (e.g., meal preparation, feeding, and changing clothing). Infants receiving low-quality caregiving were more fearful, displayed less positive joint attention, and showed greater right EEG asymmetry (Hane & Fox, 2006); these differences persisted to ages 2 and 3. Specifically, children who experienced low-quality maternal caregiving were characterized as more behaviorally inhibited, showed greater right EEG asymmetry, and had higher maternal-reported internalizing behaviors. Another line of work that demonstrates the complex relations among biological markers, environment, and behavior comes from work on maternal depression. Pre- and postnatal maternal depression has also been associated with infants' greater right EEG asymmetry (e.g., Field et al., 2004; Lusby, Goodman, Bell, & Newport, 2013). Neonates with right EEG asymmetry showed higher cortisol and lower scores on the Brazelton Neonatal Assessment Scale (Field et al., 2004). Moreover, mothers of neonates who displayed right EEG asymmetry were lower in pre- and postnatal serotonin, higher in postnatal cortisol, and displayed lower vagal tone together with greater right EEG asymmetry themselves (Field, Diego, Hernandez-Reif, Schanberg, & Kuhn, 2002). Other studies have found interactions among temperament, other biological markers, and various parenting behaviors. For instance, as reviewed above, cortisol increases to laboratory visits were found only for fearful children with an insecure attachment relationship (Nachmias et al., 1996). We have reported that fearful temperament and harsh parenting in toddlerhood interact to predict increased fearfulness and greater error-related negativity ERPs at 4.5 years (Brooker & Buss, 2014). In a study of preschoolers, Hastings and colleagues (2008) found that low baseline RSA coupled with high maternal protection predicted more internalizing symptoms (i.e., social wariness) for social-wary (i.e., inhibited) children, and they recently reported that these effects persist to age 9 (Hastings, Kahle, & Nuselovici, 2014).

Evidence is accumulating that parental–child influences at behavioral and biological levels are bidirectional. Mother–infant synchrony in physiological reactivity has been observed for cortisol (Sethre-Hofstad, Stanbury, & Rice, 2002; Bright, Granger, & Frick, 2012), salivary alpha amylase (an indicator of SNS; Davis & Granger, 2009), and heart rate reactivity (Waters, West, & Mendes, 2014), suggesting reciprocal influences between child and parent in reactivity during challenging tasks. For instance, Sethre-Hofstad and colleagues (2002) demonstrated that for high maternal-sensitivity dyads, maternal and child cortisol increases to the challenge task were correlated. These results have recently been replicated in a younger sample of mothers and infants across a variety of tasks (Atkinson et al., 2013). Moreover, maternal sensitivity was associated with more variability (interpreted as greater adaptation to threat) in cortisol responses by both infants and mothers across the different situations.

There is also evidence that a child's temperament can influence experiences of parenting as stressful. For example, mothers' heightened cortisol reactivity in parenting contexts has been associated with less sensitive care, particularly for temperamentally negative or inhibited infants, who may be more challenging for parents (Martorell & Bugental, 2006). High levels of cortisol reactivity in response to the Strange Situation procedure were found for mothers who perceived themselves as having lower power in their relationship with their child and who rated their child as temperamentally difficult (Martorell & Bugental, 2006). In addition, greater cortisol responses were associated with higher levels of harsh parenting, such as use of physical force including pushing, shoving, and hitting (Martorell & Bugental, 2006). Similarly, our work has found that a greater maternal cortisol response during the child's interactions with novel stimuli is related to greater intrusiveness during the task for mothers with inhibited toddlers (Kiel & Buss, 2013). A cortisol response under these circumstances may be associated with power assertion, which manifests as more intrusiveness and harsh parenting behavior with the child. Moreover, mothers' interpretation of their arousal in response to the infant's behavior or temperament may account for the association between maternal physiology and her behavior (e.g., Leerkes et al., 2012; Martorell & Bugental, 2006). Thus, it may also be that these mothers are more likely to interpret their stress in response to a more difficult child as frustration or anger, which promotes more controlling and aggressive behavior with the child.

Other work has shown that for mothers of children characterized by an avoidant attachment, high levels of child negativity at 6 months, and less maternal RSA suppression to challenge predicts lower levels of maternal sensitivity (Mills-Koonce et al., 2007). As this work demonstrates, the influence of child temperamental negativity or inhibition on parenting quality can be exacerbated if the parent has difficulty regulating his or her own arousal such that parents with nonadaptive physiological regulation display more negative parenting behaviors (i.e., negative intrusiveness; Mills-Koonce et al., 2009). Because a decrease in RSA allows for increases in cardiac output that support self-regulatory processes in response to external demands (Porges, 1995), together these results suggest that higher infant negativity may be particularly challenging for mothers who are not able to regulate their own arousal level in order to be sensitive to their infants.

Additional studies in older children highlight the interaction among biological, psychological, and social factors to predict socioemotional outcomes. Work from our lab has shown that shy kindergartners are more likely to display reticent and avoidant behavior with unfamiliar peers when they either receive nonsupportive maternal reactions to their negative emotions or have higher cortisol reactivity (Davis & Buss, 2012). In another study that examined the contributions of parenting, temperament, and child physiology, Hastings and colleagues found that fearful temperament and prolonged elevations in cortisol levels in response to meeting strangers in a laboratory were associated with internalizing problems in preschool girls, whereas exposure to higher levels of maternal punishment and prolonged cortisol elevations were associated with externalizing problems in preschool boys (Hastings, Ruttle, Serbin, Mills, & Stack, 2011).

Together, these findings demonstrate that a biopsychosocial model allows for a better understanding of how temperament predicts children's emotional and social lives through bidirectional interactions with context and parenting. They also highlight how assessing several indicators of children's and parents' biology and behavior, as well as the social context, might show a more complete picture of socioemotional development.

Conclusions and Future Directions

Temperament is by definition a biopsychosocial construct where individual differences are expressed across biology, behavior, and in social contexts. However, assessments of temperament almost exclusively focus on the behavioral level of analysis (either questionnaire or observationally) and, as reviewed, biological and environmental factors (e.g., parenting) are often treated as moderators or mediators of the relation between temperament and various socioemotional outcomes. The studies reviewed in this chapter highlight that assessing multiple levels of analysis provides a more comprehensive and predictive picture of children's social and emotional development. This work highlights the importance of examining parent qualities as well as child physiology and behavior simultaneously in order to more fully understand how they predict young children's socioemotional development in combination as these factors may operate in a synergistic manner that is only detectable when examined together (Hastings et al., 2011). Research is only beginning to examine these components together.

Evaluating such complex models, in which several factors interact with one another through development to shape adjustment outcomes, pose a methodological challenge. Specifically, the interactive process is not fully captured by common methodological approaches in which a factor linearly predicts another. When these models are tested via higher-order interactions that attempt to capture this complexity, the power to reliably detect these interactions requires very large samples. Given this limitation, the biopsychosocial approach of the study of temperament would benefit from recent advances in methods such as mixture models (e.g., latent profile analysis [LPA]), which are aimed at identifying groups of individuals with similar patterns across variables/characteristics. Some work studying temperament under this approach has been successful at identifying groups of children based on common temperament measures (e.g., behavior and questionnaires) by replicating theoretically derived groups (Loken, 2004) and groups that are predictive of later socioemotional outcomes (Rettew, Althoff, Dumenci, Ayer, & Hudziak, 2008). Our own work has begun using these methods to study temperament and its relation to later outcomes (e.g., Buss, 2011; Buss et al., 2013). These methods can be applied across behavioral, biological, and social factors in order to better address questions related to which children and which temperamental processes account for development socioemotional adjustment or maladjustment.

We conclude with a few recommendations for infant temperament research to move forward using biopsychosocial approaches. First, identification of temperament profiles (e.g., using LPA) should include both behavioral and biological measures. Incorporating biomarkers in the identification of temperament types will increase homogeneity of groups and will, in turn, improve prediction to socioemotional outcomes. Second, studies of temperament should always consider the contexts where behavior is observed. As we have shown in our work, eliciting context influences the range of behaviors and physiological responses that will be observed. Third, because parenting and other social processes (e.g., peers later in childhood) influence the expression of temperamental variation and trajectories, these must be incorporated into research designs and statistical models. For instance, using growth—latent class growth and growth mixture (Duchesne, Larose, Vitaro, & Tremblay, 2010; Muthen & Shedden, 1999)—models for longitudinal data will allow (1) identification of a set of distinct developmental trajectories, (2) identification of the interindividual differences in these trajectories, and (3) examination of trajectories in relation to predictors in infancy (e.g., parenting) and outcomes (e.g., internalizing or externalizing symptoms).

REFERENCES

Ainsworth, M. D. S., & Bell, S. M. (1970). Attachment, exploration, and separation: Illustrated by the behavior of one-year-olds in a strange situation. *Child Development, 41,* 49–67.

Ainsworth, M. D. S., Blehar, M. C., Waters, E., & Wall, S. (1978). *Patterns of attachment: A psychological study of the strange situation.* Hillsdale, NJ: Erlbaum.

Arcus, D. (2001). Inhibited and uninhibited children. In T. D. Wachs & G. A. Kohnstamm (Eds.), *Temperament in context* (pp. 43–60). Mahwah, NJ: Erlbaum.

Asendorpf, J. B. (1991). Development of inhibited children's coping with unfamiliarity. *Child Development, 62,* 1460–1474.

Atkinson, L., Gonzalez, A., Kashy, D. A., Santo Basile, V., Masellis, M., Pereira, J., et al. (2013). Maternal sensitivity and infant and mother adrenocortical function across challenges. *Psychoneuroendocrinology, 38*(12), 2943–2951.

Bar-Haim, Y., Lamy, D., Pergamin, L., Bakermans-Kranenburg, M. J., & van IJzendoorn, M. H. (2007). Threat-related attentional bias in anxious and nonanxious individuals: A meta-analytic study. *Psychological Bulletin, 133*(1), 1–24.

Bar-Haim, Y., Marshall, P. J., Fox, N. A., Schorr, E. A., & Gordon-Salant, S. (2003). Mismatch negativity in socially withdrawn children. *Biological Psychiatry, 54*(1), 17–24.

Bates, J. E., & Pettit, G. S. (2007). Temperament, parenting, and socialization. In J. E. Grusec & P. D. Hastings (Eds.), *Handbook of socialization: Theory and research* (pp. 153–177). New York: Guilford Press.

Beauchaine, T. (2001). Vagal tone, development, and Gray's motivational theory: Toward an integrated model of autonomic nervous system functioning in psychopathology. *Developmental Psychopathology, 13*(2), 183–214.

Bell, R. Q. (1968). A reinterpretation of the direction of effects in studies of socialization. *Psychological Review, 75*, 81–85.

Belsky, J., & Pluess, M. (2009). Beyond diathesis stress: Differential susceptibility to environmental influences. *Psychological Bulletin, 135*, 885–908.

Belsky, J., Rha, J.-H., & Park, S.-Y. (2000). Exploring reciprocal parent and child effects in the case of child inhibition in US and Korean samples. *International Journal of Behavioral Development, 24*(3), 338–347.

Bright, M. A., Granger, D. A., & Frick, J. E. (2012). Do infants show a cortisol awakening response? *Developmental Psychobiology, 54*(7), 736–743.

Brooker, R. J., & Buss, K. A. (2014). Toddler fearfulness is linked to individual differences in error-related negativity during preschool. *Developmental Neuropsychology, 39*(1), 1–8.

Buss, K. A. (2011). Which fearful toddlers should we worry about? Context, fear regulation, and anxiety risk. *Developmental Psychology, 47*, 804–809.

Buss, K. A., Davidson, R. J., Kalin, N. H., & Hill Goldsmith, H. (2004). Context-specific freezing and associated physiological reactivity as a dysregulated fear response. *Developmental Psychology, 40*(4), 583–594.

Buss, K. A., Davis, E. L., & Kiel, E. J. (2011). Allostatic and environmental load in toddlers predicts anxiety in preschool and kindergarten. *Development and Psychopathology, 23*(4), 1069–1087.

Buss, K. A., Davis, E. L., Kiel, E. J., Brooker, R. J., Beekman, C., & Early, M. C. (2013). Dysregulated fear predicts social wariness and social anxiety symptoms during kindergarten. *Journal of Clinical Child and Adolescent Psychology, 42*, 603–616.

Buss, K. A., Goldsmith, H., & Davidson, R. J. (2005). Cardiac reactivity is associated with changes in negative emotion in 24-month-olds. *Developmental Psychobiology, 46*(2), 118–132.

Buss, K. A., & Kiel, E. J. (2013). Temperamental risk factors for pediatric anxiety disorders. In R. A. Vasa & A. K. Roy (Eds.), *Pediatric anxiety disorders: A clinical guide* (pp. 47–68). New York: Springer.

Buss, K. A., Kiel, E. J., Morales, S., & Robinson, E. (2014). Toddler inhibitory control, bold response to novelty, and positive affect predict externalizing symptoms in kindergarten. *Social Development, 23*(2), 232–249.

Buss, K. A., Malmstadt Schumacher, R., Dolski, I., Kalin, N. H., Hill Goldsmith, H., & Davidson, R. J. (2003). Right frontal brain activity, cortisol, and withdrawal behavior in 6-month-old infants. *Behavioral Neuroscience, 117*(1), 11–20.

Calkins, S. D. (1997). Cardiac vagal tone indices of temperamental reactivity and behavioral regulation in young children. *Developmental Psychobiology, 31*(2), 125–135.

Calkins, S. D., Fox, N. A., & Marshall, T. R. (1996). Behavioral and physiological antecedents of inhibited and uninhibited behavior. *Child Development, 67*, 523–540.

Calkins, S. D., & Keane, S. P. (2009). Developmental origins of early antisocial behavior. *Development and Psychopathology, 21*, 1095–1109.

Champagne, F. A., & Mashoodh, R. (2009). Genes in context gene–environment interplay and the origins of individual differences in behavior. *Current Directions in Psychological Science, 18*(3), 127–131.

Chronis-Tuscano, A., Degnan, K., Pine, D., Perez-Edgar, K., Henderson, H., Diaz, Y., et al. (2009). Stable early maternal report of behavioral inhibition predicts life-time social anxiety disorder in adolescence. *Journal of the American Academy of Child and Adolescent Psychiatry, 48*, 928–935.

Cicchetti, D., & Gunnar, M. R. (2008). Integrating biological measures into the design and evaluation of preventive interventions. *Development and Psychopathology, 20*(3), 737–743.

Cipriano, E. A., & Stifter, C. A. (2010). Predicting preschool effortful control from toddler temperament and parenting behavior. *Journal of Applied Developmental Psychology, 31*, 221–230.

Dadds, M. R., & Roth, J. H. (2001). Family processes in the development of anxiety problems. In M. W. Vasey & M. R. Dadds (Eds.), *The developmental psychopathology of anxiety* (pp. 278–303). New York: Oxford University Press.

Davidson, R. J. (2004). What does the prefrontal cortex "do" in affect: Perspectives on frontal EEG asymmetry research. *Biological Psychology, 67*(1–2), 219–233.

Davis, E. L., & Buss, K. A. (2012). Moderators of the relation between shyness and behavior with peers: Cortisol dysregulation and maternal emotion socialization. *Social Development, 21*(4), 801–820.

Davis, E. P., & Granger, D. A. (2009). Developmental differences in infant salivary alpha-amylase and cortisol responses to stress. *Psychoneuroendocrinology, 34*(6), 795–804.

Degnan, K. A., Calkins, S. D., Keane, S. P., & Hill-Soderlund, A. L. (2008). Profiles of disruptive behavior across early childhood: Contributions of frustration reactivity, physiological regulation, and maternal behavior. *Child Development, 79*, 1357–1376.

Degnan, K. A., Hane, A. A., Henderson, H. A., Moas, O. L., Reeb-Sutherland, B. C., & Fox, N. A. (2011). Longitudinal stability of temperamental exuberance and social–emotional outcomes in early childhood. *Developmental Psychology, 47*, 765–780.

Degnan, K. A., Henderson, H. A., Fox, N. A., & Rubin, K. H. (2008). Predicting social wariness in middle childhood: The moderating roles of child care history, maternal personality, and maternal behavior. *Social Development, 17*, 471–487.

Diaz, A., & Bell, M. A. (2012). Frontal EEG asymmetry and fear reactivity in different contexts at 10 months. *Developmental Psychobiology, 54*(5), 536–545.

Duchesne, S., Larose, S., Vitaro, F., & Tremblay, R. E. (2010). Trajectories of anxiety in a population sample of children: Clarifying the role of children's behavioral characteristics and maternal parenting. *Development and Psychopathology, 22*, 361–373.

Eisenberg, N., Losoya, S., Fabes, R. A., Guthrie, I. K., Reiser, M., Murphy, B., et al.

(2001). Parental socialization of children's dysregulated expression of emotion and externalizing problems. *Journal of Family Psychology, 15*, 183–205.

Eisenberg, N., Smith, C. L., Sadovsky, A., & Spinrad, T. L. (2004). Effortful control: Relations with emotion regulation, adjustment, and socialization in childhood. In R. F. Baumeister & K. D. Vohs (Eds.), *Handbook of self-regulation: Research, theory, and applications* (pp. 259–282). New York: Guilford Press.

Field, T., Diego, M., Hernandez-Reif, M., Schanberg, S., & Kuhn, C. (2002). Relative right versus left frontal EEG in neonates. *Developmental Psychobiology, 41*(2), 147–155.

Field, T., Diego, M., Hernandez-Reif, M., Vera, Y., Gil, K., Schanberg, S., et al. (2004). Prenatal predictors of maternal and newborn EEG. *Infant Behavior and Development, 27*(4), 533–536.

Fox, A. S., Oler, J. A., Shelton, S. E., Nanda, S. A., Davidson, R. J., Roseboom, P. H., et al. (2012). Central amygdala nucleus (Ce) gene expression linked to increased trait-like Ce metabolism and anxious temperament in young primates. *Proceedings of the National Academy of Sciences, 109*(44), 18108–18113.

Fox, N. A., Calkins, S. D., & Bell, M. A. (1994). Neural plasticity and development in the first two years of life: Evidence from cognitive and socioemotional domains of research. *Development and Psychopathology, 6*(04), 677–696.

Fox, N. A., Henderson, H. A., Marshall, P. J., Nichols, K. E., & Ghera, M. M. (2005). Behavioral inhibition: Linking biology and behavior within a developmental framework. *Annual Review of Psychology, 56*, 235–262.

Fox, N. A., Henderson, H. A., Rubin, K. H., Calkins, S. D., & Schmidt, L. A. (2001). Continuity and discontinuity of behavioral inhibition and exuberance: Psychophysiological and behavioral influences across the first four years of life. *Child Development, 72*, 1–21.

García Coll, C., Kagan, J., & Reznick, J. S. (1984). Behavioral inhibition in young children. *Child Development, 55*, 1005–1019.

Goldsmith, H. H., Buss, A. H., Plomin, R., Rothbart, M. K., Thomas, A., Chess, S., et al. (1987). Roundtable: What is temperament? Four approaches. *Child Development, 58*, 505–529.

Goldsmith, H. H., Lemery, K. S., Aksan, N., & Buss, K. A. (2000). Temperament substrates of personality development. In V. J. Molfese & D. L. Molfese (Eds.), *Temperament and personality development across the life span* (pp. 1–32). Mahwah, NJ: Erlbaum.

Grusec, J. E., & Davidov, M. (2010). Integrating different perspectives on socialization theory and research: A domain-specific approach. *Child Development, 81*, 687–709.

Gunnar, M. R., Brodersen, L., Nachmias, M., Buss, K., & Rigatuso, R. (1996). Stress reactivity and attachment security. *Developmental Psychobiology, 29*, 191–204.

Gunnar, M. R., Talge, N. M., & Herrera, A. (2009). Stressor paradigms in developmental studies: What does and does not work to produce mean increases in salivary cortisol. *Psychoneuroendocrinology, 34*(7), 953–967.

Hane, A. A., & Fox, N. A. (2006). Ordinary variations in maternal caregiving influence human infants' stress reactivity. *Psychological Science, 17*(6), 550–556.

Hane, A. A., Fox, N. A., Henderson, H. A., & Marshall, P. J. (2008). Behavioral reactivity and approach–withdrawal bias in infancy. *Developmental Psychology, 44,* 1491–1496.

Hane, A. A., Henderson, H. A., Reeb-Sutherland, B. C., & Fox, N. A. (2010). Ordinary variations in human maternal caregiving in infancy and biobehavioral development in early childhood: A follow-up study. *Developmental Psychobiology, 52*(6), 558–567.

Hastings, P., Sullivan, C., McShane, K., Coplan, R., Utendale, W., & Vyncke, J. (2008). Parental socialization, vagal regulation, and preschoolers' anxious difficulties: Direct mothers and moderated fathers. *Child Development, 79,* 45–64.

Hastings, P. D., Kahle, S., & Nuselovici, J. M. (2014). How well socially wary preschoolers fare over time depends on their parasympathetic regulation and socialization. *Child Development, 84,* 1586–1600.

Hastings, P. D., Ruttle, P. L., Serbin, L. A., Mills, R. S. L., & Stack, D. M. (2011). Adrenocortical responses to strangers in preschoolers: Relations with parenting, temperament, and psychopathology. *Developmental Psychobiology, 53*(7), 694–710.

He, J., Degnan, K. A., McDermott, J. M., Henderson, H. A., Hane, A. A., & Fox, N. A. (2010). Anger and approach motivation in infancy: Relations to early childhood inhibitory control and behavior problems. *Infancy, 15,* 246–269.

Henderson, H. A. (2010). Electrophysiological correlates of cognitive control and the regulation of shyness in children. *Developmental Neuropsychology, 35*(2), 177–193.

Hoffman, M. L. (1982). Development of prosocial motivation: Empathy and guilt. In N. Eisenberg (Ed.), *The development of prosocial behavior* (pp. 281–313). San Diego, CA: Academic Press.

Huffman, L. C., Bryan, Y. E., Carmen, R., Pedersen, F. A., Doussard-Roosevelt, J. A., & Forges, S. W. (1998). Infant temperament and cardiac vagal tone: Assessments at twelve weeks of age. *Child Development, 69*(3), 624–635.

Insel, T., Cuthbert, B., Garvey, M., Heinssen, R., Pine, D. S., Quinn, K., et al. (2010). Research domain criteria (RDoC): Toward a new classification framework for research on mental disorders. *American Journal of Psychiatry, 167*(7), 748–751.

Janson, H., & Mathiesen, K. S. (2008). Temperament profiles from infancy to middle childhood: Development and associations with behavior problems. *Developmental Psychology, 44,* 1314–1328.

Kagan, J. (1994). *Galen's prophecy: Temperament in human nature.* Boulder, CO: Westview.

Kagan, J., Reznick, J. S., Clarke, C., Snidman, N., & García Coll, C. (1984). Behavioral inhibition to the unfamiliar. *Child Development, 55*(6), 2212.

Kagan, J., Reznik, J. S., & Gibbons, J. (1989). Inhibited and uninhibited types of children. *Child Development, 60,* 838–845.

Kagan, J., Reznick, J. S., & Snidman, N. (1987). The physiology and psychology of behavioral inhibition in children. *Child Development, 58*(6), 1459.

Kagan, J., Reznick, J. S., & Snidman, N. (1988). Biological bases of childhood shyness. *Science, 8,* 167–171.

Kagan, J., & Snidman, N. (1991). Infant predictors of inhibited and uninhibited profiles. *Psychological Science, 2,* 40–44.

Kalin, N. H., Shelton, S. E., & Davidson, R. J. (2004). The role of the central nucleus of the amygdala in mediating fear and anxiety in the primate. *Journal of Neuroscience, 24*(24), 5506–5515.

Kiel, E. J., & Buss, K. A. (2011). Prospective relations among fearful temperament, protective parenting and social withdrawal: The role of maternal accuracy in a moderated mediation framework. *Journal of Abnormal Child Psychology, 39,* 953–966.

Kiel, E. J., & Buss, K. A. (2012). Associations among context-specific maternal protective behavior, toddlers' fearful temperament, and maternal accuracy and goals. *Social Development, 21,* 742–760.

Kiel, E. J., & Buss, K. A. (2013). Toddler inhibited temperament, maternal cortisol reactivity and embarrassment, and intrusive parenting. *Journal of Family Psychology, 27,* 512–517.

Kiel, E. J., & Buss, K. A. (2014). Dysregulated fear in toddlerhood predicts kindergarten social withdrawal through protective parenting. *Infant and Child Development, 23*(3), 304–313.

Kochanska, G. (1993). Toward a synthesis of parental socialization and child temperament in early development of conscience. *Child Development, 64*(2), 325–347.

Kochanska, G. (1997a). Multiple pathways to conscience for children with different temperaments: From toddlerhood to age 5. *Developmental Psychology, 33,* 228–240.

Kochanska, G. (1997b). Mutually responsive orientation between mothers and their young children: Implications for early socialization. *Child Development, 68,* 94–112.

Kochanska, G., Aksan, N., & Carlson, J. J. (2005). Temperament, relationships, and young children's receptive cooperation with their parents. *Developmental Psychology, 41,* 648–600.

Kochanska, G., & Kim, S. (2012). Toward a new understanding of legacy of early attachments for future antisocial trajectories: Evidence from two longitudinal studies. *Development and Psychopathology, 24*(3), 783–806.

Kochanska, G., & Knaack, A. (2003). Effortful control as a personality characteristic of young children: Antecedents, correlates, and consequences. *Journal of Personality, 71,* 1087–1112.

Lee, C. L., & Bates, J. E. (1985). Mother–child interaction at age two years and perceived difficult temperament. *Child Development, 56,* 1314–1325.

Leerkes, E. M., Weaver, J. M., & O'Brien, M. (2012). Differentiating maternal sensitivity to distress and non-distress. *Parenting: Science and Practice, 12,* 175–184.

Loken, E. (2004). Using latent class analysis to model temperament types. *Multivariate Behavioral Research, 39*(4), 625–652.

Lonigan, C. J., & Vasey, M. (2009). Negative affectivity, effortful control, and attention to threat-relevant stimuli. *Journal of Abnormal Child Psychology, 37*(3), 387–399.

Lupien, S. J., Ouellet-Morin, I., Hupbach, A., Tu, M. T., Buss, C., Walker, D., et al. (2006). Beyond the stress concept: Allostatic load—a developmental biological and cognitive perspective. In D. Cicchetti & D. J. Cohen (Eds.), *Developmental psychopathology: Vol. 2. Developmental neuroscience* (2nd ed., pp. 578–628). Hoboken, NJ: Wiley.

Lusby, C. M., Goodman, S. H., Bell, M. A., & Newport, D. J. (2013).

Electroencephalogram patterns in infants of depressed mothers. *Developmental Psychobiology, 56*(3), 459–473.

Maccoby, E. E. (1983). Let's not overattribute to the attribution process: Comments on social cognition and behavior. In E. T. Higgins, D. N. Ruble, & W. W. Hartup (Eds.), *Social cognition and development: A sociocultural perspective.* Cambridge, UK: Cambridge University Press.

Maccoby, E. E. (1992). The role of parents in the socialization of children: A historical overview. *Developmental Psychology, 28,* 1006–1017.

Maccoby, E. E., & Martin, J. A. (1983). Socialization in the context of the family: Parent–child interaction. In E. M. Hetherington (Ed.) & P. H. Mussen (Series Ed.), *Handbook of child psychology: Vol. 4. Socialization, personality, and social development* (4th ed., pp. 1–102). New York: Wiley.

Marshall, P. J., Reeb, B. C., & Fox, N. A. (2009). Electrophysiological responses to auditory novelty in temperamentally different 9-month-old infants. *Developmental Science, 12*(4), 568–582.

Marshall, P. J., & Stevenson-Hinde, J. (1998). Behavioral inhibition, heart period, and respiratory sinus arrhythmia in young children. *Developmental Psychobiology, 33*(3), 283–292.

Martorell, G. A., & Bugental, D. B. (2006). Maternal variations in stress reactivity: Implications for harsh parenting practices with very young children. *Journal of Family Psychology, 20,* 641–647.

Mathew, S. J., Coplan, J. D., & Gorman, J. M. (2001). Neurobiological mechanisms of social anxiety disorder. *American Journal of Psychiatry, 158*(10), 1558–1567.

McDermott, J. M., Perez-Edgar, K., Henderson, H. A., Chronis-Tuscano, A., Pine, D. S., & Fox, N. A. (2009). A history of childhood behavioral inhibition and enhanced response monitoring in adolescence are linked to clinical anxiety. *Biological Psychiatry, 65*(5), 445–448.

McEwen, B. S., & Seeman, T. (1999). Protective and damaging effects of mediators of stress: Elaborating and testing the concepts of allostasis and allostatic load. *Annals of the New York Academy of Sciences, 896*(1), 30–47.

Meaney, M. J. (2010). Epigenetics and the biological definition of gene × environment interactions. *Child Development, 81*(1), 41–79.

Mills-Koonce, W. R., Gariepy, J.-L., Propper, C., Sutton, K., Calkins, S., Moore, G., et al. (2007). Infant and parent factors associated with early maternal sensitivity: A caregiver-attachment systems approach. *Infant Behavior and Development, 30,* 114–126.

Mills-Koonce, W. R., Propper, C., Gariepy, J. L., Barnett, M., Moore, G. A., Calkins, S., et al. (2009). Psychophysiological correlates of parenting behavior in mothers of young children. *Developmental Psychobiology, 51*(8), 650–661.

Morales, S., Perez-Edgar, K. E., & Buss, K. A. (2014). Attention biases towards and away from threat mark the relation between early dysregulated fear and the later emergence of social withdrawal. *Journal of Abnormal Child Psychology,* 1–12.

Mount, K. S., Crockenberg, S. C., Jó, P. S., & Wagar, J. L. (2010). Maternal and child correlates of anxiety in 2½-year-old children. *Infant Behavior and Development, 33,* 567–578.

Muris, P., van Brakel, A. M. L., Arntz, A., & Schouten E. (2011). Behavioral inhibition as a risk factor for the development of childhood anxiety disorders: A longitudinal study. *Journal of Child and Family Studies, 20,* 157–170.

Murray, K., & Kochanska, G. (2002). Effortful control: Factor structure and relation to externalizing and internalizing behaviors. *Journal of Abnormal Child Psychology, 30,* 503–551.

Muthen, B., & Shedden, K. (1999). Finite mixture modeling with mixture outcomes using the EM algorithm. *Biometrics, 55*(2), 463–469.

Nachmias, M., Gunnar, M., Mangelsdorf, S., Parritz, R. H., & Buss, K. (1996). Behavioral inhibition and stress reactivity: The moderating role of attachment security. *Child Development, 67*(2), 508–522.

Oler, J. A., Fox, A. S., Shelton, S. E., Rogers, J., Dyer, T. D., Davidson, R. J., et al. (2010). Amygdalar and hippocampal substrates of anxious temperament differ in their heritability. *Nature, 466*(7308), 864–868.

Olson, S. L., Sameroff, A. J., Kerr, D. C., Lopez, N. L., & Wellman, H. M. (2005). Developmental foundations of externalizing problems in young children: The role of effortful control. *Development and Psychopathology, 17,* 25–45.

Patterson, G. R. (1982). *Coercive family process: A social learning approach.* Eugene, OR: Castalia.

Pérez-Edgar, K., Bar-Haim, Y., McDermott, J. M., Chronis-Tuscano, A., Pine, D. S., & Fox, N. A. (2010). Attention biases to threat and behavioral inhibition in early childhood shape adolescent social withdrawal. *Emotion, 10*(3), 349–357.

Pérez-Edgar, K., & Fox, N. A. (2005). Temperament and anxiety disorders. *Child and Adolescent Psychiatric Clinics of North America, 14,* 681–706.

Pérez-Edgar, K., Reeb-Sutherland, B. C., McDermott, J. M., White, L. K., Henderson, H. A., Degnan, K. A., et al. (2011). Attention biases to threat link behavioral inhibition to social withdrawal over time in very young children. *Journal of Abnormal Child Psychology, 39*(6), 885–895.

Pérez-Edgar, K., Roberson-Nay, R., Hardin, M. G., Poeth, K., Guyer, A. E., Nelson, E. E., et al. (2007). Attention alters neural responses to evocative faces in behaviorally inhibited adolescents. *NeuroImage, 35*(4), 1538–1546.

Polak-Toste, C. P., & Gunnar, M. R. (2006). Temperamental exuberance: Correlates and consequences. In P. J. Marshall & N. A. Fox (Eds.), *The development of social engagement* (pp. 19–45). New York: Oxford University Press.

Porges, S. W. (1995). Cardiac vagal tone: A physiological index of stress. *Neuroscience and Biobehavioral Reviews, 19,* 225–233.

Porges, S. W. (2007). The polyvagal perspective. *Biological Psychology, 74*(2), 116–143.

Rapee, R. M. (1997). The potential role of childrearing practices in the development of anxiety and depression. *Clinical Psychology Review, 17,* 47–67.

Reeb-Sutherland, B. C., Vanderwert, R. E., Degnan, K. A., Marshall, P. J., Pérez-Edgar, K., Chronis-Tuscano, A., et al. (2009). Attention to novelty in behaviorally inhibited adolescents moderates risk for anxiety. *Journal of Child Psychology and Psychiatry, 50*(11), 1365–1372.

Rettew, D. C., Althoff, R. R., Dumenci, L., Ayer, L., & Hudziak, J. J. (2008). Latent profiles of temperament and their relations to psychopathology and wellness. *Journal of the American Academy of Child and Adolescent Psychiatry, 47*(3), 273–281.

Rothbart, M. K., Derryberry, D., & Posner, M. I. (1994). A psychobiological approach to the development of temperament. In J. E. Bates & T. D. Wachs (Eds.), *Temperament: Individual differences at the interface of biology and behavior* (pp. 83–116). Washington, DC: American Psychological Association.

Rothbart, M. K., Ellis, L. K., & Posner, M. I. (2011). Temperament and self-regulation. In K. D. Vohs & R. F. Baumeister (Eds.), *Handbook of self-regulation: Research, theory, and applications* (2nd ed., pp. 441–460). New York: Guilford Press.

Rubin, K. H., Burgess, K. B., Dwyer, K. D., & Hastings, P. (2003). Predicting preschoolers' externalizing behaviors from toddler temperament, conflict, and maternal negativity. *Developmental Psychology, 39*, 164–176.

Rubin, K. H., Burgess, K. B., & Hastings, P. D. (2002). Stability and social–behavioral consequences of toddlers' inhibited temperament and parenting behaviors. *Child Development, 73*, 483–495.

Rubin K. H., & Mills, R. S. L. (1990). Maternal beliefs about adaptive and maladaptive social behaviors in normal, aggressive, and withdrawn preschoolers. *Journal of Abnormal Child Psychology, 18*, 419–435.

Rubin, K. H., Nelson, L. J., Hastings, P. D., & Asendorpf, J. (1999). The transaction between parents' perceptions of their children's shyness and their parenting styles. *International Journal of Behavioral Development, 23*, 937–957.

Sameroff, A. J. (2009). Conceptual issues in studying the development of self-regulation. In S. L. Olson & A. J. Sameroff (Eds.), *Biopsychosocial regulatory process in the development of childhood behavior problems* (pp. 1–18). New York: Cambridge University Press.

Schmidt, L. A., Fox, N. A., Schulkin, J., & Gold, P. W. (1999). Behavioral and psychophysiological correlates of self-presentation in temperamentally shy children. *Developmental Psychobiology, 35*(2), 119–135.

Schwartz, C. E., Kunwar, P. S., Greve, D. N., Kagan, J., Snidman, N. C., & Bloch, R. B. (2011). A phenotype of early infancy predicts reactivity of the amygdala in male adults. *Molecular Psychiatry, 17*(10), 1042–1050.

Schwartz, C. E., Wright, C. I., Shin, L. M., Kagan, J., & Rauch, S. L. (2003). Inhibited and uninhibited infants "grown up": Adult amygdalar response to novelty. *Science, 300*(5627), 1952–1953.

Sethre-Hofstad, L., Stansbury, K., & Rice, M. A. (2002). Attunement of maternal and child adrenocortical response to child challenge. *Psychoneuroendocrinology, 27*(6), 731–747.

Shamir-Essakow, G., Ungerer, J. A., & Rapee, R. M. (2005). Attachment, behavioral inhibition, and anxiety in preschool children. *Journal of Abnormal Child Psychology, 33*, 131–143.

Shiner, R. L., Buss, K. A., McClowry, S. G., Putnam, S. P., Saudino, K. J., & Zentner, M. (2012). What is temperament now?: Assessing progress in temperament research on the twenty-fifth anniversary of Goldsmith et al. *Child Development Perspectives, 6*, 436–444.

Smith, C. L., & Bell, M. A. (2010). Stability in infant frontal asymmetry as a predictor of toddlerhood internalizing and externalizing behaviors. *Developmental Psychobiology, 52*(2), 158–167.

Sroufe, L. A. (2005). Attachment and development: A prospective, longitudinal study from birth to adulthood. *Attachment and Human Development, 7,* 349–367.

Stifter, C. A., & Fox, N. A. (1990). Infant reactivity: Physiological correlates of newborn and 5-month temperament. *Developmental Psychology, 26*(4), 582–588.

Stifter, C. A., Putnam, S., & Jahromi, L. (2008). Exuberant and inhibited toddlers: Stability of temperament and risk for problem behavior. *Development and Psychopathology, 20,* 401–421.

Thomas, A., Chess, S., & Birch, H. G. (1968). *Temperament and behavior disorders in children.* New York: New York University Press.

van Aken, C., Junger, M., Verhoeven, M., van Aken, M. A. G., & Dekovic, M. (2007). The interactive effects of temperament and maternal parenting on toddlers' externalizing behaviours. *Infant and Child Development, 16,* 553–572.

Waters, S. F., West, T. V., & Mendes, W. B. (2014). Stress contagion: Physiological covariation between mothers and infants. *Psychological Science, 25*(4), 934–942.

Woodward, S. A., McManis, M. H., Kagan, J., Deldin, P., Snidman, N., Lewis, M., et al. (2001). Infant temperament and the brainstem auditory evoked response in later childhood. *Developmental Psychology, 37*(4), 533–538.

Zentner, M., & Bates, J. E. (2008). Child temperament: An integrative review of concepts, research programs, and measures. *European Journal of Developmental Science, 2,* 2–37.

Zentner, M., & Shiner, R. L. (Eds.). (2012). *Handbook of temperament.* New York: Guilford Press.

CHAPTER 12

Genetic Correlates
of Early Maternal Caregiving

W. Roger Mills-Koonce, Cathi B. Propper, and Bharathi J. Zvara

Sensitive and emotionally supportive parenting is one of the most consistent and robust predictors of multiple developmental outcomes in infancy and beyond. Parental warmth and support for children's physical and emotional needs in the first year of life has been associated with the development of emotion regulation abilities (Crockenberg & Leerkes, 2000), well-functioning autonomic (Propper et al., 2008) and neuroendocrine (Blair et al., 2008) stress psychophysiology, executive functioning (Blair et al., 2011), language development (Pungello, Iruka, Dotterer, Mills-Koonce, & Reznick, 2009), later behavioral and emotional issues (Willoughby, Mills-Koonce, Propper, & Waschbusch, 2013), and academic competence (National Institute of Child Health and Human Development, Early Child Care Research Network, 1999; Rimm-Kaufman, Pianta, Cox, & Bradley, 2003). Because of its saliency as a key experiential variable during early development, a growing body of research has begun to examine the origins of sensitive caregiving behaviors, including biological, psychological, relational, contextual, and cultural influences. This chapter focuses on one of the more recent inquiries in this field: the role of genetics as a source of individual differences in early parenting behaviors. More specifically, this chapter will discuss the complexities of understanding the role of genes (including mothers', fathers', and children's genotypes) on early maternal caregiving by adopting both a biopsychosocial and a family systems approach to the study of the genetics of parenting.

Belsky (1984) proposes that caregiving is multiply determined and emerges as a joint function of the psychological processes and resources available to the parent, the contextual sources of support and stress they experience, and the characteristics of the child. This highlights the nature of parenting as a social behavior, directed toward the child but influenced by both parental characteristics and the relational and contextual environment in which those parenting behaviors are expressed. In this sense, when considering the possible sources of genetic influences on maternal care, we must focus not only on the maternal genotype but also on the genotypes of other members of the family. For example, a mother's genotype may be directly associated with her behavioral tendencies, whereas the father's and the child's genotypes may be indirectly associated with the mother's behavior via their contributions to the relational contexts within the family system.

Biopsychosocial and family systems models provide complementary frameworks for understanding the interplay between genetic and experiential influences on early parenting behaviors. A biopsychosocial model posits that biological, psychological, and social factors each play a significant role in the consolidation, maintenance, and change in parenting behaviors over time. Utilizing such a framework within this domain of study is important in that it decreases the likelihood of interpreting correlations between genotypes and phenotypes in purely reductionist terms. Furthermore, such a philosophy is conceptually compatible with and complementary to a family systems approach (Cox & Paley, 2003; Minuchin, 1974) for the study of parenting behaviors. Like the biopsychosocial model, family systems theory stresses the importance of studying persons (and phenomenon) within a hierarchy of subordinate and superordinate levels of functioning. As such, whereas the adoption of a biopsychosocial approach provides an organismic framework for the transactions between genes and environments as they influence early parenting, the adoption of a family systems approach provides a contextual framework for understanding how both the genotype of the parent as well as the genotypes of other family members may influence the parenting behaviors of mothers and fathers.

Because the study of genetic influences on human caregiving behaviors is a relatively new but growing field of research, and because technological advances have recently altered the landscape of this domain of study, there are no clear studies that effectively integrate the biopsychosocial and family systems models as currently proposed. Therefore, we first provide a description of the various methodologies that have, to date, been used for examining genetic influences on parenting behaviors. Next we offer a review of the extant literature on this topic and highlight how these findings can be integrated into a more comprehensive developmental model of parenting during infancy. Finally, we discuss the implications of such a model and possible directions for future research on these topics.

Methodologies for Exploring Genetic Influences on Parenting

The role of genetic influence on parenting behaviors was explored in the 1970s and early 1980s (Plomin, DeFries, & Loehlin, 1977; Rowe, 1981, 1983), but it was not until the 1990s that significant empirical attention was given to the role of genetics (in the form of adoption and behavioral genetic studies) in human caregiving behavior (see Plomin & Bergeman, 1991). There is now a growing literature on the roles of genetic and environmental influence on parenting in animal models (Meaney, 2001, 2007) and across the human lifespan (see McGuire, 2003; Mills-Koonce & Propper, 2011; Towers, Spotts, & Neiderhiser, 2001, for reviews), with findings indicating that both genetic and environmental influences are important for explaining individual differences in parenting. Much of this literature emerged from rigorously designed behavioral genetic twin studies and adoption studies, whereas research on the molecular genetics of parenting, though gradually coming into view, is still rather limited. The following sections provide basic descriptions of these methodologies. Each approach offers a unique perspective, each with its own strengths and weaknesses, that can help untangle the complex associations between genetics and parenting during infancy.

Behavioral Genetics

A behavioral genetics approach views parenting behaviors as "phenotypes" that can be directly influenced by the parental or child genotype (McGuire, 2003). These phenotypes can include any measured behaviors or traits, such as parental warmth or harshness, which may differ across monozygotic and dizygotic twins. By utilizing the *equal environments assumption*, which suggests that environmentally induced similarity is approximately the same for twins reared in the same family, twin studies have become a mainstay of behavioral genetics and serve as a useful methodology for establishing the heritability of a given phenotype. This is achieved by using statistical methodologies to partition phenotypic variance in parenting behaviors across monozygotic and dizygotic twins into genetic and environmental components, with the environmental portion of the variance further divided into shared and nonshared components (see Rowe, 1994). To accomplish this, twin studies take advantage of the genetic difference between monozygotic twins, who share 100% of their genes, and dizygotic twins, who typically share 50% of their genes (comparable to any full sibling pair). Such an approach assumes that if monozygotic twins are more similar than dizygotic twins for a given phenotype, then the heritability of that phenotype (or its genetic origins) may be greater than the environmental influences on the phenotype.

Two types of twin studies have been used to examine parenting behaviors. The first methodology examines the caregiving behaviors of twin parents to directly compare parenting quality across monozygotic and dizygotic adult twin pairs (each with their own children). These analyses consider the genetic effects of the parent on parenting behavior. The second approach involves comparing the caregiving behaviors of a single parent across her monozygotic or dizygotic twin pairs. These analyses consider the effects of child genotype as evocative of variations in parenting behavior. Each approach identifies the percentage of variation in caregiving behavior that is unique to genetic origins (either in the parent or the child) or environmental origin.

Although these studies have been informative for describing parenting behaviors at the population level, two criticisms have been levied against this methodology. The first is that twin studies of parenting do not adequately address individual differences in parenting behaviors; the second concern is that they do not adequately account for gene–environment interactions in the development of parenting behaviors. In addition, there have been concerns regarding the generalizability of twin studies to nontwin populations, such as having a greater likelihood of being born prematurely or low birth weight (twin newborns are typically 30% lighter than singletons) and differential in utero experiences for twins (Knickmeyer et al., 2011; Min et al., 2000; Pol et al., 2002), so findings from behavioral genetic twin studies should be interpreted with these cautions.

Adoption Studies

Adoption studies are a less common but highly informative source for understanding child genetic influences within the family system. Adoption designs include either family members reared together who are not genetically related to each other or family members who are genetically related but were adopted into different families. The most sound adoption studies include data on both the biological and adoptive parents, and preferably cases in which the adopted child has limited or no contact with the biological parents. These studies allow for children to be grouped or identified as being at elevated "genetic risk" due to the psychopathological characteristics of their biological parents (if that information is available). The caregiving behaviors across adoptive parents can then be compared as a function of child genetic risk, which is independent of any genetic risk of the adoptive parent.

Molecular Genetic Studies

The sequencing of the human genome and the growing understanding of the functions of gene pathways provide powerful tools for identifying genetic variations that contribute to human behavior. Complementary advances in biotechnological and statistical research methodologies allow for social scientists to now examine variations across individual genes (or clusters of genes) and to relate that genetic variation to individual differences in phenotypic behaviors. The benefit of molecular genetic studies is that individual differences in parenting behaviors can be directly tested as a function of specific and known differences across genotypes. The drawback of molecular genetic studies is that single-gene (and even multigene) studies are not likely to be overly informative regarding complex social behaviors such as parenting. Instead, genetic effects are likely to result from complex interactions across multiple genes and with multiple environmental experiences. Due to the complexities of such interactions, relatively large sample sizes and highly sensitive behavioral measures are required in order to achieve adequate power to detect such genetic influences.

Although each of the above methodologies have strengths and weaknesses, all three (behavioral genetics, adoption studies, and molecular genetics) offer insight into the developmental origins of variations in caregiving behaviors. Furthermore, each approach can utilize principles from both biopsychosocial and family systems theories to better ground specific findings within the multilevel dynamic system in which early caregiving behaviors occur. In the next section we highlight research on the various types of genetic influence on early maternal sensitivity and then discuss the implications and limitations of these findings.

Mechanisms of Genetic Influence on Maternal Caregiving

There are three primary mechanisms by which genetic influences within the family system may influence sensitive maternal caregiving (see Figure 12.1). The first mechanism involves direct mother gene–behavior associations or gene–environment interactions (G × E) as predictors of maternal behaviors. The second and third mechanisms involve two types of gene–environment correlations (rGEs). Evocative gene–environment correlations occur when the genotype of the child is associated with a pattern of child behavior that in turn elicits a specific type of maternal caregiving. Active gene–environment correlations occur when the genotype of the mother is associated with maternal self-selection into contexts of stress and/or support in her life (e.g., her romantic partner, social support network).* Interestingly, these three mechanisms of genetic influence on parenting behavior parallel Belsky's (1984) proposal that caregiving is the joint function of psychological processes (direct maternal genotype influence), characteristics of the child (child evocative rGE influence), and contextual sources of

---

*A third type of gene–environment correlation, the passive rGE, occurs when the association between the child's genotype and parents' caregiving is due to shared genes with the parent whose genotype is primarily responsible for her behavior. In this sense, the passive rGE is subsumed under the previously described direct effect of maternal genotype on maternal caregiving behavior.

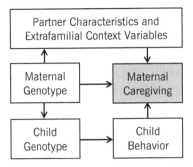

FIGURE 12.1. Conceptual model of potential family-level genetic influences on maternal caregiving, including direct effects of maternal genotype on caregiving, evocative gene–environment correlations, and active gene–environment correlations.

support and stress (maternal active rGE influence). Next we provide evidence for these three mechanisms of genetic influence on maternal caregiving as taken from twin, adoption, and molecular genetic studies.

Direct Associations between Maternal Genotype and Maternal Caregiving

Behavioral genetic studies using twin parents have identified both genetic and environmental sources of variation in parenting behaviors. Reiss (2005) reported stronger correlations in self-reported warmth, hostility, and monitoring among monozygotic than dizygotic twins, which are similar to other heritability estimates from twin studies of observed maternal warmth (Losoya, Callor, Rowe, & Goldsmith, 1997; Neiderhiser & Lichtenstein, 2008; Neiderhiser et al., 2004) and child-reported maternal monitoring (Neiderhiser et al., 2004). These studies provide evidence that, at the population level, variation in human caregiving behaviors is in part due to variations in genetic makeup. These findings are not surprising, but they provide only a glimpse into the complexity of the intricate relationship between a mother's genotype and her caregiving phenotype. Understanding caregiving behaviors that emerge from the complex interplay among biological, psychological, and experiential variables requires multilevel analyses capable of addressing individual differences in parenting behaviors. In other words, although this approach is informative, it fails to address the complexity of this phenomenon from either a biopsychosocial or family systems perspective.

There are, however, several studies identifying specific genes that may affect the development of key neurological systems associated with measurable differences in both parenting behaviors and psychological factors associated with parental functioning. To date, most of this research has focused on genetic contributions to basic individual personality and temperament characteristics (Coplan, Reichel, & Rowan, 2009; McCrae et al., 2000; Rothbart, 2007;

Rothbart, Ahadi, & Evans, 2000), and some of these characteristics, such as the "Big Five" (neuroticism, extraversion, agreeableness, conscientiousness, and openness to experience), have independently been related to parenting behaviors. For example, neuroticism has been associated with less optimal parenting, including less warmth, positive affect, nurturance, and responsiveness and more intrusiveness (Belsky, Crnic, & Woodworth, 1995; Clark, Kochanska, & Ready, 2000; Koenig, Barry, & Kochanska, 2010; ; Kochanska, Clark, & Goldman, 1997; Kochanska, Friesenborg, Lange, & Martel, 2004; Losoya et al., 1997; Metsäpelto & Pulkkinen, 2003; Prinzie et al., 2004; Spinath & O'Connor, 2003). Research has also identified associations among agreeableness and parental positive affect, sensitivity and lower levels of detachment (Belsky et al., 1995), positive interactions and more responsiveness (Clark et al., 2000; Kochanska et al., 2004), nurturance (Metsäpelto & Pulkkinen, 2003), and less overreactive parenting (Prinzie et al., 2004). Openness and conscientiousness have been associated with greater levels of sensitivity and positive expressiveness (Smith et al., 2007) and more positive emotion socialization practices (Hughes & Gullone, 2010), and negatively related to negative control in parent–child interactions (Karreman, van Tuijl, van Aken, & Deković, 2008). Extraversion has been associated with more positive affect and sensitivity (Belsky et al., 1995), lower levels of power assertion (Clark et al., 2000), more awareness of child behavior (Kochanska et al., 2004), and nurturance (Metsäpelto & Pulkkinen, 2003). Last, conscientiousness has been correlated with more responsiveness and less power assertion (Clark et al., 2000) and restrictiveness (Metsäpelto & Pulkkinen, 2003). Similarly, higher levels of parent self-regulation are also associated with more optimal parenting (Cumberland-Li, Eisenberg, Champion, Gershoff, & Fabes, 2003), whereas parents' general negative affectivity and depressive symptoms have been likewise associated with less optimal parenting (Downey & Coyne, 1990; Fish, Stifter, & Belsky, 1991). Each of these individual personality or behavioral characteristics have also been associated with specific gene variants (see Table 12.1), suggesting that such personality dimensions may be one mechanism through which an individual's genotype influences early caregiving behaviors.

There is also an emerging literature directly examining associations between molecular genetics and parenting behaviors. Whereas much of this research has occurred in animal models of offspring caregiving (see studies of maternal behavior related to the *FosB* gene in mouse mothers: Brown, Ye, Bronson, Dikkes, & Greenberg, 1996; Kuroda et al., 2007; Kuroda, Meaney, Uetani, & Kato, 2008) and the serotonin transporter gene (*5-HTTLPR*) in rhesus macaque mothers; McCormack, Newman, Higley, Maestripieri, & Sanchez, 2009), an increasing number of studies have directly examined human genetics and early caregiving behavior. One of the first studies on this topic, reported by Bakermans-Kranenburg and van IJzendoorn (2008), identified a gene × gene interaction (G × G) for mothers (a combination of the less efficient

TABLE 12.1. Adult Characteristics and Associated Gene Variants

Adult characteristics	Genes					
	DRD2	DRD4	5-HTT	COMT	OXT	MAOA
Neuroticism		✓	✓			✓
Agreeableness		✓	✓			
Extraversion	✓			✓		
Openness			✓			✓
Conscientiousness		✓	✓			
Self-regulation	✓	✓	✓	✓		✓
Negative affectivity		✓	✓	✓		
Depressive symptoms	✓		✓			
Social bonding and trust					✓	

variant of the serotonin transporter gene [5-HTT s/s] and the oxytonergic 9AA/AG system gene) that predicted lower levels of sensitive responsiveness to their infants and toddlers. This combination of genes involved a comparable variant of the serotonin transporter gene associated with less optimal care in rhesus macaques (McCormack et al., 2009) and an oxytonergic gene variant thought to be associated with circulating oxytocin, a hormone associated with bonding and caregiving behaviors in humans and nonhuman primates (Feldman, Weller, Zagoory-Sharon, & Levine, 2007). In fact, recent research on the genetics of the oxytocin system and how it relates to parenting behaviors provides further support for direct associations between maternal genotype and the parenting phenotype. On this topic, Mileva-Seitz and colleagues (2013) reported that two polymorphisms in the oxytocin peptide gene and one polymorphism in the oxytocin receptor gene were significantly associated with maternal vocalizing and eye gaze with the infant at 6-months postpartum. And perhaps more important, Feldman and colleaues (2012) have recently demonstrated a biological model for this association with a study that linked the "risk" variants of specific oxytocin receptor genes to lower levels of plasma oxytocin circulating in the body and to lower levels of parent–infant gaze synchrony.

This research is new, but quite intriguing, and demonstrates the utility of adopting a multilevel approach for identifying these associations and the mechanisms that may connect an individual's genotype and phenotype. However, although such single- and multigene studies of maternal behavior are informative of potential biological mechanisms underlying the manifestation of such maternal care, a biopsychosocial perspective also necessitates the consideration of coactional processes between genotype and environmental influences on the parenting phenotype. On this topic, van IJzendoorn, Bakermans-Kranenburg, and Mesman (2008) reported that variations in a dopamine D4 receptor

(*DRD4*) gene and a catechol-O-methyltransferase (*COMT*) gene jointly moderated mothers' vulnerability to the negative influences of daily hassles on their sensitive caregiving behavior (G × G × E interaction). Their research indicates that mothers who had the combination of the val/val or val/met *COMT* polymorphism *and* the *DRD4* 7-repeat polymorphism were observed to be less sensitive in parent–child interactions when they reported high levels of daily hassles. Interestingly, mothers in the study who had this combination of dopaminergic genes and *lower* levels of daily hassles were observed to be *more* sensitive, suggesting that this particular combination of genes resulted in a greater susceptibility to environmental stress for some mothers as a function of their genotype. As suggested by the authors of the study, this combination of genes may actually result in inefficiencies within the dopaminergic system that may leave the mother more vulnerable to the effects of environmental stress.

A separate potential association between dopaminergic system and maternal caregiving behaviors has also been identified in an examination of the dopamine transporter gene (*DAT1*) and positive and negative parenting behaviors and maternal commands (Lee et al., 2010). Across *DAT1* genotypes (9/9, 9/10, and 10/10) there were significantly higher levels of negative parenting and maternal commands observed among mothers with 9/10 and 10/10 genotypes as compared with 9/9 mothers. However, this effect was moderated by child disruptive behavior. The *DAT1* group differences in parenting were only observed under conditions of elevated child disruptive behavior such that at lower levels of child disruptive behavior there were no differences in parenting across *DAT1* genotypes. Whereas the previous study by van IJzendoorn et al. (2008) identified a potential genetic susceptibility model (in which the influence of environmental variation was dependent on maternal genotype), the findings by Lee and colleagues (2010) suggest that the influence of genetic variation on maternal parenting is constrained by environmental factors. Despite the functional difference across the G × E models, each finding is consistent with the role of dopamine in the cognitive and affective processes (particularly within the anterior cingulated cortex) that may mediate complex social behaviors such as parenting (Brunton & Russell, 2008; Fan, Hof, Guise, Fossella, & Posner, 2008).

Taken together, evidence for maternal genetic effects on caregiving behaviors from twin studies and from molecular genetics research each support the supposition that parental genetics are associated with variations in caregiving behaviors. However, these associations are often only modest to moderate in strength and there are inconsistencies across studies with regard to which caregiving dimensions or qualities show the strongest genetic correlations. For example, most of the behavioral genetic studies indicate stronger genetic correlations for negative caregiving behaviors than sensitive caregiving, whereas to date there are both correlations with sensitive and negative maternal care reported from molecular genetic studies. Furthermore, studies of individual differences using candidate genes illustrate that small genetic correlations should be expected when the direct effects of genetics are examined in isolation. In contrast, more clear effects may be present when multigene × environment interactions are considered, and to date these analyses highlight the importance of recognizing that no single gene is going to be directly responsible for a behavioral phenomenon as complex as parenting. In fact, many genes that are associated with parenting behaviors may in actuality not be directly associated with the parenting phenotype at all, but rather be associated with variation in an individual's sensitivity to environmental influence, variation in basic automatic or effortful processes such as individual reactivity, self-regulation, or executive functioning, or variation in susceptibility to psychopathology. Each of these possibilities provides a bridge that could serve as an indirect link between genotype and the early caregiving phenotype, and we are only at the tip of the iceberg in understanding these dynamic processes within individuals.

This organismic view of the etiology of parenting behavior is consistent with core tenets of a biopsychosocial approach to the study of early maternal caregiving. However, a family systems approach suggests that only examining the direct effect (and interactions) of maternal genetics is also limited because we are not examining mothers' genotypes within the embedded relationships of the family system. The next sections illustrate the utility of integrating biopsychosocial and family systems models by considering how a mother's genetics may affect the quality of her caregiving environment via the behavior of others in the family.

Evocative Gene–Environment Correlations

One process by which maternal genetics may indirectly influence her parenting behavior is through evocative gene–environment correlations (Plomin et al., 1977; Scarr & McCartney, 1983), a process by which the child elicits specific types of parenting behaviors. In this mode of transmission, the child's genotype (as inherited partially from the mother) influences child temperament and behavior, which in turn evoke responses from the environment, in this case the child's mother (Jaffee & Price, 2007). This model of child influence on parenting behavior was evidenced prior to genetically informed studies of parenting by research on child temperament and variations in maternal caregiving. For example, Mills-Koonce and colleagues (2007) and van den Boom (1994) reported that highly irritable infants received less sensitive care from their mothers and were at greater risk for developing insecure attachment relationships. Furthermore, whereas sensitive parenting can be challenged and reduced by child negativity, it can be enhanced when the child positively stimulates the mother and responds to her bids for interaction (Atkinson et al., 1999; Cox, Owen, Henderson, & Margand, 1992; Kochanska, 2001; Thompson, 1997; van den Boom, 1997). Attentive children who respond positively to their mothers tend to elicit more sensitive caring, warmth, and attention from them than children who are highly reactive and not easily soothed (Thompson, 1997; van den Boom, 1997; Shamir-Essakow, Ungerer, Rapee, & Safier, 2004).

Behavioral genetic twin studies have evidenced support for the notion that heritable characteristics of children influence measures of family environment (see Hur & Bouchard, 1995; O'Connor, Heatherington, Reiss, & Plomin, 1995), including a recent meta-analysis suggesting that genetically influenced behaviors of the child may affect and shape parental behavior (Avinun & Knafo, 2013). Previous research on identical and fraternal twins reports different child experiences of caregiving within the household that appear to be genetically mediated (on the part of the child; Rowe, 1981, 1983). Not surprisingly, differences in the care these children receive are associated with differences in their developmental outcomes (Caspi et al., 2004). On this topic, Boivin et al. (2005) reported that monozygotic twins experienced more similar levels of hostile–reactive maternal caregiving than did dizygotic twins. Furthermore, the association between child genetics and maternal hostile–reactive caregiving was primarily mediated by infant difficultness, although it should be noted that this effect was moderate in size (with approximately 31% accounted for by genetic factors as compared with 53% due to common environment effects and 16% due to unique environment effects). In addition, Forget-Dubois et al. (2007) reported a comparable child-evocative effect, but emphasized that the strength of the effect varied considerably across infancy and early toddlerhood. Indeed, in older children, similar reports of small to moderate genetically mediated child effects on parenting have also been reported, including child effects on parental negativity (Feinberg, Neiderhiser, Howe, & Hetherington, 2001; Knafo & Plomin, 2006; Larsson, Viding, Rijskijk, & Plomin, 2008; Narusyte, Andershed, Neiderhiser, & Lichtenstein, 2007) and maltreatment and neglect (Schulz-Heik et al., 2009). In addition, there is also evidence for genetically mediated child effects on sensitive caregiving. Deater-Deckard (2000) reported genetic, shared and nonshared environmental influence on variation in observations of maternal responsiveness to young children, as well as mother-reported positive and negative affect directed toward the child. In comparison to parental negativity, there is significantly less behavioral genetic research identifying genetically mediated child effects on maternal sensitivity, including research that found no genetic effects on this dimension of parenting (Roisman & Fraley, 2008).

In addition to twin studies, adoption studies provide convincing evidence that behaviors associated with a child's genetic makeup may evoke specific styles of maladaptive parenting. For example, Ge, Best, Conger, and Simons (1996) reported a significant association between biological parents' psychiatric status and adoptive parents' child-rearing behavior. This genotype–environment association was mediated by the psychopathology of the adopted child, and in the case of the mother, appeared to reflect bidirectional effects such that the antisocial behavior of the child led to the mother's harsh parenting, which in turn exacerbated the child's level of antisocial behavior. Extending these findings,

O'Connor, Neiderhiser, Reiss, Hetherington, and Plomin (1998) found that children born to antisocial mothers were more likely to receive negative parenting from their adoptive caregivers and that this association was mediated by the child's disruptive behavior. In replicating these findings, Riggins-Caspers, Cadoret, Knutson, and Langbehn (2003) found that such evocative child effects were present, but were evidenced only in high-risk families (as defined by high levels of psychopathology, legal, or marital problems among the adoptive parents).

Although adoption and twin studies have been fruitful in identifying children's genetic variability as a potential source of variation in parenting behaviors, the ability to directly examine candidate genes and their effects on the family system is a relatively new approach to examining gene–environment correlations and interactions (Rutter, 2006). To date we are aware of only two prospective studies that have reported correlations between polymorphic variants in the child and the caregiving of the parent. Propper, Willoughby, Halpern, Carbone, and Cox (2007) found that children with the long variant of a $DRD4$ gene received less sensitive caregiving (although not more harsh caregiving) than did children with the short variant of the same gene. Because this was a study of child G × E effects on the development of internalizing and externalizing behaviors, the correlation between the child gene and parenting behavior could potentially have been the result of evocative or passive genetic effects. However, variations in this gene have been associated with individual differences in infant engagement and activity levels (Cloninger, 1987; Ebstein et al., 1998), characteristics that may evoke differential responding from mothers. Another study examining a dopaminergic gene, the dopamine D2 receptor gene ($DRD2$) found that children with the A_1^+ allelic variant of the gene received significantly less sensitive caregiving than children with the A_1^- variant (Mills-Koonce et al., 2008; see also Propper, Shanahan, Russo, & Mills-Koonce, 2012). In this study, the effect of the child gene was independent of the effects of the maternal gene, suggesting that the association was indeed evocative and not passive in nature. Unfortunately, this study was not able to detect a mediating child behavioral mechanism responsible for the differences in receipt of maternal care across children with different $DRD2$ polymorphisms. Dick, Rose, and Kaprio (2006) was moderately successful in identifying a mediator of a potentially evocative gene–environment correlation between child genotype (a $DRD2$ receptor variant) and retrospective report of their receipt of care from mothers and fathers. Specifically, those with the exon 8-A $DRD2$ allele reported receipt of significantly more paternal rejection and maternal and paternal overprotectiveness; effects partially mediated by their self-report of temperament. Unfortunately, this study did not include parental genotype controls and relied on retrospective self-report (which is prone to perceptual biases) as opposed to more objective (and prospective) observations of behavior. More recently, Mileva-Seitz et al. (2012) reported associations between multiple single-nucleotide polymorphisms in the *DRD1* and *DRD2* genes and maternal responsiveness, further implicating children's dopaminergic functioning as a potential biological basis for child characteristics that evoke variation in maternal care.

Evocative gene–environment correlations provide one mechanism by which maternal genotypes indirectly influence maternal behaviors. However, the biological transmission of genetic material from parent to offspring is not the only means by which mothers' genotypes may influence their environments. In the next section, we describe how mothers' genotypes may influence their self-selection into certain environments or relationships that, in turn, influence their parenting behaviors.

Active Gene–Environment Correlations

Active gene–environment correlations refer to the processes by which genetic factors "push" or "nudge" persons (i.e., self-selection) into certain types of environments. The literature on active gene–environment correlations is the most limited of the three potential genetic mechanisms for influencing parental behaviors. This is partly due to the difficulty of disentangling active and evocative gene–environment correlations and partly due to this being a new field of research that is still in its early infancy. However, there is evidence suggesting that active maternal rGE effects on caregiving behaviors are not only possible but probable. For example, there are numerous twin studies that have examined the "genetics of experience" and subsequently identified several domains of life experience relevant to parenting behaviors that also vary according to individual genotype. Such studies include genetic correlations with life stressors (Plomin, Lichtenstein, Pedersen, McClearn, & Nesselroade, 1990), divorce (McGue & Lykken, 1992), the propensity to marry (Johnson, McGue, Krueger, & Bouchard, 2004), marital quality (Spotts et al., 2005), and social support (Bergeman, Plomin, Pedersen, & McClearn, 1990), as well as a wide array of individual interests. The active gene–environment correlation model is also consistent with assortative mating theories, which suggest nonrandom mating patterns in which individuals with similar genotypes and/or phenotypes mate with each other more frequently than what would be expected under a random mating pattern. For example, there is (1) evidence that psychopathologies such as substance abuse, antisociality, and depression in mothers may have underlying genetic influences; (2) evidence that there are correlations among these psychopathological symptoms across partners (or parents); and (3) evidence that those behaviors in the father may affect early maternal care above and beyond those behaviors in the mother. However, we are currently unaware of a single study that has pulled each of these threads together in a single specific model of active gene–environment correlations with early maternal care. Furthermore, much of the work to date has not been adequately studied or replicated (or even represented in the molecular genetics literature), but the behavioral genetics findings suggest the potential for genotypes to actively select into specific contexts or experiences that may influence the quality of maternal caregiving behaviors.

Future Directions and Considerations

As illustrated in the previous sections, a biopsychosocial approach to unraveling (to the degree possible) the genetic influences on early parenting behavior necessitates the consideration of multilevel gene–environment correlations and gene–environment interactions, as well as the interdependencies of subsystems within the family as contexts for genetic expression. Here it is important to remember the social and dyadic nature of parenting and the multiple means by which genetic influence may manifest within the family system. Figure 12.1 provides a conceptual model of the complex gene–environment interplay within and across family relationships. As is often the case for developmental researchers, translating these complex models into testable research questions is no easy feat! However, several researchers have already begun to untangle these processes, and below we highlight some new directions for future research on this topic and consider the clinical implications for the burgeoning field of study.

A Complex Model for a Complex Phenomenon: Can We Find Testable Hypotheses?

First, let us again consider why parenting behavior is such a complex phenomenon. Parenting behavior is not a simple response to stimuli, nor is it fully a conscious or automatic process. It is a biopsychosocial product of ongoing interactions among one's genetics, neurological and endocrine activity, psychological processes (including current cognitions and a history of internalized experiences from birth onward), and micro- and macroenvironmental influences ranging from interpersonal relationship qualities to cultural variations in behaviors and attitudes. Therefore, in addition to endogenous biological mechanisms that mediate genetic effects, Figure 12.1 reminds us to take an organismic approach and consider that these endogenous processes are nested within a complex family system and broader environment. As such, it is likely wise for future research to focus less on the individual as the unit of analysis (in this case, *individual* is defined as the mother with a focus solely on her genotype), and instead focus on the family system as the unit of analysis, thus allowing for simultaneous consideration of the biobehavioral connections among family members as codependent on one another. For example, as Figure 12.1 suggests, maternal parenting can be viewed as a phenotypic behavioral outcome that emerges as a function of maternal gene–environment coactions. However, maternal parenting can likewise be viewed as (1) an environmental context for children that can be manipulated by child factors; and (2) a product of her environment that the mother has self-selected into based on genetically mediated phenotypic behaviors that increase the probability of her being in a specific type of romantic relationship, social network, or exposed to certain life circumstances. In other words, inasmuch as we consider the role of mothers' genotypes as a direct influence on their phenotypic behaviors, we must equally consider the role of mothers' genotypes in the construction of their social worlds.

How might this work? Previous research has already examined the role of infant behavior on maternal parenting; now we must consider (1) the genetic correlates of those infant behaviors, (2) the linkages between those genes in the child and those in the mother, (3) whether infant behaviors mediate associations between child genes and maternal parenting, and (4) whether these mediated pathways exist above and beyond the direct associations between maternal genes and maternal parenting. This is no small task, but there is already evidence for (at least) comparable levels of child genetic effects on caregiving as there is for parent genetic effects on caregiving. Most mothers in the studies described in this chapter were between 20 and 38 years of age, meaning that their phenotypic behaviors, unlike that of their children, have been influenced by a long history of environmental experiences. Thus, it is not surprising that neither behavioral genetic studies nor single-gene association studies reveal substantial genetic effects on a behavioral system as complicated as parenting. By contrast, the interactive styles of young children in the first year of life may appear more heavily influenced by genetic variation because of a limited degree of environmental experiences and their more limited resources (i.e., physiological, cognitive) for control at that age. Thus, in the absence of complex supragenetic systems such as those available to the parent, genetic differences may more directly correlate with child behavior, and thereby have the capacity to exert an evocative influence on parenting behavior. Of course it is also possible that these two mechanisms (child and parent mediated) are not mutually exclusive and may work in tandem, thus creating a conservative and stable subsystem within the family that fosters the transgenerational transmission of caregiving from one generation to the next.

The role of child evocative effects is not new to the study of parenting behaviors, and the roles of infant and child genotypes within these processes have recently begun to receive more empirical attention, yet much less is known about the possibility of active gene–environment correlations that manifest themselves as mothers self-select into environments based on genetically mediated characteristics. Again, there is an expansive current literature on relational and contextual effects on parenting, but to our knowledge, none have considered the underlying role of maternal genetics in these social processes. As an important next step in this line of research, studies should begin to ask whether environmental experiences are randomly distributed across different genotypes, of if there is evidence of a genetically mediated selection effect, and what are the biobehavioral mechanisms explaining this linkage. For example, consider a woman with a genetic predisposition for impulsivity, thrill seeing, and reward dependence. Is it more or less likely that she would find a romantic partner who displays the same types of behaviors as compared with a partner who is phenotypically reserved, passive, and cautious? The proverb *opposites attract* for romantic relationships is often not supported empirically with studies suggesting that assortative mating patterns for humans are characterized by unions of individuals with common biobehavioral phenotypes (Thiessen & Gregg, 1980). Future research must address the question of whether the reinforcement of common biobehavioral phenotypes affects the quality of care that both parents provide to their infant, and the role of active gene–environment correlations in this process. These are testable biopsychosocial questions and hypotheses that to date have largely been unexplored.

Last, this chapter has focused exclusively on the role of the genotype as it relates to mothers' parenting of infants; however, research is quickly moving in the direction of better understanding the epigenome and the role of epigenetics as a mechanism for linking environmental experiences to long-term biological and behavioral outcomes for individuals. This is a critical new direction for the study of parenting genetics. Whereas we have discussed at length the role of the environment as a moderator, or even mediator, of genetic effects on maternal parenting, epigenetic processes offer a means by which the genome can mediate environmental experiences, both for the individual and for the individual's future offspring. In many ways, epigenetics is the new frontier of developmental biopsychosocial research It should be noted, however, that although exciting, these processes are not mutually exclusive from the previously described genetic influences on maternal parenting. As such, epigenetics should be considered as an additional process that occurs during development as opposed to an alternative.

The Implications of Genetic Studies for Parenting Interventions

The many possibilities by which genetic factors may influence parenting behaviors lead to questions regarding the implications for therapeutic and intervention programs designed to improve parent–child relationships and family functioning. Behavioral genetic studies have provided evidence to support maternally mediated genetic effects (direct and indirect) and child-mediated genetic effects on parenting behavior. More recently, molecular genetic studies have allowed researchers to identify specific genetic sources of risk for maladaptive parenting outcomes as well as heightened genetic susceptibility to environmental effects on parenting behaviors. Applying a genetic level of analysis to dysfunctional parent–child relationships may allow for a more refined understanding of the source of difficulty or pathology within the family system and thus a more tailored approach to intervention or family therapy. Of course, this research is still in its infancy, and while such therapeutic possibilities are not currently available, the potential for their future application is compelling.

Concluding Comments

Finally, as technology and analytic application progress, the possibilities for genetic studies of parenting and even broader family functioning will only increase. For example, the utilization of genome-wide association studies to examine the full human genome for correlations with phenotypic behaviors is already available for social scientists and family researchers. Although such potential is thrilling, it is not without pitfalls. Genetic "fishing expeditions" that have searched for single-gene associations with complex behaviors have often produced mixed and nonreplicated results. Nevertheless, behavioral genetic strategies, particularly when combined with new brain imaging techniques, appear very promising. The ability to characterize specific behaviorally relevant genetic polymorphism will also allow powerful tests of gene–environment interactions to further our understanding of parenting behaviors. Given our limited knowledge of how many of these processes work, a more conceptually driven approach involving joint analyses of specific gene systems (with known functional relevance) and high-quality environmental measures is likely to bear reliable and informative fruit. It stands to reason that future studies of parenting and family functioning will include a greater representation of genetically oriented analyses. However, while social scientists and family researchers should embrace this new paradigm, we should also avoid losing sight of the importance of the high-quality behavioral, relational, and contextual measures that have been developed and validated as our "bread and butter" of the past several decades. Only in the context of these experiences, and in relation to these behaviors, can truly meaningful information be extrapolated from genetic studies of family function.

REFERENCES

Atkinson, L., Chisholm, V. C., Scott, B., Goldberg, S., Vaughn, B. E., Blackwell, J., et al. (1999). Maternal sensitivity, child functional level, and attachment in Down syndrome. *Monographs of the Society for Research in Child Development, 64,* 45–66.

Avinun, R., & Knafo, A. (2014). Parenting as a reaction evoked by children's genotype: A meta-analysis of children-as-twins studies. *Personality and Social Psychology Review, 18*(1), 87–102.

Bakermans-Kranenburg, M. J., & van IJzendoorn, M. H. (2008). Gene–environment interaction of the dopamine D4 receptor (*DRD4*) and observed maternal insensitivity predicting externalizing behavior in preschoolers. *Developmental Psychobiology, 48*, 406–409.

Belsky, J. (1984). The determinants of parenting: A process model. *Child Development, 55*, 83–96.

Belsky, J., Crnic, K., & Woodworth, S. (1995). Personality and parenting: Exploring the mediating role of transient mood and daily hassles. *Journal of Personality, 63*, 905–929.

Bergeman, C., Plomin, R., Pedersen, N., & McClearn, G. (1990). Genetic and environmental influences on social support: The Swedish Adoption/Twin Study of Aging. *Journals of Gerontology, 45*, P101–P106.

Blair, C., Granger, D. A., Kivlighan, K. T., Mills-Koonce, R., Willoughby, M., Greenberg, M. T., et al. (2008). Maternal and child contributions to cortisol response to emotional arousal in young children from low-income, rural communities. *Developmental Psychology, 44*(4), 1095–1109.

Blair, C., Granger, D. A., Willoughby, M., Mills-Koonce, R., Cox, M., Greenberg, M. T., et al. (2011). Salivary cortisol mediates effects of poverty and parenting on executive functions in early childhood. *Child Development, 82*(6), 1970–1984.

Boivin, M., Pérusse, D., Dionne, G., Saysset, V., Zoccolillo, M., Tarabulsy, G., et al. (2005). The genetic–environmental etiology of parents' perceptions and self-assessed behaviours toward their 5-month-old infants in a large twin and singleton sample. *Journal of Child Psychology and Psychiatry, 46*, 612–630.

Brown, J. R., Ye, H., Bronson, R. T., Dikkes, P., & Greenberg, M. E. (1996). A defect in nurturing in mice lacking the immediate early gene fosB. *Cell, 86*, 297–309.

Brunton, P. J., & Russell, J. A. (2008). The expectant brain: Adapting for motherhood. *National Review of Neuroscience, 9*, 11–25.

Caspi, A., Moffitt, T. E., Morgan, J., Rutter, M., Taylor, A., Arseneault, L., et al. (2004). Maternal expressed emotion predicts children's antisocial behavior problems: Using monozygotic-twin differences to identify environmental effects on behavioral development. *Developmental Psychology, 40*(2), 149–161.

Clark, L. A., Kochanska, G., & Ready, R. (2000). Mothers' personality and its interaction with child temperament as predictors of parenting behavior. *Journal of Personality and Social Psychology, 79*, 274–285.

Cloninger, C. (1987). A systematic method for clinical description and classification of personality variants. *Archives of General Psychiatry, 44*, 573–588.

Coplan, R. J., Reichel, M., & Rowan, K. (2009). Exploring the associations between maternal personality, child temperament, and parenting: A focus on emotions. *Personality and Individual Differences, 46*(2), 241–246.

Cox, M. J., Owen, M. T., Henderson, V. K., & Margand, N. A. (1992). Antecedents of infant–father and infant–mother attachment. *Developmental Psychology, 28*, 474–483.

Cox, M. J., & Paley, B. (2003). Understanding families as systems. *Current Directions in Psychological Science, 12*, 193–196.

Crockenberg, S., & Leerkes, E. (2000). Infant social and emotional development in family context. In C. R. Zeanah (Ed.), *Handbook of infant mental health* (2nd ed., pp. 60–90). New York: Guilford Press.

Cumberland-Li, A., Eisenberg, N., Champion, C., Gershoff, E., & Fabes, R. A. (2003). The relation of parental emotionality and related dispositional traits to parental expression of emotion and children's social functioning. *Motivation and Emotion, 27*(1), 27–56.

Deater-Deckard, K. (2000). Parenting and child behavioral adjustment in early childhood: A quantitative genetic approach to studying family processes. *Child Development, 71*, 468–484.

Dick, D. M., Rose, R. J., & Kaprio, J. (2006). The next challenge for psychiatric genetics: Characterizing the risk associated with identified genes. *Annals of Clinical Psychiatry, 18*, 223–231.

Downey, G., & Coyne, J. C. (1990). Children of depressed parents: An integrative review. *Psychological Bulletin, 108*, 50–76.

Ebstein, R. P., Levine, J., Geller, V., Auerbach, J., Gritsenko, I., & Belmaker, R. H. (1998). Dopamine D4 receptor and serotonin transporter promoter in the determination of neonatal temperament. *Molecular Psychiatry, 3*, 238–246.

Fan, J., Hof, P. R., Guise, K. G., Fossella, J. A., & Posner, M. I. (2008). The functional integration of the anterior cingulated cortex during conflict processing. *Cerebral Cortex, 18*, 796–805.

Feinberg, M., Neiderhiser, J., Howe, G., & Hetherington, E. (2001). Adolescent, parent, and observer perceptions of parenting: Genetic and environmental influences on shared and distinct perceptions. *Child Development, 72*, 1266–1284.

Feldman, R., Weller, A., Zagoory-Sharon, O., & Levine, A. (2007). Evidence for a neuroendocrinological foundation of human affiliation: Plasma oxytocin levels across pregnancy and the postpartum period predict mother–infant bonding. *Psychological Science, 18*, 965–970.

Feldman, R., Zagoory-Sharon, O., Weisman, O., Schneiderman, I., Gordon, I., Maoz, R., et al. (2012). Sensitive parenting is associated with plasma oxytocin and polymorphisms in the *OXTR* and *CD38* genes. *Biological Psychiatry, 72*(3), 175–181.

Fish, M., Stifter, C. A., & Belsky, J. (1991). Conditions of vontinuity and discontinuity in infant negative emotionality: Newborn to five months. *Child Development, 62*, 1525–1537.

Forget-Dubois, N., Boivin, M., Dionne, G., Pierce, T., Tremblay, R., & Pérusse, D. (2007). A longitudinal twin study of the genetic and environmental etiology of maternal hostile–reactive behavior during infancy and toddlerhood. *Infant Behavior and Development, 30*, 453–465.

Ge, X., Best, K., Conger, R., & Simons, R. (1996). Parenting behaviors and the occurrence and co-occurrence of adolescent depressive symptoms and conduct problems. *Developmental Psychology, 32*, 717–731.

Hughes, E. K., & Gullone, E. (2010). Reciprocal relationships between parent and adolescent internalizing symptoms. *Journal of Family Psychology, 24*(2), 115.

Hur, Y., & Bouchard, T. (1995). Genetic influences on perceptions of childhood family environment: A reared apart twin study. *Child Development, 66*, 330–345.

Jaffee, S. R., & Price, T. S. (2007). Gene–environment correlations: A review of the evidence and implications for prevention of mental illness. *Molecular Psychiatry, 12*(5), 432–442.

Johnson, W., McGue, M., Krueger, R. F., & Bouchard, T. J., Jr. (2004). Marriage and personality: A genetic analysis. *Journal of Personality and Social Psychology, 86,* 285–294.

Karreman, A., van Tuijl, C., van Aken, M. A., & Deković, M. (2008). The relation between parental personality and observed parenting: The moderating role of pre-schoolers' effortful control. *Personality and Individual Differences, 44*(3), 723–734.

Knafo, A., & Plomin, R. (2006). Prosocial behavior from early to middle childhood: Genetic and environmental influences on stability and change. *Developmental Psychology, 42,* 771–786.

Knickmeyer, R. C., Kang, C., Woolson, S., Smith, J. K., Hamer, R. M., Lin, W., et al. (2011). Twin-singleton differences in neonatal brain structure. *Twin Research and Human Genetics: The Official Journal of the International Society for Twin Studies, 14*(3), 268.

Kochanska, G. (2001). Emotional development in children with different attachment histories: The first three years. *Child Development, 72*(2), 474–490.

Kochanska, G., Clark, L. A., & Goldman, M. S. (1997). Implications of mother's personality for their parenting and their young children's developmental outcomes. *Journal of Personality, 65,* 387–420.

Kochanska, G., Friesenborg, A. E., Lange, L. A., & Martel, M. M. (2004). Parents' personality and infants' temperament as contributors to their emerging relationship. *Journal of Personality and Social Psychology, 86*(5), 744.

Koenig, J. L., Barry, R. A., & Kochanska, G. (2010). Rearing difficult children: Parents' personality and children's proneness to anger as predictors of future parenting. *Parenting: Science and Practice, 10*(4), 258–273.

Kuroda, K. O., Meaney, M. J., Uetani, N., Fortin, Y., Ponton, A., & Kato, T. (2007). ERK-FoxB signaling in dorsal MOA neurons plans a major role in the intiation of parental behavior in mice. *Molecular and Cellular Neuroscience, 36,* 121–131.

Kuroda, K. O., Meaney, M. J., Uetani, N., & Kato, T. (2008). Neurobehavioral basis of the impaired nurturing in mice lacking the immediate early gene *FosB. Brain Research, 1211,* 57–71.

Larsson, H., Viding, E., Rijsdijk, F., & Plomin, R. (2008). Relationships between parental negativity and childhood antisocial behavior over time: A bidirectional effects model in a longitudinal genetically informative design. *Journal of Abnormal Child Psychology, 36,* 633–645.

Lee, S. S., Chronis-Tuscano, A., Keenan, K., Pelham, W. E., Loney, J., Van Hulle, C. A., et al. (2010). Association of maternal dopamine transporter genotype with negative parenting: Evidence for gene × environment interaction with child disruptive behavior. *Molecular Psychiatry, 15,* 548–558.

Losoya, S. H., Callor, S., Rowe, D. C., & Goldsmith, H. H. (1997). Origins of familial similarity in parenting: A study of twins and adoptive siblings. *Developmental Psychology, 33,* 1012–1023.

McCormack, K., Newman, T., Higley, J., Maestripieri, D., & Sanchez, M. (2009). Serotonin transporter gene variation, infant abuse, and responsiveness to stress in rhesus macaque mothers and infants. *Hormones and Behavior, 55,* 538–547.

McCrae, R. R., Costa, P. T., Jr., Ostendorf, F., Angleitner, A., Hrebíčková, M., Avia, M. D., et al. (2000). Nature over nurture: Temperament, personality, and life span development. *Journal of Personality and Social Psychology, 78,* 173–186.

McGue, M., & Lykken, D. (1992). Genetic influence on risk of divorce. *Psychological Science, 3*(6), 368–373.

McGuire, S. (2003). The heritability of parenting. *Parenting: Science and Practice, 3*(1), 73.

Meaney, M. J. (2001). Nature, nurture, and the disunity of knowledge. *Annals of the New York Academy of Sciences, 935,* 50–61.

Meaney, M. J. (2007). Environmental programming of phenotypic diversity in female reproductive strategies. *Advances in Genetics, 59,* 173–215.

Metsäpelto, R. L., & Pulkkinen, L. (2003). Personality traits and parenting: Neuroticism, extraversion, and openness to experience as discriminative factors. *European Journal of Personality, 17,* 59–78.

Mileva-Seitz, V., Fleming, A. S., Meaney, M. J., Mastroianni, A., Sinnwell, J. P., Steiner, M., et al. (2012). Dopamine receptors D1 and D2 are related to observed maternal behavior. *Genes, Brain and Behavior, 11*(6), 684–694.

Mileva-Seitz, V., Steiner, M., Atkinson, L., Meaney, M. J., Levitan, R., Kennedy, J. L., et al. (2013). Interaction between oxytocin genotypes and early experience predicts quality of mothering and postpartum mood. *PloS ONE, 8*(4), e61443.

Mills-Koonce, W. R., Gariépy, J. L., Propper, C., Sutton, K., Calkins, S., Moore, G., et al. (2007). Infant and parent factors associated with early maternal sensitivity: A caregiver-attachment systems approach. *Infant Behavior and Development, 30*(1), 114–126.

Mills-Koonce, W. R., & Propper, C. B. (2011). Within-family genetic influences on maternal caregiving. In D. W. Davis & M. C. Logsdon (Eds.), *Maternal sensitivity: A scientific foundation for practice.* Hauppauge, NY: Nova Science.

Mills-Koonce, W. R., Propper, C., Gariépy, J. L., Blair, C., Garrett-Peters, P., & Cox, M. J. (2008). Bi-directional genetic and environmental influence on mother and child behavior: The family system as the unity of analyses. *Development and Psychopathology, 19,* 1073–1087.

Min, S. J., Luke, B., Gillespie, B., Min, L., Newman, R. B., Mauldin, J. G., et al. (2000). Birth weight references for twins. *American Journal of Obstetrics and Gynecology, 182*(5), 1250–1257.

Minuchin, S. (1974). *Families and family therapy.* Cambridge, MA: Harvard University Press.

Narusyte, J., Andershed, A., Neiderhiser, J., & Lichtenstein, P. (2007). Aggression as a mediator of genetic contributions to the association between negative parent–child relationships and adolescent antisocial behavior. *European Child and Adolescent Psychiatry, 16,* 128–137.

National Institute of Child Health and Human Development, Early Child Care Research Network (1999). Chronicity of maternal depressive symptoms, maternal sensitivity, and child functioning at 36 months. *Developmental Psychology, 35*(5), 1297–1310.

Neiderhiser, J., & Lichtenstein, P. (2008). The Twin and Offspring Study in Sweden:

Advancing our understanding of genotype–environment interplay by studying twins and their families. *Acta Psychologica Sinica, 40*, 1116–1123.

Neiderhiser, J. M., Reiss, D., Pedersen, N. L., Lichtenstein, P., Spotts, E. L., Hansson, K., et al. (2004). Genetic and environmental influences on mothering of adolescents: A comparison of two samples. *Developmental Psychology, 40*, 335–351.

O'Connor, T., Hetherington, E., Reiss, D., & Plomin, R. (1995). A twin-sibling study of observed parent–adolescent interactions. *Child Development, 66*, 812–829.

O'Connor, T. G., Neiderhiser, J. M., Reiss, D., Hetherington, E. M., & Plomin, R. (1998). Genetic contributions to continuity, change, and co-occurrence of antisocial and depressive symptoms in adolescence. *Journal of Child Psychology and Psychiatry, 39*, 323–336.

Plomin, R., & Bergeman, C. S. (1991). The nature of nurture: Genetic influence on environmental measures. *Behavioral and Brain Sciences, 14*, 373–428.

Plomin, R., DeFries, J., & Loehlin, J. (1977). Genotype–environment interaction and correlation in the analysis of human behavior. *Psychological Bulletin, 84*, 309–322.

Plomin, R., Lichtenstein, P., Pedersen, N., McClearn, G., & Nesselroade, J. (1990). Genetic influence on life events during the last half of the life span. *Psychology and Aging, 5*, 25–30.

Pol, H. E. H., Posthuma, D., Baaré, W. F., De Geus, E. J., Schnack, H. G., van Haren, N. E., et al. (2002). Twin–singleton differences in brain structure using structural equation modelling. *Brain, 125*(2), 384–390.

Prinzie, P., Onghena, P., Hellinckx, W., Grietens, H., Ghesquière, P., & Colpin, H. (2004). Parent and child personality characteristics as predictors of negative discipline and externalizing problem behaviour in children. *European Journal of Personality, 18*, 73–102.

Propper, C., Moore, G., Mills-Koonce, W., Halpern, C., Hill-Soderlund, A. L., Calkins, S. D., & Cox, M. (2008). Gene–environment contributions to the development of infant vagal reactivity: The interaction of dopamine and maternal sensitivity. *Child Development, 79*(5), 1377–1394.

Propper, C., Willoughby, M., Halpern, C. T., Carbone, M. A., & Cox, M. (2007). Parenting quality, *DRD4*, and the prediction of externalizing and internalizing behaviors in early childhood. *Developmental Psychobiology, 49*, 619–632.

Propper, C. B., Shanahan, M. J., Russo, R., & Mills-Koonce, W. R. (2012). Evocative gene–parenting correlations and academic performance at first grade: An exploratory study. *Development and Psychopathology, 24*(4), 1265–1282.

Pungello, E. P., Iruka, I. U., Dotterer, A. M., Mills-Koonce, R., & Reznick, J. (2009). The effects of socioeconomic status, race, and parenting on language development in early childhood. *Developmental Psychology, 45*(2), 544–557.

Reiss, D. (2005). The interplay between genotypes and family relationships: Reframing concepts of development and prevention. *Current Directions in Psychological Science, 14*, 139–143.

Riggins-Caspers, K. M., Cadoret, R. J., Knutson, J. F., & Langbehn, D. (2003). Biology–environment interaction and evocative biology–environment correlation: Contributions of harsh discipline and parental psychopathology to problem adolescent behaviors. *Behavior Genetics, 33*, 205–220.

Rimm-Kaufman, S. E., Pianta, R. C., Cox, M. J., & Bradley, R. H. (2003). Teacher-rated family involvement and children's social and academic outcomes in kindergarten. *Early Education and Development, 14*(2), 179–198.

Roisman, G., & Fraley, R. (2008). A behavior-genetic study of parenting quality, infant attachment security, and their covariation in a nationally representative sample. *Developmental Psychology, 44*, 831–839.

Rothbart, M. K. (2007). Temperament, development, and personality. *Current Directions in Psychological Science, 16*(4), 207–212.

Rothbart, M. K., Ahadi, S. A., & Evans, D. E. (2000). Temperament and personality: Origins and outcomes. *Journal of Personality and Social Psychology, 78*, 122–135.

Rowe, D. (1981). Who controls parent–child interaction? *PsycCritiques, 26*, 744–745.

Rowe, D. (1983). Biometrical genetic models of self-reported delinquent behavior: A twin study. *Behavior Genetics, 13*, 473–489.

Rowe, D. (1994). *The limits of family influence: Genes, experience, and behavior.* New York: Guilford Press.

Rutter, M. (2006). Implications of resilience concepts for scientific understanding. *Annals of the New York Academy of Sciences, 1094*, 1–12.

Scarr, S., & McCartney, K. (1983). How people make their own environments: A theory of genotype → environment effects. *Child Development, 54*, 424–435.

Schulz-Heik, R., Rhee, S., Silvern, L., Lessem, J., Haberstick, B., Hopfer, C., et al. (2009). Investigation of genetically mediated child effects on maltreatment. *Behavior Genetics, 39*, 265–276.

Shamir-Essakow, G., Ungerer, J. A., Rapee, R. M., & Safier, R. (2004). Caregiving representations of mothers of behaviorally inhibited and uninhibited preschool children. *Developmental Psychology, 40*, 899–910.

Smith, C. L., Spinrad, T. L., Eisenberg, N., Gaertner, B. M., Popp, T. K., & Maxon, E. (2007). Maternal personality: Longitudinal associations to parenting behavior and maternal emotional expressions toward toddlers. *Parenting: Science and Practice, 7*, 305–329.

Spinath, F. M., & O'Connor, T. G. (2003). A behavioral genetic study of the overlap between personality and parenting. *Journal of Personality, 71*, 785–810.

Spotts, E. L., Lichtenstein, P., Pedersen, N., Neiderhiser, J. M., Hansson, K., Cederblad, M., et al. (2005). Personality and marital satisfaction: A behavioral genetic analysis. *European Journal of Personality, 19*(3), 205–227.

Thiessen, D., & Gregg, B. (1980). Human assortative mating and genetic equilibrium: An evolutionary perspective. *Ethology and Sociobiology, 1*(2), 111–140.

Thompson, R. A. (1997). Sensitivity and security: New questions to ponder. *Child Development, 68*, 595–597.

Towers, H., Spotts, E. L., & Neiderhiser, J. M. (2001). Genetic and environmental influences on parenting and marital relationships: Current findings and future directions. *Marriage and Family Review, 33*, 11–29.

van den Boom, D. C. (1994). The influence of temperament and mothering on attachment and exploration: An experimental manipulation of sensitive responsiveness among lower-class mothers with irritable infants. *Child Development, 65*, 1457–1477.

van den Boom, D. C. (1997). Sensitivity and attachment: Next steps for developmentalists. *Child Development, 68,* 592–594.
van IJzendoorn, M. H., Bakermans-Kranenburg, M. J., & Mesman, J. (2008). Dopamine system genes associated with parenting in the context of daily hassles. *Genes,
   Brain and Behavior, 7,* 403–410.
Willoughby, M. T., Mills-Koonce, R., Propper, C. B., & Waschbusch, D. A. (2013).
   Observed parenting behaviors interact with a polymorphism of the brain-derived
   neurotrophic factor gene to predict the emergence of oppositional defiant and
   callous–unemotional behaviors at age 3 years. *Development and Psychopathology, 25*(4), 903–917.

CHAPTER 13

A Biopsychosocial Perspective on Synchrony and the Development of Human Parental Care

Ilanit Gordon and Ruth Feldman

All actual life is encounter.
—MARTIN BUBER

Interconnection is a cornerstone of the human experience. Human affiliative bonds are formed through social interactions that entail rhythmic movements from synchronous to asynchronous exchanges. Our brain similarly functions on the basis of complex interconnections and synchronous exchanges among its ~86 billion neurons and 10^{11} synapses (Herculano-Houzel, 2009, 2012). Like synchronous interactions, which are not predetermined but emerge as a self-organizing process from the inputs of social partners (Feldman, Bamberger, & Kanat-Maymon, 2013), the immense complexity of the brain is not rooted only in its genetic code but in its self-organizing nature (Bullmore & Sporns, 2009; Bullmore & Sporns, 2012; Herculano-Houzel, 2009). What are the essential ingredients that allow our brains to develop to their full potential? It may be that the realization of the massive complexity of our brains largely depends on the richness of experience, particularly experiences occurring during early development and within the parent–infant bond. Synchronous experiences between parents and their infants provide the platform from which infants can experience their world as rich, safe, and involving multitude. Such synchronous exchanges afford the development of neural, physiological, mental, social, and behavioral systems (Feldman, 2007c, 2012b). One may argue that synchrony between the infant's physiological states and those of the caregiver during early face-to-face interactions afford a rich and safe experience that enables optimal brain development.

In order to investigate the role of parent–infant synchrony in the development of brain and behavior, we describe research applying the mechanism of *biobehavioral synchrony* to the study of human development. Biobehavioral synchrony is a process that details the ongoing coordination of physiology and behavior between attachment partners during social contact (Feldman, 2007c, 2012a, 2012b, 2012c, 2013). It implies a behavioral-based approach in which social behavior, beginning with the earliest interactions between parents and infants, are mapped onto biological processes and are tested in relation to later physiological markers and social competencies (Feldman 2012a, 2012b). *Synchrony* as a term has been coined during the early 20th century, to describe goal-directed action among groups of living organisms—ants, fish, or birds. Whether groups of ants (Wheeler, 1928), flocks of birds (Shaw, 1978), groups of fish (Greenwood, Wark, Yoshida, & Peichel, 2013), or swarms of locust (Swidbert & Rogers, 2010), animal research has demonstrated the ways by which organisms synchronize activity toward the accomplishment of social goals.

In humans, synchrony has been mostly researched within the context of affiliative bonds, which are defined by being both *selective* and *enduring*, particularly the parent–infant attachment relationship (Feldman, 2007c, 2007d). Within the parent–infant context, synchrony denotes the temporal coordinated relationship of social behaviors between partners. Inspired by an ethological framework (Lorenz, 1950; Tinbergen, 1963), which described how synchrony in mammals is moved to the intimacy of the parent–infant bond, synchrony is meticulously observed in naturalistic interactions. The building blocks of synchronous behavior are microcoded within the basic building blocks of human social behavior, including gaze, arousal, vocalizations, proximity, and touch modalities. Synchrony describes the coordination between these various dimensions of nonverbal social behavior and their physiological biomarkers.

Figure 13.1 (p. 288) presents an overall view of a biobehavioral synchrony model, depicting the integration and embeddedness of behavioral and biological components within context. The figure also delineates the components of biobehavioral synchrony that are reviewed in this chapter. We begin with a detailed description of behavioral synchrony and its ontogeny. We continue by exploring our research that has delved into the coordination of behavioral synchrony with biological function in three specific physiological pathways: the autonomic nervous system (heart rate and cardiac vagal tone measures), the endocrine system (hormonal biomarkers), and the brain (functional magnetic resonance imaging [fMRI] studies). We then describe studies that have explored biobehavioral synchrony in various psychopathologies and risk factors (premature birth, posttraumatic stress disorder, autism spectrum disorder, and maternal postpartum depression). Finally, we will outline future directions that we envision for biobehavioral synchrony research.

The Coordination of Social Behavior Begins at Birth

Following birth, a unique maternal behavioral repertoire emerges in all mammalian species and in biparental species, fathers also express a unique set of behaviors. In humans, the species-specific repertoire includes maternal gaze at infant face and body, "motherese" high-pitched vocalization, expression of positive affect, and affectionate touch (Feldman & Eidelman, 2007). These are observed repeatedly during daily experiences between parents and infants. In these repeated interactions, parent and infant continuously coregulate their physiological and behavioral states. As dyadic interaction patterns recur, infant and parent are shaped by each other's physiological and behavioral cues, leading to the formation of the attachment bond (Bowlby, 1969; Feldman, 2012a; Tronick, 2007). Such coregulated interactions facilitate the development of the infant's self-regulatory abilities (Feldman, Greenbaum, & Yirmiya, 1999; Sameroff & Fiese, 2000; Tronick, 2007). Similar to the naturally occurring variations in mammalian mothers (Champagne, 2008), the emerging human parental repertoire includes variability in patterns of eye-gaze direction toward the infant, fluctuations in affect and arousal, and the uniquely pitched sing-song "motherese" vocalization, new configurations of affectionate and functional touch, proximity position, and proprioception. These parental behaviors vary across individuals (Gordon, Zagoory-Sharon, Leckman, & Feldman, 2010a, 2010b) and cultures (Feldman, Masalha, & Alony, 2006; Feldman & Masalha, 2007), appear in unique form in mothers and fathers (Feldman, 2003; Apter-Levi, Zagoory-Sharon, & Feldman, 2014), and are sensitive to the goals of the interactive context, for instance, whether the interaction is social or exploratory in nature (Gordon, Zagoory-Sharon, Leckman, & Feldman, 2010c; Feldman, Weller, Sirota, & Eidelman, 2002).

A central feature of the human parental repertoire is that it is adaptive to the infant's online cues, provides social stimulation when infants signal their willingness to interact and limit stimulation when infant gaze averts and signals a need for rest (Feldman, 2003; Feldman & Eidelman, 2004, 2007). Already in the first postbirth day, we found that mothers provide nearly 70% of their maternal behaviors during the 7% of the time infants are in alert-scanning state, matching their social input to the infant's readiness (Feldman & Eidelman, 2007). This repertoire of maternal behavior in the immediate postbirth period and its adaptation to the infant state plays an important role in children's social development, and predicts synchrony with mother and father at 3 months (Feldman & Eidelman, 2007), neurodevelopmental maturation (Feldman & Eidelman, 2003a), and cognitive and symbolic competencies in the second year (Feldman, Eidelman, & Rotenberg, 2004). Furthermore, maternal postpartum behavior had long-term effects on physiological organization shaping autonomic regulation as measured by cardiac vagal tone, sleep patterns assessed by actigraphy across five consecutive nights, and cortisol response to social stress at 10 years of age (Feldman, Rosenthal, & Eidelman, 2014). In addition, observations conducted during the first month of life (Gordon et al., 2010a) showed that mothers and fathers engaged in unique sets of interactive behavior, including states that were characterized by gaze coordination and affectionate touch, or states in which the parent provided stimulating contact and exploratory focus, much the same as patterns observed in biparental mammals (Ahern, Hammock, & Young, 2011). These parenting styles were each continuous over time and each uniquely supported child social development and his or her social reciprocity with best friend at 3 years, pointing to the transfer of early social behavior toward other meaningful relationships in the child's life (Feldman, Gordon, Influs, Gutbir, & Ebstein, 2013). It thus appear that each social relationship provides an entire early environment, which, similar to the conceptualization of *Hidden Regulators* (Hofer, 1995), enables the integration of physiology and behavior in unique ways to support the development of self-regulatory and social skills across childhood and adolescence (Feldman, 2007a, 2007b). Despite the fact that parent–infant synchrony is considered to have gender-specific properties (Apter-Levi, Zagoory-Sharon, et al., 2014; Feldman, Gordon, Schneiderman, Weisman, & Zagoory-Sharon, 2010), both fathers and mothers show equal amounts of parent–infant synchrony (Feldman, 2003; Gordon et al., 2010a).

Parent–infant synchrony is highly sensitive to the cultural context. Our research on Israeli and Palestinian families (Feldman et al., 2006; Feldman & Masalha, 2007; Feldman, Masalha, & Derdikman-Eiron, 2010) showed that synchronous interactions are built on somewhat different building blocks in traditional and industrial societies. In traditional societies when parents interact with their infants they tend to maintain closer physical proximity, whereas in industrialized societies parents display more active parenting behavior that includes active toy presentation and touch patterns. Infants and parents match on culture-specific patterns, which reflect underlying meaning systems and cultural philosophies with regard to power hierarchies, autonomy, and gender roles. However, individual differences in synchrony—whether on active forms of social behavior or more passive physical closeness—chart culture-specific pathways to self-regulation. Infants who received more synchronous interaction, as defined by their own culture, showed greater self-regulation, higher social competence, better problem-solving skills, and more social competence in the peer group as preschoolers. Furthermore, patterns of triadic synchrony within the mother–father–child triad, as measured in the home environment, were predictive of children's ability to handle conflict with their peers with more empathy and less aggression in the preschool years (Feldman, Masalha, et al., 2010). These findings highlight the importance of including culture in our studies on synchrony and demonstrate that while the specific patterns from which synchrony is constructed may be culture specific, the universal rule applies across cultures: infants who experience greater synchrony with their attachment figures will show more optimal socioemotional and regulatory outcomes across childhood (Feldman et al., 2006).

With time and maturation, synchrony develops. With age and familiarity interactions become more coordinated and dyad specific. Psychophysiological maturation that occurs during pregnancy in the fetus (such as hormonal changes and the maturation of sleep–wake oscillatory patterns) sets the stage for the emergence of coordinated behavior at the beginning of life (Feldman, 2006). Following birth, the parental behavioral repertoire emerges and it is characterized by contingencies. As newborns experience contingencies within the context of parenting behaviors, they also respond. These early interactive patterns are considered the precursors of synchrony. The emergence of maternal behavior and its sensitive adaptation to infants' cues also activates and shapes attachment- and bonding-related neural circuits in the mother. At around 3 months of age, synchrony is first observed as infants begin to engage in face-to-face interactions and coordinated parental and infant behaviors are seen. Infants can actively take part in the world through the social exchange with their parents and they display visual, facial, and vocal behaviors in response to parental social cues. Coordinated parent–infant interactions provide critical inputs for the shaping of bonding-related neural circuits. At around 9 months of age there is a reorganization of synchronous behavior accompanied by an increased focus on joint exploration of objects and toys. During this period mutual influences of parent and infant affective states are observed as well as shorter lags to synchronous states. From 1 year onward, there is an emergence of symbol use in the infant and a development of symbolic play and complexity between infant and parent, marked by verbal components of the interaction. Nonverbally, there seems to be a level of stability and continuity in parent-specific affective contour from infancy. Affect synchrony seems to be the nonverbal component of relational systems throughout life. Social interactions between close partners contain two parallel levels: a nonverbal level, marked by sequential relations between the partners' social behaviors; and a verbal level, in which sequential relations between the symbolic expressions of the interacting partners are observed (Feldman, 2007c, 2007d).

Figure 13.1 describes multiple levels of biobehavioral synchrony and how they are embedded within one another. Behavioral synchrony (level 1), which comprises species-specific behavioral building blocks displayed by both parent and infant, has specific temporal properties that can be described. The repeated and consistent behavioral exchange between partners is solidified into patterns of synchrony. The behavioral component of synchrony is embedded within biological synchrony (level 2), which includes biomarkers such as hormones, measures of autonomic nervous system function, and brain function. The biological component of synchrony is constantly underpinning behavior, but is also constantly in conversation with behavior, as they both mutually and dynamically influence each other. Biobehavioral synchrony is embedded within a third level

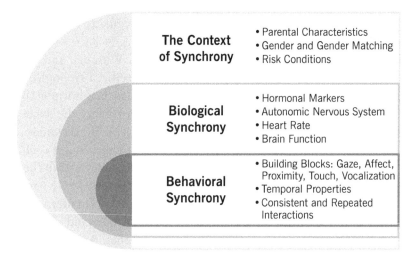

FIGURE 13.1. Building blocks of biobehavioral synchrony.

of contextual influences (level 3), including parental and child characteristics, cultural influences, and risk conditions. Levels of the biobehavioral synchrony model are embedded within one another to reflect our view that subsystems represent levels that are constantly interacting and being shaped by multiple levels of the model. While the following discussion makes a distinction among levels in the formation of biobehavioral synchrony, all subcomponents cohere into a single dynamic and complex system.

Synchrony as the Coordination of Physiology and Behavior across Multiple Physiological Systems

A hallmark of the biobehavioral synchrony model (see Figure 13.1) is that behavioral synchrony is embedded within neural and biological processes that dynamically develop as experiences occur—constantly shaping and being shaped by behavioral synchrony. Biomarkers can offer another level of representation to synchronous and coordinated exchanges. In this section we review studies that have exemplified this core component of biobehavioral synchrony in three physiological systems: the autonomic nervous system, the endocrine system, and the neural function of the brain.

The Autonomic System:
Heart Rhythms and Cardiac Vagal Tone

Research has pointed to the links between behavioral synchrony and measures of cardiac vagal tone in infant and mother (Feldman & Eidelman, 2007;

Feldman, Magori-Cohen, Galili, Singer, & Louzoun, 2011; Calkins, 1997; DeGangi, DiPietro, Greenspan, & Porges, 1991; Huffman, Bryan, Carmen, Pedersen, Doussard-Roosevelt, et al., 1998; Stifter & Corey, 2001). Cardiac vagal tone is assessed indirectly via the respiratory component in heart rate variability (respiratory sinus arrhythmia [RSA]), a measure of cardiac activity that is innervated by the vagus nerve (the 10th cranial nerve) of the parasympathetic nervous system. Both baseline levels of RSA and RSA suppression are considered as markers of adaptive coping and regulation (Porges, 1991, 1996), whereas heart rate reflects a degree of physiological arousal. Heart rate measures represent a combination of parasympathetic and sympathetic influences, as the slowing or speeding of the heart is mediated by increased or decreased activity of either branch of the autonomic nervous system or both as they coregulate activity. And thus, heart rate and vagal tone are considered to be measures of cardiac activity that represent distinct aspects of autonomic nervous system functioning (Moore & Calkins, 2004). RSA is an indicator of parasympathetic arousal, whereas heart rate is both sympathetically and parasympathetically controlled. In this way, these measures are related but provide different lenses through which we can assess the functioning of the autonomic nervous system.

Infant cardiac vagal tone at term age, representing the dispositional functionality of the system, was found to predict infant–mother and infant–father synchrony at 3 months (Feldman & Eidelman, 2007). Since infant baseline vagal tone is individually stable from birth to 10 years of age (Feldman, Rosenthal, et al., 2014), predicts the development of regulatory competencies across the first years of life (Feldman, 2009), and matures in the context of mother–infant physical contact (Feldman & Eidelman, 2003a), understanding how mother–infant interaction shapes the infant's parasympathetic response is of theoretical and clinical interest. The infant's vagal regulation in a stressful social interaction with his or her mother can differ according to the level of dyadic coordination between the mother's and infant's affective behaviors (Moore & Calkins, 2004). In this study, mothers and their 3-month-old infants were observed during the still-face paradigm. As expected, infants had more negative emotionality, decreased vagal tone, and increased heart rate during the distressing still-face episode. Infants who did not show vagal withdrawal during the still-face episode were those who experienced lower synchrony with their mothers and more vagal suppression during normal play (Moore & Calkins, 2004). In another study, mothers of 6-month-old infants who were later categorized as avoidant in their attachment (at 12 months) had an association between their vagal withdrawal and their observed sensitivity to their child's distress. No such association was found in mothers of later securely attached children (Mills-Koonce et al., 2007). Recent results of a longitudinal study highlight the possibility that early sensitive mothering is associated with increases in children's regulatory function as measured via vagal withdrawal, which in turn was associated with higher levels of sensitive parenting (Perry, Mackler, Calkins, & Keane, 2014).

Online biological synchrony of mothers' and infants' heart rhythms was found during face-to-face interactions between 3-month-old infants and their mothers. Moreover, we found that during moments of vocal or affective synchrony, the degree of heart rate coupling was stronger than during nonsynchronous episodes, suggesting a behavior-based mechanism of biological synchrony (Feldman, Magori-Cohen, et al., 2011). Similarly, maternal and infant vagal tone measures were interrelated during the most synchronous phases in the dyadic interaction (Feldman, Singer, & Zagoory, 2010).

Premature infants who received mother–infant skin-to-skin contact (kangaroo care [KC]) intervention following birth have been shown to have a more rapid maturation of the autonomic nervous system as indexed by vagal tone between 32 and 37 weeks' gestational age (Feldman & Eidelman, 2003b). This KC effect on autonomic function is accompanied by positive changes in behavioral synchrony within KC families. Mothers and fathers in families that took part in KC intervention display more affectionate touch of infant and spouse and remain in closer proximity during triadic play interactions at 3 months (Feldman, Weller, Sirota, & Eidelman, 2003). A recent summary of a longitudinal follow-up that lasted for 10 years in families of children who received KC intervention as newborns has recently been published (Feldman, Rosenthal, et al., 2014), showing that in mother–infant dyads that went through KC intervention following a premature birth, RSA and maternal behavior were dynamically interrelated over time, leading to improved physiology, executive functions, and mother–child reciprocity at 10 years of age. In this sample, KC increased RSA and maternal attachment behavior in the postpartum period, reduced maternal anxiety, and enhanced child cognitive development and executive functions from 6 months to 10 years. By 10 years of age, children receiving KC showed an attenuated stress response, improved RSA function, a more organized sleep, and better cognitive control (Feldman, Rosenthal, et al., 2014).

Beyond infancy, vagal tone has been found to relate to synchronous behavior in romantic relationships. Comparing young adults who were not romantically attached to new lovers, it was found that RSA change in response to positive and negative films was greater among singles as compared with lovers, suggesting that love enhances emotion regulation and buffers against our physiological stress response. In this study, we also demonstrated that RSA in singles decreased when viewing movies with negative emotions, whereas no such decrease was found among new lovers, pointing to a reduced stress response and a more regulated vagal regulation during the period of falling in love (Schneiderman, Zilberstein-Kra, Leckman, & Feldman, 2011).

Hormonal Markers of Biobehavioral Synchrony

Some of the most compelling support for the biobehavioral synchrony model comes from research that examines the hormonal correlates of observed synchronous behavior and describes how each hormonal system plays a unique role in supporting social behavior, as well as interacts with other neurohormonal systems and mutually coregulates social exchanges. Following a short introduction, we review studies that provide examples for the associations between synchronous interactions and the neuropeptides oxytocin (OT), vasopressin (AVP), and prolactin (PRL); the steroids cortisol (CT) and testosterone (T); and the protein enzyme salivary alpha-amylase (sAA).

The neuropeptides OT and AVP are thought to provide the neurobiological substrate that underpins sociality, social motivation, and social attunement (Carter, 1998, 2003, 2014; Gordon, Martin, Feldman, & Leckman, 2011). OT and AVP are closely related structurally and are produced in two hypothalamic nuclei in the central nervous system (CNS), as well as in multiple peripheral sites including the heart, thymus, gastrointestinal tract, ovaries, testis, epididymis, prostate and pregnant intrauterine tissue. OT receptors are widespread in the CNS and exist in brain regions known for their involvement in emotion regulation, reward and motivation, and social salience. Peripheral organs, such as the heart and kidneys, are also targets in the body for OT function (see Gimpl & Fahrenholz, 2001; Gordon et al., 2011, for a review). The means of release and production of these neuropeptides are complex and multifaceted, including not only release from the synaptic cleft but also dendritic release and perhaps axonal diffusion (Ross & Young, 2009). These various mechanisms of release can be at the basis of the dynamic coordination between central and peripheral OT activity (Pow & Morris, 1989; Ludwig & Leng, 2006). OT and AVP are systemic neuropeptides able to exert widespread and complex effects as they interact dynamically with neural systems such as the salience and reward circuits, the hypothalamic–pituitary–adrenocortical (HPA) stress response axis, the hypothalamic–pituitary–gonadal (HPG) axis, the immune system, and other peripheral organ systems (Gordon et al., 2011). OT and AVP are phylogenetically ancient hormones, known to have crucial roles in mammalian social behavior, especially within attachment and bonded relationships (Carter, 1998, 2014). Their extensive implication in sociality, in the initiation of pair bonds and in maternal behavior, makes them prime candidate biomarkers for synchrony research in humans.

Although there has been some controversy regarding the utility of peripheral measures of OT, as OT does not cross the blood–brain barrier readily, there have been several studies validating the use of peripheral OT measurement. High levels of individual stability were found in plasma OT levels across lengthy periods, for instance, from the first trimester of pregnancy to the postpartum period (Feldman, Weller, Zagoory-Sharon, & Levine, 2007), and between the first month after birth and 3 years of age (Feldman, Gordon, et al., 2013). Medium-level correlations were found between OT in plasma and saliva (Feldman, Gordon, Schneiderman, et al., 2010; Feldman, Gordon, & Zagoory-Sharon, 2011), and between salivary OT in parent and child in both mothers and fathers in infancy (Feldman, Gordon, & Zagoory-Sharon, 2010) and the preschool years (Apter-Levi, Feldman, Vakart, Ebstein, & Feldman, 2013; Feldman, Gordon, et al., 2013). Associations were found between allelic variations on the oxytocin receptor gene (*OXTR*) with peripheral levels of OT in both plasma (Feldman et al., 2012) and saliva (Apter-Levi, Feldman, et al., 2013). Finally, intranasal OT administration was found to markedly increase peripheral OT levels in humans (Weisman, Zagoory-Sharon, & Feldman, 2012), and to alter OT levels in the brain (Neumann, Maloumby, Beiderbeck, Lukas, & Landgraf, 2013). These studies demonstrate coordination between OT availability in the brain and OT levels in the periphery.

In addition to links between brain and periphery, the oxytocinergic system maintains cross-talk with multiple hormonal systems. Similar to OT, peripheral AVP concentrations have shown a high degree of individual stability. The complex cross-talk between OT and AVP is exemplified by a recent study in which intranasal administration of OT induced increases in salivary AVP concentrations in the first hour following OT manipulation (Weisman, Schneiderman, Zagoory-Sharon, & Feldman, 2012).

Similarly to OT, the neuropeptide PRL, which is also synthesized in the hypothalamus, is traditionally known for its role in lactation and its support of maternal behavior following birth (Bridges et al., 1997; Grattan, 2001; Grattan & Kokay, 2008; Mann & Bridges, 2001). Parallel to the actions of AVP in animals, PRL is also well known for its role in paternal behavior in animals (Buntin, Hnasko, Zuzick, Valentine, & Scammell, 1996; Dixson & George, 1982; Kindler, Bahr, Gross, & Philipp, 1991; Schradin & Anzenberger, 1999; Ziegler, Wegner, & Snowdon, 1996) and to a lesser extent in humans (Fleming, Corter, Stallings, & Steiner, 2002; Gordon et al., 2010c; Storey, Walsh, Quinton, & Wynne-Edwards, 2000).

Anatomically, one of the nuclei synthesizing OT and AVP in the brain—the paraventricular nucleus (PVN) of the hypothalamus—is a key structure in the HPA axis. Specifically, the PVN is also the sole site of corticotropin-releasing hormone production, leading to a cascade of events that activate the HPA axis to prompt release of CT from the adrenal gland. CT is considered a "stress hormone" and as such is highly involved in sociality. CT has been extensively implicated in the same behaviors in which OT and AVP are implicated, such as maternal behavior and responsiveness to the infant (Fleming et al., 1993; Fleming, Steiner, & Corter, 1997; Maestripieri, 2001; Stallings, Fleming, Corter, Worthman, & Steiner, 2001). However, the associations between CT and parenting are highly dependent on multiple factors such as maternal age, prior experience, and feeding patterns (Krpan, Coombs, Zinga, Steiner, & Fleming, 2005). Other markers of the HPA stress response include sAA, dehydroepiandrosterone (DHEA), and dehydroepiandrosterone sulfate (DHEA-S). Like CT, DHEA and the more stable DHEA-S are also secreted from the adrenal cortex prompted by adrenocorticotropic hormone (ACTH), most likely to protect from the neurotoxic effects of CT (Lennartsson, Kushnir, Bergquist, & Jonsdottir, 2012; Maninger, Wolkowitz, Reus, Epel, & Mellon, 2009; Morgan et al., 2004). Finally, sAA is a relatively recent addition to the array of "stress biomarkers" (Nater & Rohleder, 2009), as its secretion to the saliva is governed by the autonomic nervous system, which is characterized by increased activity during stress. Research has shown elevated levels of sAA induced by various aspects of chronic or acute psychological stress (Bosch et al., 1996, 1998; Bosch, De Geus, Veerman, Hoogstraten, & Nieuw Amerongen, 2003; Chatterton, Vogelsong, Lu, Ellman, & Hudgens, 1996; Chatterton, Vogelson, Lu, & Hudgens, 1997). The interactions between the so-called affiliation (such as OT and AVP) and stress (CT, DHEA, DHEA-S, sAA) markers are always complex and often inconsistent, leaving ample room for future scientific inquiry, for example, the literature reports on positive (Hoge, Pollack, Kaufman, Zak, & Simon, 2008; Marazziti et al., 2006; Taylor et al., 2006; Tops, van Peer, Korf, Wijers, & Tucker, 2007), negative (Altemus, Deuster, Galliven, Carter, & Gold, 1995; Heinrichs & Domes, 2008; Heinrichs & Gaab, 2007; Meinlschmidt & Heim, 2007), and nonsignificant associations between OT and CT (Gordon et al., 2008; Levine, Zagoory-Sharon, Feldman, & Weller, 2007).

Hormonal markers of affiliation and stress are highly interrelated with the activity of the gonadal steroid hormones of the HPG axis: T and estradiol (E) that regulate sexual development, function, and behavior across the lifespan (Choleris, Devidze, Kavaliers, & Pfaff, 2008; Gordon et al., 2011; Viau, 2002). T and E function is driven by the release of hypothalamic gonadotropin-releasing hormone (GRH), which in turn causes the anterior pituitary to release follicle-stimulating hormone (FSH) and luteinizing hormone (LH). HPG axis hormones exist in both sexes and figure prominently in the regulation of social behavior, partly through their interaction with OT and AVP. For instance, research shows that E potentiates the OT system, and T potentiates the AVP system and also impacts OT via the conversion of T to E (Akaishi & Sakuma, 1985; Bale, Dorsa, & Johnston, 1995; Ho & Lee, 1992; Quinones-Jenab et al., 1997; Sarkar, Frautschy, & Mitsugi, 1992). During adult life, T and E have been linked to the rapid activation of various socioemotional behavioral profiles, some of which are associated with OT and AVP, including reproductive behaviors (sexual receptivity, frequency of copulatory behavior) and aggression (Balthazart & Ball, 2006; Mehta & Beer, 2010).

It is important to note that hormones used as biomarkers of stress, affiliation, and sociality in the context of social function do not only regulate social behavior and function but are constantly and dynamically regulated by social behaviors, social context, and the experience in turn (Maruska & Fernald, 2011). Such dynamic interplay of physiology and behavior is a major component of the biobehavioral synchrony model.

Review of Our Research on Hormonal Markers of Biobehavioral Synchrony

In an attempt to examine how hormonal biomarkers of affiliation relate to behavioral synchrony in humans, several of our studies examined the effects of OT and AVP on parent–infant social synchrony. In the first study, testing maternal OT levels at early pregnancy, late pregnancy, and postpartum in relation to maternal behavior, we found that an increase in circulating OT levels during pregnancy was associated with the mother's reporting stronger attachment to her fetus (Levine et al., 2007). In addition, OT levels were highly stable across this time period (rs = .80–.96), and levels of OT in early pregnancy predicted the amount of maternal bonding behavior postpartum, including gaze at infant face and body, "motherese" high-pitched vocalization, positive affective expression, and affectionate touch, as well as coordination of these behaviors with infant state.

In the next study, we examined fathers as well as mothers of infants from birth to 6 months. We found that during the transition to parenthood OT was related to parental behavior in a gender-specific manner. Increased OT levels in mothers were related to affective maternal behavior including gaze, affectionate touch, and "motherese" vocalizations, whereas higher OT in fathers correlated with the father-specific stimulatory type of play including stimulatory touch and exploratory focus (Gordon et al., 2010a). Following parent–infant interactions at 4–6 months postpartum, we found a significant increase in parental OT levels, but only among those who provided a substantial amount of touch. Similar to the findings for the high licking-and-grooming mothers (Champagne, Diorio, Sharma, & Meaney, 2001; Meaney, 2001), among mothers who provided high levels of affectionate contact (more than two-thirds of the time) but not in mothers who displayed low levels of affectionate contact, OT levels markedly increased after interactions. Among fathers, a parallel increase in OT was observed only in those who engaged in stimulatory contact for more than two-thirds of the time (Feldman, Gordon, Schneiderman, et al., 2010).

Six months after the birth of their first child, increased levels of OT were related to triadic social synchrony among father, mother, and infant during a triadic family interaction, as measured by states of coordinated proximity and affectionate touch between the parents, and between parents and infant while both parent and child are synchronizing their social gaze. Among mothers, triadic synchrony was also independently related to lower levels of CT, which interacts in a complex manner with affiliative hormones to predict observed social behaviors (Gordon et al., 2010b). Interestingly, when paternal levels of OT were examined at 6 months postpartum in fathers, increased circulating levels of OT predicted affective synchrony (paralleling the behavioral construct that related to *maternal* OT at 1-month postpartum), whereas the neuropeptide PRL was associated with paternal facilitation of the infant's exploratory play (Gordon et al., 201c). Of interest, similar division was found between OT and

AVP. In mothers and fathers of 4-month-old infants, parents with high OT concentrations supported social engagement and displayed more affectionate touch compared with parents with low OT. In comparison, parents with high AVP levels engaged in enhanced stimulatory contact and tended to adaptively follow infants' bids to engage socially (Apter-Levi, Zagoory-Sharon, et al., 2014). OT has also been shown to underscore a level of consistency between parents' and infants' neuroendocrine system that supports a cross-generation transmission of human synchronous behavior. We have previously reported on a positive association between parents' and infants' circulating OT levels. The amount of parent–infant observed affective synchrony moderated this association, as dyads with high synchrony had the strongest correlation of parent–infant OT levels (Feldman, Gordon, & Zagoory-Sharon, 2010).

Recent studies have integrated measures of circulating OT with markers of its genetic encoding in an attempt to predict aspects of synchronous parenting. For instance, in mothers and fathers of 4- to 6-month-old infants, lower circulating levels of OT were associated with certain allelic variations on the oxytocin receptor gene (*OXTR*) and *CD38* gene (specifically, the *OXTR* rs2254298 and rs1042778 and *CD38* rs3796863 risk alleles). The combination of reduced plasma levels of OT and genetic risk was associated with reduced parental touch during parent–infant interaction (Feldman et al., 2012). Studies manipulating OT levels in parents via a single intranasal administration of OT have also supported the biobehavioral synchrony model by showing how biological alterations that occur in the parent can induce behavioral and biological effects in the parent, the infant, and the dyadic unit. OT administration to fathers, 45 minutes prior to a social interaction with their 5-month-old infant, resulted in an increase in OT, RSA, social reciprocity, and social engagement behaviors not only in the father but also in the infant, who did not receive OT (Weisman, Zagoory-Sharon, & Feldman, 2012). Employing an advanced computational analysis, researchers found that administration of OT impacted aspects of paternal motion (fathers' head speed, head acceleration, and proximity to the infant) during dyadic interaction with the infant. Most specifically, parameters of the father's head acceleration were associated with the infant's OT reactivity following OT administration to the father (Weisman, Delaherche, et al., 2013). In fathers of 5-month-olds, intranasal OT administration also had a short-term impact on salivary T levels during social interaction that predicted patterns of paternal behaviors and observed father–infant synchrony. Initially, baseline paternal T levels were inversely associated with synchronous father–infant interactive behaviors. Compared with a placebo, OT administration enhanced T production in fathers and the OT-induced change in T was correlated with parent–child social behaviors including positive affect, social gaze, touch, and vocal synchrony (Weisman, Zagoory-Sharon, & Feldman, 2014).

Intranasal OT administration to fathers prior to a "still-face" interaction with their 5-month-old infant (Tronick, Als, Adamson, Wise, & Brazelton,

1978; this paradigm includes a phase of natural face-to-face interaction followed by a dysregulating period in which the parent is nonresponsive and then a reestablishment of naturalistic interaction and parental behavior) enhanced fathers' stress response overall (as indexed by CT). In addition, alterations in paternal OT impacted infants' physiological and behavioral response as a function of observed parent–infant synchrony. When there was high dyadic parent–infant synchrony, infants' had elevated CT reactivity and increased infant social gaze to the father. In dyads with low observed social synchrony, an inverse effect was established in which the infants' CT response was reduced and infants displayed diminished social gaze toward the unavailable father (Weisman, Zagoory-Sharon, & Feldman, 2013). Interestingly, the same still-face paradigm was used to test whether parental touch can attenuate infants' reactivity to stress. Mother–infant dyads were asked to perform either the classic still-face paradigm or a version that included maternal touch during the stressful unavailability stage. Maternal and infant autonomic reactivity (vagal tone) and CT levels were sampled throughout the procedure. Stress reactivity (as indexed by CT) was lower when infants received touch during the still-face condition. Vagal tone showed a greater suppression when there was no accompanying maternal touch. Finally, touch synchrony between mother and infant during the initial free-play stage of the interaction was associated with higher infant vagal tone, whereas touch myssynchrony at that stage was correlated with higher maternal and infant CT levels (Feldman, Singer, et al., 2010).

New discoveries regarding the hormonal markers of biobehavioral synchrony in romantic partners and early friendships in children are paralleling some of the findings and insights from parent–infant research. In a 3-year longitudinal study to examine a potential cross-generation transfer of OT function from parents to child in humans, it was found that parental plasma OT was related to more efficient alleles on the OXTR. The child's social reciprocity as he or she played with a friend was associated with the child OT levels, and also specifically with *maternal* OT-related genes and hormonal levels, as well as with mother–child synchronous reciprocity (Feldman, Gordon, et al., 2013). These findings provide hormonal evidence to our longitudinal study following children from 4 months to 13 years. Children were observed interacting with their mothers and fathers at 4 months, 3 years, and 13 years. At 3 years, they were also observed in kindergarten for measures of social competence and aggression, and in early adolescence they interacted with a same-sex best friend in positive (planning joint activity in school) and conflict interactions. We found individual stability in measures of behavioral synchrony in the child's interaction with each parent across childhood. Moreover, synchronous mothering and fathering each supported a somewhat distinct line of social development. Synchronous mothering predicted greater social competence in the peer group and the capacity to dialogue joint positive interaction with friends with greater reciprocity. On the other hand, synchronous fathering predicted lower aggression in the peer group during the preschool years and adolescents' capacity to dialogue conflicts with empathy and reciprocity within an attachment relationship with their best friend (Feldman, Bamberger, et al., 2013).

To examine biobehavioral synchrony in romantic partners, 120 new lovers (60 couples) were seen in the lab during the first 3 months of their romantic bond and compared with 43 demographically matched singles. Blood was drawn for hormonal analysis and couples were seen during interactions in positive, conflict, and support-giving interactions and were interviewed regarding the emerging bond. Couples that stayed together were seen again 6 months later, approximately 9 months after the initiation of the romantic bond. We found that OT levels increased dramatically during the period of falling in love and were in fact even higher than those observed among new parents. Among couples that stayed together, OT levels did not drop at the second assessment, indicating that the OT system provides a long support for pair-bond formation in humans. Similar to the parenting context, OT correlated with the couples' reciprocity and synchronous behavior during interaction. OT levels were also associated with reported worries regarding the partner and the relationship (Schneiderman, Zagoory-Sharon, Leckman, & Feldman, 2012). In addition to OT, we also measured PRL, AVP, CT, DHEA, and T in these lovers in relation to the degree of hostility and empathy observed during the conflict dialogue. We found evidence for biobehavioral synchrony in three hormones: the individual's T level predicted higher hostility, but only when the partner also had high T. Similarly, CT predicted lower empathy and greater behavioral hostility, but only in the context of high partner's CT. The most interesting evidence of biobehavioral synchrony was found for the oxytocinergic system: the partner's OT, not the individual's OT, was predictive of the level of empathy this individual displayed toward the partner during conflict discussion, and the pattern was the same for men and women. These findings provide compelling evidence for the biobehavioral synchrony model but also demonstrates how the oxytocin system binds the biology and behavior of two individuals within a social bond (Schneiderman, Kanat-Maymon, Zagoory-Sharon, & Feldman, 2014). Finally, we computed a cumulative index of risk on the *OXTR* by combining five single nucleotide polymorphisms (SPNs) previously shown to be associated with greater susceptibility to disorders of social dysfunction such as autism or schizophrenia. We found that lovers who had lower risk on the *OXTR* showed greater empathy to their partner distress during a support-giving interaction (Schneiderman, Kanat-Maymon, Ebstein, & Feldman, 2014).

Interesting findings on OT in adults in relation to bonding-related experiences were found in two studies. Assessing OT levels in a large cohort of women and men ($N = 473$), we found that high levels of OT in women were related only to attachment anxiety, whereas in men, higher OT function had an anxiolytic effect and was associated with lower trait anxiety. These findings may relate to the different modes of stress regulation in men and women and to the close links among attachment, preoccupations, and worries in mothers (Weisman, Zagoory-Sharon, Schneiderman, Gordon, & Feldman, 2013). Finally, among romantically unattached young adults circulating levels of OT in plasma were associated with reported bonding to one's parent, and inversely correlated with reported psychological distress, most specifically depressive symptoms. In this same study, CT was also measured and was positively related to anxiety in attachment. OT and CT were not correlated with each other, and yet each predicted a unique and exclusive portion of the variance in participants' representation of their attachment to their parents as adults (Gordon et al., 2008).

Overall, these findings suggest that behavioral synchrony is intricately linked with complex endocrine processes, which involve multiple hormones mutually influencing behavior within the individual and between partners within an attachment bond. If we view hormones as one mechanism, by which epigenetic influences of experience can take place and impact development, it is clear why the continued exploration of the hormonal factors underlying synchrony is crucial.

Biological Synchrony and Brain Response

Several studies have demonstrated how the human brain responds to social synchrony. These studies allow us to incorporate brain function as another biomarker of the processes underlying coordinated interactive behavior and provide insights into the neurological basis of sociality. Novel findings from brain imaging research highlight how synchrony and interconnections exist not only within a single brain as it functions, but also in processes of brain-to-brain coupling (Hasson, Ghazanfar, Galantucci, Garrod, & Keysers, 2012). Researchers have shown that sometimes our brains have a tendency to "tick collectively" with other brains, for instance, when we watch compelling movie scenes (Hasson, Yuval, Levy, Fuhrmann, & Malach, 2004) or when we listen to music (Abrams et al., 2013). Despite the perception of a highly individualized experience, the personal experience is also a shared experience.

In a recent study at our lab, we examined mothers' brain response to synchronous interactions and tested whether her response correlated with the degree of observed synchrony between the mother and her own infant. Healthy mothers were asked to view three video vignettes depicting synchronous interactions between mother and infant and two myssynchronous interactions, one of a clinically depressed mother containing no maternal behavior and no synchrony, the other of a clinically anxious mother, including high amounts of maternal behaviors that were uncoordinated with infant cues. Interactions between mother and own infant were microcoded for synchrony. We found that synchronous interactions elicited greater activity in reward-related areas, including the nucleus accumbens (NAcc) and dorsal anterior cingulate cortex (dACC), as well as in "mirror neuron" embodiment-related areas—inferior parietal lobule (IPL) and supplementary motor area. Furthermore, mothers' behavioral synchrony with her own infant correlated with her dACC response to synchrony in others. These findings are consistent with models of embodiment, simulation, and mirroring that highlight how social action is underlaid by social recognition. As both mother and infant embody, coordinate, and coregulate each other's socioaffective states they can share in biobehavioral synchrony (Atzil, Hendeler, & Feldman, 2014).

In another fMRI study, we were able to chart distinct profiles of limbic and cortical activity, as well as their functional connectivity, which differentiated mothers whose caregiving style was synchronous from mothers whose behaviors were marked by intrusiveness and miscoordination. Mothers of 4- to 6-month-olds who were rated (using microanalysis of behavior) as being synchronous while interacting with their infant showed enhanced brain activations in the left NAcc, whereas mothers who interacted intrusively with their infant exhibited higher activations in the right amygdala. Among synchronous mothers, researchers found enhanced functional connectivity among the left NAcc, the right amygdala, and neural circuits that are involved with empathy, emotion modulation, and theory of mind. In intrusive mothers, left NAcc and right amygdala were functionally correlated with brain regions that are implicated in proaction. Associations between peripheral concentrations of OT and neural activations in the left NAcc and right amygdala were found only in mothers rated as synchronous. Sorting points into neighborhood (SPIN) analysis—complex mathematical analysis that tests the temporal organization of activity in a brain nucleus—demonstrated that in the synchronous group, left NAcc and right amygdala activations showed clearer temporal organization, whereas among intrusive mothers, activations of these nuclei exhibited greater cross-time disorganization (Atzil, Hendler, & Feldman, 2011).

While mothers' and fathers' of 4- to 6-month-old infants viewed videos of their own infants versus those of unfamiliar infants during solitary play in the fMRI scanner, baseline OT and AVP levels were measured. Results indicate that neural networks implicated in mentalizing and empathy, including premotor and motor cortices, IPL, inferior frontal gyrus, and insula are coordinated between mothers and fathers as they view videos of their own child. Results also show a differential gender-based association between the levels of the neuropeptides OT and AVP and mothers' and fathers' brain response. Mothers showed higher amygdala activations and an association between OT levels and amygdala response, whereas fathers showed greater activation in social brain regions that was associated with circulating AVP levels (Atzil, Hendler, Zagoory-Sharon, Winetraub, & Feldman, 2012). To address the issue of the neural basis of the parenting experience and its hormonal biomarkers in fathers, a recent study assessed brain activations via fMRI and circulating OT levels in three groups of parents: heterosexual primary-caregiving mothers, homosexual primary-caregiving fathers, and homosexual secondary-caregiving fathers.

Results indicated that parenting is underlaid by a global "parental-caregiving" network that integrates two neural circuits: a subcortical and paralimbic emotional processing network and a cortical mentalizing network (which includes frontopolar–medial–prefrontal and temporo–parietal brain regions). Primary-caregiving mothers had greater activation in the emotion processing network that was associated with increased OT levels and enhanced parent–infant synchrony, whereas increased OT and synchrony were associated with increased activation in the mentalizing network for secondary-caregiving fathers. Interestingly, primary-caregiving fathers had enhanced functional connectivity of the amygdala and the superior temporal sulcus (STS). These fathers' amygdala activation was similar to amygdala activations observed in mothers, yet coupled with high activation of the STS comparable to secondary-caregiving fathers. Among all fathers, the degree of amygdala–STS connectivity was associated with the amount of time fathers spent in direct child care (Abraham et al., 2014).

Biobehavioral Synchrony in Pathology

Several pathological conditions can provide unique windows to study the associations between hormones and behavior in conditions when the bonding process is disrupted or is not provided consistently. In the following, we review our research on OT and other hormonal systems in relation to behavioral synchrony in various psychopathologies.

Prematurity

Previous research has shown that premature birth can be associated with reduced infant alertness, decreased maternal behaviors, and a diminished coordination of maternal behavior with infant alertness in the weeks following birth. We found that indeed, at 3 months following a premature birth, father–infant and mother–infant interactions were less synchronous. The combination of a premature birth with a diminished maturation of autonomic nervous system (as indexed by cardiac vagal tone) was related to the lowest amounts of maternal behavior in the postpartum period and the lowest levels of maternal touch at 3 months (Feldman & Eidelman, 2007). Longitudinal associations were also found between disorganized and delayed pattern of development of biological rhythms during the last weeks of gestation, including weekly assessment of sleep–wake cyclicity and vagal tone, and these impacted the development of synchronous mother–infant behavior (Feldman, 2006). When we examined visual synchrony in mother–infant dyads of typically developing and prematurely born infants when the infants were 3 months old, we found that preterm infants and their mothers displayed short and frequent episodes of gaze synchrony that were quickly terminated following initiation, whereas full-term infants and their mothers were able to maintain shared gaze for longer periods (Harel, Gordon,

Geva, & Feldman, 2011). In the first study to demonstrate the long-term effects of KC, a touch-based intervention given for 2 consecutive weeks following a premature birth, researchers found benefiting impacts on child's physiology and cognition, and on parental mental health and mother–child relational patterns across the first decade of the child's life (Feldman, Rosenthal, et al., 2014). In the postpartum period KC enhanced infants' autonomic function as well as maternal behavior. From 6 months to 10 years, KC increased measures of child development and reduced anxiety in the mother. By 10 years of age, children who had received KC showed a more regulated stress response (indexed by CT), more organized sleep patterns, improved autonomic function, organized sleep, and better cognitive function. The combination of enhanced autonomic function in the child and sensitive maternal behavior were dynamically interrelated over time, and led to improved physiology, executive functions, and mother–child reciprocity at 10 years (Feldman, Rosenthal, et al., 2014).

Autism Spectrum Disorders

Social interactions of preschoolers with autism spectrum disorders (ASD) with their mother and father were compared with those of typically developing (TD) preschoolers with the parent in the home ecology. Four saliva measures of OT were collected from parent and child. Children with ASD engaged less frequently in gaze synchrony, touch synchrony, and in joint attention with their parents. Children with ASD also showed lower baseline OT levels. However, during social interaction with mother or father, OT level normalized after 25 minutes of interaction and remained high as long as the social contact was maintained. However, OT levels dropped to the initial diminished levels 10 minutes after parent–child contact was terminated. OT levels in the children correlated with the amount of parent–child social synchrony (Feldman, Golan, Hirschler-Guttenberg, Ostfeld-Etzion, & Zagoory-Sharon, 2014), showing consistency with the biobehavioral synchrony model in this group.

Maternal Depression

Maternal depression in the postpartum period, particularly when persistent over time, can have detrimental effects on infant development. Already during the first postpartum year, infants of depressed mothers exhibit reduced regulatory function, negative emotionality, and low social engagement during dyadic interaction. These infants also exhibit high CT reactivity (Feldman et al., 2009). In a longitudinal study following infants of depressed mothers from birth to 6 years, we found effects of maternal depression on several hormonal systems. At 6 years old, children of mothers who have been diagnosed as chronically depressed across the first years of life showed increased propensity to develop psychopathology. The biobehavioral synchrony model was supported by findings showing how salivary OT was lower in mothers, fathers, and children in depressed families and the associations between low OT with low levels of empathy and social engagement observed in children of depressed mothers. Family members were tested not only for circulating salivary OT levels but also for allelic variation in the *OXTR* gene (rs2254298 single-nucleotide polymorphism). A certain allelic variation (the rs2254298 GG homozygous genotype) was found to be overrepresented in depressed mothers and their families, and it correlated with lower salivary oxytocin. However, presence of a single rs2254298 A allele in depressed mothers markedly decreased risk of child psychopathology (Apter-Levi, Feldman, et al., 2013). In addition to the OT system, we also found alteration in mothers' and children's CT response. Children of depressed mothers had higher diurnal CT levels and lower CT diurnal variability. Their mothers, in turn, showed lower DHEA diurnal levels and flatter diurnal DHEA curves. Following stressors, children of depressed mothers—particularly those who were diagnosed with internalizing disorder—did not return to baseline levels at recovery but continued to increase, indicating that sessions with mother causes stress rather than provide a stress-regulating mechanism. Consistent with the model, higher CT levels in the children were mediated by maternal and child social behavior, specifically, lower maternal sensitivity and higher child withdrawal during interactions.

Posttraumatic Stress Disorder

To assess patterns of maternal and child behavior and hormonal production under condition of severe environmental adversity, we evaluated hormones and behavior in 232 families. These included 158 children living in Sderot, a town located 10 kilometers from the Gaza border and exposed to repeated and unpredictable missile attacks and 86 demographically matched controls. Children were divided into three groups: controls; exposed children diagnosed with posttraumatic stress disorder (PTSD); and exposed children who, despite the fact of living in a continuous war zone, showed greater resilience (exposed-no-PTSD). CT and sAA were measured before and after stressors in mother and child. Whereas control children showed the typical increase–decrease CT response, exposed children exhibited diminished variability. Children with PTSD showed very low and flat CT and sAA, whereas exposed-no-PTSD children had consistently high response. These were associated with the level of mother–child reciprocity during interactions. Behaviorally, children with PTSD tended to employ more strategies of behavioral withdrawal compared with children who did not have PTSD who tended to display more comfort-seeking behaviors (Feldman, Vengrober, Eidelman-Rothman, & Zagoory-Sharon, 2013).

We also measured cumulative risk on multiple genetic markers of OT and AVP in mother, father, and child and how these interact with social behavior to predict PTSD in war-exposed children. Maternal sensitive support during stressful simulation of the child's war experience reduced the effects of war exposure on the child's propensity to develop Axis I disorder in general, and PTSD in particular. Furthermore, the chronicity of PTSD from infancy to middle childhood (ages 7–8 years) in war-exposed children was related to higher genetic risk in the child and his or her parents, as well as low maternal support and greater initial avoidance symptoms in the child (Feldman, Vengrober, & Ebstein, 2014).

Future Research

Considering that synchrony is inherent to the human social experience and neurophysiology—especially in the context of our earliest bonds with our parents—it is crucial to deepen our understanding of the dyadic interplay of coordinated behavior with biology. It seems that there is a need to include and develop new and yet unexplored biomarkers, for instance, those arising from the fields of imaging and neurogenetics. We believe that the future of microanalysis will see new and exciting associations between microbehavioral measures and eye-tracking data or measures of brain function and genetic expression. The rich and comprehensive nature of these types of data will allow scientists to create more compelling and accurate descriptions of biobehavioral connections.

Within microanalysis, there is still a need to develop better and more advanced building blocks of behavior to describe subtleties and idiosyncrasies. Perhaps new and advanced tools from engineering and computer sciences could be incorporated to better describe behavior and synchronous experiences, in ways that have not yet been captured by the existing behavioral building blocks of microanalysis. Aspects of behavior that can tap into the subtleties of our social essence, such as velocity and force of movement, may need to be included in future coding schemes.

Finally, it is surprising how little research has tapped into the neurophysiological basis of synchrony beyond the parent–infant dyad to include triadic family interactions, and even larger family groups that include siblings, grandparents, and others. We are born into the family group and are set to "join" others very early in life. Groups comprise a hugely important part of how we function in society, and a description of the continuity of synchrony in the family group and in other groups throughout life could contribute greatly to the biobehavioral synchrony literature. We expect future research paradigms to describe and examine what form synchrony takes in groups as they dynamically form and interact. Following, we will be able to delve into the biological basis of such shared states, whether it is by measuring hormonal or autonomic nervous system markers during group interactions or by manipulating levels of hormones and neuropeptides prior to group interactions and measuring changes in observed synchronous behavior.

REFERENCES

Abraham, E., Hendeler, T., Shapira-Lichter, I., Kanat-Maymon, Y., Zagoory-Sharon, O., & Feldman, R. (2014). Father's brain is sensitive to childcare experiences. *Proceedings of the National Academy of Sciences, 111*(27), 9792–9797.

Abrams, D. A., Ryali, S., Chen, T., Chordia, P., Khouzam, A., Levitin, D. J., et al. (2013). Inter-subject synchronization of brain responses during natural music listening. *European Journal of Neuroscience, 37*(9),1458–1469.

Ahern, T. H., Hammock, E. A., & Young, L. J. (2011). Parental division of labor, coordination, and the effects of family structure on parenting in monogamous prairie voles (*Microtus ochrogaster*). *Developmental Psychobiology, 53*(2), 118–131.

Akaishi, T., & Sakuma, Y. (1985). Estrogen excites oxytocinergic, but not vasopressinergic cells in the paraventricular nucleus of female rat hypothalamus. *Brain Research, 335*(2), 302–305

Altemus, M., Deuster, P. A., Galliven, E., Carter, C. S., & Gold, P. W. (1995). Suppression of hypothalmic–pituitary–adrenal axis responses to stress in lactating women. *Journal of Clinical Endicrinology and Metabolism, 80*(10), 2954–2959.

Apter-Levi, Y., Feldman, M., Vakart, A., Ebstein, R. P., & Feldman, R. (2013). Impact of maternal depression across the first 6 years of life on the child's mental health, social engagement, and empathy: The moderating role of oxytocin. *American Journal of Psychiatry, 170*, 1161–1168.

Apter-Levi, Y., Zagoory-Sharon, O., & Feldman, R. (2014). Oxytocin and vasopressin support distinct configurations of social synchrony. *Brain Research, 1580*, 124–132.

Atzil, S., Hendeler, T., & Feldman, R. (2011). Specifying the neurobiological basis of human attachment: Brain, hormones, and behavior in synchronous and intrusive mothers. *Neuropsychopharmacology, 36*, 2603–2615.

Atzil, S., Hendeler, T., & Feldman, R. (2014). The brain basis of social synchrony. *Social Cognitive and Affective Neuroscience, 9*(8), 1193–1202.

Atzil, S., Hendler, T., Zagoory-Sharon, O., Winetraub, Y., & Feldman, R. (2012). Synchrony and specificity in maternal and the paternal brain: Relations to oxytocin and vasopressin. *Journal of the American Academy of Child and Adolescent Psychiatry, 51*, 798–811.

Bale, T. L., Dorsa, D. M., & Johnston, C. A. (1995). Oxytocin receptor mRNA expression in the ventromedial hypothalamus during the estrous cycle. *Journal of Neuroscience, 15*(7-1), 5058–5064.

Balthazart, J., & Ball, G. F. (2006). Is brain estradiol a hormone or a neurotransmitter? *Trends in Neurosciences, 29*(5), 241–249.

Bosch, J. A., Brand, H. S., Ligtenberg, T. J., Bermond, B., Hoogstraten, J., & Nieuw Amerongen, A. V. (1996). Psychological stress as a determinant of protein levels and salivary-induced aggregation of *Streptococcus gordonii* in human whole saliva. *Psychosomatic Medicine, 58*, 374–382.

Bosch, J. A., Brand, H. S., Ligtenberg, A. J., Bermond, B., Hoogstraten, J., & Nieuw Amerongen, A. V. (1998). The response of salivary protein levels and S-IgA to an academic examination are associated with daily stress. *Journal of Psychophysiology, 12*, 384–391.

Bosch, J. A., De Geus, E. J., Veerman, E. C., Hoogstraten, J., & Nieuw Amerongen, A. V. (2003). Innate secretory immunity in response to laboratory stressors that evoke distinct patterns of cardiac autonomic activity. *Psychosomatic Medicine, 65,* 245–258.

Bowlby, J. (1969). *Attachment and loss: Vol.1. Attachment.* New York: Basic.

Bridges, R. S., Robertson, M. C., Shiu, R. P., Sturgis, J. D., Henriquez, B. M., & Mann, P. E. (1997). Central lactogenic regulation of maternal behavior in rats: Steroid dependence, hormone specificity, and behavioral potencies of rat prolactin and rat placental lactogen I. *Endocrinology, 138,* 756–763.

Bullmore, E. T., & Sporns, O. (2009). Complex brain networks: Graph theoretical analysis of structured and functional systems. *Nature Reviews Neuroscience, 10*(4), 312.

Bullmore, E. T., & Sporns, O. (2012). The economy of brain network organization. *Nature Reviews Neuroscience, 13,* 336–349.

Buntin, J. D., Hnasko, R. M., Zuzick, P. H., Valentine, D. L., & Scammell, J. G. (1996). Changes in bioactive prolactin-like activity in plasma and its relationship to incubation behavior in breeding ring doves. *General and Comparative Endocrinology, 102,* 221–232.

Calkins, S. D. (1997). Cardiac vagal tone indices of temperamental reactivity and behavioral regulation in young children. *Developmental Psychobiology, 31*(2), 125–135.

Carter, C. S. (1998). Neuroendocrine perspectives on social attachment and love. *Psychoneuroendocrinology, 23*(8), 779–818.

Carter, C. S. (2003). Developmental consequences of oxytocin. *Physiology and Behavior, 79*(3), 383–397.

Carter, C. S. (2014). Oxytocin pathways and the evolution of human behavior. *Annual Review of Psychology, 65,* 17–39.

Champagne, F., Diorio, J., Sharma, S., & Meaney, M. J. (2001). Naturally occurring variations in maternal behavior in the rat are associated with differences in estrogen-inducible central oxytocin receptors. *Proceedings of the National Academy of Sciences, 98*(22), 12736–12741.

Champagne, F. A. (2008). Epigenetic mechanisms and the transgenerational effects of maternal care. *Frontiers in Neuroendocrinology, 29,* 386–397.

Chatterton, R. T., Jr., Vogelsong, K. M., Lu, Y. C., Ellman, A. B., & Hudgens, G. A. (1996). Salivary alpha-amylase as a measure of endogenous adrenergic activity. *Clinical Physiology, 16,* 433–448.

Chatterton, R. T., Jr., Vogelsong, K. M., Lu, Y. C., & Hudgens, G. A. (1997). Hormonal responses to psychological stress in men preparing for skydiving. *Journal of Clinical Endocrinology and Metabolism, 82,* 2503–2509.

Choleris, E., Devidze, N., Kavaliers, M., & Pfaff, D. W. (2008). Steroidal/neuropeptide interactions in hypothalamus and amygdala related to social anxiety. *Progress in Brain Research, 170,* 291–303.

DeGangi, G. A., DiPietro, J. A., Greenspan, S. I., & Porges, S. W. (1991). Psychophysiological characteristics of the regulatory disordered infant. *Infant Behavior and Development, 14,* 37–50.

Dixson, A. F., & George, L. (1982). Prolactin and parental behaviour in a male new world primate. *Nature, 299,* 551–553.

Feldman, R. (2003). Infant–mother and infant–father synchrony: The coregulation of positive arousal. *Infant Mental Health Journal, 24*(1), 1–23.

Feldman, R. (2006). From biological rhythms to social rhythms: Physiological precursors of mother–infant synchrony. *Developmental Psychology, 42,* 175–188.

Feldman, R. (2007a). Mother–infant synchrony and the development of moral orientation in childhood and adolescence: Direct and indirect mechanisms of developmental continuity. *American Journal of Orthopsychiatry, 77*(4), 582–597.

Feldman, R. (2007b). On the origins of background emotions: From affect synchrony to symbolic expression. *Emotion, 7*(3), 601.

Feldman, R. (2007c). Parent–infant synchrony and the construction of shared timing: Physiological precursors, developmental outcomes, and risk conditions. *Journal of Child Psychology and Psychiatry, 48,* 329–354.

Feldman, R. (2007d). Parent–infant synchrony biological foundations and developmental outcomes. *Current Directions in Psychological Science, 16*(6), 340–345.

Feldman, R. (2009). The development of regulatory functions from birth to five years; Insights from premature infants. *Child Development, 80,* 544–561.

Feldman, R. (2012a). Bio–behavioral synchrony: A model for integrating biological and microsocial behavioral processes in the study of parenting. *Parenting, 12*(2–3), 154–164.

Feldman, R. (2012b). Oxytocin and social affiliation in humans. *Hormones and Behavior, 61*(3), 380–391.

Feldman, R. (2012c). Parent–infant synchrony: A bio–behavioral model of mutual in?uences in the formation of affiliative bonds. *Monographs of the Society for Research in Child Development, 77,* 42–51.

Feldman, R. (2013). Synchrony and the neurobiological basis of social affiliation. In M. Mikulincer, & P. R. Shaver (Eds.), *Mechanisms of social connection: From brain to group* (pp. 145–166). Washington, DC: American Psychological Association.

Feldman, R., Bamberger, E., & Kanat-Maymon, Y. (2013). Parent-specific reciprocity from infancy to adolescence shapes children's social competence and dialogical skills. *Attachment and Human Development, 15,* 407–423.

Feldman, R., & Eidelman, A. I. (2003a). Direct and indirect effects of breast milk on the neurobehavioral and cognitive development of premature infants. *Developmental Psychobiology, 43,* 109–119.

Feldman, R., & Eidelman, A. I. (2003b). Skin-to-skin contact (kangaroo care) accelerates autonomic and neurobehavioural maturation in preterm infants. *Developmental Medicine and Child Neurology, 45*(4), 274–281.

Feldman, R., & Eidelman, A. I. (2004). Parent–infant synchrony and the social-emotional development of triplets. *Developmental Psychology, 40*(6), 1133.

Feldman, R., & Eidelman, A. I. (2007). Maternal postpartum behavior and the emergence of infant–mother and infant–father synchrony in preterm and full-term infants: The role of neonatal vagal tone. *Developmental Psychobiology, 49*(3), 290–302.

Feldman, R., Eidelman, A. I., & Rotenberg, N. (2004). Parenting stress, infant emotion regulation, maternal sensitivity, and the cognitive development of triplets: A model for parent and child influences in a unique ecology. *Child Development, 75,* 1774–1791.

Feldman, R., Golan, O., Hirschler-Guttenberg, Y., Ostfeld-Etzion, S., & Zagoory-Sharon, O. (2014). Parent–child interaction and oxytocin production in preschoolers with autism spectrum disorder. *British Journal of Psychiary, 205*(2), 107–112.

Feldman, R., Gordon, I., Influs, M., Gutbir, T., & Ebstein, R. (2013). Parental oxytocin and early caregiving jointly shape childen's oxytocin response and social reciprocity. *Neuropsychopharmacology, 38*, 1154–1162.

Feldman, R., Gordon, I., Schneiderman, I., Weisman, O., & Zagoory-Sharon, O. (2010). Natural variations in maternal and paternal care are associated with systemic changes in oxytocin following parent–infant contact. *Psychoneuroendocrinology, 35*, 1133–1141.

Feldman, R., Gordon, I., & Zagoory-Sharon, O. (2010). The cross-generation transmission of oxytocin in humans. *Hormones and Behavior, 58*, 669–676.

Feldman, R., Gordon, I., & Zagoory-Sharon, O. (2011). Maternal and paternal plasma, salivary, and urinary oxytocin and parent–infant synchrony: Considering stress and affiliation components of human bonding. *Developmental Science, 14*(4), 752–761.

Feldman, R., Granat, A., Pariente, C., Kanety, H., Kuint, J., & Gilboa-Schechtman, E. (2009). Maternal depression and anxiety across the postpartum year and infant social engagement, fear regulation, and stress reactivity. *Journal of the American Academy of Child and Adolescence Psychiatry, 48*, 919–927.

Feldman, R., Greenbaum, C. W., & Yirmiya, N. (1999). Mother–infant affect synchrony as an antecedent to the emergence of self-control. *Developmental Psychology, 35*, 223–231.

Feldman, R., Magori-Cohen, R., Galili, G., Singer, M., & Louzoun, Y. (2011). Mother and infant coordinate heart rhythms through episodes of interaction synchrony. *Infant Behavior and Development, 34*, 569–577.

Feldman, R., & Masalha, S. (2007). The role of culture in moderating the links between early ecological risk and young children's adaptation. *Development and Psychopathology, 19*(1), 1–21.

Feldman, R., Masalha, S., & Alony, D. (2006). Microregulatory patterns of family interactions: Cultural pathways to toddlers' self-regulation. *Journal of Family Psychology, 20*(4), 614.

Feldman, R., Masalha, S., & Derdikman-Eiron, R. (2010). Conflict resolution in the parent–child, marital, and peer contexts and children's aggression in the peer group: A process-oriented cultural perspective. *Developmental Psychology, 46*(2), 310.

Feldman, R., Rosenthal, Z., & Eidelman, A. I. (2014). Maternal–preterm skin-to-skin contact enhances child physiologic organization and cognitive control across the first 10 years of life. *Biological Psychiatry, 75*, 56–64.

Feldman, R., Singer, M., & Zagoory, O. (2010). Touch attenuates infants' physiological reactivity to stress. *Developmental Science, 13*, 271–278.

Feldman, R., Vengrober, A., & Ebstein, R. P. (2014). Affiliation buffers stress: Cumulative genetic risk in oxytocin–vasopressin genes combines with early caregiving to predict PTSD in war-exposed young children. *Transcultural Psychiatry, 4*, e370.

Feldman, R., Vengrober, A., Eidelman-Rothman, M., & Zagoory-Sharon, O. (2013).

Stress reactivity in war-exposed young children with and without PTSD: Relations to maternal stress hormones, parenting, and child emotionality and regulation. *Development and Psychopathology, 25*, 942–955.

Feldman, R., Weller, A., Sirota, L., & Eidelman, A. I. (2002). Skin-to-skin contact (kangaroo care) promotes self-regulation in premature infants: Sleep–wake cyclicity, arousal modulation, and sustained exploration. *Developmental Psychology, 38*(2), 194.

Feldman, R., Weller, A., Sirota, L., & Eidelman, A. I. (2003). Testing a family intervention hypothesis: The contribution of mother–infant skin-to-skin contact (kangaroo care) to family interaction, proximity, and touch. *Journal of Family Psychology, 17*, 94–107.

Feldman, R., Weller, A., Zagoory-Sharon, O., & Levine, A. (2007). Evidence for neuroendocrinological foundation of human affiliation: Plasma oxytocin levels across pregnancy and the postpartum period predict mother–infant bonding. *Psychological Science, 18*(11), 965–970.

Feldman, R., Zagoory-Sharon, O., Weisman, O., Schneiderman, I., Gordon, I., Maoz, R., et al. (2012). Sensitive parenting is associated with plasma oxytocin and polymorphisms in the *OXTR* and *CD38* genes. *Biological Psychiatry, 72*, 175–181.

Fleming, A. S., Corter, C., Franks, P., Surbey, M., Schneider, B., & Steiner, M. (1993). Postpartum factors related to mother's attraction to newborn infant odors. *Developmental Psychobiology, 26*, 115–132.

Fleming, A. S., Corter, C., Stallings, J., & Steiner, M. (2002). Testosterone and prolactin are associated with emotional responses to infant cries in new fathers. *Hormones and Behavior, 42*, 399–413.

Fleming, A. S., Steiner, M., & Corter, C. (1997). Cortisol, hedonics, and maternal responsiveness in human mothers. *Hormones and Behavior, 32*, 85–98.

Gimpl, G., & Fahrenholz, F. (2001). The oxytocin receptor system: Structure, function, and regulation. *Physiological Reviews, 81*(2), 629–683.

Gordon, I., Martin, C., Feldman, R., & Leckman, J. F. (2011) Oxytocin and social motivation. *Developmental Cognitive Neuroscience, 1*(4), 471–493.

Gordon, I., Zagoory-Sharon, O., Leckman, J. F., & Feldman, R. (2010a). Oxytocin and the development of parenting in humans. *Biological Psychiatry, 68*, 377–382.

Gordon, I., Zagoory-Sharon, O., Leckman, J. F., & Feldman, R. (2010b). Oxytocin, cortisol, and triadic family interactions. *Physiology and Behavior, 101*, 679–684.

Gordon, I., Zagoory-Sharon, O., Leckman, J. F., & Feldman, R. (2010c). Prolactin, oxytocin, and the development of paternal behavior across the first six months of fatherhood. *Hormones and Behavior, 58*(3), 513–518.

Gordon, I., Zagoory-Sharon, O., Schneiderman, I., Leckman, J. F., Weller, A., & Feldman, R. (2008). Oxytocin and cortisol in romantically unattached young adults: Associations with bonding and psychological distress. *Psychophysiology, 45*, 349–352.

Grattan, D. R. (2001). The actions of prolactin in the brain during pregnancy and lactation. *Progress in Brain Research, 133*, 153–171.

Grattan, D. R., & Kokay, I. C. (2008). Prolactin: A pleiotropic neuroendocrine hormone. *Journal of Neuroendocrinology, 20*, 752–763.

Greenwood, A. K., Wark, A. R., Yoshida, K., & Peichel, C. L. (2013). Genetic and neural modularity underlie the evolution of schooling behavior in threespine sticklebacks. *Current Biology, 23*(19), 1884–1888.

Harel, H., Gordon, I., Geva, R., & Feldman, R. (2011). Gaze behaviors of preterm and full-term infants in nonsocial and social contexts of increasing dynamics: Visual recognition, attention regulation, and gaze synchrony. *Infancy, 16*(1), 69–90.

Hasson, U., Ghazanfar, A. A., Galantucci, B., Garrod, S., & Keysers, C. (2012). Brain-to-brain coupling: A mechanism for creating and sharing a social world. *Trends in Cognitive Sciences, 16,* 114–121.

Hasson, U., Yuval, N., Levy, I., Fuhrmann, G., & Malach, R. (2004). Intersubject synchronization of cortical activity during natural vision. *Science, 303*(5664), 1634–1640.

Heinrichs, M., & Domes, G. (2008). Neuropeptides and social behaviour: Effects of oxytocin and vasopressin in humans. *Progress in Brain Research, 170,* 337–350.

Heinrichs, M., & Gaab, J. (2007). Neuroendocrine mechanisms of stress and social interaction: Implications for mental disorders. *Current Opinion in Psychiatry, 20*(2), 158–162.

Herculano-Houzel, S. (2009). The human brain in numbers: A linearly scaled-up primate brain. *Frontiers in Human Neuroscience, 3,* 1–11.

Herculano-Houzel, S. (2012). The remarkable, yet not extraordinary, human brain as a scaled-up primate brain and its associated cost. *Proceedings of the National Academy of Sciences, 109,* 1066–10668.

Ho, M. L., & Lee, J. N. (1992). Ovarian and circulating levels of oxytocin and arginine vasopressin during the estrous cycle in the rat. *Acta Endocrinologica, 26*(6), 530–534

Hofer, M. A. (1995). Hidden regulators. In S. Goldberg, R. Muir, & J. Kerr (Eds.), *Attachment theory: Social, developmental and clinical perspectives* (pp. 203–230). Hillsdale, NJ: Analytic Press.

Hoge, E. A., Pollack, M. H., Kaufman, R. E., Zak, P. J., & Simon, N. M. (2008). Oxytocin levels in social anxiety disorder. *CNS Neuroscience and Therapuetics, 14*(3), 165–170.

Huffman, L. C., Bryan, Y. E., Carmen, R., Pedersen, F. A., Doussard-Roosevelt, J. A., & Forges, S. W. (1998). Infant temperament and cardiac vagal tone: Assessments at twelve weeks of age. *Child Development, 69*(3), 624–635.

Kindler, P. M., Bahr, J. M., Gross, M. R., & Philipp, D. P. (1991). Hormonal-regulation of parental care behavior in nesting male bluegills: Do the effects of bromocriptine suggest a role for prolactin? *Physiological Zoology, 64,* 310–322.

Krpan, K. M., Coombs, R., Zinga, D., Steiner, M., & Fleming, A. S. (2005). Experiential and hormonal correlates of maternal behavior in teen and adult mothers. *Hormones and Behavior, 47,* 112–122.

Lennartsson, A. K., Kushnir, M. M., Bergquist, J., & Jonsdottir, I. H. (2012). DHEA and DHEA-S response to acute psychosocial stress in healthy men and women. *Biological Psychology, 90*(2), 143–149.

Levine, A., Zagoory-Sharon, O., Feldman, R., & Weller, A. (2007). Oxytocin during preganancy and early postpartum: Individual patterns and maternal-fetal attachment. *Peptides, 28,* 1162–1169.

Lorenz, K. (1950). The comparative method in studying innate behavior patterns. *Symposia of the Society for Experimental Biology, 4*, 221–268.

Ludwig, M., & Leng, G. (2006). Dendritic peipitide release and peptide-dependent behaviors. *Nature Reviews Neuroscience, 7*, 126–136.

Maestripieri, D. (2001). Biological bases of maternal attachment. *Current Directions in Psychological Science, 10*, 79–83.

Maninger, N., Wolkowitz, O. M., Reus, V. I., Epel, E. S., & Mellon, S. H. (2009). Neurobiological and neuropsychiatric effects of dehydroepiandrosterone (DHEA) and DHEA sulfate (DHEAS). *Frontiers in Neuroendocrinology, 30*(1), 65–91.

Mann, P. E., & Bridges, R. S. (2001). Lactogenic hormone regulation of maternal behavior. *Progress in Brain Research, 133*, 251–262.

Marazziti, D., Dell'Osso, B., Baroni, S., Mungai, F., Catena, M., Rucci, P., et al. (2006). A relationship between oxytocin and anxiety of romantic attachment. *Clinical Practice and Epidemology in Mental Health, 2*, 28.

Maruska, K. P., & Fernald, R. D. (2011). Social regulation of gene expression in the hypothalamic–pituitary–gonadal axis. *Physiology, 26*(6), 412–423.

Meaney, M. J. (2001). Maternal care, gene expression, and the transmission of individual differences in stress reactivity across generations. *Annual Review of Neuroscience, 24*, 1161–1192.

Mehta, P. H., & Beer, J. (2010). Neural mechanisms of the testosterone–aggression relation: The role of orbitofrontal cortex. *Journal of Cognitive Neuroscience, 22*(10), 2357–2368.

Meinlschmidt, G., & Heim, C. (2007). Sensitivity to intranasal oxytocin in adult men with early parental separation. *Biological Psychiatry, 61*(9), 1109–1111.

Mills-Koonce, W. R., Gariépy, J. L., Propper, C., Sutton, K., Calkins, S., Moore, G., et al. (2007). Infant and parent factors associated with early maternal sensitivity: A caregiver-attachment systems approach. *Infant Behavior and Development, 30*(1), 114–126.

Moore, G. A., & Calkins, S. D. (2004). Infants' vagal regulation in the still-face paradigm is related to dyadic coordination of mother–infant interaction. *Developmental Psychology, 40*(6), 1068–1080.

Morgan, C. A., III, Southwick, S., Hazlett, G., Rasmusson, A., Hoyt, G., Zimolo, Z., et al. (2004(. Relationships among plasma dehydroepiandrosterone sulfate and cortisol levels, symptoms of dissociation, and objective performance in humans exposed to acute stress. *Archives of General Psychiatry, 61*(8), 819–825.

Nater, U. M., & Rohleder, N. (2009). Salivary alpha-amylase as a non-invasive biomarker for the sympathetic nervous system: Current state of research. *Psychoneuroendocrinology, 34*, 486–496.

Neumann, I. D., Maloumby, R., Beiderbeck, D. I., Lukas, M., & Landgraf, R. (2013). Increased brain and plasma oxytocin after nasal and peripheral administration in rats and mice. *Psychoneuroendocrinology, 38*(10), 1985–1993.

Perry, N. B., Mackler, J. S., Calkins, S. D., & Keane, S. P. (2014). A transactional analysis of the relation between maternal sensitivity and child vagal regulation. *Developmental Psychology, 50*(3), 784

Porges, S. W. (1991). Vagal tone: An autonomic mediator of affect. In J. Garber & K. A. Dodge (Eds.), *The development of emotion regulation and dysregulation:*

Cambridge studies in social and emotional development (pp. 111–128). New York: Cambridge University Press.

Porges, S. W. (1996). Physiological regulation in high-risk infants: A model for assessment and potential intervention. *Development and Psychopathology, 8,* 29–42.

Pow, D. V., & Morris, J. F. (1989). Dendrites of hypothalamic magnocellular neurons release neurohypophysial peptides by exocytosis. *Neuroscience, 32,* 435–439.

Quinones-Jenab, V., Jenab, S., Ogawa, S., Adan, R. A., Burbach, J. P., & Pfaff, D. W. (1997). Effects of estrogen on oxytocin receptor messenger ribonucleic acid expression in the uterus, pituitary, and forebrain of the female rat. *Neuroendocrinology, 65*(1), 9–17.

Ross, H. E., & Young, L. J. (2009). Oxytocin and the neural mechanisms regulating social cognition and affiliative behavior. *Frontiers in Neuroendocrinology, 30*(4), 534–547.

Sameroff, A. J., & Fiese, B. H. (2000). Transactional regulation: The developmental ecology of early intervention. In J. P. Shonkoff & S. J. Meisels (Eds.), *Handbook of early childhood intervention* (2nd ed., pp. 135–159). Cambridge, UK: Cambridge University Press.

Sarkar, D. K., Frautschy, S. A., & Mitsugi, N. (1992). Pituitary portal plasma levels of oxytocin during the estrous cycle, lactation, and hyperprolactinemia. *Annals of the New York Academy of Sciences, 652,* 397–410.

Schneiderman, I., Kanat-Maymon, Y., Ebstein, R. P., & Feldman, R. (2014). Cumulative risk on the oxytocin receptor gene (*OXTR*) underpins empathic communication difficulties at the first stages of romantic love. *Social Cognitive and Affective Neuroscience, 9*(10), 1524–1529.

Schneiderman, I., Kanat-Maymon, Y., Zagoory-Sharon, O., & Feldman, R. (2014). Mutual influences between partners' hormones shape conflict dialog and relationship duration at the initiation of romantic love. *Social Neuroscience, 9*(4), 337–351.

Schneiderman, I., Zagoory-Sharon, O., Leckman, J. F., & Feldman, R. (2012). Oxytocin during the initial stages of romantic attachment: Relations to couples' interactive reciprocity. *Psychoneuroendocrinology, 37,* 1277–1285.

Schneiderman, I., Zilberstein-Kra, Y., Leckman, J. F., & Feldman, R. (2011). Love alters autonomic reactivity to emotions. *Emotion, 11*(6), 13–14.

Schradin, C., & Anzenberger, G. (1999). Prolactin, the hormone of paternity. *News in Physiological Sciences, 14,* 223–231.

Shaw, E. (1978). Schooling fishes: The school, a truly egalitarian form of organization in which all members of the group are alike in influence, offers substantial benefits to its participants. *American Scientist, 66*(2), 166–175.

Stallings, J., Fleming, A. S., Corter, C., Worthman, C., & Steiner, M. (2001). The effects of infant cries and odors on sympathy, cortisol, and autonomic responses in new mothers and nonpostpartum women. *Parenting, 1,* 71–100.

Stifter, C. A., & Corey, J. M. (2001). Vagal regulation and observed social behavior in infancy. *Social Development, 10*(2), 189–201.

Storey, A. E., Walsh, C. J., Quinton, R. L., & Wynne-Edwards, K. E. (2000). Hormonal correlates of paternal responsiveness in new and expectant fathers. *Evolution and Human Behavior, 21,* 79–95.

Swidbert, O. R., & Rogers, S. M. (2010). Gregarious desert locusts have substantially larger brains with altered proportions compared with the solitarious phase. *Proceedings of the Royal Society of London B, 277*(1697), 3087–3096.

Taylor, S. E., Gonzaga, G. C., Klein, L. C., Hu, P., Greendale, G. A., & Seeman, T. E. (2006). Relation of oxytocin to psychological stress responses and hypothalamic–pituitary–adrenocortical axis activity in older women. *Psychosomatic Medicine, 68*(2), 238–245.

Tinbergen, N. (1963). On aims and methods in ethology. *Zeitschrift fur Tierpsychologie, 20,* 410–433.

Tops, M., van Peer, J. M., Korf, J., Wijers, A. A., & Tucker, D. M. (2007). Anxiety, cortisol, and attachment predict plasma oxytocin. *Psychophysiology, 44*(3), 444–449.

Tronick, E. (2007). *The neurobehavioral and social-emotional development of infants and children.* New York: Norton.

Tronick, E., Als, H., Adamson, L., Wise, S., & Brazelton T. B. (1978). The infant's response to entrapment between contradictory messages in face-to-face interaction. *Journal of the American Academy of Child and Adolescent Psychiatry, 17,* 1–13.

Viau, V. (2002). Functional cross-talk between the hypothalamic–pituitary–gonadal and adrenal axes. *Journal of Neuroendocrinology, 14*(6), 506–513.

Weisman, O., Delaherche, E., Rondeau, M., Chetouani, M., Cohen, D., & Feldman, R. (2013). Oxytocin shapes parental motion during father–infant interaction. *Biology Letters, 9*(6), 20130828.

Weisman, O., Schneiderman, I., Zagoory-Sharon, O., & Feldman, R. (2012). Salivary vasopressin increases following intranasal oxytocin administration. *Peptides, 40,* 99–103.

Weisman, O., Zagoory-Sharon, O., & Feldman, R. (2012). Oxytocin administration to parent enhances physiological and behavioral readiness for social engagement. *Biological Psychiatry, 72,* 982–989.

Weisman, O., Zagoory-Sharon, O., & Feldman, R. (2013). Oxytocin administration alters HPA reactivity in the context of parent–infant interaction. *European Neuropsychopharmacology, 23*(12), 1724–1731.

Weisman, O., Zagoory-Sharon, O., & Feldman, R. (2014). Oxytocin administration, salivary testosterone, and father–infant social behavior. *Progress in Neuropsychopharmacology and Biological Psychiatry, 49,* 47–52.

Weisman, O., Zagoory-Sharon, O., Schneiderman, I., Gordon, I., & Feldman, R. (2013). Plasma oxytocin distributions in a large cohort of women and men and their gender-specific associations with anxiety. *Psychoneuroendocrinology, 38,* 694–701.

Wheeler, W. M. (1928). *The social insects.* New York: Harcourt.

Ziegler, T. E., Wegner, F. H., & Snowdon, C. T. (1996). Hormonal responses to parental and nonparental conditions in male cotton-top tamarins, *Saguinus oedipus,* a new world primate. *Hormones and Behavior, 30,* 287–297.

PART IV

ADVERSITY AND RISK

IMPLICATIONS FOR INFANT DEVELOPMENT

CHAPTER 14

Introduction to Part IV

Current Directions in the Study of Risk and Adversity in Infancy

Charles H. Zeanah and Kathryn L. Humphreys

Current research in infant development and psychopathology has begun to focus more intently on understanding the impact of early experiences, particularly exposure to stressful experiences and subsequent responses to those events. Biopsychosocial approaches, as illustrated throughout this volume, are attempting to delineate the complex interactions among social contexts, psychological processes, and biological reactions that mediate the effect of experience on outcomes. There is clear evidence that brain structure and functioning are significantly affected by infants' experiences—both positive and negative. In addition, there is considerable interest in cellular and molecular processes activated by exposure to adverse experiences, and how these processes may relate to pathological outcomes.

These new frameworks, building on established approaches, are to some degree changing the questions being asked about risk and adversity in infancy. In recent years, there has been a shift from identifying risk factors to exploring risk mechanisms or processes more specifically. This has always been a goal of risk research, of course, but because of advances in the science of brain development and functioning, gene regulation, and cellular and molecular processes, significant advances in studying the impact of adversity have been possible.

In this chapter, we selectively illustrate rather than comprehensively review relevant studies for purposes of highlighting current trends, as a full review of all relevant studies is beyond the scope in this brief overview. We begin with a brief primer on the behavioral manifestations of disorder and risk for disorder in early life. Next, we consider risk factors from three models of the association between stress and developmental outcomes: (1) the widely accepted cumulative risk approach, (2) the diathesis–stress model, and (3) the differential susceptibility model. These topics shift the focus from solely on environmental risk factors to the complex interactions between environmental risk and developmental and individual differences. Next, recent characterizations of the environmental risk factors for infant and child development are considered, including toxic stress and exploring the specific types of deviations from the expectable environment that can occur in this crucial developmental period. These approaches are concerned with targeting how the environment exerts effects on the developing infant, and some also explicitly consider how individual infant factors may increase susceptibility to both positive and negative environments. We then discuss relevant developmental processes that may mediate and moderate the effects of adversity on outcomes, including sensitive periods in brain development, developmental programming, allostatic load, and epigenetic processes. Next, we highlight the protective qualities of parent–infant relationships for infants in adverse environmental contexts. We conclude by identifying the potential future areas for research in order to continue to move the field forward.

Disorder and Risk for Disorder in Early Life

Zero to Three, an advocacy organization focused on promoting well-being in infants and toddlers, created a task force to develop the *Diagnostic Classification of Mental Health and Developmental Disorders of Infancy and Early Childhood* (DC: 0–3; Zero to Three, 1994) in order to establish a diagnostic system specific to the developmental level of young children. Other nosological approaches (e.g., *Diagnostic and Statistical Manual of Mental Disorders* [DSM-5]; American Psychiatric Association, 2013) have thus far been unable to adequately include diagnostic criteria relevant for very young children. The second edition of DC: 0–3R (Zero to Three, 2005) is currently in use, which includes a multiaxial approach, with clinical disorders on Axis I, relationship disorders on Axis II, medical and developmental disorders on Axis III, psychosocial stressors on Axis IV, and emotional and social functioning on Axis V. There is debate about whether we can accurately diagnose infants with "within-the-person psychiatric disorders" (Lyons-Ruth, Zeanah, Benoit, Madigan, & Mills-Koonce, 2014).

Infants and young children are completely dependent on caregivers for survival. Thus, when considering the behaviors of young children, it is important to understand the role of the caregiver in shaping, sustaining, or amplifying maladaptive behaviors. A common observation in young children is that problematic behaviors or symptoms may be evident in one relationship but not in others, suggesting that disorders may exist between the young child and his or her caregiver rather than within the young child. Sroufe (1989) emphasized that although poignantly expressed as child behavior problems, most psychopathology in the first 3 years of life is best conceptualized as relationship disturbances.

Nevertheless, some disorders that present in early childhood have little to no relational contributors (e.g., autism spectrum disorders), whereas others have a required relational component to their etiology (e.g., disinhibited social engagement disorder [DSED]). In between are the majority of disorders in which child contributors interact with parent contributors to lead to disturbed child behavior, such as sleep disruptions, aggression, or emotional dysregulation.

Psychiatric disorders in preschool children are conceptualized similarly to those in older children (see Egger & Angold, 2006), whereas for children younger than 2 years, other disorders predominate, including sensory processing or regulatory disorders, feeding–eating disorders, sleep–wake disorders, posttraumatic stress disorder, attachment disorders (i.e., reactive attachment disorder and DSED), and relationship disorders. Still, disorders defined in current diagnostic systems for infants and toddlers are mostly not well validated, and there remains considerable debate about how best to conceptualize the relational components of most behaviors observed in this age range (Sameroff & Emde, 1989).

Exploring Risk Factors

Cumulative Risk

One of the most consistent findings in research in developmental psychopathology is that risk factors and outcomes are often neither specifically nor directly linked. Multifinality describes when a single risk factor increases the probability of a variety of adverse outcomes. For example, maternal depression increases risk in infants for insecure attachment (Shaw & Vondra, 1993), language and cognitive problems (Murray, 1992), and social interactive problems (Tronick & Reck, 2009). Equifinality describes when many different risk conditions increase the risk for a single outcome. For example, parental conflict (Shaw, Vondra, Hommerding, Keenan, & Dunn, 1994), insecure attachment (Fearon, Bakermans-Kranenburg, Van IJzendoorn, Lapsey, & Roisman, 2010), maternal depression (Goodman et al., 2011), and difficult infant temperament (Miner & Clarke-Stewart, 2008) have all been shown to increase the risk of externalizing behavior problems.

One illustration of lack of specificity in risk to outcome relations is the cumulative risk model, in which the number of risk factors is more predictive of poor outcomes than any particular risk factor. An influential recent example of this model is the Adverse Childhood Experiences Study (Felitti et al., 1998). In this study, more than 17,000 middle-class adults were asked to complete questionnaires about 10 types of stressful or traumatic experiences in their childhood: psychological abuse, physical abuse, sexual abuse, emotional neglect, physical neglect, divorce/loss of parent, substance use in the home, depression or mental illness in the home, mother treated violently, or someone in the home was imprisoned. By summing the number of different types of adverse experiences, investigators assigned a score from 0 to 10 to all participants, and found a linear relationship between the number of adverse experiences and a variety of health outcomes, including psychiatric disorders (e.g., depression), biomedical conditions (e.g., heart disease, chronic obstructive pulmonary disease, liver disease), and high-risk behaviors (e.g., smoking, sexual promiscuity, suicide attempts). Lack of specificity was the rule rather than the exception. For example, 9 of the 10 types of adverse childhood experiences were linked to risk for heart disease as an adult (Felitti & Anda, 2014).

Many studies have also shown the cumulative risk model to be useful in linking early experiences to child development outcomes. Cumulative risks predicted externalizing and internalizing behavior problems in 4-year-olds (Trentacosta, Hyde, Goodlett, & Shaw, 2013). In another study, Appleyard and colleagues examined child maltreatment, intimate partner violence, family disruption, low socioeconomic status, and high parental stress in early and middle childhood on child behavior outcomes in adolescence among 171 children (Appleyard, Egeland, van Dulmen, & Sroufe, 2005). Increasing numbers of these risks in early childhood linearly predicted increases in behavior problems in adolescence. Underscoring the importance of early experiences, multiple risks during infancy and early childhood better explained variance in adolescent behavior than risks in middle childhood. Though the focus is typically on exposure to negative events, Evans and colleagues also highlighted the importance of cumulative resources, noting that as assets accumulate, the probability of positive outcomes increases (Evans, Li, & Whipple, 2013). Consideration of both positive and negative exposures is a promising area for further exploration.

Diathesis–Stress

The diathesis–stress model provides an explanation of how risks and outcomes might be linked. The basic premise is that the presence of a stressor results in negative outcomes only among individuals with a vulnerability to the stressor. The vulnerability, which might be a genetic polymorphism, a pattern of stress reactivity, or even a temperamental disposition, is considered to render an individual more susceptible to the stressful experience than those without the vulnerability. This model helps to explain why only some individuals develop disorders following similar stressors and also why all individuals who share a specific vulnerability do not succumb to an adverse outcome.

This model has led to a variety of gene × environment interaction studies. For example, Hill and colleagues (2013) found that the presence of the low-activity, but not the high-activity, variant of the monoamine oxidase A (*MAOA*) functional promoter polymorphism (*MAOA-LPR*) involved in the regulation of neurotransmitters including serotonin and dopamine, interacted with stressful life events during pregnancy to lead to higher infant negative emotionality at 5 weeks of age. Both the diathesis (infant genotype of the low-activity *MAOA-LPR*) and the stress (stressful events during pregnancy) appeared to be necessary to predict negative emotionality in infants.

Differential Susceptibility

From an evolutionary perspective, however, it is unclear why genetic polymorphisms that create *only* vulnerability would be preserved. Belsky and Pluess (2009) have proposed a differential susceptibility model as an alternative to the diathesis–stress model. This hypothesis predicts that rather than some individuals being vulnerable only to negative outcomes, these individuals may simply be more sensitive to environmental context "for better and for worse," such that susceptible individuals will show more positive outcomes when they grow up in favorable environments in addition to more negative outcomes in adverse environments (i.e., "orchid children"). Conversely, some individuals may be relatively unaffected by the range of potential rearing environments (i.e., "dandelion children").

For example, Bakermans-Kranenburg and van IJzendoorn (2006) demonstrated the moderating effect of a variant within the dopamine receptor *D4* gene, which is involved in the regulation of dopamine and has been linked to a number of psychiatric disorders, on the association between maternal sensitivity and externalizing behavior problems in young children. Children with the 7-repeat allele and insensitive mothers had the highest levels of externalizing behaviors, whereas children with the same allele but with sensitive mothers had the least externalizing behaviors, suggesting that the 7-repeat allele may confer increased sensitivity to one's environment. Intermediate levels of externalizing behaviors were found for those who lacked the allele, regardless of how sensitive or insensitive their mothers were.

Another example of differential susceptibility comes from the Bucharest Early Intervention Project (BEIP; Nelson, Fox, & Zeanah, 2014). It is well known that young children reared in institutions are at increased risk for indiscriminate social behavior, though not all children who experience institutional rearing develop indiscriminate behavior. The BEIP prospectively followed infants between 6 and 30 months of age who had been abandoned at or soon after birth and placed in large impersonal institutions. These infants were comprehensively assessed and then randomized to foster care (which had not existed previously) or to care as usual (i.e., institutional care). This randomized controlled trial of foster care as an alternative to institutional care provided an opportunity to examine the differential susceptibility hypothesis. Children with the *short/short* (*s/s*) genotype in the serotonin-transporter-linked polymorphic region (*5HTTLPR*) that codes for the serotonin transporter, and *met* carriers (as opposed to *val/val* individuals) in the brain-derived neurotrophic factor (*BDNF*) gene, a well-studied gene involved in learning and development, demonstrated the lowest levels of indiscriminate behavior in foster care and the highest levels in the care-as-usual condition. Children without these genotypes demonstrated little difference in levels of indiscriminate behaviors over time (Drury, Gleason, et al., 2012). In a separate study of this sample, the *5HTTLPR* genotype was also found to moderate the association between institutional care and external-izing symptomatology. Again, the *s/s* individuals were most susceptible to the negative environment (i.e., continued institutionalization) and most receptive to a positive environmental change (i.e., high-quality foster care), whereas the *long* (*l*) carriers were intermediate in terms of externalizing signs with no differences based on treatment group (Brett et al., 2015).

Davies and Cicchetti (2014) examined the potential mechanism behind their finding of differential susceptibility in a study that also examined the *5HTTLPR* gene in relation to early care and externalizing. Specifically, they studied the association between maternal unresponsiveness and child external-izing behaviors in disadvantaged 2-year-old children. Maternal unresponsive-ness significantly predicted increases in externalizing behaviors 2 years later, but only for children possessing the *l/l* genotype. Responsive mothers of chil-dren with the *l/l* genotype had the lowest scores for externalizing behaviors. A mediated moderation analysis found that young children's angry reactivity to maternal negativity partly accounted for the greater susceptibility of *l/l* carriers to variations in maternal unresponsiveness.

Exploring Adverse Environments

Toxic Stress

Links between adverse early experiences and later maladaptive outcomes have increasingly focused on brain and biological systems that may mediate negative outcomes resulting from exposure to severe stress and trauma (Humphreys & Zeanah, 2015). In fact, the experience of stress resulting from adverse events, especially early in development, has provided an organizing framework for understanding psychopathology in childhood, even in infants and young chil-dren. For example, the concept of "toxic stress," the cumulative and pernicious effect of multiple, chronic environmental adversities, has been used to pro-vide a framework for understanding the long-term physical and mental health consequences of stress on developing brain circuitry and other organ systems (Shonkoff & Garner, 2012). Inherent in this construct is the notion that an individual's immediate responses to stress are designed to be adaptive, but if chronically activated, stress response systems may be maladaptive.

For example, diurnal cortisol, an important product of the body's stress response, has been shown to be disrupted in children who have experienced maltreatment (Bernard, Butzin-Dozier, Rittenhouse, & Dozier, 2010; Dozier et al., 2006; Fisher, Stoolmiller, Gunnar, & Burraston, 2007). Persistent exposure to adverse environments is associated with flattened diurnal variation, with morning values lower and afternoon and evening values higher in children who have not experienced adversity.

Though a useful model for highlighting differences between typical and atypical stress, toxic stress as a construct has not been defined carefully, and its predictions about maladaptive outcomes are broad, universal, and post hoc. Furthermore, it is not obvious why similar patterns of stress dysregulation, for example, would derive both from deprivation, as occurs in children raised in institutions, and from chronic trauma, as occurs in children exposed to repeated intimate partner violence.

Deviations from the Expectable Environment

Although adverse experiences, including stress and trauma, seem to overwhelm children's abilities to function effectively, what has not been done consistently in research is to distinguish between the effects of two different types of input: inadequate input (e.g., neglect/deprivation) and harmful input (e.g., abuse/trauma), on brain and biological development. Importantly, each type of deviation from the "expectable environment" for an infant has been associated with a broad array of maladaptive outcomes, including various domains of psychopathology (National Research Council, 2013). Approaches to outlining the specific etiology for negative outcomes, as well as creating or selecting prevention and intervention programs may be informed by considering the unique consequences of inadequate and harmful input in early childhood (Humphreys & Zeanah, 2015).

Brain plasticity is greatest in the earliest years, but the impact of early experience on brain development "cuts both ways," given that the quality of the environmental input has a direct impact on the result of such plasticity. Deviations from the expectable caregiving environment have potentially harmful effects on a range of important skills, including the development of cognitive, affective, and social abilities that take shape in the earliest years of life. Consistent and nurturing caregivers play a crucial part in helping children develop emotion regulation abilities (Field, 1994), and the lack of appropriate caregiving due to abuse or neglect is linked to poor emotion regulation skills (Kim & Cicchetti, 2010). Though both harmful input and inadequate input in infancy are associated with negative outcomes, the differing impact of these deviations may be seen in specific neurobiological and behavioral sequelae.

For example, excessive and prolonged activation of fear circuitry during exposure to a trauma would be expected to increase the individual's risk for posttraumatic stress disorder symptomatology. Children who have experienced abuse demonstrate a lower threshold for detecting angry faces than children who were not abused (Pollak & Sinha, 2002), indicating an attentional bias toward threatening stimuli. Children who have been physically abused also have greater difficulty disengaging from angry faces (Pollak & Tolley-Schell, 2003). The specifc focus on anger, presumably because of its salience in abuse, illustrates hypervigilance, a key symptom of posttraumatic stress disorder, and extends to enhanced ability to identify angry facial expressions (Pollak, Klorman, Thatcher, & Cicchetti, 2001).

Lack of input may also have long-term deleterious effects. For example, several studies indicate a four- to fivefold increase in risk for inattention and hyperactivity/impulsivity in children raised in conditions of deprivation compared with children unexposed to deprivation. Although attention-deficit/hyperactivity disorder (ADHD) is typically conceptualized as primarily genetic in origin, infants who have been neglected and placed in foster care (dosReis, Zito, Safer, & Soeken, 2001), and those raised in institutions (Kreppner, O'Connor, & Rutter, 2001; Roy, Rutter, & Pickles, 2004; Zeanah et al., 2009), are at increased risk for inattention and hyperactvity/impuslivity. A recent study of school-age children with histories of institutional rearing in infancy found that teacher ratings of signs of ADHD demonstrated patterns of thinning in the cerebral cortex comparable to those with ADHD and no institutional rearing (McLaughlin et al., 2013), suggesting that inadequate input in early infancy may be another pathway into the phenotype we define as ADHD.

Deviations from the expectable environment, both in the form of harmful input and lack of necessary input, are clearly associated with increased risks for subsequent psychopathology. Contemporary research is beginning to explore brain structure and function associated with various psychopathological profiles, but a gap remains between identifying descriptive accounts of aberrant behaviors and types of symptoms. Specific lines of inquiry are needed in order to understand the mechanisms by which experiences in differing environmental conditions lead to different patterns of function.

Exploring Developmental Processes in the Context of Adversity

Timing and Sensitive Periods

Human brain development is currently understood to involve three different processes (see Nelson et al., 2014, for more details). The basic architecture or blueprint for brain structure is provided by genetics. Many of the aspects of brain development are open to influences by individual experiences, however, allowing for adaptation to vastly different and often unpredictable environmental experiences. Two types of experience—experience-dependent and experience-expectant development—have been described as sculpting details of brain development beyond the basic blueprint (Greenough, Black, & Wallace, 1987).

Experience-dependent development involves acquisition of information and learning from distinct individual experiences, and necessarily, is ongoing throughout the lifespan. Most likely, this involves active creation of new synaptic connections and development of new circuitry. Learning new skills and developing perspectives are examples of experience-dependent development.

Experience-expectant development is a form of neural development that encompasses experiences anticipated to be present for virtually all members of a species. Input of an experience-expectant kind is also anticipated to occur at certain times in development, when the brain "anticipates" the input and is able to make use of the information. An example to illustrate the differences between experience-dependent and experience-expectant development is the acquisition of verbal language by human infants. The predisposition to develop verbal language is experience-expectant, but the specific language an infant acquires is experience-dependent. At 6 months of age infants can readily discriminate among the sounds of languages from around the world, however, by 12 months of age this ability diminishes as infants begin to lose the ability to distinguish between some sounds not present in their native language. Increased efficiency in native language processing required for further specialization comes at the cost of the reduced ability to process other languages. Infants who experience minimal or no language exposure, on the other hand, are at risk for long-term problems because the input did not occur at the expected time in development (Fox, Zeanah, & Nelson, 2014).

Given that human infants are an altricial species, having a caregiver is an experience-expectant stimulus (Tottenham, 2014). Infants are predisposed to form attachments to caregiving adults, even to parents who mistreat them (Cicchetti, Rogosch, & Toth, 2006). The formation of an experience-expectant attachment to a caregiver requires only minimal input during the sensitive period. On the other hand, variability in an infant's experiences with a caregiver seem to be importantly related to the qualitative type of attachment that develops—secure, avoidant, resistant, or disorganized (NICHD Early Care Research Network, 2006). The type of attachment formed by an infant–caregiver dyad is therefore likely to constitute an experience-dependent process.

Closely related to the notion of experience-expectant development is the concept of sensitive periods. For development to proceed normally, certain kinds of experience or input must occur at certain times, specifically when brain circuitry is maximally able to make use of the input (Nelson et al., 2014). The period during which the brain is most likely to respond to incoming information is called a sensitive period. Input during the prior period before a sensitive period opens or after it closes will have little effect on brain development. Although we are often most concerned about sensitive periods in behavioral development, sensitive periods are actually properties of neural circuits (Knudsen, 2004). Complex behavioral constructs such as IQ, emotion regulation, and attachment involve many different levels of neural circuits, each of which may have different sensitive periods. This cascading time line protects the individual against a single moment in time being essential.

At the level of infant behavior, sensitive periods have been studied with regard to timing of interventions designed to ameliorate infants who are experiencing adversity. Two longitudinal studies of infants raised in impersonal, depriving institutions illustrate these approaches. In the English and Romanian Adoptees Study (ERAS; Rutter, Sonuga-Barke, & Castle, 2010), children were adopted into middle-class English families following abandonment by their birth parents and placement in depriving institutions in Romania. They were followed from infancy through adolescence and investigators tracked persistence of four deprivation-specific maladaptive patterns of behavior at age 15 years: cognitive impairment, inattention/overactivity, disinhibited attachment, and quasi-autism. Children adopted prior to 6 months were extremely unlikely to show persistence of these patterns—less than 5% of children adopted prior to 6 months showed persistence of any of these four deprivation-specific patterns (Rutter, Sonuga-Barke, Beckett, et al., 2010).

As discussed above, another study of Romanian abandoned children who were placed in institutions is the BEIP (Zeanah et al., 2003). This is the first ever, randomized controlled trial of foster care as an alternative to institutional care. In this study, sensitive periods were demonstrated at various ages. Infants placed in foster care prior to 12 months were protected from developing motor stereotypies (Bos, Zeanah, Smyke, Fox, & Nelson, 2010), before 15 months were protected from language delays (Windsor et al., 2011), and those placed before 24 months were more likely to form secure attachments (Smyke, Zeanah, Fox, Nelson, & Guthrie, 2010), and have higher IQs (Nelson et al., 2007). At age 8 years, BEIP investigators demonstrated that teacher-rated social skills and electroencephalography (EEG) alpha power (brain activity associated with attention and thought to reflect higher cortical functioning) were significantly greater in children placed in foster care before 24 months of age (Almas et al., 2012; Vanderwert, Marshall, Nelson, Zeanah, & Fox, 2010).

These studies suggest a disparate range of ages that seem to reflect behavioral sensitive periods across different domains of development. On the other hand, if we were to apply these findings to the question of timing of interventions, a more circumspect conclusion is necessary. That is, the weight of evidence from a broad range of relevant studies indicates that the earlier a child experiencing environmental adversity is removed and placed in an enhanced environment, the more likely the child will recover and the fuller the recovery is likely to be (Fox et al., 2014; Zeanah, Gunnar, McCall, Kreppner, & Fox, 2011). Certainly, there may be important treatment gains provided by later interventions, but the probability of full recovery appears to lessen as brain plasticity diminishes.

Developmental Programming

The fetal environment exerts a significant influence on physiological functioning and subsequent risk for disease, including diseases that emerge in adulthood (Davis & Thompson, 2014). *Developmental programming, fetal programming,* and *biological programming* are all terms referring to the calibration early in life of various bodily systems and processes to environmental conditions, especially extreme conditions. Stressors during pregnancy, such as poor nutrition, more than one fetus, or excessive steroid exposure, may impact appropriate adaptation. When there is a mismatch between the environment expected by the fetus due to stressors in pregnancy and the later environment, problems may ensue because earlier programming may limit the infant's ability to adapt. The original study in this area demonstrated links between low birth weight infants and risk for heart disease in adulthood. Reviewing records kept by nurse home visitors in the United Kingdom in the early 20th century of birth and infancy weights, Barker (2003) compared these records with death records of the same individuals who had been seen by the nurses in infancy. Individuals who had been born with low birth weight were significantly more likely to develop coronary disease as adults.

Evidence from numerous animal studies and increasing evidence from studies of humans suggest that impaired fetal growth followed by rapid catch-up in infancy is a strong predictor of many diseases in adults, including obesity, hypertension, non-insulin-dependent diabetes, and heart disease (Davis & Thompson, 2014). Relative undernutrition "programs" physiological and metabolic systems, and when followed by overnutrition leads to disease (Barker, 2012). Both the undernutrition early and the overnutrition later are necessary to confer increased risk.

How developmental programming might affect other behaviors and brain development is less clearly elucidated. Implicit in the programming hypothesis is the idea of a phenotypic plasticity in which outcomes can be calibrated by experiences in utero and following birth. The maternal neuroendocrine system provides information to the developing fetus about the current maternal environment, and as such may shape fetal development to prepare the infant for a similar environment at birth. Studies have implicated hypothalamic–pituitary–adrenocortical (HPA) axis (part of the neuroendocrine system that is crucial in regulating the stress response) programming prenatally (O'Connor et al., 2005), and the impact of both maternal cortisol (a hormone that fluctuates throughout the day and spikes in response to stress) and pregnancy anxiety in early gestation predicted infant mental development measured at age 12 months (Davis & Sandman, 2010). Though the effect of maternal stress on long-term child outcomes has been traditionally characterized from a "risk factor" perspective, evolutionary–developmental theory has been used to consider the adaptive aspects of programming from maternal stress (e.g., Del Giudice, 2012). Intense maternal stress during pregnancy has been linked to a host of psychopathologi-cal profiles, including anxiety, inattention, and aggression (Glover, 2011), and some of these behaviors may be considered to be adaptive in high-stress con-texts, much as the prenatal calibration to undernutrition may be adaptive in low food resource environments.

Allostatic Load

Allostatic load is a similar construct to toxic stress (McEwen & Stellar, 1993). Allostasis refers to maintaining homeostasis or physiological stability through changing environmental circumstances and conditions. Maintaining physi-ological regulation within a relative narrow range has survival value. Nervous, endocrine, and immune system mediators are triggered by various stressors to ensure that the individual responds adaptively. However, if these systems are activated repeatedly or chronically, allostatic load theory postulates that mal-adaptive consequences will ensue. Allostatic load refers to cumulative negative costs (wear and tear) that the body experiences due to repeated or prolonged activation in response to stressors (Danese & McEwen, 2012). Overexposure to neural, endocrine, and immune stress mediators can compromise function-ing in various organ systems and lead to disease. McEwen (2000) has described four patterns of allostatic load: (1) excessive stress and repeated, novel events that cause repeated elevations of stress mediators over long periods of time; (2) failure to habituate or adapt to the same stressor, leading to overexposure to stress mediators when the body fails to deactivate hormonal stress response to a repeated event; (3) failure to regulate stress responses or to display the normal diurnal regulation of cortisol; and (4) inadequate hormonal stress response that allows other systems, such as the inflammatory cytokines, proteins induced by oxidant stress, to become overactive.

Measuring allostatic load is complex, potentially including systolic and dia-stolic blood pressure (indexing cardiovascular health), waist to hip ratio (index-ing more chronic levels of metabolism and adipose tissue deposition), serum high-density lipoprotein (HDL) and total cholesterol (indexing atherosclerosis), blood levels of glycosylated hemoglobin (indexing glucose metabolism over sev-eral days' time), serum dihydroepiandrosterone sulfate (DHEA-S, a functional HPA axis antagonist), overnight urinary cortisol excretion (indexing 12-hour HPA axis activity), and overnight urinary norepinephrine and epinephrine excretion levels (indexing indices of 12-hour sympathetic nervous system activ-ity; McEwen, 2000).

In one of the few studies in early childhood, an allostatic load index was created in a sample of 2-year-old children from measures of low birth weight, short naps, reduced sleep time, high cortisol laboratory reactivity to novel epi-sodes, and flat home diurnal cortisol slope over the day (Buss, Davis, & Kiel, 2011). The allostatic load index and an environmental load index were summed to create a cumulative load index that ranged from 0 to 11. Concurrent associations were found between load indices and internalizing and externalizing problem behaviors in the children. When extremes in this low-risk sample were examined, they found that the load indices were more predictive of internalizing problems that continued to increase over the next 3 years. Early indicators of allostatic load could provide a more specific means of identifying children for whom early intervention is indicated within high-risk groups.

Epigenetics

Epigenetics refers to functionally relevant modifications to the genome that do not involve a change in nucleotide sequence. These changes impact gene expression, and to date, three processes have most studied: telomere shortening, gene methylation, and histone modification. Most of this work has been conducted in animals, but studies in humans are beginning to appear and signal an important new direction for understanding the mechanisms by which adverse experiences may change developmental trajectories. The study of epigenetics has provided insight into how environmental exposures to stress can impact health through changes in gene expression. The process behind developmental programming, for example, likely involves both methylation and demethylation, a process that affects the expression of genes (Seckl & Holmes, 2007). Increased deoxyribonucleic acid (DNA) methylation of the glucocorticoid receptor, which is involved in regulating stress responsivity, as well as increased lethargic behavior, was found in newborns whose mothers reported depression during their pregnancy compared with infants whose mothers were not depressed (Conradt, Lester, Appleton, Armstrong, & Marsit, 2013). Mapping potential epigenetic changes that link experience to gene expression and behavior is an exciting area of research in the field of infant development.

Another epigenetic process, the study of telomere shortening as an index of stress, is also beginning to be explored. Telomeres are specialized nucleotide repeats located at the end of chromosomes that confer chromosomal stability (Blackburn, 2000; Chan & Blackburn, 2004). Telomeres often shorten with replication and, when telomeres become too short, cellular senescence is triggered. Therefore, telomere length (TL) is considered a biological marker of cellular aging (Epel et al., 2004) that may also reflect cumulative stress exposure; indeed, shorter TL has been associated with a number of age-related health problems, including cardiovascular disease, cancer, stroke, and diabetes (Price, Kao, Burgers, Carpenter, & Tyrka, 2013). Oxidative stress shortens telomeres, and recent studies have demonstrated that children who have experienced various types of adversity (e.g., maltreatment, exposure to violence, institutional rearing) have shorter telomeres than less stressed children.

Drury and colleagues examined exposure to deprivation among children from the BEIP and operationalized as a percentage of the time each child at baseline (range of 6 to 30 months, mean age 22 months) and at 54 months of age had lived in an institution (Drury, Theall, et al., 2012). Children with greater exposure to institutional care had significantly shorter relative TL in middle childhood, with an important moderation by gender. For girls, more institutional rearing at baseline was associated with shorter telomeres in middle childhood. For boys, more institutional care through 54 months of age was associated with shorter telomeres in middle childhood. Asok et al. extended these findings by demonstrating that responsive parenting moderated the effect of maltreatment on TL, after controlling for household income, birth weight, gender, and minority status (Asok, Bernard, Roth, Rosen, & Dozier, 2013). Taken together, these findings suggest that negative early experiences in the form of deprivation or abuse may result in increased cellular aging. On the other hand, responsive parenting may have protective benefits on telomere shortening for young children exposed to early-life stress. If so, these findings have significant implications for early parenting interventions.

Exploring Infant–Caregiver Relationships

Human infants require caregivers' protection and support to ensure survival for years after birth (Tottenham, 2014). Beyond providing basic instrumental needs and physical protection, however, relationships between infants and caregivers also provide an essential role in helping infants regulate responses to stressors and other experiences of adversity. Implicit in the studies cited in previous sections is that the proximal social context for infant development is the infant's relationship(s) with caregiver(s). For better or worse, infant experiences of environmental risk conditions will be experienced through a relatively small number of relationships with caregivers. As an example, poverty is one of the most studied and best documented risk factors for outcomes across a range of developmental domains (Brooks-Gunn & Duncan, 1997). Still, a 12-month-old infant does not know what it means to be poor except as experienced through his or her primary caregiving relationships. Poor infants who have secure attachments, for example, are likely to be protected from adverse outcomes compared with nonsecurely attached infants. Secure attachment has been found to buffer the impact of parental stress (Tharner et al., 2012), indicating the importance of infant–caregiver relationship in protecting the developing child from salient risk factors.

The protective effects of these relationships are often most evident in the extremes of environmental adversity. For example, in BEIP, caregiving quality at 30 months of age was associated with psychopathology 2 years later. This association was mediated by security of attachment at 42 months (McGoron et al., 2012). These findings indicate that having a secure attachment relationship with a caregiver, even among children with histories of extreme deprivation, can protect against the risk of later psychopathology.

Future Directions

We have outlined in this chapter several current directions in the study of risk and adversity in infancy. We expect that these lines of research will be continued in the future, and with the seemingly ever-expanding technical advances and understanding of genetics and the brain, much can be gained by further study. Particularly innovative areas for future work include the biological embedding of early environmental experiences. Identifying the mechanisms by which early adversity confers broad risk for a number of mental and physical difficulties may provide promising avenues for prevention and intervention, and promises to bring studies of the precursors of mental and physical health into increasingly closer alignment. Additionally, further study of individual differences in response to early experience may allow for specific tailoring of interventions, as well as refinement in our diagnostic system. The National Institute of Mental Health Research Domain Criteria (RDoC) project (Insel et al., 2010) was created to guide the study of psychopathology by linking specific behavioral phenotypes (as opposed to disorder-level approaches) to underlying pathophysiology. This effort is ongoing and is expected to generate research that deviates from current diagnostic systems that have not explicitly considered etiology in the formulation of most disorders (e.g., DSM-5; American Psychiatric Association, 2013). The RDoC framework will provide a substantial push for researchers to consider the genetic and neural underpinnings of psychopathology. We believe that this approach, particularly when accompanied by careful consideration of how the environment dynamically interacts with the developing brain, is likely to contribute to mechanistic understandings of disease onset and progression. Last, in concert with recent calls for further action linking neuroscience with clinical practice (Holmes, Craske, & Graybiel, 2014), we believe an important area for future research is in studying the impact of extant effective psychological interventions. By studying the mechanisms of change underpinning proven interventions, we can improve existing interventions as well as develop new techniques for treating and preventing psychopathology.

Conclusions

Infancy is a period when the environment is of great importance due to the heightened plasticity, presence of sensitive periods, and the experience-expectant and experience-dependent nature of the developing brain. Adverse experiences during this period have been linked to a myriad of negative outcomes, and current biopsychosocial frameworks are beginning to delineate the specific impact of various types of negative experiences and the mechanisms by which these experiences result in psychopathology and other outcomes. Individual differences, in the form of genetics and temperament, seem to moderate the impact of such negative events. Additionally, caregivers are critical for providing children with the basic necessities for survival, and relationships with caregivers may buffer infants from stress and foster positive experiences that provide a strong foundation for future development. Longitudinal studies can identify trajectories of children based on specific forms of adverse early experiences, considering both developmental and individual differences, and the role of infant–caregiver relationships. Though there is much yet to learn, there are already clear implications from research on infant development. Specifically, supporting programs and policies that work to help caregivers be consistent and sensitive to their infants is essential for promoting infant mental health.

REFERENCES

Almas, A. N., Degnan, K. A., Radulescu, A., Nelson, C. A., Zeanah, C. H., & Fox, N. A. (2012). Effects of early intervention and the moderating effects of brain activity on institutionalized children's social skills at age 8. *Proceedings of the National Academy of Sciences of the United States of America, 109*(Suppl.), 17228–17231.

American Psychiatric Association. (2013). *Diagnostic and statistical manual of mental disorders* (5th ed.). Arlington, VA: Author.

Appleyard, K., Egeland, B., van Dulmen, M. H. M., & Sroufe, L. A. (2005). When more is not better: The role of cumulative risk in child behavior outcomes. *Journal of Child Psychology and Psychiatry, 46*, 235–245.

Asok, A., Bernard, K., Roth, T. L., Rosen, J. B., & Dozier, M. (2013). Parental responsiveness moderates the association between early-life stress and reduced telomere length. *Development and Psychopathology, 25*(3), 577–585.

Bakermans-Kranenburg, M. J., & van IJzendoorn, M. H. (2006). Gene–environment interaction of the dopamine D4 receptor (*DRD4*) and observed maternal insensitivity predicting externalizing behavior in preschoolers. *Developmental Psychobiology, 48*, 406–409.

Barker, D. J. P. (2003). Developmental origins of adult health and disease. *European Journal of Epidemiology, 18*(8), 733–736.

Barker, D. J. P. (2012). Human growth and chronic disease: A memorial to Jim Tanner. *Annals of Human Biology, 39*(5), 335–341.

Belsky, J., & Pluess, M. (2009). Beyond diathesis stress: Differential susceptibility to environmental influences. *Psychological Bulletin, 135*, 885–908.

Bernard, K., Butzin-Dozier, Z., Rittenhouse, J., & Dozier, M. (2010). Cortisol production patterns in young children living with birth parents vs. children placed in foster care following involvement of Child Protective Services. *Archives of Pediatrics and Adolescent Medicine, 164*, 438–443.

Blackburn, E. H. (2000). Telomere states and cell fates. *Nature, 408*, 53–56.

Bos, K. J., Zeanah, C. H., Smyke, A. T., Fox, N. A., & Nelson, C. A. (2010). Stereotypies in children with a history of early institutional care. *Archives of Pediatrics and Adolescent Medicine, 164*, 406–411.

Brett, Z. H., Humphreys, K. L., Smyke, A. T., Gleason, M. M., Nelson, C. A., Zeanah, C. H., et al. (2015). *5HTTLPR* genotype moderates the longitudinal impact of early caregiving on externalizing behavior. *Development and Psychopathology, 27*, 7–18.

Brooks-Gunn, J., & Duncan, G. J. (1997). The effects of poverty on children. *The Future of Children, 7*, 55–71.

Buss, K. A., Davis, E. L., & Kiel, E. J. (2011). Allostatic and environmental load in toddlers predicts anxiety in preschool and kindergarten. *Development and Psychopathology, 23*, 1069–1087.

Chan, S. R. W. L., & Blackburn, E. H. (2004). Telomeres and telomerase. *Philosophical Transactions of the Royal Society of London B: Biological Sciences, 359*, 109–121.

Cicchetti, D., Rogosch, F. A., & Toth, S. L. (2006). Fostering secure attachment in infants in maltreating families through preventive interventions. *Development and Psychopathology, 18*, 643–649.

Conradt, E., Lester, B. M., Appleton, A. A., Armstrong, D. A., & Marsit, C. J. (2013). The role of DNA methylation of NR3C1 and 11β-HSD2 and exposure to maternal mood disorder in utero on newborn neurobehavior. *Epigenetics, 8*, 1321–1329.

Danese, A., & McEwen, B. S. (2012). Adverse childhood experiences, allostasis, allostatic load, and age-related disease. *Physiology and Behavior, 106*, 29–39.

Davies, P. T., & Cicchetti, D. (2014). How and why does the *5-HTTLPR* gene moderate associations between maternal unresponsiveness and children's disruptive problems? *Child Development, 85*, 484–500.

Davis, E. P., & Sandman, C. A. (2010). The timing of prenatal exposure to maternal cortisol and psychosocial stress is associated with human infant cognitive development. *Child Development, 81*, 131–148.

Davis, E. P., & Thompson, R. A. (2014). Prenatal foundations: Fetal programming of health and development. *Zero to Three, 34*, 6–11.

Del Giudice, M. (2012). Fetal programming by maternal stress: Insights from a conflict perspective. *Psychoneuroendocrinology, 37*, 1614–1629.

dosReis, S., Zito, J. M., Safer, D. J., & Soeken, K. L. (2001). Mental health services for youths in foster care and disabled youths. *American Journal of Public Health, 91*, 1094–1099.

Dozier, M., Manni, M., Gordon, M. K., Peloso, E., Gunnar, M. R., Stovall-McClough, K. C., et al. (2006). Foster children's diurnal production of cortisol: An exploratory study. *Child Maltreatment, 11*(2), 189–197.

Drury, S. S., Gleason, M. M., Theall, K. P., Smyke, A. T., Nelson, C. A., Fox, N. A., et al. (2012). Genetic sensitivity to the caregiving context: The influence of *5HTTLPR* and *BDNF* val66met on indiscriminate social behavior. *Physiology and Behavior, 106*, 728–735.

Drury, S. S., Theall, K., Gleason, M., Smyke, A. T., De Vivo, I., Wong, J., et al. (2012). Telomere length and early severe social deprivation: Linking early adversity and cellular aging. *Molecular Psychiatry, 17*(7), 719–727.

Egger, H. L., & Angold, A. (2006). Common emotional and behavioral disorders in preschool children: Presentation, nosology, and epidemiology. *Journal of Child Psychology and Psychiatry, 47*(3–4), 313–337.

Epel, E. S., Blackburn, E. H., Lin, J., Dhabhar, F. S., Adler, N. E., Morrow, J. D., et al. (2004). Accelerated telomere shortening in response to life stress. *Proceedings of the National Academy of Sciences of the United States of America, 101,* 17312–17315.

Evans, G. W., Li, D., & Whipple, S. S. (2013). Cumulative risk and child development. *Psychological Bulletin, 139,* 1342–1396.

Fearon, R. P., Bakermans-Kranenburg, M. J., Van IJzendoorn, M. H., Lapsey, A. M., & Roisman, G. I. (2010). The significance of insecure attachment and disorganization in the development of children's externalizing behavior: A meta-analytic study. *Child Development, 81*(2), 435–456.

Felitti, V. J., & Anda, R. F. (2014). The lifelong effects of adverse childhood experiences. In D. L. Chadwick, R. Alexander, A. P. Giardino, D. Esernio-Jenssen, & J. D. Thackeray (Eds.), *Chadwick's child maltreatment* (4th ed., pp. 203–216). St. Louis, MO: STM Learning.

Felitti, V. J., Anda, R. F., Nordenberg, D., Williamson, D. F., Spitz, A. M., Edwards, V., et al. (1998). Relationship of childhood abuse and household dysfunction to many of the leading causes of death in adults: The Adverse Childhood Experiences (ACE) Study. *American Journal of Preventive Medicine, 14,* 245–258.

Field, T. (1994). The effects of mother's physical and emotional unavailability on emotion regulation. *Monographs of the Society for Research in Child Development, 59,* 208–227.

Fisher, P. A., Stoolmiller, M., Gunnar, M. R., & Burraston, B. O. (2007). Effects of a therapeutic intervention for foster preschoolers on diurnal cortisol activity. *Psychoneuroendocrinology, 32,* 892–905.

Fox, N. A., Zeanah, C. H., & Nelson, C. A. (2014). A matter of timing: Enhancing positive change for the developing brain. *Zero to Three, 34*(3), 4–9.

Glover, V. (2011). Prenatal stress and the origins of psychopathology: An evolutionary perspective. *Journal of Child Psychology and Psychiatry, 52*(4), 356–367.

Goodman, S. H., Rouse, M. H., Connell, A. M., Broth, M. R., Hall, C. M., & Heyward, D. (2011). Maternal depression and child psychopathology: A meta-analytic review. *Clinical Child and Family Psychology Review, 14,* 1–27.

Greenough, W. T., Black, J. E., & Wallace, C. S. (1987). Experience and brain development. *Child Development, 58,* 539–559.

Hill, J., Breen, G., Quinn, J., Tibu, F., Sharp, H., & Pickles, A. (2013). Evidence for interplay between genes and maternal stress in utero: Monoamine oxidase A polymorphism moderates effects of life events during pregnancy on infant negative emotionality at 5 weeks. *Genes, Brain, and Behavior, 12,* 388–396.

Holmes, E. A., Craske, M. G., & Graybiel, A. M. (2014). Psychological treatments: A call for mental-health science. *Nature, 511*(7509), 287–289.

Humphreys, K. L., & Zeanah, C. H. (2015). Deviations from the expectable environment in early childhood and emerging psychopathology. *Neuropsychopharmacology, 40,* 154–170.

Insel, T., Cuthbert, B., Garvey, M., Heinssen, R., Pine, D. S., Quinn, K., et al. (2010). Research domain criteria (RDoC): Toward a new classification framework for research on mental disorders. *American Journal of Psychiatry, 167,* 748–751.

Kim, J., & Cicchetti, D. (2010). Longitudinal pathways linking child maltreatment, emotion regulation, peer relations, and psychopathology. *Journal of Child Psychology and Psychiatry, 51*(6), 706–716.

Knudsen, E. I. (2004). Sensitive periods in the development of the brain and behavior. *Journal of Cognitive Neuroscience, 16,* 1412–1425.

Kreppner, J. M., O'Connor, T. G., & Rutter, M. (2001). Can inattention/overactivity be an institutional deprivation syndrome? *Journal of Abnormal Child Psychology, 29*(6), 513–528.

Lyons-Ruth, K., Zeanah, C. H., Benoit, D., Madigan, S., & Mills-Koonce, W. R. (2014). Disorder and risk for disorder during infancy and toddlerhood. In E. J. Mash & R. A. Barkley (Eds.), *Child psychopathology* (3rd ed., pp. 673–736). New York: Guilford Press.

McEwen, B. S. (2000). Allostasis and allostatic load: Implications for neuropsychopharmacology. *Neuropsychopharmacology, 22,* 108–124.

McEwen, B. S., & Stellar, E. (1993). Stress and the individual: Mechanisms leading to disease. *Archives of Internal Medicine, 153,* 2093–2101.

McGoron, L., Gleason, M. M., Smyke, A. T., Drury, S. S., Nelson, C. A., Gregas, M. C., et al. (2012). Recovering from early deprivation: Attachment mediates effects of caregiving on psychopathology. *Journal of the American Academy of Child and Adolescent Psychiatry, 51,* 683–693.

McLaughlin, K. A., Sheridan, M. A., Winter, W., Fox, N. A., Zeanah, C. H., & Nelson, C. A. (2013). Widespread reductions in cortical thickness following severe early-life deprivation: A neurodevelopmental pathway to attention-deficit/hyperactivity disorder. *Biological Psychiatry, 76,* 629–638.

Miner, J. L., & Clarke-Stewart, K. A. (2008). Trajectories of externalizing behavior from age 2 to age 9: Relations with gender, temperament, ethnicity, parenting, and rater. *Developmental Psychology, 44,* 771–786.

Murray, L. (1992). The impact of postnatal depression on infant development. *Journal of Child Psychology and Psychiatry, 33,* 543–561.

National Research Council. (2013). *New directions in child abuse and neglect research.* Washington, DC: National Academies Press.

Nelson, C. A., Fox, N. A., & Zeanah, C. H. (2014). *Romania's abandoned children.* Cambridge, MA: Harvard University Press.

Nelson, C. A., Zeanah, C. H., Fox, N. A., Marshall, P. J., Smyke, A. T., & Guthrie, D. (2007). Cognitive recovery in socially deprived young children: The Bucharest Early Intervention Project. *Science, 318,* 1937–1940.

NICHD Early Care Research Network. (2006). Infant–mother attachment classification: Risk and protection in relation to changing maternal caregiving quality. *Developmental Psychology, 42*(1), 38–58.

O'Connor, T. G., Ben-Shlomo, Y., Heron, J., Golding, J., Adams, D., & Glover, V. (2005). Prenatal anxiety predicts individual differences in cortisol in pre-adolescent children. *Biological Psychiatry, 58,* 211–217.

Pollak, S. D., Klorman, R., Thatcher, J. E., & Cicchetti, D. (2001). P3b reflects maltreated children's reactions to facial displays of emotion. *Psychophysiology, 38*(2), 267–274.

Pollak, S. D., & Sinha, P. (2002). Effects of early experience on children's recognition of facial displays of emotion. *Developmental Psychology, 38*(5), 784–791.

Pollak, S. D., & Tolley-Schell, S. A. (2003). Selective attention to facial emotion in physically abused children. *Journal of Abnormal Psychology, 112*(3), 323–338.

Price, L. H., Kao, H. T., Burgers, D. E., Carpenter, L. L., & Tyrka, A. R. (2013). Telomeres and early-life stress: An overview. *Biological Psychiatry, 73*, 15–23.

Roy, P., Rutter, M., & Pickles, A. (2004). Institutional care: Associations between overactivity and lack of selectivity in social relationships. *Journal of Child Psychology and Psychiatry, 45*, 866–873.

Rutter, M., Sonuga-Barke, E. J., Beckett, C., Bell, C. A., Kreppner, J., Kumsta, R., et al. (2010). Deprivation-specific psychological patterns: Effects of institutional deprivation by the English and Romanian Adoptee Study team. *Monographs of the Society for Research in Child Development, 75*(1), 1–252.

Rutter, M., Sonuga-Barke, E. J., & Castle, J. (2010). I. Investigating the impact of early institutional deprivation on development: Background and research strategy of the English and Romanian Adoptees (ERA) Study. *Monographs of the Society for Research in Child Development, 75*(1), 1–20.

Sameroff, A. J., & Emde, R. N. (Eds.). (1989). *Relationship disturbances in early childhood: A developmental approach.* New York: Basic Books.

Seckl, J. R., & Holmes, M. C. (2007). Mechanisms of disease: Glucocorticoids, their placental metabolism and fetal "programming" of adult pathophysiology. *Nature Clinical Practice: Endocrinology and Metabolism, 3*, 479–488.

Shaw, D. S., & Vondra, J. I. (1993). Chronic family adversity and infant attachment security. *Journal of Child Psychology and Psychiatry, 34*, 1205–1215.

Shaw, D. S., Vondra, J. I., Hommerding, K. D., Keenan, K., & Dunn, M. (1994). Chronic family adversity and early child behavior problems: A longitudinal study of low income families. *Journal of Child Psychology and Psychiatry, 35*, 1109–1122.

Shonkoff, J. P., & Garner, A. S. (2012). The lifelong effects of early childhood adversity and toxic stress. *Pediatrics, 129*(1), e232–e246.

Smyke, A. T., Zeanah, C. H., Fox, N. A., Nelson, C. A., & Guthrie, D. (2010). Placement in foster care enhances quality of attachment among young institutionalized children. *Child Development, 81*(1), 212–223.

Sroufe, L. A. (1989). Relationship and relationship disturbances. In A. J. Sameroff & A. J. Emde (Eds.), *Relationship disturbances in early childhood* (pp. 97–205). New York: Basic Books.

Tharner, A., Luijk, M. P. C. M., van IJzendoorn, M. H., Bakermans-Kranenburg, M. J., Jaddoe, V. W. V., Hofman, A., et al. (2012). Infant attachment, parenting stress, and child emotional and behavioral problems at age 3 years. *Parenting, 12*, 261–281.

Tottenham, N. (2014). The importance of early environments for neuro-affective development. *Current Topics in Behavioral Neurosciences, 16*, 109–129.

Trentacosta, C. J., Hyde, L. W., Goodlett, B. D., & Shaw, D. S. (2013). Longitudinal prediction of disruptive behavior disorders in adolescent males from multiple risk domains. *Child Psychiatry and Human Development, 44,* 561–572.

Tronick, E., & Reck, C. (2009). Infants of depressed mothers. *Harvard Review of Psychiatry, 17,* 147–156.

Vanderwert, R. E., Marshall, P. J., Nelson, C. A., Zeanah, C. H., & Fox, N. A. (2010). Timing of intervention affects brain electrical activity in children exposed to severe psychosocial neglect. *PLoS ONE, 5*(7), e11415.

Windsor, J., Benigno, J. P., Wing, C. A., Carroll, P. J., Koga, S. F., Nelson, C. A., et al. (2011). Effect of foster care on young children's language learning. *Child Development, 82,* 1040–1046.

Zeanah, C. H., Egger, H. L., Smyke, A. T., Nelson, C. A., Fox, N. A., Marshall, P. J., et al. (2009). Institutional rearing and psychiatric disorders in Romanian preschool children. *American Journal of Psychiatry, 166*(7), 777–785.

Zeanah, C. H., Gunnar, M. R., McCall, R. B., Kreppner, J. M., & Fox, N. A. (2011). Children without permanent parents: Research, practice, and policy: VI. Sensitive periods. *Monographs of the Society for Research in Child Development, 76,* 147–162.

Zeanah, C. H., Nelson, C. A., Fox, N. A., Smyke, A. T., Marshall, P., Parker, S. W., et al. (2003). Designing research to study the effects of institutionalization on brain and behavioral development: The Bucharest Early Intervention Project. *Development and Psychopathology, 15,* 885–907.

Zero to Three. (1994). *Diagnostic classification of mental health and developmental disorders of infancy and early childhood.* Washington, DC: Author.

Zero to Three. (2005). *Diagnostic classification of mental health and developmental disorders of infancy and early childhood* (rev. ed.). Washington, DC: Author.

CHAPTER 15

Adversity in
Early Social Relationships

Mary Dozier, Caroline K. P. Roben, and Julie R. Hoye

Infants' relationships with their parents provide critical input for developing brain and behavioral systems. The role of parents in infants' psychobiological development has been most clearly studied in cases in which infants are deprived of parental care, such as with institutionalized children (Nelson, Fox, & Zeanah, 2014), and in experimental animal studies of social isolation or deprivation (see Harlow, Dodsworth, & Harlow, 1965; Suomi, 1997). Animal studies have also illuminated how variations in parenting behavior have lasting effects on the development of offspring (e.g., Francis, Diorio, Liu, & Meaney, 1999; Weaver et al., 2004). Behavioral, neurobiological, and epigenetic parenting findings from animal studies can be compared to the variations of parenting in human populations of children at risk for adversity. In this chapter, we examine how variations in parenting, specifically in the form of abuse and neglect, influence psychobiological development. We also discuss psychosocial intervention as a means of experimentally manipulating parenting and the resulting influences on child development.

Early on, parents serve as coregulators for infants, with infants gradually taking over regulation of biological and behavioral systems themselves. When parents are responsive to children's cues, infants receive input that is critical to brain and behavioral development. Such experiences are key to children's developing adequate self-regulatory capabilities. Many parents fail to respond in consistent and predictable ways, however, which can adversely affect young children's developing adequate self-regulatory systems. In the case of some caregivers, this is seen in neglect, with parents providing inadequate input. In the case of others, this is seen in abuse, with parents providing aversive input. Children who lack a caregiver, as in the case of institutionalized children, experience the most extreme conditions of privation (Nelson et al., 2014). Given infants' dependence on caregiver input for developing self-regulatory capabilities at the biological, behavioral, and emotional levels, this lack of input or aversive input has consequences that can be cascading (Institute of Medicine [IOM], 2013). Recovery is nonetheless possible when parenting changes as the result of intervention. Plasticity of brain and behavioral systems makes the developing child vulnerable to problematic environments, but also receptive to remediation. There are consequences of neglect and abuse on young children's developing biological and behavioral systems, and the possibility for recovery.

Why Is Parenting So Important?

Human infants are evolutionarily prepared to depend upon caregivers. Humans are a highly altricial species, with a quite protracted period of immaturity. Infants are reliant on parents for help regulating a wide range of functions, from neuroendocrine and temperature regulation to feelings of safety and security (Hofer, 1994, 2006). When caregivers cannot be depended on for protection and security, as in the case of neglect or abuse, there are problematic consequences for infants.

Children may experience any number of types of adversity, including neglect, abuse, institutional care, and exposure to domestic or neighborhood violence, among other things. Experiencing one type of adversity often increases the risk of other types of adversity, with the co-occurrence of multiple types of adversity common (e.g., Dong, Anda, Dube, Giles, & Felitti, 2003; Dong et al., 2004; Hillis et al., 2004). Although attempts have been made to isolate the effects of different types of adversity, the strongest statements can be made with regard to cumulative risk, with the greater number of risk factors predicting more problematic outcomes (Appleyard, Egeland, van Dulmen, & Sroufe, 2005; Sameroff, Bartko, Baldwin, Baldwin, & Seifer, 1998). This is a phenomenon that was identified by Sameroff and colleagues several decades ago (Sameroff & Chandler, 1975), which has attracted attention in recent years as the Adverse Childhood Experiences Study (ACES) results were published (e.g., Chapman et al., 2004).

While acknowledging the importance of cumulative risk, we also consider the specific types of adversity—neglect, abuse, and institutional care—in more detail below.

Maltreatment

In the United States, about 700,000 children are documented as maltreated annually (out of about 3 million referrals for possible maltreatment; U.S. Department of Health and Human Services [US DHHS], 2013). Infants are disproportionately represented among these numbers. Of the total documented as maltreated in 2012, 12.8% were children under the age of 1, 7% between the ages of 1 and 2, and 7% between the ages of 2 and 3 (US DHHS, 2013). Many more parents behave in ways that are harmful to children through acts of commission or omission than those who are formally charged with abuse or neglect.

By far the most common form of maltreatment is neglect, representing about three-quarters of all maltreatment cases (US DHHS, 2013; IOM, 2013). Neglect is a failure to care for or protect a child in a way that places the child in danger (Child Abuse Prevention and Treatment Act [CAPTA], 2010). Often, neglect involves a parent leaving a child or children unattended, or otherwise failing to meet needs at a level that is noticeable.

There are far fewer documented cases of abuse than neglect, with abuse making up about 18% of all maltreatment cases in the United States (US DHHS, 2013). Abuse refers to physical harm of children at the hands of caregivers. Among infants, abusive head trauma (previously termed *shaken baby syndrome*) is often the result of young children experiencing shaking and/or blunt impact (Christian, Block, & the Committee on Child Abuse and Neglect, 2009). Infants under the age of 4 months, the age that corresponds with the longest periods of crying, experience such injury at the highest rates (Barr, Trent, & Cross, 2006; Lee, Barr, Catherine, & Wicks, 2007).

Parental frightening behavior often does not meet the threshold for abusive behavior, but is relatively common, especially among highly stressed parents, and has problematic effects on the development of infants and young children (Hesse & Main, 2006; Schuengel, Bakermans-Kranenburg, & Van IJzendoorn, 1999). When parents behave in frightening ways, infants have difficulty depending on them effectively for help regulating behavior.

Institutional Care

Orphanages and other institutional settings represent the most extremely neglecting conditions (Dozier et al., 2014; Nelson et al., 2014; Pinheiro, 2006). In the last several centuries, institutional care has become commonplace in many countries for the care of children who lose their parents, are abandoned, or are taken away by authorities (Hrdy, 1999; Smith, 1995). In such facilities, young children often do not have a primary caregiver. Typically staff members work shifts, with children experiencing many caregivers over time. The staff–child ratio is often very low, such that there is little chance that children receive individualized attention or contingent responding. In these contexts, routines are established to enhance efficiency (such as feeding or diapering), but not with individual child needs in mind (Dozier, Zeanah, Wallin, & Shauffer, 2012; Leiden Conference on the Development and Care of Children without Permanent Parents, 2012; Nelson et al., 2014; Smith, 1995). Not surprisingly, children under these conditions often show global deficits across all domains of functioning that are not highly canalized.

Conditions of neglect and abuse are rarely as extreme as conditions of institutional care, and children do not typically show the pervasive deficits seen in institutional settings. Nonetheless, in less extreme conditions of neglect and/or abuse, deficits are often seen in attachment relationships and regulation of behavior and physiology, with these outcomes often having cascading effects.

Remediation and Recovery

It is hard to imagine an intervention more powerful than changing the caregiving environment of children who experience adversity. Fundamental changes in parenting can be accomplished through adoption or foster care, or through interventions that help birth parents interact in qualitatively different ways.

Whereas foster care is designed to be a temporary caregiving situation, adoption is intended to be permanent. There are exceptions of course, with foster caregivers sometimes adopting children in their care, and more rarely adoptive parents disrupting the adoption. An enhanced system of foster care was used in the Bucharest Early Intervention Project (BEIP). In the BEIP, children were randomly assigned from Romanian orphanages to care as usual or to enhanced foster care. In enhanced foster care, parents were permanent caregivers who were dedicated to raising the children, although parental rights were not terminated. In general, adoption has dramatic effects on child outcomes, with children showing advantages in attachment security, physiological regulation, and regulation of emotions and behaviors (Johnson et al., 2010; Nelson et al., 2007; Smyke, Zeanah, Fox, Nelson, & Guthrie, 2010). Although the timing of the adoption (and/or the length of time in extremely adverse conditions) matters in terms of child outcomes, adoption can be seen to have robust effects. Foster care can also result in dramatic improvements in children's ability to regulate attachment, behavior, and physiology (Bernard, Butzin-Dozier, Rittenhouse, & Dozier, 2010; Dozier, Stovall, Albus, & Bates, 2001). These effects are described in more detail in specific sections below.

Although parenting interventions for maltreating parents do not represent the "sledgehammer effect" of adoption, they can help change the environments infants are experiencing in fundamental ways when parents successfully develop different parenting approaches. Interventions have been found to have pervasive effects (e.g., Bernard, Dozier, Bick, & Gordon, 2014; Bernard, Hostinar, &

Dozier, 2015; Cicchetti, Rogosch, & Toth, 2006; Hoffman, Marvin, Cooper, & Powell, 2006; Meade, Weston-Lee, Haggerty, & Dozier, 2014). Several interventions are described later in this chapter.

Effects of Adversity on Attachment, Emotion Regulation, and Hypothalamus–Pituitary–Adrenocortical Regulation

Experiences of early adversity such as neglect, abuse, and institutional care have their most pronounced effects on early developing behavioral and biological systems that are most highly reliant on environmental input. The attachment system, the system of regulating emotions, and the hypothalamus–pituitary–adrenocortical (HPA) axis are among these systems most affected.

Attachment

Infants organize their attachment systems around the availability of caregivers (Bowlby, 1969/1982). When caregivers are available and responsive, infants typically develop secure, organized attachments (Ainsworth, Blehar, Waters, & Wall, 1978). When caregivers reject infants' bids for reassurance, infants often develop avoidant attachments, and when caregivers are inconsistent in availability, infants often develop resistant attachments. Avoidant and resistant attachments represent organized strategies; such strategies are both organized around the availability of the caregiver and provide the child an organized approach to dealing with distress.

Attachment and Maltreatment

When children are maltreated or experience other types of significant adversity, they are at increased risk for developing disorganized attachments (Bernard et al., 2010; Carlson, Cicchetti, Barnett, & Braunwald, 1989; Cicchetti et al., 2006; Cyr, Euser, Bakermans-Kranenburg, & van IJzendoorn, 2010; van IJzendoorn, Schuengel, & Bakermans-Kranenburg, 1999). Disorganized attachments reflect a lack of strategy or breakdown in strategy when children are distressed and in their parents' presence. Hesse and Main (2000) have suggested that, when children have frightening caregivers, they experience an unsolvable dilemma. Because such children are frightened of the caregivers on whom they need to depend, they experience a conflict (Hesse & Main, 2000). This dilemma is manifested behaviorally in the Strange Situation when children behave in ways that seem paradoxical (e.g., moving toward the caregiver and then moving sharply away, or crying while falling to the floor), or in ways that directly reflect their conflict or apprehension (e.g., freezing or stilling when reuniting with parent; Main & Solomon, 1990). These disorganized attachments are particularly concerning because they are predictive of a range of later problems, including externalizing behavior problems, dissociative symptoms, and future psychopathology (Carlson, 1998; Fearon, Bakermans-Kranenburg, van IJzendoorn, Lapsley, & Roisman, 2010; Lyons-Ruth, Easterbrooks, & Cibelli, 1997; Lyons-Ruth, Connell, Zoll, & Stahl, 1987; van IJzendoorn et al., 1999).

Cyr et al. (2010) conducted a meta-analysis that included the 10 studies of attachment quality with maltreated samples. The effect size was large for both disorganized attachment and insecure attachment (d = 2.19 and 2.10, respectively). Although neglect was more strongly related to insecure attachment and abuse to disorganized attachment, both neglect and abuse were predictive of disorganized and insecure attachments.

Attachment and Institutional Care

Under almost all conditions, children form attachments to their parents or caregivers. In terms of our evolutionary history, maintaining attachments was key to survival for infants, with attachment appearing highly canalized under most conditions. The only apparent exception is that some institutionalized children fail to develop fully formed attachments, and some postinstitutionalized children may take some period of time before they show a fully formed attachment after being placed with adoptive parents (Zeanah, Smyke, Koga, & Carlson, 2005). Indeed, Zeanah et al. found that, whereas all children who had lived continuously with birth parents showed fully developed attachments, only 3.2% of institutionalized children showed fully developed attachments.

Attachment Following Adversity: Foster and Adoptive Care

Stovall-McClough and Dozier examined the process by which children form attachments to new foster parents. Foster parents were asked to describe incidents when children were distressed (i.e., hurt, separated, and frightened) each day immediately following placements. Children younger than about a year of age showed secure behaviors when placed with nurturing caregivers quite quickly, typically within the first week to two of placement. Children placed after about a year tended to show avoidant or resistant behaviors even when placed in the care of nurturing parents, and over a period of several months (Stovall & Dozier, 2000; Stovall-McClough & Dozier, 2004). Nonetheless, even though longer periods of time were required for consolidation among older than younger infants, eventually both groups formed secure attachments when placed with nurturing caregivers, as assessed in the Strange Situation. However, when placed with non-nurturing caregivers, children were at high risk for disorganized attachments (Stovall-McClough & Dozier, 2004).

Van den Dries, Juffer, van IJzendoorn, and Bakermans-Kranenburg (2009) conducted a meta-analysis of adopted children's attachment quality relative to nonadopted children and foster children. Children adopted before the age of 1 showed secure attachments at rates similar to nonadopted children. Although children adopted after the age of 1 showed secure attachments at rates lower than low-risk birth children, these rates were comparable to the rates of foster children. Similarly to foster children, disorganized attachments were elevated among adopted children relative to nonadopted children. Although being adopted later than 12 months of age confers some disadvantage for children, such children fare surprisingly well given their early history of disadvantage.

Emotion Regulation

In early childhood, infants are limited in their abilities to regulate their own emotions and are dependent on caregivers for managing their distress (Sroufe, 1996; Tronick, 1989). Emotion regulation, defined as the process responsible for monitoring, evaluating, and modifying emotional reactions (Thompson, 1994), is a critical component of socioemotional competence and mental health (e.g., Eisenberg & Fabes, 1992; Shonkoff & Phillips, 2000). Development of adequate emotion regulation is dependent on parenting and experience, as well as internal biological predispositions (Calkins, 1994). Early attachment relationships and experiences shape the rapidly developing limbic system using an environmentally driven process (Cassidy, 1994). Due to rapidly changing biology and interactions with the environment, emotion regulation skills develop dramatically across the first few years of life, as children shift from being dependent on coregulation with their caregiver to being able to utilize independent strategies to decrease the intensity and duration of negative emotions (Calkins, Gill, Johnson, & Smith, 2001; Cole et al., 2011; Kopp, 1982).

Caregivers promote and scaffold emotion regulation development in several ways. Very young infants are highly attuned and responsive to their caregivers' emotions and use parental emotional signals to guide their own behavior (Klinnert, Campos, Sorce, Emde, & Svejda, 1983; Lelwica & Haviland, 1987; Malatesta & Izard, 1984). Mutual, reciprocal interactions between caregivers and infants may consolidate infant emotion regulation skills (Panksepp, 2001), with links between putative biological rhythms indicative of regulation in 3-month-olds and mother–infant synchrony (Feldman, 2006; Moore & Calkins, 2004). Moreover, affect synchrony and contingent responsiveness in infancy predict self-regulation in toddlerhood (Feldman & Eidelman, 2004; Feldman & Greenbaum, 1997; Shaw, Keenan, & Vondra, 1994; Shaw et al., 1998), suggesting that caregiving responsiveness is a mechanism in the development of independent regulation skills. As children grow older and as they develop the ability to use language, they communicate their needs to their parents through both verbal and nonverbal expressions, but still need parental support in the service of developing emotion regulation skills (Cole, Armstrong, & Pemberton, 2010;

Kopp, 1989). Discussion, support, and labeling of emotions can help children learn about how to manage negative emotions on their own (e.g., Gottman, Katz, & Hooven, 1997; Kopp, 2009; Lunkenheimer, Shields, & Cortina, 2007; Saarni, 1999; Shipman et al., 2007).

The quality and history of the parent–child relationship is important in this scaffolding process. Cassidy (1994) has described emotion regulation as an adaptive strategy that functions to maintain the infant's relationship with his or her caregiver. Securely attached children could be more likely to freely and flexibly share emotions with their parents if they believe those emotions will be responded to sensitively than children who believe their emotions will be dismissed, ignored, or responded to inappropriately (e.g., with anger). Taken from this view, infant emotions are expressed based on the degree to which the infant expects others to respond to his or her emotional signals. This theory is supported by research that finds associations among attachment, children's emotion regulation, and parents' responses to child negative emotion (Berlin & Cassidy, 2003; Diener, Mangelsdorf, McHale, & Frosch, 2002; Volling, McElwain, Notaro, & Herrera, 2002; Vondra, Shaw, Swearingen, Cohen, & Owens, 2001).

Children in environments without nurturing, responsive caregivers could thus struggle to develop the skills necessary for regulating their emotions. Children could either receive little or no response to their negative emotions, as in the case of neglect, or harsh, threatening, and inconsistent responses, as in the case of maltreatment (Milner, 2000). Such environments can be doubly detrimental, for children who are maltreated may not only experience the lack of supportive and responsive caregiving to their distress, but they may also endure abusive or neglecting caregiving that can be the source of distress (Shipman & Zeman, 2001). Consistent with this line of reasoning, Cicchetti and colleagues (Cicchetti, Ackerman, & Izard, 1995; Kim & Cicchetti, 2010; Rogosch, Cicchetti, & Aber, 1995) have found that maltreated children may struggle to understand, develop strategies for, and regulate emotions.

In the most extreme example of poor caregiving environments, prolonged institutional care, young children are at a high risk for profound negative effects on emotional development. Late adoption from institutional care was associated with poorer emotion regulation than earlier adoption from the institutional environment, and with larger amygdala volume (Tottenham et al., 2010). In addition, young children in Romanian institutional care were less likely to show positive emotion and more likely to show negative emotion during a puppet task than children who had never been institutionalized (Smyke et al., 2007).

Maladaptive emotion regulation strategies, or emotion dysregulation, can have cascading effects on the development of psychopathology (Cole, Michel, & Teti, 1994). Problems in regulating emotion are diffuse and long lasting, associated with externalizing behaviors, such as aggression and behavior problems

(Eisenberg et al., 2001; Kim & Cicchetti, 2010), internalizing behaviors, such as depression (Cole, Luby, & Sullivan, 2008; Maughan & Cicchetti, 2002), and challenges in peer relations (Kim & Cicchetti, 2010; Rogosch et al., 1995).

HPA Axis and Biological Regulation

As the infant brain develops, early experiences shape morphological and functional changes (Gunnar & Donzella, 2002). The HPA axis is especially sensitive to such adversity (Bernard et al., 2010; Bruce, Fisher, Pears, & Levine, 2009; Gunnar, Fisher, & The Early Experience, Stress, and Prevention Network, 2006; Gunnar & Vasquez, 2001; Levine, Wiener, & Coe, 1993). The HPA axis performs two orthogonal functions. First, the HPA axis mounts a biological response to perceived stress, ultimately resulting in the production of glucocorticoids (cortisol in humans, corticosterone in rats). This cascade diverts resources away from processes associated with long-term survival, such as reproduction, immune functioning, growth, and storage of energy. Instead, these resources are used to quickly increase available energy to address the immediate stressor (Gunnar & Cheatham, 2003; Gunnar & Quevedo, 2007). Second, the HPA axis plays an important role in maintaining and regulating the circadian patterns, such as waking, sleeping, and metabolism (Gunnar & Cheatham, 2003). Humans exhibit a diurnal pattern of cortisol, with cortisol peaking soon after wake-up, reflecting the metabolism of glucose into energy resources for the day. Cortisol levels decrease sharply midmorning and gradually decrease until bedtime (Gunnar & Donzella, 2002).

These functions are sensitive to the effects of early adversity and the quality of maternal care (e.g., Bernard et al., 2010; Bernard & Dozier, 2010; Gunnar & Donzella, 2002; Gunnar & Vasquez, 2001; Hane & Fox, 2006; Levine, 2005). Frightening maternal behavior (commonly seen in cases of abuse) or inadequate input (such as in cases of neglect and institutionalization) may result in dysregulation of the HPA axis. Gunnar and Vazquez (2001) have argued that, similar to the hyporesponsive period seen among rodent pups, human infants and young children experience a hyporeactive period, during which the developing brain is protected from high levels of circulating glucocorticoids. When experiencing challenge, the presence of a trusted caregiver buffers the infant from an increase in the production of cortisol and the downstream effects of high levels of circulating glucocorticoids. However, when the infant does not have a trusted caregiver or the caregiver is unavailable for some reason, infants show an increase in cortisol.

This hyporesponsive period is evident in infants' cortisol responses in the Strange Situation. The Strange Situation procedure (Ainsworth et al., 1978) elicits a strong behavioral response in infants through a series of separations between infant and mother. Only infants who have difficulty relying on their caregivers, as in the case of infants with disorganized (Bernard & Dozier, 2010; Hertsgaard, Gunnar, Erickson, & Nachmias, 1995; Spangler & Grossmann, 1993) or insecure (Spangler & Grossmann, 1993) attachments, show a cortisol response. Children with secure attachments failed to show a cortisol response to the Strange Situation despite typically showing strong behavioral reactions (Bernard & Dozier, 2010; Hertsgaard et al., 1995).

Maltreatment and adverse early experiences have also been shown to affect the diurnal pattern of cortisol. Bruce et al. (2009) found that children in foster care exhibit lower morning levels of cortisol than low-income, nonmaltreated children. Similarly, children in foster care typically show a flatter diurnal slope than low-risk children (Fisher, Gunnar, Dozier, Bruce, & Pears, 2006). Bernard et al. (2010) compared children living with neglecting birth parents, children in foster care, and low-risk children. Children living with neglecting birth parents exhibited the flattest diurnal slopes and the lowest levels of morning cortisol, whereas low-risk children exhibited the steepest slopes and highest levels of morning cortisol, and foster children showed levels intermediate to these two groups (Bernard et al., 2010).

Dysregulation of the HPA system is also seen among children who have experienced institutional care, though findings are varied. The most robust findings are that children often show blunted cortisol levels while institutionalized. Young children in Eastern European orphanages exhibited lower morning levels of cortisol and flatter diurnal slopes than nonadopted children living with their birth parents and institutionalized children adopted before 8 months of age (Carlson & Earls, 1997; Kroupina, Gunnar, & Johnson, 1997). This pattern was seen as children were placed in foster or adoptive homes, though cortisol patterns appeared to normalize as children spend more time in an enriched environment (Bruce, Kroupina, Parker, & Gunnar, 2000).

Cortisol has received much attention in recent years as an indicator of biological functioning. This attention has come partly because cortisol is easily collected through saliva sampling, assays can be completed by many different labs, and differences in levels have been associated with adversity. Nonetheless, there are many other rich measures that are emerging as potentially of interest.

Other Biological Indicators of Early Adversity

A number of studies have explored the effects of early adversity on later biological functioning in adolescents and adults. Differences between children who experienced adversity and comparison children have emerged in brain structure, brain function, and in epigenetic signatures of maltreatment. Several examples of such findings are provided here.

Internationally adopted adolescents who experienced severe social deprivation in early childhood were found to have larger amygdalae than nonadopted adolescents (Mehta et al., 2009; Tottenham et al., 2010), with larger amygdalae associated with difficulties in emotion regulation. Differences in amygdala volume among children adopted internationally are associated with the severity of deprivation, with children who spent a longer period of time in institutional care having larger amygdalae than children who spent a shorter period of time in institutional care (Mehta et al., 2009; Tottenham et al., 2010). Differences related to adversity have also emerged in prefrontal cortex functioning. Through functional magnetic resonance imaging (fMRI) during a behavioral inhibition task, Mueller et al. (2010) found that children who experienced early maltreatment showed greater activation of the inferior frontal cortex, striatum, and dorsal anterior cingulate cortex (dACC) than children without histories of maltreatment. This difference was observed during tasks that required increased executive functioning to correctly respond, suggesting impaired impulse and behavioral control. In fact, children who experienced early maltreatment exhibited longer reaction times when inhibiting a prepotent response than children without histories of maltreatment (Lewis, Dozier, Ackerman, & Sepulveda-Kozakowski, 2007; Mueller et al., 2010).

Through postmortem analyses, McGowan et al. (2009) examined levels of epigenetic regulation in the brain within groups of maltreated and nonmaltreated adult suicide completers, as well as a control group that died of natural causes. Adults who experienced childhood abuse exhibited unique regulation of the glucocorticoid receptor in the hippocampus, receptors associated with the regulation of the HPA axis, than nonmaltreated suicide completers and those who died of natural causes. Suicide completers who experienced childhood abuse were found to have increased cytosine methylation of the exon $1_F NR3C1$ promoter, which is associated with the expression of glucocorticoid receptors, than nonmaltreated suicide completers and those who died of natural causes. Increased methylation of the exon $1_F NR3C1$ promoter was associated with decreased hippocampal $NR3C1$ gene expression (McGowan et al., 2009). Similarly, Romens et al. (2015) found that adolescents who experienced physical maltreatment also had more methylation of the exon $1_F NR3C1$ promoter in whole blood. Overall, these findings suggest that early adversity has a lasting impact on the hippocampus and HPA axis.

Telomere length has also been associated with early adversity and maternal care. Telomeres are short deoxyribonucleic acid (DNA) regions located at the ends of the chromosome that primarily serve to protect genomic DNA during replication (Blackburn, 2001). Under normative conditions, telomere length will decrease with each replication cycle (McEachern, Krauskopf, & Blackburn, 2000). However, various cellular stressors, such as oxidative stress, increase the rate of telomere attrition (von Zglinicki, 2002). Telomere length in adulthood has been associated with early life stress, such as retrospective reports of maltreatment, trauma, familial mental illness, and parental unemployment (Kananen et al., 2010; Kiecolt-Glaser et al., 2011; O'Donovan et al., 2011; Tyrka et al., 2010).

In childhood, increased exposure to violence is associated with shorter telomere length (Shalev et al., 2012). In a study of Romanian adoptees, Drury et al. (2011) found that length of time spent in institutional care was inversely associated with telomere length. Asok, Bernard, Roth, Rosen, and Dozier (2013) found that children living with high-risk birth parents had shorter telomeres than low-risk children. In fact, findings from Asok et al. (2013) emphasize the buffering ability of maternal care. High-risk children who had sensitive, responsive mothers had longer telomeres than high-risk children who did not experience responsive parenting. These methodologies demonstrate that early adversity results in pervasive changes across behavioral and biological systems.

Interventions

When infants experience early adversity, they are at risk for problems developing organized attachments, and for challenges in developing adequate self-regulatory capabilities. Several evidence-based interventions have been developed that explicitly target these issues among infants and young children. Given infants' dependence on caregivers, these early intervention programs always focus on the caregiver–infant relationship as the mechanism of change to a greater or lesser extent.

Attachment and Biobehavioral Catch-up (ABC) specifically works to enhance attachment organization and children's regulatory capabilities through a 10-session in-home intervention for children ages 6 months to 2 years who have experienced early adversity (Dozier & The Infant Caregiver Project, 2013). Attachment is targeted through helping parents behave in nurturing ways when their children are distressed (Ainsworth et al., 1978), and regulatory capabilities are targeted through helping parents follow the lead of their children effectively (Calkins, 1994; Calkins & Keane, 2009; Calkins, Smith, Gill, & Johnson, 1998). The intervention has proven effective through several randomized clinical trials. Parents in the ABC intervention group follow infants' lead more, delight more in their children, and are less intrusive than parents in the control intervention group (Bick & Dozier, 2013; Meade et al., 2014). Infants randomly assigned to the ABC intervention showed lower levels of disorganized attachment and higher levels of secure attachment than infants randomly assigned to Developmental Education for Families (DEF) (Bernard et al., 2012). Indeed, of the ABC children, only 32% had disorganized attachments, as contrasted with 57% of the children in the control intervention group.

Infants in the ABC intervention also showed more normative diurnal cortisol production than infants in the DEF intervention (Bernard, Dozier, et al., 2014; Bernard, Hostinar, & Dozier, 2015). More specifically, ABC children showed high wake-up values and a steeper slope from morning to evening than children in the treatment control group when assessed shortly after the intervention's completion (Bernard, Dozier, et al., 2014). These effects were sustained more than 2 years after the intervention when children were assessed at the age of 4 (Bernard, Hostinar, et al., 2015). Again, children in the ABC group showed higher wake-up values and steeper slope than children in the control intervention group. These differences parallel those seen by Fisher, Stoolmiller, Gunnar, and Burraston (2007) among older children.

Differences are also seen in affect expression, with children in the ABC group showing less anger in a frustrating task than children in the control group (Lind, Bernard, Ross, & Dozier, 2014). Finally, children in the ABC group show better executive functioning than children in the control group, shifting between categorizing by dimensions of shape or color more effectively when required (Lewis-Morrarty, Dozier, Bernard, Terraciano, & Moore, 2012).

Child–parent psychotherapy (CPP) is a more time-intensive intervention than ABC that targets some of the same intervention goals, including children's attachment organization and, perhaps more indirectly, self-regulation for children from birth through age 5 (Lieberman, Ippen, & Van Horn, 2006). Although often delivered in the home, CPP can also be delivered in an office or clinic setting. CPP focuses more on parents' experiences of trauma and earlier attachment experiences as a mechanism for parental behavioral change than does ABC. CPP was more effective than a control in reducing disorganized attachments (Cicchetti et al., 2006). Children who received CPP showed more positive self-representations and fewer posttraumatic stress disorder symptoms than children in a control condition (Lieberman et al., 2006; Toth, Maughan, Manly, Spagnola, & Cicchetti, 2002).

A third intervention that targets key attachment and self-regulation issues in children 0 to 5 is Circle of Security (Hoffman et al., 2006). Circle of Security is typically implemented in groups in an office-based setting. Assessments of children's attachments are conducted at the beginning of treatment, which guide the work conducted during the intervention. A premise of the intervention is that parents typically have difficulty in either nurturing their distressed child, or supporting their child in exploration. Parents are helped to see, through observations of their behavior with their child and through discussion of past challenges in life, which challenge is more salient for them. A pre-/post-intervention test of the intervention's effectiveness has been conducted (Hoffman et al., 2006). More of the children showed secure attachments at post-intervention than at pre-intervention. To make the intervention more accessible and affordable than the full version, the developers designed a DVD version that does not require as high a level of training and supervision as the original.

There are other interventions that have been developed for infants who have experienced adversity that have effects on infant attachment or self-regulation, or associated variables. The interventions described here, though, present examples of the range of interventions, and generally have the strongest evidence base.

Conclusions

Early adversity has significant deleterious effects on infants' ability to organize attachment, as well as on their ability to regulate biology, emotions, and behavior. Caregivers are essential coregulators for children, and when they cannot function effectively in that capacity, there are serious consequences for infants and young children. Effects are seen especially in systems that are highly dependent on input from caregivers during early development, such as attachment, emotion regulation, and HPA regulation. Plasticity in these systems is apparent in effects of adversity, and in effects of remediation.

The next generation of research on early neglect and maltreatment is likely to continue to examine the effects of social environments on biological development in infancy. Due to advances in biological methodologies, including increasingly accessible sampling techniques, the field of infant research can incorporate novel biomarkers of stress into research on early adversity. Such biomarkers include gene expression, immune function, and epigenetic change, including DNA methylation and microribonucleic acid (RNA) regulation. Whereas these markers have been shown to be affected by neglect and maltreatment in studies involving rodents, nonhuman primates, and human adults (Caspi et al., 2002; Roth, Lubin, Funk, & Sweatt, 2008; Szyf & Bick, 2013), research among human infants is sparse. By including these various forms of measurement in future projects, the importance of issues such as early adversity, enhanced parenting, and timing will provide important insights on infants' and young children's developing biological and brain systems.

Whereas various preventative interventions have been shown to be effective in changing parent behaviors and child outcomes, many questions remain. One such question involves the duration of positive outcomes from such treatments. Longitudinal research is under way to examine the effects of ABC on key developmental tasks in middle childhood, including peer relations, executive functioning, and emotion regulation. Additional questions surround processes and mechanisms of change during early attachment interventions. Meade et al. (2014) found that when interventionists provided more active feedback regarding key parental behaviors, parents showed more change than when interventionists provided less frequent feedback (Meade et al., 2014). Such findings will help the field optimize the delivery of early interventions.

REFERENCES

Ainsworth, M. D. S., Blehar, M. C., Waters, E., & Wall, S. (1978). *Patterns of attachment: A psychological study of the Strange Situation.* Hillsdale, NJ: Erlbaum.

Appleyard, K., Egeland, B., van Dulmen, M. H. M., & Sroufe, L. A. (2005). When more is not better: The role of cumulative risk in child behavior outcomes. *Journal of Child Psychology and Psychiatry, 46,* 235–245.

Asok, A., Bernard, K., Roth, T. L., Rosen, J. B., & Dozier, M. (2013). Parental responsiveness moderates the association between early-life stress and reduced telomere
length. *Development and Psychopathology, 25*(3), 577–585.

Barr, R. G., Trent, R. B., & Cross, J. (2006). Age-related incidence curve of hospitalized
shaken baby syndrome cases: Convergent evidence for crying as a trigger to shaking. *Child Abuse and Neglect, 30*(1), 7–16.

Berlin, L. J., & Cassidy, J. (2003). Mothers' self-reported control of their preschool children's emotional expressiveness: A longitudinal study of associations with infant–
mother attachment and children's emotion regulation. *Social Development, 12*,
477–495.

Bernard, K., Butzin-Dozier, Z., Rittenhouse, J., & Dozier, M. (2010). Young children
living with neglecting birth parents show more blunted daytime patterns of cortisol production than children in foster care and comparison children. *Archives of
Pediatrics and Adolescent Medicine, 164*, 438–443.

Bernard, K., & Dozier, M. (2010). Examining infants' cortisol responses to laboratory
tasks among children varying in attachment disorganization: Stress reactivity or
return to baseline? *Developmental Psychology, 46*(6), 1771.

Bernard, K., Dozier, M., Bick, J., & Gordon, K. M. (2014). Normalizing blunted diurnal cortisol rhythms among children at risk for neglect: The effects of an early
intervention. *Development and Psychopathology, 8*, 1–13.

Bernard, K., Dozier, M., Bick, J., Lewis-Morrarty, E., Lindhiem, O., & Carlson, E.
(2012). Enhancing attachment organization among maltreated infants: Results of
a randomized clinical trial. *Child Development, 83*, 623–636.

Bernard, K., Hostinar, C., & Dozier, M. (2015). Intervention effects on diurnal cortisol
rhythms of CPS-referred infants persist into early childhood: Preschool follow-up
results of a randomized clinical trial. *JAMA Pediatrics, 169*, 112–119.

Bick, J., & Dozier, M. (2013). The effectiveness of an attachment-based intervention in
promoting foster mothers' sensitivity toward foster infants. *Infant Mental Health
Journal, 34*, 95–103.

Blackburn, E. H. (2001). Switching and signaling at the telomere. *Cell, 106*(6), 661–673.

Bowlby, J. (1969/1982). *Attachment and loss* (Vol. 1). London: Hogarth Press.

Bruce, J., Fisher, P. A., Pears, K. C., & Levine, S. (2009). Morning cortisol levels in
preschool-aged foster children: Differential effects of maltreatment type. *Developmental Psychobiology, 51*, 14–23.

Bruce, J., Kroupina, M., Parker, S., & Gunnar, M. (2000). *The relationships between
cortisol patterns, growth retardation, and developmental delays in postinstitutionalized children.* Paper presented at the International Conference on Infant
Studies, Brighton, UK.

Calkins, S. D. (1994). Origins and outcomes of individual differences in emotion regulation. *Monographs of the Society for Research in Child Development, 59*, 53–72.

Calkins, S. D., Gill, K. L., Johnson, M. C., & Smith, C. L. (2001). Emotional reactivity
and emotion regulation strategies as predictors of social behavior with peers during toddlerhood. *Social Development, 8*, 310–334.

Calkins, S. D., & Keane, S. P. (2009). Developmental origins of early antisocial behavior. *Development and Psychopathology, 21*, 1095–1109.

Calkins, S. D., Smith, C. L., Gill, K. L., & Johnson, M. C. (1998). Maternal interactive style across contexts: Relations to emotional, behavioral and physiological regulation during toddlerhood. *Social Development, 7*, 350–369.

Carlson, E. A. (1998). A prospective longitudinal study of attachment disorganization/disorientation. *Child Development, 69*(4), 1107–1128.

Carlson, M., & Earls, F. (1997). Psychological and neuroendocrinological sequelae of early social deprivation in institutionalized children in Romania. *Annals of the New York Academy of Sciences, 807*(1), 419–428.

Carlson, V., Cicchetti, D., Barnett, D., & Braunwald, K. (1989). Disorganized/disoriented attachment relationships in maltreated infants. *Developmental Psychology, 25*(4), 525.

Caspi, A., McClay, J., Moffitt, T. E., Mill, J., Martin, J., Craig, I. W., et al. (2002). Role of genotype in the cycle of violence in maltreated children. *Science, 297*, 851–854.

Cassidy, J. (1994). Emotion regulation: Influences of attachment relationships. *Monographs of the Society for Research in Child Development, 59*, 228–249.

Chapman, D. P., Anda, R. F., Felitti, V. J., Dube, S. R., Edwards, V. J., & Whitfield, C. L. (2004). Adverse childhood experiences and the risk of depressive disorders in adulthood. *Journal of Affective Disorders, 82*, 217–225.

Child Abuse Prevention and Treatment Act of 2010, Pub. L. No. 93-247. (2010). Reauthorization Act of 2010. Retrieved March 9, 2014, from *www.govtrack.us/congress/bills/111*

Christian, C. W., Block, R., & The Committee on Child Abuse and Neglect. (2009). Abusive head trauma in infants and children. *Pediatrics, 123*, 1409–1411.

Cicchetti, D., Ackerman, B. P., & Izard, C. E. (1995). Emotions and emotion regulation in developmental psychopathology. *Development and Psychopathology, 7*, 1–10.

Cicchetti, D., Rogosch, F. A., & Toth, S. L. (2006). Fostering secure attachments in infants in maltreating families through preventive interventions. *Development and Psychopathology, 18*, 623–649.

Cole, P. M., Armstrong, L. M., & Pemberton, C. K. (2010). Language and emotion. In M. A. Bell & S. D. Calkins (Eds.), *Child development at the intersection of emotion and cognition*. Washington, DC: American Psychological Association.

Cole, P. M., Luby, J., & Sullivan, M. W. (2008). Emotions and the development of childhood depression: Bridging the gap. *Child Development Perspectives, 2*, 141–148.

Cole, P. M., Michel, M. K., & Teti, L. O. (1994). The development of emotion regulation and dysregulation: A clinical perspective. *Monographs of the Society for Research in Child Development, 59*, 73–100.

Cole, P. M., Tan, P. Z., Hall, S. E., Zhang, Y., Crnic, K. A., Blair, C. B., et al. (2011). Developmental changes in anger expression and attention focus: Learning to wait. *Developmental Psychology, 47*, 1078–1089.

Cyr, C., Euser, E. M., Bakermans-Kranenburg, M. J., & van IJzendoorn, M. H. (2010). Attachment security and disorganization in maltreating and high-risk families: A series of meta-analyses. *Development and Psychopathology, 22*, 87–108.

Diener, M. L., Mangelsdorf, S. C., McHale, J. L., & Frosch, C. A. (2002). Infants' behavioral strategies for emotion regulation with fathers and mothers: Associations with emotional expressions and attachment quality. *Infancy, 3*, 153–174.

Dong, M., Anda, R. F., Dube, S. R., Giles, W. H., & Felitti, V. J. (2003). The relationship of exposure to childhood sexual abuse to other forms of abuse, neglect, and household dysfunction during childhood. *Child Abuse and Neglect, 27*(6), 625–639.

Dong, M., Anda, R. F., Felitti, V. J., Dube, S. R., Williamson, D. F., Thompson, T. J., et al. (2004). The interrelatedness of multiple forms of childhood abuse, neglect, and household dysfunction. *Child Abuse and Neglect, 28*(7), 771–784.

Dozier, M., & The Infant Caregiver Project. (2013). *Attachment and Biobehavioral Catch-up.* Unpublished manuscript, University of Delaware.

Dozier, M., Kaufman, J., Kobak, R. R., O'Connor, T. G., Sagi-Schwartz, A., Scott, S., et al. (2014). Consensus statement on group care for children and adolescents. *American Journal of Orthopsychiatry, 84,* 219–225.

Dozier, M., Stovall, K. C., Albus, K. E., & Bates, B. (2001). Attachment for infants in foster care: The role of caregiver state of mind. *Child Development, 72,* 1467–1477.

Dozier, M., Zeanah, C. H., Wallin, A. R., & Shauffer, C. (2012). Institutional care for young children: Review of literature and policy implications. *Social Issues and Policy Review, 6,* 1–25.

Drury, S. S., Theall, K., Gleason, M. M., Smyke, A. T., De Vivo, I., Wong, J. Y. Y., et al. (2011). Telomere length and early severe social deprivation: Linking early adversity and cellular aging. *Molecular Psychiatry, 17*(7), 719–727.

Eisenberg, N., & Fabes, R. A. (Eds.). (1992). *Emotion and its regulation in early development: New directions for child development: No. 55.* San Francisco: Jossey-Bass.

Eisenberg, N., Gershoff, E. T., Fabes, R. A., Shepard, S. A., Cumberland, A. J., Losoya, S. H., et al. (2001). Mother's emotional expressivity and children's behavior problems and social competence: Mediation through children's regulation. *Developmental Psychology, 37*(4), 475.

Fearon, R. P., Bakermans-Kranenburg, M. J., van IJzendoorn, M. H., Lapsley, A. M., & Roisman, G. I. (2010). The significance of insecure attachment and disorganization in the development of children's externalizing behavior: A meta-analytic study. *Child Development, 81,* 435–456.

Feldman, R. (2006). From biological rhythms to social rhythms: Physiological precursors of mother–infant synchrony. *Developmental Psychology, 42,* 175–188.

Feldman, R., & Eidelman, A. I. (2004). Parent–infant synchrony and the social-emotional development of triplets. *Developmental Psychology, 40,* 1133–1147.

Feldman, R., & Greenbaum, C. W. (1997). Affect regulation and synchrony in mother–infant play as precursors to the development of symbolic competence. *Infant Mental Health Journal, 18,* 4–23.

Fisher, P. A., Gunnar, M. R., Dozier, M., Bruce, J., & Pears, K. C. (2006). Effects of therapeutic interventions for foster children on behavioral problems, caregiver attachment, and stress regulatory neural systems. *Annals of the New York Academy of Sciences, 1094*(1), 215–225.

Fisher, P. A., Stoolmiller, M., Gunnar, M. R., & Burraston, B. O. (2007). Effects of a therapeutic intervention for foster preschoolers on diurnal cortisol activity. *Psychoneuroendocrinology, 32,* 892–905.

Francis, D., Diorio, J., Liu, D., & Meaney, M. J. (1999). Nongenomic transmission across generations of maternal behavior and stress responses in the rat. *Science, 286,* 1155–1158.

Gottman, J. M., Katz, L. F., & Hooven, C. (1997). *Meta-emotion: How families communicate emotionally.* Mahwah, NJ: Earlbaum.

Gunnar, M., & Quevedo, K. (2007). The neurobiology of stress and development. *Annual Review of Psychology, 58,* 145–173.

Gunnar, M. R., & Cheatham, C. L. (2003). Brain and behavior interface: Stress and the developing brain. *Infant Mental Health Journal, 24*(3), 195–211.

Gunnar, M. R., & Donzella, B. (2002). Social regulation of the cortisol levels in early human development. *Psychoneuroendocrinology, 27*(1), 199–220.

Gunnar, M. R., Fisher, P. A., & The Early Experience, Stress, and Prevention Network. (2006). Bringing basic research on early experience and stress neurobiology to bear on preventive interventions for neglected and maltreated children. *Development and Psychopathology, 18,* 651–677.

Gunnar, M. R., & Vazquez, D. M. (2001). Low cortisol and a flattening of expected daytime rhythm: Potential indices of risk in human development. *Development and Psychopathology, 13*(3), 515–538.

Hane, A. A., & Fox, N. A. (2006). Ordinary variations in maternal caregiving influence human infants' stress reactivity. *Psychological Science, 17,* 550–556.

Harlow, H. F., Dodsworth, R. O., & Harlow, M. K. (1965). Total social isolation in monkeys. *Proceedings of the National Academy of Sciences of the United States of America, 54,* 90–97.

Hertsgaard, L., Gunnar, M., Erickson, M. F., & Nachmias, M. (1995). Adrenocortical responses to the Strange Situation in infants with disorganized/disoriented attachment relationships. *Child Development, 66*(4), 1100–1106.

Hesse, E., & Main, M. (2000). Disorganized infant, child and adult attachment: Collapse in behavioral and attentional strategies. *Journal of the American Psychoanalytic Assocation, 48,* 1097–1127.

Hesse, E., & Main, M. (2006). Frightening, threatening, and dissociative behavior in low-risk parents: Description, discussion, and interpretations. *Development and Psychopathology, 18,* 309–343.

Hillis, S. D., Anda, R. F., Dube, S. R., Felitti, V. J., Marchbanks, P. A., & Marks, J. S. (2004). The association between adverse childhood experiences and adolescent pregnancy, long-term psychosocial outcomes, and fetal death. *Pediatrics, 113,* 320–327.

Hofer, M. (1994). Hidden regulators in attachment, separation, and loss. *Monographs of the Society for Research in Child Development, 59,* 192–207.

Hofer, M. (2006). Psychobiological roots of early attachment. *Current Directions in Psychological Science, 15,* 84–88.

Hoffman, K. T., Marvin, R. S., Cooper, G., & Powell, B. (2006). Changing toddlers' and preschoolers' attachment classifications: The Circle of Security intervention. *Journal of Consulting and Clinical Psychology, 74*(6), 1017.

Hrdy, S. B. (1999). *Mother nature: Maternal instincts and how they shape the human species.* New York: Ballantine Books.

Institute of Medicine. (2013). *New directions in child abuse and neglect research.* Washington DC: National Academies Press.

Johnson, D. E., Guthrie, D., Smyke, A. T., Koga, S. F., Fox, N. A., Zeanah, C. H., et al. (2010). Growth and associations between auxology, caregiving environment, and cognition in socially deprived Romanian children randomized to foster vs. ongoing institutional care. *Archives of Pediatrics and Adolescent Medicine, 164*(6), 507–516.

Kananen, L., Surakka, I., Pirkola, S., Suvisaari, J., Lönnqvist, J., Peltonen, L., et al. (2010). Childhood adversities are associated with shorter telomere length at adult age both in individuals with an anxiety disorder and controls. *PLoS ONE, 5*(5), e10826.

Kiecolt-Glaser, J. K., Gouin, J. P., Weng, N. P., Malarkey, W. B., Beversdorf, D. Q., & Glaser, R. (2011). Childhood adversity heightens the impact of later-life caregiving stress on telomere length and inflammation. *Psychosomatic Medicine, 73*(1), 16–22.

Kim, J., & Cicchetti, D. (2010). Longitudinal pathways linking child maltreatment, emotion regulation, peer relations, and psychopathology. *Journal of Psychology and Psychiatry, 51*, 706–716.

Klinnert, M. D., Campos, J. J., Sorce, J. F., Emde, R. N., & Svejda, M. (1983). Emotions as behavior regulators: Social referencing in infancy. In R. Plutchik & H. Kellerman (Eds.), *Emotion: Theory, research and experience* (Vol. 2, pp. 57–86). New York: Academic Press.

Kopp, C. B. (1982). Antecedents of self-regulation: A developmental perspective. *Developmental Psychology, 18*, 199–215.

Kopp, C. B. (1989). Regulation of distress and negative emotions: A developmental view. *Developmental Psychology, 25*(3), 343–354.

Kopp, C. B. (2009). Emotion-focused coping in young children: Self and self-regulatory processes. *New Directions for Child and Adolescent Development, 124*, 33–46.

Kroupina, M., Gunnar, M. R., & Johnson, D. E. (1997). *Report on salivary cortisol levels in a Russian baby home.* Minneapolis: University of Minnesota, Institute of Child Development.

Lee, C., Barr, R. G., Catherine, N., & Wicks, A. (2007). Age-related incidence of publicly reported shaken baby syndrome cases: Is crying a trigger for shaking? *Journal of Developmental and Behavioral Pediatrics, 28*, 288–293.

Leiden Conference on the Development and Care of Children without Permanent Parents. (2012). The development and care of institutionally reared children. *Child Development Perspectives, 6*, 174–180.

Lelwica, J. M., & Haviland, M. (1987). The induced affect response: 10-week-old infants' responses to three emotion expressions. *Developmental Psychology, 23*, 97–104.

Levine, S. (2005). Developmental determinants of sensitivity and resistance to stress. *Psychoneuroendocrinology, 30*(10), 939–946.

Levine, S., Wiener, S. G., & Coe, C. L. (1993). Temporal and social factors influencing behavioral and hormonal responses to separation in mother and infant squirrel monkeys. *Psychoneuroendocrinology, 18*(4), 297–306.

Lewis, E., Dozier, M., Ackerman, J., & Sepulveda-Kozakowski, S. (2007). The effect of placement instability on adopted children's inhibitory control abilities and oppositional behavior. *Developmental Psychology, 43*, 1415–1427.

Lewis-Morrarty, E., Dozier, M., Bernard, K., Terraciano, S., & Moore, S. (2012). Cognitive flexibility and theory of mind outcomes among foster children: Preschool follow-up results of a randomized clinical trial. *Journal of Adolescent Health, 52,* S17–S22.

Lieberman, A. F., Ippen, C. G., & Van Horn, P. (2006). Child–parent psychotherapy: 6-month follow up of a randomized controlled trial. *Journal of the American Academy of Child and Adolescent Psychiatry, 45,* 913–918.

Lind, T., Bernard, K., Ross, E., & Dozier, M. (2014). Interaction effects on negative affect of CPS-referred children: Results of a randomized clinical trial. *Child Abuse and Neglect, 38,* 1459–1467.

Lunkenheimer, E. S., Shields, A. M., & Cortina, K. S. (2007). Parental emotion coaching and dismissing in family interaction. *Social Development, 16,* 232–248.

Lyons-Ruth, K., Connell, D. B., Zoll, D., & Stahl, J. (1987). Infants at social risk: Relations among infant maltreatment, maternal behavior, and infant attachment behavior. *Developmental Psychology, 23,* 223–232.

Lyons-Ruth, K., Easterbrooks, M. A., & Cibelli, C. D. (1997). Infant attachment strategies, infant mental lag, and maternal depressive symptoms: Predictors of internalizing and externalizing problems at age 7. *Developmental Psychology, 33,* 681–692.

Main, M., & Solomon, J. (1990). Procedures for identifying infants as disorganized/disoriented during the Ainsworth Strange Situation. In M. T. Greenberg, D. Cicchetti, & E. Cummings (Eds.), *Attachment in the preschool years: Theory, research, and intervention* (pp. 161–182). Chicago: University of Chicago Press.

Malatesta, C. A., & Izard, C. E. (1984). The ontogenesis of human signals: From biological imperative to symbol utilization. In N. A. Fox & R. J. Davidson (Eds.), *The psychobiology of affective development* (pp. 161–206). Hillsdale, NJ: Erlbaum.

Maughan, A., & Cicchetti, D. (2002). Impact of child maltreatment and interadult violence on children's emotion regulation abilities and socioemotional adjustment. *Child Development, 73,* 1525–1542.

McEachern, M. J., Krauskopf, A., & Blackburn, E. H. (2000). Telomeres and their control. *Annual Review of Genetics, 34*(1), 331–358.

McGowan, P. O., Sasaki, A., D'Alessio, A. C., Dymov, S., Labonté, B., Szyf, M., et al. (2009). Epigenetic regulation of the glucocorticoid receptor in human brain associated with childhood abuse. *Nature Neuroscience, 12,* 342–348.

Meade, E. B., Weston-Lee, P., Haggerty, D., & Dozier, M. (2014). *Effectiveness of community implementation of Attachment and Biobehavioral Catch-up.* Unpublished manuscript, University of Delaware.

Mehta, M. A., Golembo, N. I., Nosarti, C., Colvert, E., Mota, A., Williams, S. C. R., et al. (2009). Amygdala, hippocampal and corpus callosum size following severe early institutional deprivation: The English and Romanian Adoptees Study pilot. *Journal of Child Psychology and Psychiatry, 50,* 943–951.

Milner, J. S. (2000). Social information processing and child physical abuse: Theory and research. In D. J. Hansen (Ed.), *Motivation and child maltreatment* (pp. 39–84). Lincoln: University of Nebraska Press.

Moore, G. A., & Calkins, S. D. (2004). Infants' vagal regulation in the still-face paradigm is related to dyadic coordination of mother–infant interaction. *Developmental Psychology, 40,* 1068–1080.

Mueller, S. C., Maheu, F. S., Dozier, M., Peloso, E., Mandell, D., Leibenluft, E., et al.

(2010). Early-life stress is associated with impairment in cognitive control in adolescence: An fMRI study. *Neuropsychologia, 48,* 3037–3044.

Nelson, C. A., Fox, N. A., & Zeanah, C. H. (2014). *Romania's adopted children: Deprivation, brain development, and the struggle for recovery.* Boston: Harvard University Press.

Nelson, C. A., Zeanah, C. H., Fox, N. A., Marshall, P. J., Smyke, A. T., & Guthrie, D. (2007). Cognitive recovery in socially deprived young children: The Bucharest Early Intervention Project. *Science, 318,* 1937–1940.

O'Donovan, A., Epel, E., Lin, J., Wolkowitz, O., Cohen, B., Maguen, S., et al. (2011). Childhood trauma associated with short leukocyte telomere length in posttraumatic stress disorder. *Biological Psychiatry, 70*(5), 465–471.

Panksepp, J. (2001). The long-term psychobiological consequences of infant emotions: Prescriptions for the twenty-first century [Special issue]. *Infant Mental Health Journal, 22,* 132–173.

Pinheiro, P. S. (2006). *World report on violence against children: United Nations secretary-general's study on violence against children.* New York: United Nations.

Rogosch, F. A., Cicchetti, D., & Aber, J. L. (1995). The role of child maltreatment in early deviations in cognitive and affective processing abilities and later peer relationship problems [Special issue]. *Development and Psychopathology, 7,* 591–609.

Romens, S. E., McDonald, J., Svaren, J., & Pollak, S. D. (2015). Associations between early life stress and gene methylation in children. *Child Development, 86,* 303309.

Roth, T. L., Lubin, F. D., Funk, A. J., & Sweatt, J. D. (2008). Lasting epigenetic influence of early-life adversity on the BDNF gene. *Biological Psychiatry, 65,* 760–769.

Saarni, C. (1999). *The development of emotional competence.* New York: Guilford Press.

Sameroff, A. J., Bartko, W. T., Baldwin, A., Baldwin, C., & Seifer, R. (1998). Family and social influences on the development of child competence. In M. Lewis & C. Feiring (Eds.), *Families, risk, and competence* (pp. 161–185). Mahwah, NJ: Erlbaum.

Sameroff, A. J., & Chandler, M. J. (1975). Reproductive risk and the continuum of caretaking casualty. In. F. D. Horowitz, M. Hetherington, S. Scarr-Salapatek, & G. Sigel (Eds.), *Review of child development research* (Vol. 4, pp. 187–244). Chicago: University of Chicago Press.

Schuengel, C., Bakermans-Kranenburg, M. J., & Van IJzendoorn, M. H. (1999). Frightening maternal behavior linking unresolved loss and disorganized infant attachment. *Journal of Consulting and Clinical Psychology, 67,* 54–63.

Shalev, I., Moffitt, T. E., Sugden, K., Williams, B., Houts, R. M., Danese, A., et al. (2012). Exposure to violence during childhood is associated with telomere erosion from 5 to 10 years of age: A longitudinal study. *Molecular Psychiatry, 18*(5), 576–581.

Shaw, D. S., Keenan, K., & Vondra, J. I. (1994). Developmental precursors of externalizing behavior: Ages 1 to 3. *Developmental Psychology, 30,* 355–364.

Shaw, D. S., Winslow, E. B., Owens, E. B., Vondra, J. I., Cohn, J. F., & Bell, R. Q. (1998). The development of early externalizing problems among children from low-income families: A transformational perspective. *Journal of Abnormal Child Psychology, 26,* 95–107.

Shipman, K. L., Schneider, R., Fitzgerald, M. M., Sims, C., Swisher, L., & Edwards, A. (2007). Maternal emotion socialization in maltreating and non-maltreating families: Implications for children's emotion regulation. *Social Development, 16*(2), 268–285.

Shipman, K. L., & Zeman, J. (2001). Socialization of children's emotion regulation in mother–child dyads: A developmental psychopathology perspective. *Development and Psychopathology, 13*, 317–336.

Shonkoff, J., & Phillips, D. (Eds.). (2000). *From neurons to neighborhoods: Science of early childhood development.* Washington, DC: National Academy Press.

Smith, E. P. (1995). Bring back the orphanges: What policymakers of today can learn from the past. *Child Welfare, 74*, 115–142.

Smyke, A. T., Koga, S. F., Johnson, D. E., Fox, N. A., Marshall, P. J., Nelson, C. A., et al. (2007). The caregiving context in institution-reared and family-reared infants and toddlers in Romania. *Journal of Child Psychology and Psychiatry, 48*, 210–218.

Smyke, A. T., Zeanah, C. H., Fox, N. A., Nelson, C. A., & Guthrie, D. (2010). Placement in foster care enhances quality of attachment among young institutionalized children. *Child Development, 81*(1), 212–223.

Spangler, G., & Grossmann, K. E. (1993). Biobehavioral organization in securely and insecurely attached infants. *Child Development, 64*(5), 1439–1450.

Sroufe, L. A. (1996). *Emotional development.* New York: Cambridge University Press.

Stovall, K. C., & Dozier, M. (2000). The development of attachment in new relationships: Single subject analyses for 10 foster infants. *Development and Psychopathology, 12*, 133–156.

Stovall-McClough, K. C., & Dozier, M. (2004). Forming attachments in foster care: Infant attachment behaviors during the first 2 months of placement. *Development and Psychopathology, 16*, 253–271.

Suomi, S. J. (1997). Early determinants of behaviour: Evidence from primate studies. *British Medical Bulletin, 53*, 170–184.

Szyf, M., & Bick, J. (2013). DNA methylation: A mechanism for embedding early life experiences in the genome. *Child Development, 84*(1), 49–57.

Thompson, R. A. (1994). Emotion regulation: A theme in search of definition. *Monographs of the Society for Research in Child Development, 59*, 250–283.

Toth, S. L., Maughan, A., Manly, J. T., Spagnola, M., & Cicchetti, D. (2002). The relative efficacy of two interventions in altering maltreated preschool children's representational models: Implications for attachment theory. *Development and Psychopathology, 14*(4), 877–908.

Tottenham, N., Hare, T. A., Quinn, B. T., McCarry, T. W., Nurse, M., Gilhooly, T., et al. (2010). Prolonged institutional rearing is associated with atypically larger amygdala volume and difficulties in emotion regulation. *Developmental Science, 13*, 46–61.

Tronick, E. Z. (1989). Emotions and emotional communication in infants [Special issue]. *American Psychologist, 44*, 112–119.

Tyrka, A. R., Price, L. H., Kao, H. T., Porton, B., Marsella, S. A., & Carpenter, L. L. (2010). Childhood maltreatment and telomere shortening: Preliminary support for an effect of early stress on cellular aging. *Biological Psychiatry, 67*(6), 531–534.

U.S. Department of Health and Human Services, Administration on Children, Youth and Families. (2013). *Trends in foster care and adoption*. Washington, DC: U.S. Government Printing Office.

van den Dries, L., Juffer, F., van IJzendoorn, M. H., & Bakermans-Kranenburg, M. J. (2009). Fostering security?: A meta-analysis of attachment in adopted children. *Child and Youth Services Review, 31*, 410–421.

van IJzendoorn, M. H., Schuengel, C., & Bakermans-Kranenburg, M. J. (1999). Disorganized attachment in early childhood: Meta-analysis of precursors, concomitants, and sequelae. *Development and Psychopathology, 11*, 225–249.

Volling, B. L., McElwain, N. L., Notaro, P. C., & Herrera, C. (2002). Parents' emotional availability and infant emotional competence: Predictors of parent–infant attachment and emerging self-regulation. *Journal of Family Psychology, 16*, 447–465.

von Zglinicki, T. (2002). Oxidative stress shortens telomeres. *Trends in Biochemical Sciences, 27*(7), 339–344.

Vondra, J. I., Shaw, D. S., Swearingen, L., Cohen, M., & Owens, E. B. (2001). Attachment stability and emotional and behavioral regulation from infancy to preschool age. *Development and Psychopathology, 13*, 13–33.

Weaver, I. C. G., Cervoni, N., Champagne, F. A., D'Alessio, A. C., Sharma, S., Seckl, J. R., et al. (2004). Epigenetic programming by maternal behavior. *Nature Neuroscience, 7*, 847–854.

Zeanah, C. H., Smyke, A. T., Koga, S. F., & Carlson, E. (2005). Attachment in institutionalized and community children in Romania. *Child Development, 76*, 1015–1028.

CHAPTER 16

The Social Ecology of Infant Sleep

Structural and Qualitative Features of Bedtime and Nighttime Parenting and Infant Sleep in the First Year

Douglas M. Teti, Lauren Philbrook, Mina Shimizu,
Jon Reader, Hye-Young Rhee, Brandon McDaniel, Brian Crosby,
Bo-Ram Kim, and Ni Jian

Good sleep plays a vitally important role in promoting physical and mental health and is essential for optimal child development (Lemola & Richter, 2013; El-Sheikh & Buckhalt, 2015). Persistent sleep problems in childhood are linked with child dysfunction across a broad spectrum, including concurrent daytime externalizing and internalizing behavioral problems (Sheridan et al., 2013), daytime sleepiness attentional and memory problems (Li et al., 2014; Huber & Born, 2014), and poor academic performance (Buckhalt & Staton, 2011). In addition, sleep disturbances in the preschool years predict heightened risk for alcohol and substance abuse in adolescence (Wong, Brower, Fitzgerald, & Zucker, 2004), and proneness to anxiety and depression in adulthood (Gregory, Caspi, Eley, Moffitt, & O'Connor, 2005).

Quality of sleep in childhood can also directly impact the larger family system. Although sleep regulation develops rapidly across the first year and proceeds well for many infants, for some infants it does not (Lee & Rosen, 2012). When it does not, it can have a profound and negative impact on parental well-being and the health of the family system. Sleep disturbances among infants are a chief complaint of parents during pediatric office visits (Boyle & Cropley,

2004), primarily because dysregulated infant sleep almost invariably leads to dysregulated sleep in at least one and frequently both parents. That in turn can place families in turmoil (Byars, Yeomans-Maldonado, & Noll, 2011; Mindell, 1999). Prevalence estimates of sleep problems range from less than 10 to 52% among children in the infancy and preschool years (Sadeh, Mindell, & Rivera, 2011), depending on who is doing the reporting and how sleep problems are defined.

There is evidence that sleep patterns observed in later childhood are rooted in sleep patterns first established in infancy (Scher, Epstein, & Tirosh, 2004), and that sleep in infancy and at later points in development is multiply determined by maturational, constitutional, and environmental forces (El-Sheikh & Sadeh, 2015). We provide in this chapter a detailed analysis of an important environmental influence—parenting—on sleep development in infancy. We do so, however, with explicit acknowledgment that infant sleep is complexly determined, with psychosocial influences in continual transaction with biological factors to shape infant sleep.

Development of Sleep in Infancy

Sleep development in the first year follows a predictable course. Whether measured objectively (e.g., actigraphy, polysomnogaphy, videosomnography) or via parent report, infant sleep shows dramatic consolidation across the first 4 months, as defined by (1) sharp decreases in frequency and duration of night awakenings; (2) increases in overall amounts of nighttime sleep and in the duration of individual sleep bouts; and (3) the development of the ability to "sleep through the night," a phrase commonly used by parents to denote the ability to (apparently) sleep continuously from the point of sleep onset at bedtime to the point of morning wake-up, without parental intervention (Henderson, France, & Blampied, 2011). This nocturnal period typically coincides with the period of nocturnal sleep of the parents. As the work of Anders (Anders, Halpern, & Hua, 1992) and others (e.g., Henderson, France, Owens, & Blampied, 2010) have shown, however, infants who sleep through the night have in reality developed self-regulated sleep, or the capacity to put themselves back to sleep after one or more nocturnal awakenings without signaling (i.e., crying or calling out) to the parents. By 6 months of age, this capacity is regularly observed in many infants, although sleep continues to develop and consolidate throughout infancy (and beyond) as evidenced by decreases across age in overall amounts of sleep (15–17 hours in the first month of life to about 14 hours by 12 months; Wolfson, 1996), by gradual decreases in the frequency and duration of daytime naps (Crosby, LeBourgeois, & Harsh, 2005), and by proportional increases in quiet sleep (akin to nonrapid eye movement [NREM] sleep) and decreases in active sleep (akin to rapid eye movement [REM] sleep) across the first year (So, Adamson, & Horne, 2007).

Central and autonomic nervous system maturation accounts for much of the consolidation of sleep across the first year (El-Sheikh, Erath, & Bagley, 2012; Huber & Born, 2014; Sheldon, 2014). At the same time, despite the strong influence of brain maturation on sleep development, sleep development does not always progress smoothly. Many infants, for example, are not sleeping through the night by 6 months of age, and it is estimated that between 25 and 33% of infants show sleep problems throughout the first year, ranging from frequent, signaled night awakenings to difficulties setting to sleep at bedtime or throughout the night (Mindell, Kuhn, Lewin, Meltzer, & Sadeh, 2006). Some of this variation can be traced directly to differences in brain development, as evidenced by elevated sleep problems among children with neurological disorders (Cotton & Richdale, 2006; Williams, Sears, & Allard, 2004). Infant sleep quality, however, has also been reliably linked with aspects of the physical environment, such as ambient noise and light levels (Franco et al., 1998; Harrison, 2004), and more complexly with features of the infant's social environment (Sadeh, Tikotsky, & Scher, 2010; Teti, Kim, Mayer, & Countermine, 2010). Indeed, like many developmental domains in early life, infant sleep can be placed at the center of broader social–ecological forces and can be influenced, directly and indirectly, by factors that are both "distal" (e.g., culture, socioeconomic status) and "proximal" (e.g., specific parenting practices, parenting quality) to the infant (Teti, Shimizu, Crosby, Kim, & Whitesell, 2014). In addition, infant sleep patterns may also strongly influence qualitative and structural aspects of family processes, as evidenced by the impact infant sleep difficulties can have on coparenting quality (McDaniel & Teti, 2012) and on parents' choices about how to structure infant sleep arrangements (Countermine & Teti, 2010; Ramos, Youngclarke, & Anderson, 2007). Sadeh and Anders (1993) proposed a transactional model of child sleep that emphasizes dynamic linkages among distal sociocultural factors, proximal parental factors, and child sleep outcomes, noting that infant sleep can be the outcome as well as a cause of family interactional patterns.

In the sections to follow, we explore the impact of what is emerging as a critically important proximal influence on infant sleep: parenting during infant bedtime and throughout the night. This chapter focuses on parenting practices, or *what* parents do, and parenting quality, or *how competently* parents do what they do. We discuss the relative impact of bedtime/nighttime practices on nighttime infant sleep quality as well as interlinkages between parenting quality and practices. We then broaden the focus to discuss bedtime/nighttime parenting in the context of the larger family system, with a discussion of how individual and marital distress may shape how parents structure infant sleep, what parents do with their infants at night, and how well they do it.

Bedtime and Nighttime Parenting: Practices, Quality, and Infant Sleep

Parental Involvement and Infant Self-Soothing

One of the major methodological limitations of extant research on parenting at bedtime and nighttime is an overreliance on parent report. This is likely due to the difficulties encountered in conducting bedtime and nighttime observations in the home. However, a relatively small but consistent body of literature, using direct observation, has examined associations between parenting practices and infant sleep in infancy, and we review those findings here. In their study of 21 infants across the first 8 months of life, Anders et al. (1992) used time-lapse video observations and found that infants who were put into their cribs at bedtime while still awake were more likely to put themselves back to sleep without parental intervention, following a night awakening, compared with infants who were asleep when put into their cribs at bedtime. Further, the 3-month-old infants who were asleep when put into their cribs at bedtime were likely to be removed from their cribs by their parents if they awakened during the night, compared with infants who were put into their cribs while still awake. By 8 months of age, 7 of the 21 infants (all male) were identified by parents as having sleep difficulties, and at bedtime all 7 of these infants were always put into their cribs after they had fallen asleep. These findings suggested that the act of placing an infant down to sleep while still awake promoted an ability in the infants to soothe themselves to sleep without parental intervention, not just when first going to sleep at night but throughout the night. The infants in Anders et al.'s study were all solitary sleepers, and it was unclear if this ability could be promoted equally well when infants and parents bed shared. Also unclear was whether the appearance of this ability early in life was developmentally significant, perhaps serving as a precursor of later (improved) capacities for behavioral and emotion regulation. This is an important question that to date has not been empirically examined.

In a later longitudinal study of 80 solitary-sleeping infants across the first year, Burnham, Goodlin-Jones, Gaylor, and Anders (2002) found that infants' capacity for self-soothing to sleep by 12 months was improved when parents' latency to respond to infant night awakenings at 3 months of age was longer, and when the time infants spent out of their crib decreased across the first year. These findings, along with those of Anders et al. (1992), suggested that self-regulated sleep in infants was best promoted by parenting that provided infants multiple opportunities to soothe themselves to sleep on their own, by putting them down to sleep at bedtime while still awake, by refraining from responding immediately to infant night awakenings, particularly early in life, and by structuring infant sleep so that infants spend the bulk of their time in their own cribs. These findings were supported by a later, large Internet-based study of over 5,000 U.S. and Canadian families with children 0–3 years of age, which reported that better consolidated and longer periods of nighttime infant sleep were associated with bedtime/nighttime parenting that encouraged infant self-soothing and independent sleep, compared with parenting characterized by frequent bouts of nighttime intervention and parent–child interaction (Sadeh, Mindell, Luedtke, & Wiegand, 2009).

We emphasize, however, that conclusions about whether or not parents should be structuring independent infant sleep, promoting infants' ability to soothe themselves to sleep, and so on are not without controversy. The efficacy of such practices may depend on context, cultural prescriptions, and parental beliefs and goals (Burnham, 2013; Giannotti & Cortesi, 2009; McKenna, Ball, & Gettler, 2007; Teti, Crosby, McDaniel, Shimizu, & Whitesell, 2015; Worthman, 2011). It may also depend on how infant sleep quality is actually assessed (i.e., whether it is measured using parental report or by some other means; Teti et al., 2014). We return to this point later in this chapter. At the least, however, these results called attention to the importance of examining patterns of parental behavior that take place between the infant at bedtime and throughout the night, patterns that may begin early in the first year, persist across time, and in turn may organize different patterns of sleep regulation in infants that are stable over time.

Bedtime Routines

A separate line of research has underscored the efficacy of bedtime structure and routines in promoting sleep quality and consolidation in infancy and early childhood. Hale, Berger, LeBourgeois, and Brooks-Gunn (2011) demonstrated that parents' use of "language-based" routines, such as storytelling, book reading, or singing, was predictive of longer sleep durations among 3-year-old children, and (interestingly) was associated with improved cognitive and socioemotional outcomes. The efficacy of bedtime routines is not limited, however, to routines that are exclusively language based. Using two separate samples (an infant, 7- to 18-month-old sample, $n = 206$; and a toddler–preschool 18- to 36-month-old sample, $n = 199$) and following a 1-week baseline data-gathering period (Week 1), Mindell, Telofski, Wiegand, and Kurtz (2009) assigned two-thirds of each sample to a 30-minute bedtime routine that was implemented nightly for the next 2 weeks (Week 2 and Week 3). For the infants, this routine consisted of (in order) a bath, a massage, then quiet activities (cuddling, singing a lullaby), followed by lights out. For the toddler–preschool group, the routine consisted of a bath, applying a body lotion, and then quiet activities, followed by lights out. Control children continued to receive their normal bedtime procedures.

Findings from this study were rather dramatic. From parent-reported daily diary data, children in both age groups assigned to the bedtime routine condition had significant decreases in latency to fall asleep and in frequency and duration of night awakenings, and increases in the longest sleep bout of the night, between baseline and either Week 2 or Week 3. Parents in the routine condition also rated their children as sleeping better, and in a better mood in the morning, than parents in the control condition. In addition, improvements in the mood states of mothers in the bedtime routine conditions (e.g., reduced tension, depression, anger, and fatigue) coincided with the improvements reported in their children's sleep. No changes, by contrast, were observed across the 3-week period in the sleep behavior of the control children, or in the mood states of their mothers. Collectively, these findings are consistent with other literature showcasing the benefits of predictable, daily routines on young children's capacity to engage with, understand, and predict their environment (Spagnola & Fiese, 2007). Daily nurturing routines practiced in sleep contexts likely foster children's perceptions that their sleep environment is predictable, controllable, and free of potential threats. It is perhaps not surprising that sleep quality, which requires one to relinquish consciousness and vigilance to achieve a state of deep sleep, is likely to be promoted under such conditions (Dahl & El-Sheikh, 2007; Teti et al., 2010), even in infancy, and that improvements in infant sleep quality are associated with improvements in maternal well-being.

Bedtime Parenting Quality, Parenting Practices, and Their Interaction

Surprisingly few studies have examined linkages between quality of parenting (i.e., warmth, sensitivity, emotional availability [EA]) and infant sleep, and only one published study, to our knowledge, has examined parenting quality at bedtime and infant sleep quality. That particular study, one of several emerging from the SIESTA research program (Teti, Principal Investigator), involved 45 infants and mothers, video recorded mothers' EA from video recordings of parenting during infant bedtimes, using a cross-sectional sample of infants at 1, 3, 6, 12, and 24 months of age (Teti et al., 2010). Small "bullet" video cameras (up to four per household) and accompanying microphones were channeled through a central digital video recorder, with one camera suspended above the infant's sleeping surface, another trained on the door of the room where the infant slept to ascertain who entered and exited the room, a third trained on any area of the infant's room that the parent had designated as a place he or she took the infant if the infant awakened during the night, and a fourth camera (if needed) set up in a separate room (e.g., the parent's room) the parent indicated was a room he or she used during nighttime infant awakenings. Parents were asked to start the recording approximately 1 hour before they began bedtime with their infant, and to end it when the infant woke up in the morning.

Teti et al.'s (2010) study drew from attachment theory (Ainsworth, Blehar, Waters, & Wall, 1978) and EA theory (Biringen, Derscheid, Vliegen, Closson, & Easterbrooks, 2014), proposing that sensitive, emotionally attuned parenting when putting infants to bed should promote in infants feelings of safety, security, and trust in their sleep environments, and in turn the ability to settle into and enjoy better-quality sleep than insensitive, emotionally unavailable parenting. It was thus predicted that emotionally available mothering during infant bedtimes would predict better-quality infant sleep throughout the night and greater infant capacities for soothing oneself to sleep, compared with emotionally unavailable mothering. Mothers' EA, which was a composite measure that combined ratings of maternal sensitivity, structuring, hostility (reverse scored), and intrusiveness (reverse scored) during infant bedtimes, was scored by two observers who were blind to all other data obtained on the mothers and infants. Infant sleep quality was assessed each day for 7 consecutive days using an infant sleep diary that asked mothers to report each morning on the frequency and duration of their infants' night awakenings the night before, and on the frequency with which parents had to return to tend to their infants before their infants fell asleep. Mothers were also asked to respond to the question "Do you think that your infant has sleeping difficulties?" using a 4-point scale (0 = *no*; 1 = *yes, mild*; 2 = *yes, moderate*; 3 = *yes, severe*).

As predicted, maternal EA at bedtime was inversely associated with the frequency of infant night awakenings and mothers' ratings of whether their infants had a sleep difficulty. These findings were consistent with predictions that emotionally available parenting at bedtime would predict improved sleep quality in infants (i.e., fewer awakenings) during the night, which appeared to spill over into maternal perceptions of their infants as good versus poor sleepers. Also consistent with predictions was the finding of the inverse association between emotionally available mothering and the frequency with which mothers had to return to their infants at bedtime, which we took as an index of the ease with which infants could go to sleep at bedtime on their own, without parental intervention.

To our knowledge, Teti et al. (2010) is the first study to assess linkages among parenting quality *at bedtime*, from direct observations, and infant sleep quality. Interestingly, other work that has assessed linkages between parenting quality in daytime contexts and infant sleep has not reported significant results. In a study of sleep patterns of 12-month-olds, Scher (2001) assessed mothers' EA during a daytime observation of mother–infant free play and found no association between EA and infant sleep regulation. In addition, Bordeleau, Bernier, and Carrier (2012) found no direct associations between a naturalistic, home assessment of maternal sensitivity, using the Maternal Behavior Q-Set (Pederson & Moran, 1995) and infant nighttime sleep duration assessed from a parent-reported infant sleep diary. The reasons for these discrepancies are unclear. Perhaps quality of daytime parenting in nonsleep contexts is not strongly linked to quality of parenting at infant bedtimes. Alternatively, infant bedtimes are clearly more temporally proximal to infant sleep behavior during the night, and thus bedtime parenting might be expected to have a stronger impact on infants' nighttime sleep behavior than parenting that occurs earlier in the day.

In a longitudinal study that has emerged from the SIESTA research program, bedtime parenting practices and parenting quality, again from direct observations obtained at infant bedtimes and throughout the night, were jointly examined as predictors of infant sleep quality across the infant ages of 1, 3, and 6 months (Philbrook et al., 2015). In this study of 95 infants and their parents, parenting practices and parenting quality (maternal EA) at infant bedtimes were scored to high levels of interrater reliability by separate teams of coders, and a third team of coders scored infant sleep from video recordings of infant sleep behavior throughout the ensuing night. All three teams of coders (bedtime parenting practices, bedtime parenting quality, and infant nighttime sleep behavior) were fully blind to the data being produced by the other coding teams. Bedtime practices that were scored included parental presence with the infant, parent–infant close physical contact, quiet activities (e.g., soft singing, book reading), arousing activities (highly verbal/physical stimulation of the infant), nursing, and parents' exclusive focus on the infant.

Noteworthy in this study was the finding that mothers' EA was highly stable across the first 6 months of life, and EA was significantly and positively associated with several parenting practices, including quiet activities (1 and 3 months) and exclusive focus on the infant (3 and 6 months; $ps < .05$). Maternal EA was inversely associated with the amount of arousing activities at 3 months and the amount of close parent–infant contact at 6 months ($ps < .05$). Thus, emotionally available mothers at bedtime were more likely to make use of quiet activities, to give their infants quality time and attention, and to refrain from overly stimulating their infants. Multilevel modeling analyses further demonstrated that infants of emotionally available mothers across the three time points spent less of the night distressed on average ($p < .001$) and spent more of the night asleep ($p < .01$). Additionally, infants of mothers who used less close contact at bedtime spent more time asleep ($p < .05$). There were also two interactions between maternal EA and parenting practices. Infants of mothers who were more emotionally available and used less close contact spent more of the nighttime asleep ($p < .05$), whereas infants of mothers who used more close contact spent less time asleep regardless of EA. Infants of mothers who were more emotionally available and less arousing at bedtime also spent more time asleep at night ($p < .01$), whereas infants of mothers who engaged in more arousing activities showed similar, lower nighttime sleep percentages regardless of EA.

To our knowledge, this study extends previous work and is the first to examine the joint contributions of parenting practices and parenting quality (scored from the same data stream) at bedtimes to infant sleep quality throughout the night. Replicating Teti et al. (2010), Philbrook et al. (2015) found that higher bedtime parenting quality was generally associated with better infant sleep quality, but especially so when mothers engaged in less close contact and arousing activities with their infants at bedtime.

Structuring Infant Sleep:
Sleep Arrangements and Infant–Parent "Risk"

No particular set of parenting practices with infants at night has been more controversial than parents' choices about how best to structure infant sleep. The controversy in particular relates to whether infants should sleep alone in a separate room from parents (solitary sleep), or with the parents, either in the same room but on a separate sleeping surface (room sharing) or in the same bed with the parents (bed sharing). Separate literatures indicate, on the one hand, the benefits of cosleeping, in particular bed sharing, for infants' survival and physical health, but on the other, the apparent risks of cosleeping to the marital and parenting subsystems. In a series of laboratory experiments using polysomnography to assess infant and maternal nighttime sleep, McKenna and colleagues (McKenna et al., 2007; McKenna & McDade, 2005; Mosko, Richard, & McKenna, 1997) demonstrated that cosleeping facilitated breast-feeding, which has important health benefits to infants (Ball, 2003; Godfrey & Meyers, 2009). Cosleeping also appeared to protect against sudden infant death syndrome (SIDS) by increasing the amount of time infants spend in lighter stages of sleep, reducing the amount of time spent in deeper sleep states (from which it is more difficult to arouse from a respiratory anomaly), and increasing the frequency of synchronized mother–infant arousals, which promoted mothers' ability to monitor the infant during the night. Drawing from biological anthropology, McKenna et al. (2007) proposed that bed sharing is a sleep arrangement that infants and mothers are biologically prepared to use and that, compared with other sleep arrangements, is most conducive to infant survival. Importantly, these conclusions, and their recommendations to engage in safe bed sharing, are in direct opposition to recommendations from the American Academy of Pediatrics (2005) not to cosleep because of concerns about increased risk of SIDS and other dangers (e.g., suffocation) to infants who share a bed with a parent.

At the same time, studies of parenting and child sleep have also linked cosleeping with family and developmental risk. Children who cosleep, for example, have been found to be at higher risk for sleep disturbances, compared with children who sleep in separate rooms (DeLeon & Karraker, 2007; Lozoff, Askew, & Wolf, 1996; Madansky & Edelbrock, 1990; Ong, Yang, Wong, alSiddiq, & Khu, 2010; Ramos et al., 2007; Sourander, 2000). This appears to be true even in cultures (e.g., China) that are supportive of cosleeping (Liu, Liu, & Wang, 2003; Tan, Marfo, & Dedrick, 2009; Wang et al., 2013) and has raised concerns about the wisdom of cosleeping because of other work showing that nighttime sleep disruption in childhood is associated with socioemotional, behavioral, and attentional problems (Cortesi, Fiannotti, Sebastiani, Vagnoni, & Marioni, 2008; Liu et al., 2003; Simard, Nielsen, Tremblay, Boivin, & Montplaisir, 2008; Sourander, 2000; Wang et al., 2013). Further, parents who cosleep with infants beyond the first few months of life appear to be at risk for marital discord and personal distress (Cortesi et al., 2008; Countermine & Teti, 2010), which themselves are known risk factors for socioemotional and behavioral problems in young children (Gelfand & Teti, 1990; Teti, Gelfand, Messinger, & Isabella, 1995).

Thus, whereas early cosleeping, and in particular bed sharing, carries clear health benefits to the infant if safely practiced, persistent cosleeping has been associated with family dysfunction and infant sleep disruption, both of which are predictive of cognitive and social developmental problems in early childhood. Importantly, it is unclear from this work whether persistent cosleeping plays a causal role in any of this, or whether it is symptomatic of preexisting family problems. There is some evidence for the latter perspective. For example, Teti et al. (2015) found that coparenting distress when infants were 1 month of age was associated with cosleeping that persisted across the infants' first 6 months of life, whereas positive coparenting at 1 month predicted a move out of cosleeping arrangements and into solitary sleeping arrangements by 6 months. Further, Teti and Crosby (2012) reported that elevated depressive symptoms and worries about infant night waking in mothers appeared to lead mothers to seek out and spend more time with their infants at night, independent of any sign of infant distress, and that this in turn was associated with mothers' reports of increased infant night waking. These two studies are of particular relevance to the well-established but heretofore unexplained findings of linkages between maternal depressive symptoms and infant night awakenings (Bayer, Hiscock, Hampton, & Wake, 2007; Messer & Richards, 1993; Warren, Howe, Simmens, & Dahl, 2006). Based on their video observations, Teti and Crosby (2012) proposed that the maternal depressive symptom–infant night-waking link may be both infant driven (i.e., frequent nighttime infant sleep problems lead to chronic sleep loss in mothers, leading to maternal dysphoria) and mother driven (i.e., elevated depressive symptoms and anxieties about infant nighttime sleep behavior lead mothers to spend more time with infants at night and, intentionally or not, perturb their infants' sleep).

Sleep Arrangements, Parenting, and Family Functioning: Contributions from Project SIESTA

Overview of Project SIESTA

In an attempt to shed some light on the sleep arrangement controversy, Teti and his Project SIESTA colleagues have been examining linkages among sleep arrangement use across the infants' first year, infant–parent sleep, parenting, and parental functioning. Families during infants' first year were visited at home when infants were 1, 3, 6, 9, 12, 18, and 24 months of age, and at each age point, parent and infant sleep quality was measured across 7 consecutive nights.

We note at the outset that this study was done using a U.S., central Pennsylvania sample, a sample that is part of a culture that supports the use of solitary infant sleep over parent–infant cosleeping (Anuntaseree et al., 2008; Mindell, Sadeh, Kohyama, & How, 2010). Thus, these findings are not generalizable to cultures that are more supportive of infant–parent cosleeping. This caveat notwithstanding, this study builds on earlier work in several ways. To begin, it made use of *patterns* of sleep arrangement use across the infants' first year, rather than sleep arrangements being used at a single point in time. Second, this study used both objective (actigraphy) and a maternal-report measure of infant nighttime sleep (a daily infant sleep diary), each of which were averaged across 7 consecutive days, each of which provides different information about infant sleep quality. Infant sleep diary information is limited to infant nighttime awakenings that the parent actually notices and thus more likely to be associated with infant vocalizations and signaling to the parent, whereas actigraphy takes into account all nighttime awakenings (i.e., nighttime activity that occurs above a set threshold that is used to demarcate wake time), whether or not they are associated with infant vocalizations. Third, unlike virtually all prior work to date examining correlates of infant sleep arrangements, this study examined linkages among sleep arrangements, parental functioning, and parental sleep quality in both mothers and fathers. Finally, Teti et al. (2014) assessed relations between sleep arrangements and both parenting quality and parenting practices during infant bedtimes, using video-recorded observations of parenting across the first year, and household chaos, from direct, in-home observations. The inclusion of household chaos, conceptualized in terms of the physical organization of the home, management of intrusions, and adherence to schedules and routines (Matheny, Wachs, Ludwig, & Phillips, 1995; Weisner, 2010), stemmed from an interest in determining whether sleep arrangements were associated with overall family functioning, using an index that was independent of parental report.

The data to be reported here pertain to those collected during the infants' first year of life. One hundred sixty-seven families were recruited into this study at 1 month; by 12 months, 149 families remained in the study. Dropouts did not differ from completers in marital adjustment, positive and negative coparenting, household chaos, parental adjustment to infant nighttime sleep, bedtime parenting quality, and in the sleep arrangements being used at 1 month of infant age. Dropouts were, however, less likely than completers to be White and to breast-feed their infants at 1 month of age. There were 80 female and 69 male infants in the 149 families that completed the study through 12 months. Ninety-five percent of parents were married or living with a partner. Thirty-seven percent of mothers were primiparous, and 86% of mothers and 85% of fathers were White, with the remaining evenly split among African American, Asian American, Latino, or "Other." Eighty percent of mothers were breast-feeding their infants, either full- or part-time, at 1 month of age. That dropped to 33% by

12 months. Sixty-two percent and 65% of mothers were employed full- or part-time at 1 and 12 months, respectively. The sample was fairly well educated. Ninety-nine percent of mothers had completed high school, and 60% of mothers had a bachelor's degree or higher. Eighty-six percent of fathers had completed high school, with 61% completing a bachelor's degree or higher. Ninety-five percent of fathers and 62% of mothers were employed full- or part-time at 1 month; 98% of fathers and 65% of mothers were employed full- or part-time at 12 months. Median yearly family income was $60,000.

Assessment Measures

Home visits were conducted when infants were 1, 3, 6, 9, and 12 months of age. At each age point, family assessments were done across 7 consecutive days, with some assessments occurring once and others across multiple days at each age point. Once at each occasion, mothers and fathers completed questionnaire measures pertaining to their infants' sleep arrangements, marital adjustment, and coparenting quality. An observational assessment of the quality of parental behavior during infant bedtimes was also made from a video recording during 1 night at each age point. Assessments made across multiple days at each age point included (1) household chaos, which was obtained from observations of household organization during three separate visits to the home; and (2) infant and parent sleep quality, which was assessed daily across 7 consecutive days in the assessment week using actigraphy for mothers, fathers, and infants, and a mother-reported sleep diary for infants.

Determining Sleep Arrangement Use in the First Year

Sleep arrangements in SIESTA were assessed using the Sleep Practices Questionnaire (SPQ; Goldberg & Keller, 2007), a measure broadly designed to tap into parental perceptions about their infants' sleep behavior. At each infant age point, mothers responded to the SPQ item: "Where does your baby usually sleep at night?" and at each age point, four sleep arrangement categories were scored: solitary sleep (infant slept in a separate room), room sharing (infant slept in the same room as parents, but on a separate sleeping surface), bed sharing (infant slept in the same bed as the parents), and combination (infant's sleep arrangement varied across the night among solitary sleep, room sharing, and/or bed sharing). Complete sleep arrangement data were available on 139 families through 12 months. These data were aggregated across all five age points to create five sleeping arrangement categories across the first year: consistent solitary sleep (infant slept in a separate room all night from 1 through 12 months, $n = 34$), early switch to solitary sleep (infant switched to solitary sleep arrangement by 3 or 6 months, $n = 52$), late switch to solitary sleep (infant switched to solitary sleep arrangement by 9 or 12 months, $n = 13$), consistent cosleeping (room sharing or bed sharing from 1 through 12 months, $n = 21$), and inconsistent (no discernible infant sleep arrangement pattern across the first year, $n = 19$). The frequency of sleep arrangements used at 1, 3, 6, 9, and 12 months in the five aggregate groups is presented in Table 16.1. Note that in the consistent cosleeping group, only three families engaged in consistent bed sharing through 12 months, and only five had engaged in consistent bed sharing through 6 months. In addition, in the consistent cosleeping group, only one family engaged in consistent room sharing through 12 months. Thus, the majority of these families switched back and forth between room sharing and bed sharing throughout the infants' first year.

TABLE 16.1. Distribution of Sleep Arrangements in the Five Aggregate Sleep Arrangement Groups in SIESTA

	Infant age (months)				
	1	3	6	9	12
Consistent solitary sleep					
Solitary sleep	34	34	34	34	34
Room sharing	0	0	0	0	0
Bed sharing	0	0	0	0	0
Combination[a]	0	0	0	0	0
Early switchers					
Solitary sleep	0	28	52	52	52
Room sharing	39	16	0	0	0
Bed sharing	4	2	0	0	0
Combination[a]	9	6	0	0	0
Late switchers					
Solitary sleep	0	0	0	7	13
Room sharing	9	9	9	4	0
Bed sharing	1	2	1	0	0
Combination[a]	3	2	3	2	0
Consistent cosleeping					
Solitary sleep	0	0	0	0	0
Room sharing	7	8	4	6	6
Bed sharing[b]	10	6	11	9	8
Combination[a]	4	7	6	6	7
Inconsistent					
Solitary sleep	3	14	9	9	7
Room sharing	12	3	3	4	4
Bed sharing	1	0	0	1	1
Combination[a]	3	2	7	5	7

[a]Infants' sleep is divided among bed sharing, room sharing, and solitary sleep.
[b]The majority of families in the consistently cosleeping group switched back and forth between room sharing and bed sharing throughout the infants' first year. Only three families engaged in consistent bed sharing throughout the full year, and only five families engaged in consistent bed sharing between 1 and 6 months of age.

Quality of Coparenting

An additional questionnaire measure used at all age points in SIESTA was the Coparenting Relationship Scale (CRS; Feinberg, Brown, & Kan, 2012), which assessed a parent's perception of how well he or she and his or her partner worked together as a child-rearing team. The CRS measured interparental agreement, closeness, exposure of child to conflict, coparenting support, undermining, endorsement of partner's parenting, and division of labor. Positive coparenting dimensions (agreement, closeness, support, endorsement, and division of labor) were summed to create a positive coparenting composite at all age points. In addition, the two dimensions of negative coparenting (competition–undermining and exposure to conflict) were summed to create a negative coparenting composite at each age point. Internal reliability of the positive and negative coparenting composites was very high.

Household Chaos

Also measured in SIESTA at each age point was household chaos, from direct observations of the home environment during each weeklong home visit and from phone interviews with each parent. Our approach was consistent with conceptualizations and measurement systems used in prior work, which typically has depicted chaos in terms of physical organization of the home, management of intrusions, and adherence to schedules and routines (Matheny et al., 1995; Weisner, 2010). The measure included 11 items that assessed physical disorganization in the home (e.g., cleanliness, clutter, physical condition of the home) and noncompliance with study protocol (e.g., rescheduling or arriving late to appointments, promptness in completion of study measures). Each item was scored on a 1- to 3-point scale where 1 reflected no or very little chaos and 3 reflected high chaos. This measure was internally reliable and highly stable across time. This was consistent with earlier work finding strong longitudinal stability in assessments of chaos in the home (Deater-Deckard et al., 2009; Matheny et al., 1995).

Parents' EA and Parenting Practices at Bedtime

Parents' EA (Biringen et al., 2014) with infants during bedtimes was scored from the digital video recordings of bedtime, using a camera setup similar to that used in Teti et al. (2010). From the videos, it was clear that mothers were much more likely to be putting infants to bed than fathers and that mothers interacted more with their infants than did fathers. Bedtime EA on mothers and infants was obtained much more frequently from mothers ($Ns > 100$ at each age point) than from fathers ($Ns < 45$ at each age point). These numbers, when further subdivided by sleep arrangement groupings, yielded cell sizes that were too small for meaningful analyses of fathers' EA, and thus analyses of linkages between EA and sleep arrangements were conducted only for maternal EA. All EA coding was done by a rater who was trained and certified on the EA system. At each age point, the four maternal EA scales (sensitivity, structuring, nonintrusiveness, and nonhostility) for mothers were standardized and summed to create a composite measure of maternal EA that was highly reliable in terms of internal reliability and interrater reliability.

From the same video streams, separate coders, blind to all EA data, recorded parenting practices during infant bedtimes, using an interval (30-seconds) sampling technique that involved indicating the presence or absence of particular parenting practices observed during bedtime and throughout the night. These practices included infant sleep location (infant's room, parent's room, other), parental presence (with the infant), close parent–infant contact, nursing, quiet activities with the infant, arousing/stimulating activities, interparental conflict, and infant state of arousal (awake and nondistressed, awake and distressed, and asleep). Also scored were the number of parental interventions to infant distress and infant nondistress (either when awake or asleep) throughout the night.

Actigraphy (to Assess Parent and Infant Sleep Quality)

For 7 consecutive days at each age point, infants, mothers, and fathers wore a Respironics/Mini Mitter actiwatch (model AW-64) to assess sleep–wake activity across each night. Infants wore the actiwatch on their upper ankle (affixed with a soft elastic band), and mothers and fathers wore it on their wrists. For each infant and parent on each of the 7 nights, actigraphs provided data on fragmented sleep and the number of minutes awake after sleep onset (WASO). The mean of each of these measures was obtained for the full week of data collection. In addition, a daily sleep diary (the 24-Hour Sleep Patterns Interview [24-HSPI]; Meltzer, Mindell, & Levandoski, 2007) was used to confirm with each parent when he or she went to bed and when he or she fell asleep the previous night, as a cross-check with actigraph data.

Infant Sleep Diary

Mothers also completed an infant sleep diary (adapted from Burnham et al., 2002) every morning across the full week of data collection at each age that asked the mother to record when the infant was put down to sleep and when he or she fell asleep the previous night, and also the frequency of infant night waking during the previous night. This diary was used to cross-check each infant's actigraphy record to confirm the onset of sleep time and morning wake time for the infant. In addition, however, this diary provided information from mothers directly about infant night-waking frequency during the week. This index was obtained for each infant by summing across the full 7 nights of data collection at each age.

Sleep Arrangement Patterns and Infant–Parent Sleep

All analyses of sleep arrangement linkages with outcome measures used covariance pattern analysis. Infant fragmented sleep, and the number of minutes infants spent in WASO, was found to decrease sharply across the first year (ps < .0001), particularly between 1 and 6 months of age, reflecting the expected rapid consolidation of infant nighttime sleep with maturation during the first year of life (Henderson et al., 2011; see Figure 16.1 for infant sleep fragmentation). However, contrary to expectations, infant sleep arrangement patterns across the first year were found to be unrelated to infant sleep fragmentation and WASO, nor was the interaction of sleep arrangements and infant age significant for either of these two dependent variables. This was unexpected in light of earlier work linking cosleeping, and in particular bed sharing, with elevated infant night waking (DeLeon & Karraker, 2007; Lozoff et al., 1996; Ong et al., 2010; Ramos et al., 2007; Sourander, 2000), although it should be noted that these studies used maternal report to assess infant sleep quality, not actigraphy.

Additional analyses on mothers' sleep fragmentation and WASO revealed that, similar to infant sleep, mothers sleep fragmentation and WASO decreased significantly across the infants' first year (ps < .0001), indicating improved maternal sleep across the year, although this decrease was more gradual and

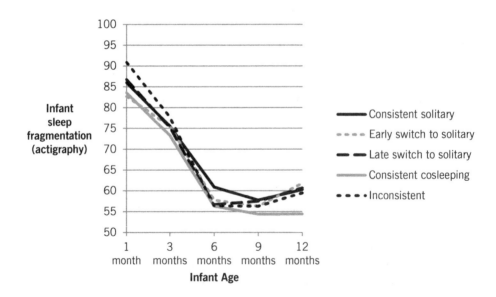

FIGURE 16.1. Infant sleep fragmentation, from actigraphy, across the infants' first year for the five different sleep arrangements groups.

linear compared with that observed for infant sleep fragmentation (see Figure 16.2 for maternal sleep fragmentation). However, in contrast to infant sleep, mothers' sleep fragmentation was significantly associated with sleep arrangements ($p < .0001$). Post hoc analyses revealed that mothers who used consistent solitary sleeping arrangements across the first year had less fragmented sleep compared with mothers of infants in consistent cosleeping arrangements (adjusted $p = .0004$), mothers in late-switching arrangements (mothers who did not switch their infants into solitary sleep until 9–12 months; adjusted $p = .02$), and mothers of infants in inconsistent sleep arrangements across the first year (adjusted $p = .007$). In addition, mothers whose infants switched into solitary sleep arrangements between 3 and 6 months had less fragmented sleep than mothers of infants in consistent cosleeping arrangements (adjusted $p = .02$). The interaction of sleep arrangements × infant age on mothers' sleep fragmentation was not significant. Similar results were obtained for mothers' WASO data. Interestingly, no linkages were found among sleep arrangement patterns, infant age and their interaction, and fathers' sleep fragmentation and fathers' WASO.

Collectively, these results revealed that, using actigraph measures of sleep quality, mothers, but not infants or fathers, in persistent cosleeping arrangements (i.e., persisting beyond 6 months of infant age) were more likely to experience sleep disruptions, compared with mothers of infants in consistent solitary arrangements and mothers whose infants switched into solitary sleep before 6 months. Interestingly, similar analyses conducted on mothers' reports of the frequency of infant night waking from the infant sleep diary revealed results that

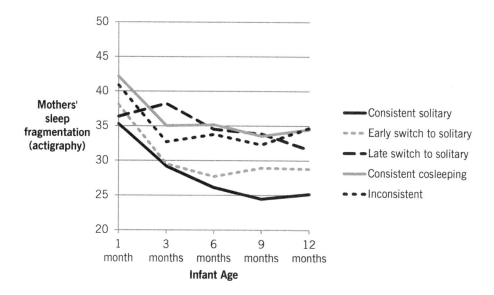

FIGURE 16.2. Mothers' sleep fragmentation, from actigraphy, across the infants' first year for the five different sleep arrangements groups.

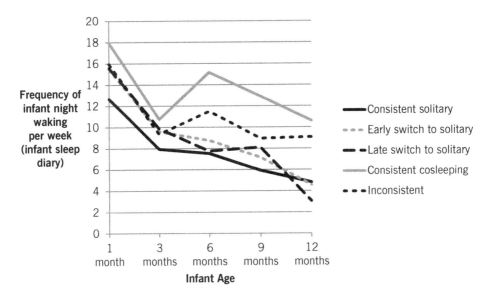

FIGURE 16.3. Mother reports of infant nighttime awakenings, from daily infant sleep diaries, across the infants' first year for the five different sleep arrangements groups.

were more consistent with those obtained with mothers' actigraph data than with infant actigraph data (see Figure 16.3). Specifically, infant night-waking frequency decreased across the first year ($p < .0001$; as expected), and was significantly associated with sleep arrangements ($p = .0009$). Post hoc pairwise comparisons showed that mothers of infants in consistent cosleeping arrangements reported significantly more infant night awakenings than mothers of infants in consistent solitary sleep arrangements (adjusted $p = .0005$), and mothers of infants who switched into solitary sleep before 6 months ($p = .007$). In sum, mothers' perceptions of their infants' sleep quality coincided much more closely with actigraphy measures of *mothers'* own sleep quality than with actigraphy measures of *infants'* sleep quality.

Sleep Arrangement Patterns, Coparenting, Household Chaos, and Bedtime Parenting

A significant association was seen between mothers' reports of negative coparenting and sleep arrangements ($p = .0002$), but not with infant age or the interaction of sleep arrangements by infant age. Post hoc pairwise comparisons indicated that mothers of infants in consistent cosleeping arrangements reported higher levels of negative coparenting than mothers of infants in consistent solitary sleep (adjusted $p < .0001$), mothers of early-switching infants (adjusted $p = .008$), mothers of late-switching infants (adjusted $p = .03$), and mothers of infants in inconsistent sleep arrangements throughout the first year (adjusted

$p = .01$). These differences were evident from 1 month of infant age onward and did not show differential change with different sleep arrangements over time. Mothers' positive coparenting was also associated with sleep arrangements ($p = .01$). Post hoc pairwise comparisons revealed that mothers of infants in consistent cosleeping arrangements reported less positive coparenting than mothers of infants in consistent solitary sleeping arrangements (adjusted $p = .005$). No other pairwise comparison was significant. No associations were found between fathers' coparenting and sleep arrangements.

Additional analyses revealed that household chaos increased across the first year in all groups ($p = .018$), and was significantly associated with sleep arrangements ($p = .0005$). Pairwise comparisons showed that families using consistent solitary infant sleeping arrangements were less chaotic than families using consistent cosleeping arrangements (adjusted $p = .015$) and late-switching families (adjusted $p = .001$). In addition, early-switching families were less chaotic than late-switching families (adjusted $p = .04$). Similar analyses on mothers' EA with infants at bedtime revealed a significant association with infant sleep arrangements ($p = .0002$), but not with infant age or the interaction of infant age with sleep arrangement patterns. Post hoc comparisons revealed that mothers of infants in consistent solitary sleeping arrangements were more emotionally available with their infants at bedtime than mothers of infants in consistent cosleeping arrangements (adjusted $p = .0001$) and mothers in late-switching arrangements (adjusted $p = .03$). In addition, early-switching mothers were more emotionally available to their infants at bedtime than mothers of infants in consistent cosleeping arrangements (adjusted $p = .004$).

Analyses on parenting practices revealed a variety of associations with sleep arrangement patterns. As expected, infants whose parents indicated that they slept in separate rooms throughout the first year (consistent solitary sleepers) spent significantly more time, both at bedtime and throughout the night, in their own rooms than infants in consistent cosleeping, late-switching infants, and infants in inconsistent sleep arrangements. In addition, infants in early-switching families were observed to spend more time in their own room after 3 months of age, and infants in late-switching families began to spend more time in their own room after 9 months. Thus, mothers' reports of infants' sleep arrangement patterns coincided nicely with the video observations. Parents of infants in persistent cosleeping arrangements (i.e., consistent cosleepers, late switchers, and inconsistent cosleepers) were observed to intervene more frequently to bouts of infant distress at night, when infants were awake but not distressed, and when infants were sound asleep, compared with parents of infants in consistent solitary sleep.

Correlational analyses were then conducted to explore associations between parenting quality (mothers' EA) and bedtime and nighttime parenting practices. A number of statistically significant associations emerged. Maternal EA at bedtime was positively associated with the time infants spent in their own rooms at bedtime, and negatively associated with the time infants spent in their parents' room and their parents' bed. Similar associations were found between bedtime EA and nighttime infant sleep locations. Bedtime EA correlated positively with the amount of time infants spent in their own separate rooms during the night and negatively with the amount of time infants spent in their parents' room during the night and in their parents' bed. These findings are consistent with the results, reported above, that EA among mothers of infants in consistent solitary sleep or who switched into solitary sleep early in the first year was significantly higher than mothers of infants in cosleeping arrangements that persisted throughout the first year.

Sleep Arrangement Patterns and Sociodemographics

A final set of analyses were conducted to examine any associations between first-year infant sleep arrangement patterns and sample sociodemographics. No associations were found among sleep arrangement patterns and mothers' and fathers' education, mothers' and fathers' age, yearly family income, family size, partner status (i.e., living with a partner vs. not), and breast-feeding, at any age. One difference that was found was that the proportion of nonWhites in the consistent cosleeping group was greater (42%) compared with that proportion in the other sleep arrangement groups (< 15%). However, race was not associated with any other sociodemographic variable, nor was race associated with any of the outcome measures in the consistent cosleeping group.

Interpreting SIESTA Findings

These findings, along with those from earlier work (Anders et al., 1992; Burnham et al., 2002; Mindell et al., 2006; Teti et al., 2010), converge on the point that both *what parents do* in infant sleep contexts (bedtime and nighttime parenting practices) and *how parents do what they do* (parenting quality) relate, in theoretically predictable ways, to infants' ability to put themselves to sleep, and to develop self-regulated sleep, across the first year. Infant sleep quality is compromised by high amounts of parental presence and close physical contact at night, and by parenting that is poorly structured, unresponsive, and insensitive. Conversely, bedtime parenting that is well structured, follows a routine, is sensitive and affectively attuned to infant needs, and provides infants ample opportunities to soothe themselves to sleep on their own at bedtime and throughout the night, appears to promote the development of self-regulated infant sleep. It is important to note that the associations above derive from samples from the United States and other Western industrialized societies that endorse the practice of solitary infant sleep, particularly by the end of the infant's first year when developmental issues pertaining to the establishment of day–night sleeping rhythms and sleep consolidation have largely resolved. It is not clear how well they converge with samples from non-Western cultures that are more likely to endorse various forms of infant–parent cosleeping, although we note that similar linkages between cosleeping and disrupted child sleep have been reported (from parent-report measures of child sleep) in Chinese samples (Liu et al., 2003; Tan et al., 2009; Wang et al., 2013), a country in which cosleeping occurs at substantially higher rates than in the United States (Wang et al., 2013). What has yet to be done in cosleeping-friendly cultures is an examination of individual differences in how cosleeping arrangements are structured (e.g., with vs. without father presence in the same room), and whether such individual differences are linked with marital and individual well-being and, in turn, infant–parent relationships and infant development.

Sleep Arrangements, Infant–Parent Sleep, and Parental and Interparental Dynamics

Further examination of SIESTA data, however, raises questions about the degree to which cosleeping, and in particular bed sharing, puts infants at risk for higher amounts of nighttime awakenings compared with solitary sleep. Mothers of infants in consistent cosleeping arrangements reported more night awakenings in their infants compared with mothers of infants in consistent solitary sleep and early-switching mothers, which is in line with earlier work that made use of maternal reports of infant sleep quality (DeLeon & Karraker, 2007; Lozoff et al., 1996; Ong et al., 2010; Ramos et al., 2007; Sourander, 2000). However, these differences were not supported by actigraph recordings of infant sleep. Indeed, actigraphy data revealed that it was *mothers', but not infants' or fathers' sleep*, that was disrupted in cosleeping arrangements, and only for cosleeping that lasted beyond the infant age of 6 months.

We propose that the tendency of mothers in persistent cosleeping arrangements to report higher frequencies of infant night awakenings may be related to other, family-based and personal factors. Mothers' reports of positive coparenting were lower in the consistent cosleeping group compared with the mothers in the consistent solitary sleep group; and mothers' reports of negative coparenting were higher in the consistent cosleeping group compared with all other groups. These "main effect" differences, which particularly disfavored mothers of infants in consistent cosleeping arrangements, were apparent as early as 1 month of infant age and persisted throughout the full year. In addition, analyses of household chaos, which was obtained from independent observations of family organization and compliance with study protocol, yielded a pattern of findings similar to that obtained for mothers' coparenting adjustment, with the lowest levels of household chaos found in families with infants in consistent solitary sleep arrangements and in early-switching families, compared with late-switching families and families of infants in consistent solitary sleep. Again, sleep arrangement group differences in household chaos were evident as early as 1 month of infant age. Collectively, these findings do not support the premise that sleeping arrangements were causal to mothers' coparenting quality and household chaos during the infant's first year, given that these differences were evident very early in the infants' life (1 month). Instead, these data suggest that persistent cosleeping throughout the infant's first year, particularly in a culture in which persistent cosleeping is not supported, may be symptomatic of preexisting heightened marital and family stress that is evident early in the life of the infant. This heightened distress, which appears to be particularly felt by mothers in the marital and coparenting domains, may predispose mothers to structure infant sleeping arrangements to allow them to spend more time with their infants at night. Indeed, the overall pattern of findings leads us to speculate that distressed mothers may be more likely to do this as a way of compensating for a perceived lack of closeness and intimacy in their marriages, and to maintain these arrangements in the face of continuing coparenting distress, which as reported above was found to be highly stable over time. These findings support and extend the earlier work of Teti et al. (2015), who reported that maritally distressed mothers who coslept with their infants at 1 month were more likely to maintain these cosleeping arrangements through 6 months, compared with nondistressed cosleeping mothers at 1 month, who by contrast were more likely to move their infants into solitary sleep by 6 months. The present findings also extend the findings of Teti and Crosby (2012), who found that mothers with elevated depressive symptoms and excessive worries about their infants' nighttime sleep behavior were more likely to seek out and spend time with their infants during the night than mothers with low symptom levels, and that distressed mothers' propensity for doing so was largely unrelated to whether or not their infants were distressed.

The question remains, however, why mothers of infants in consistent cosleeping arrangements reported higher levels of night awakenings in their infants relative to the other sleep arrangement groups, when similar analyses of actigraphy data revealed no sleep arrangement differences in infant sleep. One possible explanation is that mothers who sleep in close proximity to their infants notice their infant nighttime arousals more than mothers who sleep separately from their infants and thus are more likely to report infant arousals than mothers in solitary sleeping arrangements. If this were the case, stronger and more consistent associations would be expected between mothers' reports of infant night waking and actigraph reports of mothers' sleep disruption in consistent cosleeping arrangements than in consistent solitary sleep arrangements. This hypothesis was not supported: Instead, more consistent, positive correlations were found between mothers' reports of infant night waking and actigraph reports of mothers' sleep disruption in consistent solitary sleeping arrangements than in consistent cosleeping arrangements. We offer the following alternative hypothesis: If persistent cosleeping in a culture that does not support it is a marker of family and maternal distress (as it appeared to be in this sample), maternal distress may be manifested by a hypersensitivity to and hypervigilance about infant night awakenings, leading distressed mothers to perceive even very brief infant arousals and postural shifts as night awakenings. These very brief infant arousals may go unnoticed by nondistressed mothers, and they may be too brief and below threshold to be identified as wake activity by actigraphy. The question of whether distressed mothers and/or mothers who cosleep with their infants overreport infant night awakenings has, to date, rarely been addressed in the mother–infant sleep literature, and emphasizes the need to corroborate parent reports of infant/child sleep with objective assessments of infant sleep, such as actigraphy.

Sleep Arrangements and Mothers' Bedtime Parenting

There was no theoretical or empirical basis for expecting linkages between sleep arrangements and mothers' bedtime EA. Finding such linkages was not surprising, however, in light of the fact that mothers in persistent cosleeping arrangements had more fragmented sleep (and thus at risk for cumulative sleep debt), were more maritally stressed, and had more chaotic households. Indeed, sleep deprivation and fatigue is known to disrupt the quality of social relationships, including the parent–child relationship (Giallo, Rose, Cooklin, & McCormack, 2013; Kahn-Greene, Lipizzi, Conrad, Kamimori, & Killgore, 2006). In turn, marital maladjustment, poor coparenting quality, and household chaos are well established as predictors of parenting difficulties (Cabrera, Shannon, & La Taillade, 2009; Coldwell, Pike, & Dunn, 2006; Coln, Jordan, & Mercer, 2013; McCoy, George, Cummings, & Davies, 2013). Of special interest were the negative associations obtained between mothers' bedtime EA and nighttime maternal interventions with infants when infants were not distressed. Stated differently, mothers identified as emotionally unavailable to their infants at bedtime were more likely than emotionally available mothers at bedtime to intervene with their infants at night when their infants did not appear to need intervention. Bedtime EA and nighttime parenting were scored by separate coding teams that were blind to each other's data, and thus shared method variance cannot account for this link. These findings suggest that, in cultures that support independent infant sleep, one aspect of competent nighttime parenting of infants is the understanding that nighttime interventions are warranted only when infants are distressed, but not warranted when infants are not distressed, whether they are awake or not. Subsequent research needs to replicate this association, preferably using observational data, and in so doing address the broader question of what constitutes competent parenting with infants at night, how such parenting is conditioned by culture, and determining parenting competence not simply in terms of infant sleep quality but also in terms of infant socioemotional and cognitive developmental milestones.

Again, sleep arrangement patterns across the first year did not moderate longitudinal patterns of EA from 1 to 12 months, and thus there was no evidence that differences in sleep arrangement patterns caused differences in mothers' bedtime EA. These findings raise additional questions about whether persistent cosleeping in a culture that does not endorse it is not just a risk marker for maternal sleep loss and family stress but also for early socioemotional problems in children. If this were the case, we would expect that such risks would be realized only to the extent that persistent cosleeping was associated with persistent family and parenting stress across the first year. In the absence of such stress, we would expect no ill effects of persistent cosleeping on parenting and children's early development. Clearly, this is a topic for further research.

Sleep Arrangements and Fathers

In contrast to mothers, fathers' sleep and perceptions of coparenting quality were remarkably unrelated to sleep arrangement patterns. We note that mothers in this sample were almost exclusively the primary caregivers for their infants, and much more likely than fathers to take primary responsibility for putting their infants to bed. This was corroborated by our bedtime video data, which almost always involved mothers but sporadically involved fathers in bedtime activities. We suspect that, whereas mothers' involvement with their infants at bedtime and throughout the night was a constant, fathers' involvement in these activities varied widely. We would expect stronger linkages between infant sleep arrangements and fathers' sleep quality under conditions of high father involvement. This is an important question for further research.

Conclusions

This chapter addressed the role of parenting practices and parenting quality, particularly at bedtime and during the night, as predictors of infant and early childhood sleep and that place children at risk for poor sleep and, in turn, for adjustment difficulties in socioemotional and cognitive developmental domains (Bates, Viken, Alexander, Beyers, & Stockton, 2002). Parenting that provides infants opportunities to soothe themselves to sleep, follows regular and predictable bedtime routines, limits parental presence and close physical contact with infants at night, that is emotionally attuned and sensitive to infant needs at bedtime, and not overly solicitous of infants during the night is associated with the development of self-regulated, quality sleep during the first year. SIESTA findings further indicate that, contrary to most available reporting linkages between cosleeping and increased infant nighttime awakenings (relying primarily on parent reports), cosleeping, especially if persistent beyond the infants' age of 6 months, was more clearly associated with disruptions in mothers' sleep, but not infants' or fathers' sleep (using actigraph data), and was also associated with coparenting distress and more chaotic households. We propose that persistent cosleeping may be a marker, but not necessarily a cause of, family distress, and that further research should delve more deeply into the interlinkages that exist between family distress and sleep arrangements and their impact on infant and family outcomes over time.

If mothers who engage in persistent cosleeping do so because they are distressed, and if persistent cosleeping places mothers at risk for sleep disruption, cumulative sleep debt, and relationship difficulties with their infants, such mothers comprise a high-risk group in need of intervention. The primary goal of such an intervention should not be, in our view, to advise against cosleeping with one's infant, but instead to improve the marital and coparenting relationship, particularly around but not limited to decisions parents make about infant sleep arrangements, and to make certain that parents who wish to cosleep think carefully about and discuss with each other the reasons they wish to do it, and ideally to be in full agreement if the decision to cosleep is made. We believe such an intervention should aim to make parents fully aware of the perks and pitfalls of cosleeping and help parents understand that whereas cosleeping, if practiced safely, can facilitate breast-feeding and parents' ability to monitor the infant during the night, persistent cosleeping can lead to parent sleep disruption and cumulative sleep debt, which could detrimentally impact the marital and parent–infant relationships over the long term (e.g., McDaniel & Teti, 2012). Cosleeping, in other words, should be done with full knowledge and support of both parenting partners. It should not be practiced as a way of compensating for a lack of marital intimacy or because parents harbor unrealistic anxieties about their infants' nighttime sleep–wake behavior.

It is important to note that virtually all data available on the role of parenting on infant sleep derive from cultures in which persistent parent–infant cosleeping is not the norm. In a cosleeping culture, we would not expect persistent cosleeping during the infant's first year to be a marker of risk, nor is it clear if the practices identified to date as putting infants at risk for poor sleep would be the same in a cosleeping culture. It would nevertheless be important to examine, in cultures in which persistent cosleeping is more highly endorsed, whether distressed parents and in particular mothers are more likely to prolong the practice of cosleeping and/or to seek out and spend more time with infants in contexts other than sleep contexts, compared with mothers of infants of solitary sleeping infants. It is also tempting to speculate about whether parents in cosleeping cultures who decide not to cosleep with their infants are more likely to experience criticism from others and, in turn, elevations in marital, personal, and parenting distress.

More broadly, although this chapter is dedicated to a review and discussion of parenting practices and parenting quality in child sleep contexts and their link to infant sleep, it remains the case that precious little is known about parenting of infants and young children in bedtime contexts. Direct observation, and not just parent report, of bedtime/nighttime parenting is needed to redress this dearth, not simply to determine how parenting in such contexts organize child sleep, but also how it predicts developmental outcomes in early childhood and beyond, and how it relates to the quality with which parents interact with each other. We argue that there are distinct "perks" in engaging in direct observations of parenting in child sleep contexts. One is that parenting in these contexts qualifies in every respect as naturalistic. It is not structured by an observer, yet it is goal-directed and involves a context that is universal to all parents. It is critical to understand what individual differences in parenting looks like, both in terms of what parents do (practices) and how well they do it (quality) in child sleep contexts, and what those individual differences portend for children's development, both short- and long term. It is also important to examine how bedtime and nighttime parenting compares with parenting observed in more traditional daytime contexts, both structured (e.g., free play, feeding, teaching) and unstructured, and whether parenting in particular contexts is a stronger predictor of children's development. Second, observations of parenting in child sleep contexts, particularly during bedtimes, frequently involves both parents to varying degrees, and any other children in the family. As such, it provides a rare window for examining multiple subsystems in the family (parent–child, parent–parent, siblings, etc.), and how well or poorly these subsystems coordinate as parents work to put their children to bed. From our video recordings of bedtime parenting, we have observed some highly organized, well-coordinated families, and others that were poorly organized and coordinated, replete with marital discord that appeared to spill over into parents' interactions with individual children. We would thus argue that observations of bedtime and nighttime parenting provide researchers with opportunities to study not just parenting but also the coparenting relationship and the overall health and integrity of the family system.

Finally, it behooves social scientists interested in the role of parenting in child sleep to incorporate characteristics of the child that have direct or indirect theoretical relevance to sleep quality. What immediately comes to mind in this regard is infant temperament, given evidence that connects infant temperamental characteristics, such as negative affectivity, inversely with infant sleep quality (Halpern, Anders, Garcia Coll, & Hua, 1994; Spruyt et al., 2008). Interestingly, relatively few studies have examined infant temperament as a potential moderator of linkages between bedtime/nighttime parenting and infant sleep. We believe this is a fruitful area of inquiry, given recent findings from SIESTA that infant surgency (characterized by high activity, positive affect, high levels of approach, and perceptual sensitivity; Gartstein & Rothbart, 2003) moderated associations between maternal EA at bedtime and infant sleep duration such that a positive association was found only for highly surgent infants, but not for infants low in surgency (Jian, Kim, Crosby, & Teti, 2014). We propose that additional infant "characteristics" that index regulatory capacities in infants, such as vagal regulation and stress reactivity measured very early in life, may also prove to be important moderators of the effects of parenting practices and quality on infant sleep development and thus worthy of systematic study.

We have just scratched the surface in understanding the role of parenting in organizing sleep in infancy, and how parenting, infant sleep patterns, and parent sleep patterns mutually influence one another over time. Future research is needed to further explore these linkages, and to better understand how the effects of parenting on child sleep are conditioned by child characteristics, individual parental beliefs, and cultural belief systems. Such work should contribute importantly to the field of parenting in its own right. In addition, however, we expect such work to contribute to a greater appreciation of the impact of bedtime/nighttime parenting on infant sleep regulation, and of the independent and joint effects of parenting and child sleep on cognitive and socioemotional development in the early years.

ACKNOWLEDGMENTS

We thank the many undergraduate and graduate students who have contributed to Project SIESTA, and to the talented project coordinating efforts of Corey Whitesell, Renee Stewart, and Cori Reed. Special thanks are given to the participating families. The research base on linkages among bedtime and nighttime parenting and sleep in infancy has been growing and is a particular focus of Project SIESTA (Study of Infants' Emergent Sleep TrAjectories), a research program funded by the National Institutes of Health (No. R01 HD052809) awarded to D. M. T. that examines parenting practices and parenting quality in infant sleep contexts and their links with sleep and development among infants during the first 2 years.

REFERENCES

Ainsworth, M. D. S., Blehar, M. C., Waters, E., & Wall, S. (1978). *Patterns of attachment: A psychological study of the Strange Situation.* Hillsdale, NJ: Erlbaum.

American Academy of Pediatrics. (2005). The changing concept of sudden infant death syndrome: Diagnostic coding shifts, controversies regarding the sleeping environment, and new variables to consider in reducing risk. *Pediatrics, 116,* 1245–1255.

Anders, T. F., Halpern, L. F., & Hua, J. (1992). Sleeping through the night: A developmental perspective. *Pediatrics, 90*(4), 554–560.

Anuntaseree, W., Mo-suwan, L., Vasiknanonte, P., Kuasirikul, S., Ma-a-lee, A., & Choprapawon, C. (2008). Factors associated with bed sharing and sleep position in Thai neonates. *Child, Care, Health and Development, 34*(4), 482–490.

Ball, H. L. (2003). Breastfeeding, bed-sharing, and infant sleep. *Birth: Issues in Perinatal Care, 30*(3), 181–188.

Bates, J. E., Viken, R. J., Alexander, D. B., Beyers, J., & Stockton, L. (2002). Sleep and adjustment in preschool children: Sleep diary reports by mothers relate to behavior reports by teachers. *Child Development, 73*(1), 62–74.

Bayer, J. K., Hiscock, H., Hampton, A., & Wake, M. (2007). Sleep problems in young infants and maternal mental and physical health. *Journal of Paediatrics and Child Health, 43*(1–2), 66–73.

Biringen, Z., Derscheid, D., Vliegen, N., Closson, L., & Easterbrooks, M. A. (2014). Emotional availability (EA): Theoretical background, empirical research using the EA scales, and clinical applications. *Developmental Review, 34*(2), 114–167.

Bordeleau, S., Bernier, A., & Carrier, J. (2012). Maternal sensitivity and children's behavior problems: Examining the moderating role of infant sleep duration. *Journal of Clinical Child and Adolescent Psychology, 41*(4), 471–481.

Boyle, J., & Cropley, M. (2004). Children's sleep: Problems and solutions. *Journal of Family Health, 14*(3), 61–63.

Buckhalt, J. A., & Staton, L. E. (2011). Children's sleep, cognition, and academic performance in the context of socioeconomic status and ethnicity. In M. El-Sheikh (Ed.), *Sleep and development: Familial and socio-cultural considerations* (pp. 245–264). New York: Oxford University Press.

Burnham, M. M. (2013). Co-sleeping and self-soothing during infancy. In A. R. Wolfson & H. E. Montgomery-Downs (Eds.), *The Oxford handbook of infant, child, and adolescent sleep and behavior* (pp. 127–139). New York: Oxford University Press.

Burnham, M. M., Goodlin-Jones, B. L., Gaylor, E. E., & Anders, T. F. (2002). Nighttime sleep– wake patterns and self-soothing from birth to one year of age: A longitudinal intervention study. *Journal of Child Psychology and Psychiatry, 43*(6), 713–725.

Byars, K. C., Yeomans-Maldonado, G., & Noll, J. G. (2011). Parental functioning and pediatric sleep disturbance: An examination of factors associated with parenting stress in children clinically referred for evaluation of insomnia. *Sleep Medicine, 12*(9), 898–905.

Cabrera, N. J., Shannon, J. D., & La Taillade, J. J. (2009). Predictors of coparenting in Mexican American families and links to parenting and child social emotional development. *Infant Mental Health Journal, 30*(5), 523–548.

Coldwell, J., Pike, A., & Dunn, J. (2006). Household chaos—links with parenting and child behaviour. *Journal of Child Psychology and Psychiatry, 47*(11), 1116–1122.

Coln, K. L., Jordan, S. S., & Mercer, S. H. (2013). A unified model exploring parenting practices as mediators of marital conflict and children's adjustment. *Child Psychiatry and Human Development, 44*(3), 419–429.

Cortesi, F., Fiannotti, F., Sebastiani, T., Vagnoni, C., & Marioni, P. (2008). Cosleeping versus solitary sleeping in children with bedtime problems: Child emotional problems and parental distress. *Behavioral Sleep Medicine, 6*, 89–105.

Cotton, S., & Richdale, A. (2006). Brief report: Parental descriptions of sleep problems in children with autism, Down syndrome, and Prader–Willi syndrome. *Research in Developmental Disabilities, 27*(2), 151–161.

Countermine, M. S., & Teti, D. M. (2010). Sleep arrangements and maternal adaptation in infancy. *Infant Mental Health Journal, 31*(6), 647–663.

Crosby, B., LeBourgeois, M. K., & Harsh, J. (2005). Racial differences in reported napping and nocturnal sleep in 2- to 8-year-old children. *Pediatrics, 115,* 225.

Dahl, R. E., & El-Sheikh, M. (2007). Considering sleep in a family context: Introduction to the special issue. *Journal of Family Psychology, 21,* 1–3.

Deater-Deckard, K., Mullineaux, P. Y., Beekman, C., Petrill, S. A., Schatschneider, C., & Thompson, L. A. (2009). Conduct problems, IQ, and household chaos: A longitudinal multi-informant study. *Journal of Child Psychology and Psychiatry, 50*(10), 1301–1308.

DeLeon, C. W., & Karraker, K. H. (2007). Intrinsic and extrinsic factors associated with night waking in 9-month-old infants. *Infant Behavior and Development, 30,* 596–605.

El-Sheikh, M., & Buckhalt, J. (2015). Moving sleep and child development research forward: Priorities and recommendations from the SRCD-sponsored forum on sleep and child development. *Monographs of the Society for Research in Child Development, 80*(1), 15–32.

El-Sheikh, M., Erath, S. A., & Bagley, E. J. (2013). Parasympathetic nervous system activity and children's sleep. *Journal of Sleep Research, 22,* 282–288.

El-Sheikh, M., & Sadeh, A. (2015). Sleep and development: Introduction to the monograph. *Monographs of the Society for Research in Child Development, 80*(1), 1–14.

Feinberg, M. E., Brown, L. D., & Kan, M. L. (2012). A multi-domain self-report measure of coparenting. *Parenting, 12,* 1–21.

Franco, P., Pardou, A., Hassid, S., Lurquin, P., Groswasser, J., & Kahn, A. (1998). Auditory arousal thresholds are higher when infants sleep in the prone position. *Journal of Pediatrics, 132*(2), 240–243.

Gartstein, M. A., & Rothbart, M. K. (2003). Studying infant temperament via the Revised Infant Behavior Questionnaire. *Infant Behavior and Development, 26*(1), 64–86.

Gelfand, D. M., & Teti, D. M. (1990). The effects of maternal depression on children. *Clinical Psychology Review, 10,* 329–353.

Giallo, R., Rose, N., Cooklin, A., & McCormack, D. (2013). In survival mode: Mothers and fathers' experiences of fatigue in the early parenting period. *Journal of Reproductive and Infant Psychology,31*(1), 31–45.

Giannotti, F., & Cortesi, F. (2009). Family and cultural influences on sleep development. *Child and Adolescent Psychiatric Clinics of North America, 18,* 849–861.

Godfrey, J. R., & Meyers, D. (2009). Toward optimal health: Maternal benefits of breastfeeding. *Journal of Women's Health, 18*(9), 1307–1310.

Goldberg, W. A., & Keller, M. A. (2007). Co-sleeping during infancy and early childhood: Key findings and future directions. *Infant and Child Development, 16,* 457–469.

Gregory, A. M., Caspi, A., Eley, T. C., Moffitt, T., & O'Connor, T. G. (2005). Prospective longitudinal associations between persistent sleep problems in childhood and anxiety and depression disorders in adulthood. *Journal of Abnormal Child Psychology, 33*(2), 157–163.

Hale, L., Berger, L. M., LeBourgeois, M. K., & Brooks-Gunn, J. (2011). A longitudinal study of preschoolers' language-based bedtime routines, sleep duration, and well-being. *Journal of Family Psychology, 25*(3), 423–433.

Halpern, L. F., Anders, T. F., Garcia Coll, C., & Hua, J. (1994). Infant temperament: Is there a relation to sleep–wake states and maternal nighttime behavior? *Infant Behavior and Development, 17*(3), 255–263.

Harrison, Y. (2004). The relationship between daytime exposure to light and night-time sleep in 6–12-week-old infants. *Journal of Sleep Research, 13,* 345–352.

Henderson, J. M. T., France, K. G., & Blampied, N. M. (2011). The consolidation of infants' nocturnal sleep across the first year of life. *Sleep Medicine Reviews, 15,* 211–220.

Henderson, J. M. T., France, K. G., Owens, J. L., & Blampied, N. M. (2010). Sleeping through the night: The development of self-regulated nocturnal sleep during infancy. *Pediatrics, 126*(5), e1081–e1087.

Huber, R., & Born, J. (2014). Sleep, synaptic connectivity, and hippocampal memory during early development. *Trends in Cognitive Science, 18*(3), 141–152.

Jian, N., Kim, B.-R., Crosby, B., & Teti, D. M. (2014). *Infant temperament, maternal emotional availability at bedtime, and infant sleep from 3 to 6 months.* Manuscript in preparation.

Kahn-Greene, E. T., Lipizzi, E. L., Conrad, A. K., Kamimori, G. H., & Killgore, W. D. S. (2006). Sleep deprivation adversely affects interpersonal responses to frustration. *Personality and Individual Differences, 41*(8), 1433–1443.

Lee, K. A., & Rosen, L. A. (2012). Sleep and human development. In C. M. Morin & C. A. Espie (Eds.), *The Oxford handbook of sleep and sleep disorders* (pp. 75–94). New York: Oxford University Press.

Lemola, S., & Richter, D. (2013). The course of subjective sleep quality in middle and old adulthood and its relation to physical health. *Journals of Gerontology, Series B: Psychological Sciences and Social Sciences, 68*(5), 721–729.

Li, L., Ren, J., Shi, L., Jin, X., Yan, C., Jiang, F., et al. (2014). Frequent nocturnal awakening in children: Prevalence, risk factors, and associations with subjective sleep perception and daytime sleepiness. *BMC Psychiatry, 14,* 204.

Liu, X., Liu, L., & Wang, R. (2003). Bed sharing, sleep habits, and sleep problems among Chinese school-aged children. *Sleep: Journal of Sleep and Sleep Disorders Research, 26*(7), 839–844.

Lozoff, B., Askew, G. L., & Wolf, A. W. (1996). Cosleeping and early childhood sleep problems: Effects of ethnicity and socioeconomic status. *Developmental and Behavioral Pediatrics, 17*(1), 9–15.

Madansky, D., & Edelbrock, C. (1990). Cosleeping in a community sample of 2- and 3-year-old children. *Pediatrics, 86*(2), 197–203.

Matheny, A. P., Wachs, T. D., Ludwig, J. L., & Phillips, K. (1995). Bringing order out of chaos: Psychometric characteristics of the confusion, hubbub, and order scale. *Journal of Applied Developmental Psychology, 16*(3), 429–444.

McCoy, K. P., George, M. R. W., Cummings, E. M., & Davies, P. T. (2013). Constructive and destructive marital conflict, parenting, and children's school and social adjustment. *Social Development, 22*(4), 641–662.

McDaniel, B. T., & Teti, D. M. (2012). Coparenting quality during the first three months after birth: The role of infant sleep quality. *Journal of Family Psychology, 26*(6), 886–895.

McKenna, J. J., Ball, H. L., & Gettler, L. T. (2007). Mother–infant cosleeping, breast-feeding and sudden infant death syndrome: What biological anthropology has discovered about normal infant sleep and pediatric sleep medicine. *Yearbook of Physical Anthropology, 50*, 133–161.

McKenna, J. J., & McDade, T. (2005). Why babies should never sleep alone: A review of the co-sleeping controversy in relation to SIDS, bedsharing and breast feeding. *Paediatric Respiratory Reviews, 6*, 134–152.

Meltzer, L. J., Mindell, J. A., & Levandoski, L. J. (2007). The 24-hour sleep patterns interview: A pilot study of validity and feasibility. *Behavioral Sleep Medicine, 5*(4), 297–310.

Messer, D., & Richards, M. (1993). The development of sleeping difficulties. In I. St. James-Roberts, G. Harris, & D. Messer (Eds.), *Infant crying, feeding, and sleeping: Development, problems and treatments. The developing body and mind* (pp. 150–173). Hertfordshire, UK: Harvester Wheatsheaf.

Mindell, J. A. (1999). Empirically supported treatments in pediatric psychology: Bedtime refusal and night wakings in young children. *Journal of Pediatric Psychology, 24*(6), 465–481.

Mindell, J. A., Kuhn, B., Lewin, D. S., Meltzer, L. J., & Sadeh, A. (2006). Behavioral treatment of bedtime problems and night wakings in infants and young children. *Sleep, 29*, 1263–1276.

Mindell, J. A., Sadeh, A., Kohyama, J., & How, T. H. (2010). Parental behaviors and sleep outcomes in infants and toddlers: A cross-cultural comparison. *Sleep Medicine, 11*(4), 393–399.

Mindell, J. A., Telofski, L. S., Wiegand, B., & Kurtz, E. (2009). A nightly bedtime routine: Impact on sleep in young children and maternal mood. *Journal of Sleep and Sleep Disorders Research, 32*(5), 599–606.

Mosko, S., Richard, C., & McKenna, J. (1997). Infant arousals during mother–infant bed sharing: Implications for infant sleep and sudden infant death syndrome research. *Pediatrics, 100*(5), 841–849.

Ong, L. C., Yang, W. W., Wong, S. W., alSiddiq, F., & Khu, Y. S. (2010). Sleep habits and disturbances in Malaysian children with epilepsy. *Journal of Paediatrics and Child Health, 46*, 80–84.

Philbrook, L. E., Jian, N., Kim, B.-R., McDaniel, B. T., Reader, J. M., Rhee, H.-Y., et al. (2015, March). *Influences and interactions of parenting practices and quality at bedtime on infant sleep quality across the first 6 months.* Paper presented at the biennial meeting of the Society for Research in Child Development, Philadelphia, PA.

Ramos, K. D., Youngclarke, D., & Anderson, J. E. (2007). Parental perceptions of sleep problems among co-sleeping and solitary sleep children. *Infant and Child Development, 16*, 417–431.

Sadeh, A., & Anders, T. F. (1993). Infant sleep problems: Origins, assessment, interventions. *Infant Mental Health Journal, 14*(1), 17–34.

Sadeh, A., Mindell, J., & Rivera, L. (2011). "My child has a sleep problem": A cross-cultural comparison of parental definitions. *Sleep Medicine, 12*(5), 478–482.

Sadeh, A., Mindell, J. A., Luedtke, K., & Wiegand, B. (2009). Sleep and sleep ecology in the first 3 years: A web-based study. *Journal of Sleep Research, 18*, 60–73.

Sadeh, A., Tikotzky, L., & Scher, A. (2010). Parenting and infant sleep. *Sleep Medicine Reviews, 14*(2), 89–96.

Scher, A. (2001). Mother–child interaction and sleep regulation in one-year olds. *Infant Mental Health Journal, 22*(5), 515–528.

Scher, A., Epstein, R., & Tirosh, E. (2004). Stability and changes in sleep regulation: A longitudinal study from 3 months to 3 years. *International Journal of Behavioral Development, 28*(3), 268–274.

Sheldon, S. H. (2014). The function, phylogeny, and ontogeny of sleep. In S. H. Sheldon, R. Ferber, M. H. Kryger, & D. Gozal (Eds.), *Principles and practice of pediatric sleep medicine* (2nd ed., pp. 3–12). London: Elsevier/Saunders.

Sheridan, A., Murray, L., Cooper, P. J., Evangeli, M., Byram, V., & Halligan, S. L. (2013). A longitudinal study of child sleep in high and low risk families: Relationship to early maternal settling strategies and child psychological functioning. *Sleep Medicine, 14*(3), 266–273.

Simard, V., Nielsen, T. A., Tremblay, R. E., Boivin, M., & Montplaisir, J. Y. (2008). Longitudinal study of preschool sleep disturbance: The predictive role of maladaptive parental behaviors, early sleep problems, and child/mother psychological factors. *Archives of Pediatric Adolescent Medicine, 162*(4), 360–367.

So, K., Adamson, T. M., & Horne, R. S. C. (2007). The use of actigraphy for assessment of the development of sleep/wake patterns in infants during the first 12 months of life. *Journal of Sleep Research, 16*(2), 181–187.

Sourander, A. (2000). Emotional and behavioural problems in a sample of Finnish three-year-olds. *European Child and Adolescent Psychiatry, 10*, 98–104.

Spagnola, J., & Fiese, B. H. (2007). Family routines and rituals: A context for development in the lives of young children. *Infants and Young Children, 20*(4), 284–299.

Spruyt, K., Aitken, R. J., So, K., Charlton, M., Adamson, T. M., & Horne, R. S. C. (2008). Relationship between sleep/wake patterns, temperament and overall development in term infants over the first year of life. *Early Human Development, 84*(5), 289–296.

Tan, T. X., Marfo, K., & Dedrick, F. (2009). Preschool-age adopted Chinese children's sleep problems and family sleep arrangements. *Infant and Child Development, 18*, 422–440.

Teti, D. M., & Crosby, B. (2012). Maternal depressive symptoms, dysfunctional cognitions, and infant night waking: The role of maternal nighttime behavior. *Child Development, 83*(3), 939–953.

Teti, D. M., Crosby, B., McDaniel, B., Shimizu, M., & Whitesell, C. (2015). Marital and emotional adjustment in mothers and infant sleep arrangements during the first six months. *Monographs of the Society for Research in Child Development, 80*(1), 160–176.

Teti, D. M., Gelfand, D. M., Messinger, D., & Isabella, R. (1995) Maternal depression and the quality of early attachment: An examination of infants, preschoolers, and their mothers. *Developmental Psychology, 31*, 364–376.

Teti, D. M., Kim, B.-R., Mayer, G., & Countermine, M. (2010). Maternal emotional availability at bedtime predicts infant sleep quality. *Journal of Family Psychology, 24*(3), 307–331.

Teti, D. M., Shimizu, M., Crosby, B., Kim, B.-R., & Whitesell, C. (2014). *Sleep arrangements, parent infant sleep during the first year, and parenting at risk.* Manuscript in preparation.

Wang, G. H., Xu, G. X., Liu, Z. J., Lu, N., Ma, R., & Zhang, E. T. (2013). Sleep patterns and sleep disturbances among Chinese school-aged children: Prevalence and associated factors. *Sleep Medicine, 14*, 45–52.

Warren, S. L., Howe, G., Simmens, S. J., & Dahl, R. E. (2006). Maternal depressive symptoms and child sleep: Models of mutual influence over time. *Development and Psychopathology, 18*(1), 1–16.

Weisner, T. S. (2010). Well-being, chaos, and culture: Sustaining a meaningful daily routine. In G. Evans & T. Wachs (Eds.), *Chaos and its influence on children's development: An ecological perspective* (pp. 221–224). Washington, DC: American Psychological Association.

Williams, P. G., Sears, L. L., & Allard, A. (2004). Sleep problems in children with autism. *Journal of Sleep Research, 13*, 265–268.

Wolfson, A. R. (1996). Sleeping patterns of children and adolescents: Developmental trends, disruptions, and adaptations. *Child and Adolescent Psychiatric Clinics of North America, 5*, 549–568.

Wong, M. M., Brower, K. J., Fitzgerald, H. E., & Zucker, R. A. (2004). Sleep problems in early childhood and early onset of alcohol and other drug use in adolescence. *Alcoholism: Clinical and Experimental Research, 28*(4), 578–587.

Worthman, C. M. (2011). Developmental cultural ecology of sleep. In M. El-Sheikh (Ed.), *Sleep and development* (pp. 167–194). New York: Oxford University Press.

CHAPTER 17

Infant Vulnerability
to Psychopathology

Sherryl H. Goodman

The notion of vulnerability to the development of psychopathology has a long and honored history. Among the most seminal early contributors to understanding vulnerability were Lois Murphy, Norman Garmezy, and Emmy Werner. Beginning in the 1930s, Lois Murphy carefully characterized the development of a group of children from early infancy through adolescence, focusing on biological, psychological, and environmental processes as vulnerabilities (Murphy & Moriarty, 1976). Norman Garmezy also recognized the potential value of vulnerabilities in understanding pathways to disorder (or competence) and in designing preventive interventions (Garmezy, 1971). This work, carried on in particular by Ann Masten, has led to many important new findings (beginning with Masten & Garmezy, 1985). Emmy Werner's exquisitely detailed longitudinal study further provided strong evidence that vulnerabilities are not inevitably associated with succumbing to the development of psychopathology (Werner & Smith, 1977). Indeed, it is important to note that all three of these seminal contributors to the understanding of early vulnerabilities are equally well known for their work on resilience (Masten & Garmezy, 1985; Werner & Smith, 1982). Overall, this early work introduced not only the concept of vulnerability, but also the biopsychosocial perspective on vulnerability and the need to understand divergent pathways both to vulnerability and from vulnerability to disorder (or competence). One might say both that we have come a long way since this early work and that current work on studies of vulnerability strongly benefits from the contributions of these seminal leaders.

In this chapter, the focus is on understanding vulnerabilities to the development of psychopathology as they occur in infancy, which is important for several reasons. First, infancy is a period during which influences on development may be strongest (Bornstein, 2014). Second, from a developmental psychopathology perspective, it is understood that prior development influences later development (Cicchetti & Schneider-Rosen, 1986). That is, infants who have adapted well to the challenges of infancy will likely face future developmental challenges with greater resources relative to those who emerge from infancy with biological and/or behavioral vulnerabilities. Infants with early vulnerabilities, on the other hand, may be at a greater risk of experiencing later problems given that such individuals would face the challenges of later developmental stages with less optimal resources. Third, as discussed later, given this developmental perspective, infancy is clearly an essential time period for experimental or clinical interventions that may potentially alter developmental trajectories. Changes in the environment and/or in the individual's internal vulnerabilities may enhance the infant's ability to adapt to later developmental challenges. Intervening in vulnerabilities, whether through prevention or treatment, whether targeting the infant or the parents or the larger social system, has the potential to decrease the likelihood of the psychopathology that might otherwise later develop (Sroufe & Rutter, 1984).

The chapter begins with an overview of infant vulnerability to psychopathology, followed by a review of relevant research, emphasizing both the methods and the findings. Finally, the chapter concludes with indications of next steps for continuing along these important lines of study. Throughout, the phenomenon of infant vulnerability to psychopathology is described from a biopsychosocial perspective, with a focus on early experiences, including during fetal development.

Infant Vulnerability to Psychopathology: An Overview

Psychopathology in infancy is rare. Thus the focus of this chapter is on infant vulnerability to the *later* development of psychopathology. Such "later" psychopathology may occur as early as during the toddler years or not until adulthood. Although both are concerning, researchers have increasingly been contributing to the understanding of early onset psychopathology (e.g., Egger & Angold, 2006). Indeed, specialized classification systems have been developed, such as the *Diagnostic Classification of Mental Health and Developmental Disorders of Infancy and Early Childhood* (DC: 0–3; Zero to Three, 2005). For example, when developmentally informed assessment and "translation" of symptom criteria are considered, major depressive disorder (MDD) has been reliably and validly identified among preschool-age children (Luby, Heffelfinger, et al., 2003; Luby, Mrakotsky, et al., 2003). MDD among preschool-age children is characterized by not only sadness, anhedonia (loss of interest or pleasure in everyday activities), and appetite and weight problems, all of which are typical of older children or adults with MDD, but also by age-specific symptoms such as being grouchy, whining or crying frequently, and play or talk that focuses on death or suicide (Luby, Heffelfinger, et al., 2003). Anxiety disorders, including separation anxiety disorder (SAD), specific phobias, and generalized anxiety disorder (GAD), have also been identified in toddlers and preschool-age children (Shamir-Essakow, Ungerer, & Rapee, 2005). For example, young children with SAD have unrealistic and persistent worry about something bad happening to themselves or their caregiver. Disruptive behavior disorders, specifically oppositional defiant disorder (ODD) and attention-deficit/hyperactivity disorder (ADHD), typically first onset in the preschool years (Lavigne, LeBailly, Hopkins, Gouze, & Binns, 2009). Young children with ODD show symptoms of uncooperative, defiant, and hostile behavior that is frequent and serious enough to significantly interfere with daily functioning. Toddlers with ADHD typically show signs of hyperactivity and impulsivity that is sufficiently frequent and intense as to distinguish it from typical toddler behavior. It is also important to consider that disorders in young children often are comorbid, evidenced by the co-occurrence of two or more disorders (Luby, Heffelfinger, et al., 2003).

Although psychopathology to this point has been described in categorical/diagnostic terms, describing and understanding psychopathology in dimensional terms is at least as important. The well-validated Child Behavior Checklist (CBCL) uses a dimensional approach to understanding psychopathology and yields scores on internalizing and externalizing problems in children as young as age 18 months (Ivanova et al., 2010). Another reliable and valid assessment tool, the Infant–Toddler Social and Emotional Assessment (ITSEA; Carter, Briggs-Gowan, Jones, & Little, 2003), similarly yields scores on internalizing and externalizing, but also on dysregulation and extends down to 12-month-olds (and up to 36-month-olds; see Bagner, Rodríguez, Blake, Linares, and Carter, 2012, for a review of assessment tools for young children's psychopathology).

This basic overview of early-onset psychopathology underscores the need to understand infant vulnerabilities to the development of psychopathology. Vulnerabilities are defined here as qualities or characteristics of the infant or the environment that increase the likelihood of the later development of psychopathology. Potential sources of vulnerability are numerous. They include genetic and other biological factors, family characteristics (e.g., depression in a parent or marital conflict), and other environmental qualities (e.g., the stressors and deprivations associated with poverty). Broadly, the understanding of vulnerability has the potential to reveal key mechanisms in the development of psychopathology (Ingram & Price, 2010).

An important conceptual distinction is between vulnerabilities and early signs or symptoms of disorder. For example, in addition to knowledge of onset of disorders as early as toddlerhood, as just reviewed, it is beginning to be understood that infants can display symptoms of depression or other disorders

(Brief-ITSEA: Briggs-Gowan & Carter, 2007). These early signs of disorder may or may not be continuous with later manifestations of disorders (as reviewed in Ingram & Price, 2010). Nonetheless, the focus of this chapter is on characteristics or qualities that are conceptualized to precede the onset of psychopathology.

One illustration of this distinction is in the Goodman and Gotlib integrative model (see Figure 17.1), which seeks to explain the transmission of risk for the development of psychopathology from depression in mothers to their children (Goodman & Gotlib, 1999). In this model, the offspring of mothers with depression are predicted to develop vulnerabilities in one or more domain of functioning. The domains of infant functioning that index vulnerabilities may be psychobiological (e.g., the hypothalamic–pituitary–adrenocortical [HPA] axis), cognitive (e.g., biased attention), affective (e.g., difficulties in emotion regulation such as reward processing), and behavioral or interpersonal (e.g.,

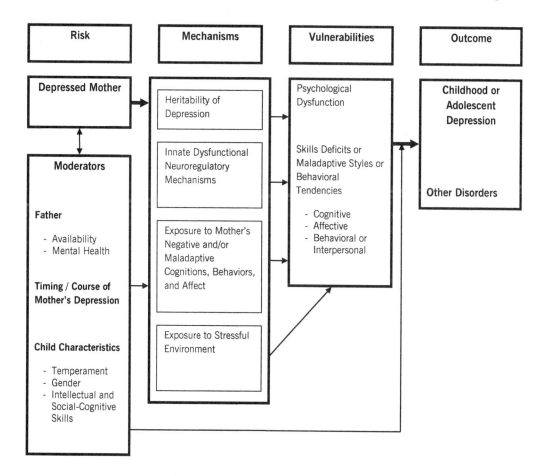

FIGURE 17.1. Integrative model for the transmission of risk to children of depressed mothers. From Goodman and Gotlib (1999). Copyright 1999 by the American Psychological Association. Reprinted by permission.

inadequate social skills). Moreover, the vulnerabilities are thought to interact and, in particular, to exacerbate one another. In this way, the model is meant to capture key features of biobehavioral organisms in the sense that biological and psychological aspects of functioning are inextricably linked. Finally, it is these vulnerabilities that may subsequently lead to the development of depression or other disorders.

The word *may* in the previous sentence is captured in the model by a set of proposed moderators. A moderating variable is one that changes the direction (i.e., positive or negative) or strength of association between two other variables. The idea of moderation is highly relevant to the understanding of vulnerabilities in that their degree of presence would increase or decrease the likelihood of infants either showing vulnerabilities or of vulnerabilities progressing into disorders. As an example, within the Goodman and Gotlib (1999) model, only a subset of infants born to depressed mothers are expected to have vulnerabilities or, even in the presence of vulnerabilities, go on to develop psychopathology as evidence has supported. For example, in a review of that evidence, we found that the association between depression in mothers' and children's internalizing problems was stronger in girls than in boys and in families living in poverty relative to middle- or higher-income families (Goodman et al., 2011).

Other concepts that are helpful to understand in the context of considering infant vulnerability are *trait markers*, *biological markers*, or *endophenotypes*, three terms that are often used interchangeably. Indeed, the construct of endophenotypes was developed to capture the hypothesized pathways from genotype to disorder (Gottesman & Gould, 2003) and thus is very compatible with the notion of vulnerability. Endophenotypes go beyond routine use of the term *vulnerability* in that they are defined as being state independent (present prior to and between episodes of a disorder), heritable (possibly inferred from rates of disorder in relatives), associated with the disorder of concern in the population, and present at higher rates in family members without the disorder than in the general population. These are useful specifications to consider in interpreting the findings reviewed in this chapter.

Often conceptualized as antonyms to vulnerability, competence and protective factors are also important to understand in the context of infant vulnerabilities to the development of psychopathology. Protective factors, internal or external, may promote competent development and alter trajectories toward the development of psychopathology. Examples include the parenting qualities that have been found to be associated with healthy infant development in well-replicated studies (Sroufe, Coffino, & Carlson, 2010), including sensitive parenting (Bakermans-Kranenburg, van IJzendoorn, & Juffer, 2003), positive family relationships (Rosenblum, Dayton, & Muzik, 2009), and secure attachment (Rutter, 1987). Broadly speaking, competence as an individual difference variable is viewed as one's ability to benefit from resources, both internal and external, in order to facilitate healthy development (Waters & Sroufe, 1983). It is essential that they be included in models of vulnerabilities to the development of psychopathology.

Relatedly, developmental psychopathologists early on recognized the importance of understanding the development of individuals who do not advance toward psychopathology despite the presence of vulnerabilities or risks. Early notions of a subset of at-risk children being invulnerable were replaced with a focus on coping and resilience (Anthony, 1974). Masten (2001) makes a strong case for understanding resilience processes rather than a static construct and for models of the likely dynamic, transactional associations among variables in the prediction of psychopathology or adaptation. Cicchetti (2013) also argues for a multilevel approach in his research on the role of resilience in the association between childhood maltreatment and psychopathology. Such approaches recognize the importance of considering coping and resilience in models of vulnerability to the development of psychopathology.

In addition to the notion that not all individuals with vulnerabilities will develop psychopathology, multifinality also applies to consideration of infants' vulnerabilities to the development of psychopathology (Cicchetti & Rogosch, 1996). Even within a group of infants with similar vulnerabilities, some will manage to embark on a healthy pathway and others will develop disorder, and even the specific disorder they develop may vary. Despite the reviewed evidence for vulnerabilities in infants as precursors to disorder, links between particular vulnerabilities and particular disorders are relatively weak. Thus, understanding the development of psychopathology requires complex models, attempting to explain the processes involved in these widely varying trajectories.

Theoretical Models

Multidimensional Models

It is essential to place the work reviewed here in the context of understanding that no single biological or environmental factor—maternal depression, prenatal exposures, a particular genetic polymorphism, and so on—is likely to explain the development of psychopathology. Moreover, any single vulnerability likely does not account for the later development of psychopathology; such univariate predictor models are almost certainly inadequate and require consideration of the influences of additive or interacting vulnerabilities. Further, vulnerabilities, even in combination, are not invariably associated with the development of psychopathology (e.g., Rutter, 1990). In general terms, vulnerabilities will more likely be associated with the development of psychopathology when they are numerous, in the context of risk factors, and when protective factors are absent or inadequate (Cicchetti & Schneider-Rosen, 1986). The constructs, processes, and mechanisms reviewed in this chapter have all been brought to bear to address this complexity.

Diathesis–Stress Models

Gottesman and Shields (1972) introduced diathesis–stress models to describe how biological vulnerabilities to the development of psychopathology might be expressed only under certain environmental conditions. Later interpretations of the model also considered the reverse roles of biology and environment (Monroe & Simons, 1991). Gene–environment interaction models are one example (Rutter, 2007), such as the now classic Caspi et al. studies (Caspi, Hariri, Holmes, Uher, & Moffitt, 2010), which have provided substantial evidence for an interaction between the serotonin transporter gene (*5-HTT*) and exposure to stress in predicting depression, such that individuals with a specific variant of this gene appeared to be more sensitive to stressors, and therefore, more vulnerable to the development of depression. As valuable as they have been, most of the gene–environment models have been replaced with or modified in light of transactional models or differential susceptibility models.

Transactional Models of Risk or Vulnerability

Sameroff's seminal work on transactional models challenges ideas about main-effect causes of psychopathology (Sameroff, 1975, 2009). The emphasis is on the mutual, bidirectional influences between infants' domains of functioning (e.g., biological) and qualities of the environment (e.g., parent responsiveness), and how these influences play out over the course of development.

As one example, as was touched on in the section on temperament, infants who are high in the temperament construct of negative affectivity (NA) may shape their environments by evoking negative responses from their caregivers. These transactional processes may, in turn, contribute to the infants' later development of psychopathology. Indeed, in a study beginning in infancy and proceeding over 5 years, Pesonen and colleagues (2008) found that although the effect of maternal perceived stress on changes in infant negative and positive affectivity was greater, evidence was also found for the reverse: increases in offspring's NA and decreases in positive affectivity contributed to increases in levels of maternal stress. Similarly, research has suggested that adolescents' past disorders increased the likelihood (and number) of future maternal depression episodes (Raposa, Hammen, & Brennan, 2011). This research highlights the importance of acknowledging the dynamic interplay that exists between infant and environment in the development and maintenance of psychopathology.

Differential Susceptibility Models

Diathesis–stress models may place undue emphasis on individuals' vulnerability. In recent findings, individuals with the same allelic variation have been found to demonstrate different outcomes dependent on their early environmental exposures. Interestingly, it is not just early exposure to adverse environments that matters but also exposure to enriched environments (Pluess & Belsky, 2013). Differential susceptibility models shift the emphasis away from vulnerability to adverse experiences toward a notion of developmental plasticity (Belsky, 1997; Brune, 2012). The advantage of this approach is that it accounts for not only negative consequences from exposure to adverse environments, but also the possibility of positive consequences from supportive environments, as well as the idea that some individuals may be less susceptible to both negative and positive influences. Stress response systems play a key role in such models, referred to as biological sensitivity to context (Boyce & Ellis, 2005; Ellis, Essex, & Boyce, 2005).

Origins of Infant Vulnerabilities

Up to this point in the chapter, the focus has been on theoretical and conceptual understandings of infant vulnerabilities. The following sections outline evidence for various sources of influence on infant vulnerabilities, beginning with the earliest: during fetal development. Genetic and postnatal influences are then discussed.

Fetal Influences on Infant Vulnerabilities

Several infant vulnerabilities may have their origins in fetal development. That is, both intra- and extrauterine experiences are increasingly understood to influence fetal neural system development in ways that may contribute to the development of psychopathology. Although such experiences include the mother's drug or alcohol use and environmental toxins (Huizink & Mulder, 2006), this chapter focuses on maternal stress and psychopathology. What are the mechanisms that might explain associations between these prenatal exposures and infant vulnerabilities? This question has proved to be challenging and findings are still emerging. Proposed mechanisms that have received the strongest empirical support include reduced hippocampal volume alterations in the stress response system and in systems involved in the capacity to adaptively respond to environmental changes, including epigenetic programing of stress regulation systems and alterations of the placenta (Bale, 2011; Coussons-Read, 2013; Matthews & Phillips, 2012; O'Donnell et al., 2012).

Building on prospective longitudinal animal studies linking prenatal stress to the later development of psychopathology (e.g., Schneider, Moore, & Kraemer, 2003), studies of prenatal stress and psychopathology exposures in humans have yielded important findings related to infant vulnerabilities to psychopathology. For example, depression in mothers during pregnancy has been associated with risk for infants' premature delivery (Grigoriadis et al., 2013), which is concerning given that premature delivery is associated with risk for the later development of internalizing behavior problems and attention problems (Talge et al., 2010), ADHD (Galéra et al., 2011), and even predicted adolescent depressive disorders in a case-control prospective cohort study (Patton, Coffey, Carlin, Olsson, & Morley, 2004).

In the study of prenatal exposures to maternal psychopathology, researchers have been challenged to understand the specificity of associations to particular disorders, or even whether it is general maternal distress that matters. Part of the challenge is the high rate of comorbidity between depression and anxiety, and the co-occurrence of both depression and anxiety with stress, including, as we have found, during pregnancy (Goodman & Tully, 2009). Thus, understanding the separate influences of prenatal depression, stress, and anxiety has been difficult, and may not be feasible given the challenges of either finding sufficiently large samples of women without the comorbid disorder or correlated stress, or of interpreting findings from statistical controls of one such variable for the other. Moreover, among disorders in mothers, prenatal depression is not alone in its association with prematurity or low birth weight. Anorexia nervosa has been found to have similar associations, although inconsistently (see Micali & Treasure, 2009, for a review), as has schizophrenia (Nilsson et al., 2008).

In terms of other infant vulnerabilities, beyond prematurity and low birth weight, prenatal depression has been found to be associated with infants' higher negative affective temperament (Davis et al., 2007; Rouse & Goodman, 2014). Prenatal depression, anxiety, and drinking have been associated with infants' patterns of dampened cortisol reactivity to stressors (Grant et al., 2009; Haley, Handmaker, & Lowe, 2006; Keenan, Gunthorpe, & Grace, 2007). More broadly, mothers' cortisol levels during pregnancy, which were associated with psychosocial stress exposure, predicted infants' cortisol levels (Karlén, Frostell, Theodorsson, Faresjö, & Ludvigsson, 2013). Higher prenatal maternal cortisol levels also predicted infants' more negative behavior (crying and fussing during bath sessions) through 5 months of age (de Weerth, van Hees, & Buitelaar, 2003). Further, we found prenatal depression to be associated with infants' disorganized attachment (Hayes, Goodman, & Carlson, 2013). This is just a sampling of findings on prenatal influences on infant vulnerabilities, with an emphasis on prenatal depression.

A closely related topic is fetal exposure to psychotropic medication. About half of all pregnancies are unplanned (Finer & Kost, 2011), and rates of antidepressant usage among childbearing-age women are high. Thus, women taking medications may not realize that they are pregnant, resulting in many fetuses having at least early medication exposure. Recent reviews reveal that antidepressant exposure is significantly associated with neonatal outcomes such as gestational age and birth weight, but effect sizes are small, and appropriate comparison groups are not always studied (Ross et al., 2013). Thus it may be that women's history (e.g., age of onset) or severity of depression, both of which may be correlated with patterns of medication use, matter more for understanding associations with infant vulnerabilities than the medication exposure per se.

Genetic Influences on Infant Vulnerabilities

Several vulnerabilities to the development of psychopathology are at least moderately heritable. Support for heritability has been found, typically from twin studies, for psychobiological vulnerabilities such as neuromotor abnormalities (Gamma et al., 2013), vagal tone (Snieder, van Doornen, Boomsma, & Thayer, 2007), cortisol levels (see Bartels, Van den Berg, Sluyter, Boomsma, & de Geus, 2003, for a review), cortisol reactivity (Steptoe, van Jaarsveld, Semmler, Plomin, & Wardle, 2009), and frontal electroencephalogram (EEG) asymmetry (Anokhin, Heath, & Myers, 2006), as well as for behavioral vulnerabilities such as social withdrawal or behavioral inhibition (BI), and negative affectivity (NA) (Dilalla, Kagan, & Reznick, 1994). Moving beyond behavior genetics studies, candidate gene studies have identified specific polymorphisms associated with withdrawn behavior (Rubin et al., 2013). An important caveat is that many studies of the heritability of these trait-level vulnerabilities have been conducted on adults or older children and may not be accurate for infants. It is not unusual for researchers to find different levels of heritability of a trait for different ages of children, with heritability sometimes being stronger for younger children, but more often stronger for older children. For example, temperament as measured in neonates (irritability, resistance to soothing, activity level, reactivity, and reinforcement value) has been found to have negligible heritability (Riese, 1990), whereas changes in BI (a component of temperament) from 12 to 30 months, were more highly heritable, based on higher concordance for monozygotic than dizygotic twins (Matheny, 1989).

Yet it is now well understood that environmental influences profoundly alter pathways from vulnerabilities to the emergence of disorder, regardless of heritability, and that gene–environment interactions and correlations play essential roles (Beauchaine & Gatzke-Kopp, 2013). Moreover, epigenetic research has highlighted the importance of considering these environment–genome interactions in the study of infant vulnerabilities. For example, prenatal stress has been found to decrease placental 11β hydroxysteroid dehydrogenase 2 (11B-HSD2) and reduce deoxyribonucleic acid (DNA) methylation in the hippocampus and amygdala at the corticotrophin-releasing hormone (CRH) gene (Mueller, Brocke, Fries, Lesch, & Kirschbaum, 2010; O'Donnell et al., 2012). In turn, both have been found to alter responsiveness of the HPA axis, which is discussed in the next section as a vulnerability to the later development of psychopathology (Kofink, Boks, Timmers, & Kas, 2013).

Postnatal Influences on Infant Vulnerabilities

Inadequate parenting is the postnatal influence most often cited as imposing vulnerabilities to the development of psychopathology on infants. Inadequate parenting may be one of the strongest mediators of the association between depression and other disorders or stressors in parents and their infant's vulnerabilities to the later development of psychopathology (e.g., Goodman & Gotlib, 1999). Although I focus here on depression in mothers, it is important to also be aware of similar literatures, such as parenting qualities as mediators of the association between marital (interparental) conflict and the development of psychopathology (Davies, Sturge-Apple, Cicchetti, Manning, & Vonhold, 2012).

Depression in mothers has reliably been shown to be associated with inadequate parenting, albeit often with small effect sizes. For example, we found that, among depressed mothers, higher symptom levels were significantly associated with less accuracy in interpreting babies' facial expressions, particularly positive facial expressions, with a moderate effect size (Broth, Goodman, Hall, & Raynor, 2004). In a meta-analytic review of 46 observational studies of parenting and depression in mothers, small but significant effect sizes were found for associations between depression in mothers and more disengaged and negative behavior, as well as lower levels of positive behavior (Lovejoy, Graczyk, O'Hare, & Neuman, 2000). Moreover, child age moderated the association between depression and positive behaviors. Specifically, and most relevant for this chapter, the association was significant only for infants under 1 year of age and not for children ages 1 to 5 years.

Some researchers have taken the next step of directly testing the mediational model, that inadequate parenting explains at least part of the variance in associations between depression in mothers and infant vulnerabilities. In this model, researchers propose that as depression symptom levels increase, mothers subsequently engage in fewer of the parenting qualities associated with healthy infant development (e.g., sensitive, warm parenting) and more of the parenting qualities known to interfere with healthy infant development (e.g., disengaged or harsh/intrusive parenting). These changes in parenting qualities are then expected to be associated with infant vulnerabilities. Most important, the purported mediational role of parenting would be supported by findings that the changes in parenting qualities statistically account, at least in part, for associations between maternal depressive symptoms and infant vulnerabilities.

The model has been supported in several studies of associations between depression in mothers and youth psychopathology (e.g., Elgar, Mills, McGrath, Waschbusch, & Brownridge, 2007; Goodman & Tully, 2006), but not all studies find support for mediation (e.g., Hoffman, Crnic, & Baker, 2006). However, most of the studies of the mediational role of parenting in associations between depression in mothers and child psychopathology have studied older children and not infant vulnerabilities per se. Additional studies are needed.

Models of qualities of early parenting as vulnerabilities to the development of psychopathology are not limited to depression. For example, Linehan's (1993) developmental model of borderline personality disorder implicates parents' insensitive response to children's emotions, especially negative emotions. Other strong examples come from social learning theory models for the development of ODD and conduct disorder (Patterson, 1982). The effectiveness of interventions to enhance parenting qualities in reducing child conduct problems provides further support for the role of parenting qualities (Beauchaine, Webster-Stratton, & Reid, 2005).

A more general construct to account for postnatal influences on infant vulnerabilities is stress. Stress may explain associations between parenting qualities and infant vulnerabilities. More broadly, stress is an essential construct for understanding the context in which infant vulnerabilities emerge (Hammen, 2002).

Specific Vulnerabilities

What follows is a brief overview of some specific vulnerabilities to the development of psychopathology. The focus here is on systems that have been reliably measured in infancy and have strong links to later development of psychopathology, although evidence for the latter varies across the vulnerabilities. This is not meant to be a comprehensive list.

Neuroendocrine Systems

At the core of the neuroendocrine system is the HPA axis. Among its numerous functions, the HPA axis regulates mood, emotions, and responses to stress. In typically developing infants and children, based on studies of cortisol levels as an index of HPA activity, it is now well understood that elevations in cortisol associated with short-term stressors are an adaptive stress response and function to reestablish homeostasis. Moreover, beginning early in life, social relationships play key roles as buffers of stress responses (Hostinar, Sullivan, & Gunnar, 2014).

HPA axis activity is strongly associated with the development of depression and other disorders. Dysfunctional neuroregulatory systems in infants of depressed mothers have been proposed as a mechanism to explain risk for the later development of psychopathology (Goodman & Gotlib, 1999). By the age of 3 months, human infants have adult-equivalent levels of cortisol, the primary steroid hormone produced by the HPA system in response to stress, and are capable of responding to stress. The infant HPA axis has been found to be relatively unresponsive to many acute psychological stressors, but moderately responsive to acute physical stressors, although it is important to note that effect sizes decrease over the course of infancy, as infants develop a range of stress-regulation abilities (Jansen, Beijers, Riksen-Walraven, & de Weerth, 2010).

At least two models have been proposed for the HPA axis system as an infant vulnerability to psychopathology. First, early exposure to stressors, whether pre- or postnatal, may predispose children to alterations in their stress response systems, which is a vulnerability given implications for later ability to adaptively respond to stressors (Gunnar, Porter, Wolf, & Rigatuso, 1995).

Second, early stressors, again pre- or postnatal, may reprogram HPA system regulation through epigenetic processes. Such processes may alter the expression of genes involved in the functioning of the HPA system (Booij, Wang, Levesque, Tremblay, & Szyf, 2013), with similar implications for the later development of psychopathology.

Consistent with these models, researchers have found some support for HPA axis dysregulation in infants as a vulnerability to the development of psychopathology (Gunnar & Quevedo, 2007b). In terms of predictors within infancy, higher cortisol reactivity to a heel stick in newborns predicted lower scores on "distress-to-limitations" temperament at age 6 months (Gunnar et al., 1995). In terms of longer-term predictions, Gunnar reminds us of some important cautions. First, it is essential to take into account normative decreases in cortisol reactivity known to occur over infancy, at least among healthy infants in low-risk environments (see Keenan, 2000, for a review). Second, HPA axis dysregulation associated with early experiences may remit once the adverse experience is resolved, explaining at least some of the circumstances in which early vulnerabilities may not predict the later development of psychopathology (Gunnar & Quevedo, 2007a). Third, among children at relatively low risk for the development of psychopathology, individual differences in cortisol reactivity are likely of low predictive value (Gunnar, Brodersen, Krueger, & Rigatuso, 1996). Thus cortisol may be most productively studied in infants in high-risk environments or who have additional qualities or characteristics imposing risk for the development of psychopathology.

Brain Function

It is well established that the left hemisphere is involved in the management and expression of positive, approach-related emotional responses to positive stimuli and reward and the right hemisphere with negative, withdrawal-directed emotional responses (Fox, 1991). Much attention has been devoted to the study of asymmetrical brain functioning, given long-standing evidence for associations between relatively greater activation of the right prefrontal cortevx (negative asymmetry values) and lower levels of positive affect, higher levels of approach-related deficits, and greater vulnerability to depression (Davidson, 1994; Davidson & Fox, 1982). These ideas have fueled numerous studies that included measures of EEG, the recording of electrical activity along the scalp, to index this vulnerability, including in infancy (Marshall, Bar-Haim, & Fox, 2002). Specifically, EEG has been used to measure differential activation of the left and right cerebral hemispheres either as a baseline measure or while processing positive and negative emotions. In typically developing populations of infants, the left frontal region is relatively more active in relation to positive emotions, whereas the right frontal region is more active in relation to negative emotions (as reviewed in Fox, 1991).

Studies of resting or baseline EEG asymmetry in infants have also been found to reveal individual differences in the tendency to become distressed or to show a "depressed" affective style (Fox, 1991). For example, an early study found that frontal EEG asymmetry in 10-month-old infants predicted the extent to which infants cried in response to a brief separation from their mothers (Davidson & Fox, 1989). Attempts to explain those individual differences implicate adverse rearing environments (McLaughlin, Fox, Zeanah, & Nelson, 2011). For example, Field and colleagues found elevated depression symptom levels to be associated with EEG asymmetry in infants as early as 1 month of age (Jones, Field, Fox, Lundy, & Davalos, 1997). A meta-analytic review of the studies of EEG asymmetry in infants of depressed mothers revealed that the association is stronger for younger, relative to older, infants (Thibodeau, Jorgensen, & Kim, 2006).

In addition to attempts to predict EEG asymmetry in infants, researchers have also examined the predictive validity of these asymmetries, with a focus on predicting indices of the development of psychopathology. First, EEG patterns are found to be relatively stable both within infancy (Lusby, Goodman, Bell, & Newport, 2014) and from infancy to early childhood (Jones, Field, Davalos, & Pickens, 1997). Second, EEG asymmetry patterns identified in infants have been found to be prospectively associated with the emergence of early indices or precursors of psychopathology. For example, infants with relative right-frontal EEG asymmetry displayed more stable observed BI over the first 4 years of life (Fox, Henderson, Rubin, Calkins, & Schmidt, 2001). Further, children with greater left-frontal asymmetry scores at 36 months of age were observed to display disruptive behavior with an unknown peer at 5 years of age (Degnan et al., 2011). Given evidence for the stability in EEG asymmetry scores from infancy to at least early childhood, it is also relevant that greater right EEG asymmetry measured in 4-year-olds was associated with 9-year-olds' lower levels of mother-reported emotion regulation skills and higher levels of physiological arousal (heart rate and heart rate variability) during a speech task (Hannesdóttir, Doxie, Bell, Ollendick, & Wolfe, 2010). Additional support for predictive validity comes from a quasi-experimental study in which earlier age at which orphaned children were placed into foster care was correlated with increased EEG alpha power at 42 months of age (Marshall, Reeb, Fox, Nelson, & Zeanah, 2008).

Another index of brain functioning that can be reliably measured in infants is the orienting response from event-related potential (ERP) brain recordings. Interest has particularly, although not exclusively, focused on the P3 (or P300) ERP component, which is hypothesized to reflect attention to stimuli in the environment. Even as early as 3 months of age, infants orient to novel stimuli (Friedman, Cycowicz, & Gaeta, 2001). In adults, P3 amplitude reductions are hypothesized to reflect a genetic vulnerability to a range of externalizing problem behaviors, and have been associated with children's disruptive behavior disorders. Additionally, P3 amplitude reductions have been found in offspring of parents with externalizing disorders (Iacono, Malone, & McGue, 2003). Consistent with the idea that early experiences alter the functioning of neural systems, maltreated 15-month-old infants were found to differ from nonmaltreated infants on ERP responses (P260, P1, and Nc components) to angry relative to happy facial expressions (Curtis & Cicchetti, 2013).

Autonomic Functioning

Research on the parasympathetic nervous system (PNS), which is a neuroregulatory process, has yielded consistent findings in support of the PNS as an index of vulnerability to the development of psychopathology, particularly in terms of emotion dysregulation. Broadly speaking, the PNS is responsible for the "resting state" actions of the autonomic nervous system (ANS). The primary component of the PNS is the vagal system, which is understood to play a key role in the regulation, expression, and experience of emotion (Porges, 2011). Vagal tone is quantified by measuring the amplitude of respiratory sinus arrhythmia (RSA), the patterns of increases and decreases in heart rate across the respiratory cycle (Beauchaine, 2012; Porges, 2007). Higher amplitude of RSA reflects greater cardiac vagal tone. Three key indices of RSA are of concern: (1) low baseline RSA, (2) lower RSA suppression (less responsiveness to stimuli, especially emotionally evocative stimuli), and (3) lower recovery. More broadly, RSA reflects one's ability to regulate internal physiological states while responding appropriately to external stimuli. In adults, RSA is concurrently and prospectively associated with major depressive disorder (Rottenberg, Clift, Bolden, & Salomon, 2007; Rottenberg, Wilhelm, Gross, & Gotlib, 2002).

Vagal tone has also been found to be a reliable index of individual differences in infants' reactivity (Fracasso, Porges, Lamb, & Rosenberg, 1994) and consistent with lab-based observations and maternal report of negative reactivity (Porges, Doussard-Roosevelt, Portales, & Suess, 1994; Stifter & Fox, 1990). Even in 3-month-old infants, patterns of RSA activity are associated with behavioral indices of recovery from stress (Bazhenova, Plonskaia, & Porges, 2001). In 9-month-old infants, high baseline vagal tone was found to be associated with more behavioral reactivity. In terms of consistency over time, findings vary. Specifically, although no significant changes were found in baseline and poststress vagal tone in infants prospectively studied at 5, 7, 10, and 13 months of age (Fracasso et al., 1994), in a study of 2-month-olds who were seen again at 5 years of age, baseline vagal tone was not continuous (there was a significant increase), whereas the change from baseline-to-task change (suppression) was continuous (Bornstein & Suess, 2000).

Most consistent with the concerns of this chapter, long-standing evidence supports vagal tone as an index of vulnerability to the development of psychopathology (Porges, Doussard-Roosevelt, Portales, & Greenspan, 1996).

Specifically, vagal tone in 9-month-olds predicted maternal reports of more difficult temperament in 3-year-olds, beyond the contribution of temperament measured at 9 months (Porges et al., 1994). Further, lower magnitude of the vagal tone change score (from baseline to during a challenging task) at 9 months of age (less decrease) was significantly prospectively associated with higher levels of behavior problems at 36 months of age on CBCL/2–3 scales indexing social withdrawal, depression, and aggression (Porges et al., 1996). At a follow up of this sample, when the children were 54 months old, those with behavior problem scores (total, internalizing, and externalizing) in the clinically significant range were less likely to have shown the expected suppression of RSA during the challenging task relative to those in the low behavior problem group, although small sample sizes precluded finding statistical significance of these group differences (Dale et al., 2011).

Temperament

Temperament is commonly defined as biologically based, early emerging, stable individual differences (Rothbart & Derryberry, 1981). Although several prominent researchers in this area have proposed somewhat distinct dimensions of temperament, the common themes are activity level, affectivity/emotionality, attention, and reactivity (or, conversely, self-regulation) (Frick, 2004; Rothbart & Goldsmith, 1985; Shiner et al., 2012). In typically developing infants and children, temperament has been a key construct in understanding early emerging individual differences. Moreover, temperament, especially reactivity and regulation, may even originate in fetal development, as evidenced by patterns of fetal heart rate and movement (DiPietro et al., 2002).

Of most relevance to infant vulnerability to psychopathology is the idea proposed by temperament theorists that some infants may be biologically predisposed to negative emotionality (e.g., Kagan & Snidman, 1999) or to react to novelty with excessive fear and autonomic hyperarousal (see Lonigan, Phillips, Wilson, & Allan, 2011, for a review). Among the infant vulnerabilities that are the focus of this chapter, temperament is the one that has been most often studied for its predictive associations with the development of psychopathology. For example, observed approach and inhibition in reaction to a set of low- and high-intensity toys, measured with a lab-based task at 6 and 12 months, predicted both internalizing and externalizing behavior problems at 2 years of age, especially for the high-intensity toys (Putnam & Stifter, 2005). In a large prospective longitudinal study, internalizing and externalizing problems at 18 and 30 months and 4–5 and 8–9 years of age were predicted by profiles that classified children's temperament over the developmental period (Janson & Mathiesen, 2008). For example, children whose temperament scores designated them to be in an "undercontrolled" profile had significantly higher levels of externalizing problems at each age relative to children with other temperament profiles. Similarly, higher NA, measured in the first year of life, was associated with more externalizing problems in preschool-age children, although some aspects of NA were also associated with preschoolers' internalizing problems (Gartstein, Putnam, & Rothbart, 2012). In the same sample, lower levels of infant regulatory capacity/orienting (but not NA) predicted toddlers' higher levels of depression-like symptoms, although high NA in the subsample of infants of mothers with elevated depression symptoms showed higher levels of depressive symptoms as toddlers (Gartstein & Bateman, 2008). Higher NA in infants at 9 months of age also predicted 4-year-olds' higher withdrawal (a composite score including lab observations and maternal report), although in boys only (Perez-Edgar, Schmidt, Henderson, Schulkin, & Fox, 2008). Showing remarkable evidence of infant vulnerability to psychopathology, infant temperament, specifically the tendency to express negative emotions, has been found to predict behavior problems and psychopathology as far forward as middle childhood (Bates, Bayles, Bennett, Ridge, & Brown, 1991; Sayal, Heron, Maughan, Rowe, & Ramchandani, 2014) and even adolescence (Guerin, Gottfried, & Thomas, 1997; Teerikangas, Aronen, Martin, & Huttunen, 1998).

In considering temperament of infants as a vulnerability, it is important to consider not only how each infant is disposed to experience the world (e.g., degree of distress proneness), but also the mediating factors involved in the pathway to possible psychopathology. The effects of temperament on the development of psychopathology, as with other vulnerabilities, is likely to be dependent on how caregivers (and, later, others) respond to the child's temperament rather than on the direct effects of temperament alone. Although the Goodman and Gotlib (1999) model proposes a mediational model whereby mechanisms such as inadequate parenting would explain associations between depression in mothers and adverse outcomes in offspring, other mediational models have also been tested. For example, support was found for children's internalizing problems (mother reported at 4, 7, and 15 years of age) being explained by the co-occurrence of negative parenting styles and children's BI (observed in the lab at ages 14 and 24 months; Williams et al., 2009). Infants and toddlers with higher BI, who also had mothers with higher permissive parenting style, had the highest levels of internalizing problems at age 4 years, although there were no significant interactions between BI and parenting in the prediction of change in internalizing problems from 4 to 15 years of age. No significant interactions were found between BI and parenting in the prediction of externalizing problems. Studies of transactional processes are particularly needed to better understand how early temperament and caregiving environments relate to each other over time.

Consideration of temperament as a vulnerability to the later development of psychopathology raises some intriguing questions. For example, abnormalities in circadian rhythms are implicated in the pathophysiology of bipolar disorders (Milhiet et al., 2014). Thus, it is possible that key temperament constructs may reveal early vulnerabilities for the later development of bipolar and other disorders.

Associations among Vulnerabilities

Having introduced several different infant vulnerabilities to the development of psychopathology, it is important to consider how they might relate to one another. One potential unifying construct is emotion regulation (or, conversely, dysregulation). Although researchers use different words, phrases, and definitions to capture the construct, a general consensus is that emotion regulation refers to the regulatory processes by which emotions facilitate adaptive functioning, both within the child and between the child and others or, conversely, that emotion dysregulation will be associated with maladaptive functioning (Cole, Martin, & Dennis, 2004). Given this definition, it is clear that many of the vulnerabilities relate to the construct of emotion dysregulation, which, despite diversity in definitions and measures, has been broadly recognized for its associations with the development of psychopathology (Cole et al., 2004; Keenan, 2000). Thus, it is not surprising that researchers have been interested in how the vulnerabilities relate to one another. Several questions about relationships within and among vulnerabilities have been addressed.

A few researchers have included two or more measures of infant vulnerabilities within the same study, in order to test hypotheses of their interrelationships. Support has been mixed. For example, baseline vagal tone and salivary cortisol, measured both at baseline and in response to a heel stick, were not significantly associated in newborns, although behavioral state (e.g., crying) was significantly associated with the physiological measures during both the stress and recovery periods (Gunnar et al., 1995). During the heel stick, both lower vagal tone and higher cortisol were associated with more crying. Other researchers have found that individual differences in infants' responses to mild frustrations were found to be associated with vagal tone (more easily frustrated infants showed higher RSA at baseline and less task reactivity) and with mother-rated temperament (more easily frustrated infants were rated as more active and less easily soothed, having higher distress to limitations and to novelty, and showing shorter orienting; Calkins, Dedmon, Gill, Lomax, & Johnson, 2002).

Researchers have also tested models in which two vulnerabilities are in a moderated relationship with each other in the prediction of later outcomes. For example, negative reactivity, measured at 9 months of age by maternal report, predicted 4-year-olds' social wariness only for those who had right-frontal EEG asymmetry, also measured at 9 months of age, but not for those with left-frontal EEG asymmetry (also interesting: the association was for boys only; Henderson, Fox, & Rubin, 2001). Similarly, Degnan and colleagues (2011) found a significant interaction between temperament and EEG asymmetry in the prediction of social competence with peers at 5 years of age. Specifically, children who showed high, stable exuberance in infancy and when toddlers, based on a lab task, were observed to have greater social competence with unfamiliar peers at age 5 only if they had left- and not right-frontal EEG asymmetry, as measured at 36 months. Moreover, having been high in exuberance across infancy and toddlerhood was only significantly associated with externalizing problems among those with greater left-frontal EEG asymmetry. Temperament and cortisol have also been found to be in a moderated relationship (Perez-Edgar et al., 2008). Withdrawal behavior at 4 years of age was predicted by an interaction between negative affect at 9 months of age and concurrent cortisol. Specifically, among those who had been high in NA as infants, cortisol and withdrawal were significantly, positively, and concurrently correlated, whereas for those who had been low in NA there was no significant association.

Another index of infant well-being, attachment security, may also play a moderating (or mediating) role in associations between adversities and vulnerabilities. As one example of evidence for moderated relationships, higher levels of depressive symptoms in mothers, measured when infants were 2 months of age, were associated with lower resting RSA, but only in infants who showed disorganized attachment (Tharner et al., 2013). As an example of a mediated relationship, maternal history of major depression since the child's birth was indirectly associated with 48-month-old toddlers' dysregulation problems through the toddlers' attachment insecurity, measured at 20 and 36 months of age (Gonzalez, 2010). Crittenden (2009) has written more broadly on the various pathways from infant attachment style to the development of psychopathology and offers suggestions for future work in this area.

In general, researchers find that combinations of measures of vulnerabilities increase the strength of predictions of the development of psychopathology, relative to single indices. For example, among 8-year-olds, those with both higher cortisol levels and higher RSA levels showed the lowest symptom levels of depression and anxiety (El-Sheikh, Arsiwalla, Hinnant, & Erath, 2011). Equally important is combining indices within a vulnerability. As an example, the interaction of resting/baseline RSA and RSA reactivity (to a sad film) predicted depression in adults with childhood-onset depressive disorder history and in controls with no history of major mental disorder (Yaroslavsky, Rottenberg, & Kovacs, 2013). Further studies are needed to understand whether infants who show multiple vulnerabilities not only are at higher risk for the development of psychopathology but also whether the predicted psychopathology is more severe relative to infants with a single vulnerability.

Next Steps in the Study of Infant Vulnerabilities

Early on in this chapter, it was suggested that vulnerabilities precede the onset of psychopathology. However, building on the important work on classification and measurement of disorders that may emerge in infancy, it is essential that studies test such a model. That is, more studies are needed to test three questions. First, what is the extent to which vulnerabilities precede the onset of psychopathology? Second, what models explain clinically meaningful portions of variance in the onset of psychopathology? Third, to what extent do vulnerabilities explain (mediate) associations between risk factors and the emergence of psychopathology? Embedded in each of these questions is an emphasis on effect sizes, which allow for consideration that even "small" effect sizes can have clinical and public health significance, regardless of statistical significance. In addition to this general call, the following are more specific suggestions for future research.

Understanding Comorbidities and Correlates

Another challenge noted earlier is how to understand potentially unique influences of prenatal depression, stress, and anxiety on infant vulnerabilities. This has been difficult because of the high levels of comorbidity between depression and anxiety, and knowledge that both disorders co-occur in the context of high stress levels. For example, in the National Comorbidity Survey, approximately 75% of adults with lifetime or recent depression also had at least one additional mental health or substance abuse diagnosis (Kessler et al., 2005). Thus, large samples would be needed in order to identify individuals with depression disorder and no anxiety disorder and vice versa, while also including those individuals with comorbid depression and anxiety as a third group to be studied. Similarly, large samples would be needed to ensure a broad range of stress/distress levels in the latter three groups. A common alternative approach, to measure multiple predictors and parse them apart statistically, raises other concerns. Researchers grappling with these issues of comorbidity and correlates may benefit from considering qualities that underlie multiple disorders, such as those suggested within the research domain criteria (Cuthbert & Kozak, 2013; Sanislow et al., 2010).

Future studies should also take into consideration additional common comorbidities, such as depression with substance use or abuse, given findings such as Kessler et al. (2005), as noted. Also needed are studies that parse out the relative contribution of prenatal exposure to antidepressant medication relative to mothers' depression characteristics, such as age of onset and pregnancy levels of severity.

The Role of Fathers

It is abundantly clear that the role of fathers has been understudied and, despite some recent attention, important questions remain unanswered. More study is needed of psychopathology in fathers as an independent variable and also as a potential moderator of associations between disorder in mothers and infant out-comes (see Edward, Castle, Mills, Davis, & Casey, 2015, for a recent review). Also important to understand is the role of father involvement in association with depression in mothers, with the potential to buffer the development of infant vulnerabilities or interfere with the development of psychopathology even in the presence of vulnerabilities. This is only a small sample of the important questions to be asked about the role of fathers in relation to better understanding infant vulnerabilities to the development of psychopathology.

Longitudinal Studies

Many of our most pressing questions concern the potential for prenatal and/or genetic influences to be modified by postnatal exposures/experiences (Laurent, 2014). To address these questions, such as the extent to which early experiences "program" stress sensitivity or other vulnerabilities, it is essential to conduct studies beginning in pregnancy.

An even more basic question that requires longitudinal designs is the short- and long-term consistency and predictive validity of the indices of vulnerability that we have introduced. Such studies have yielded promising findings. For example, individual differences in patterns of change across repeated administrations of the Neonatal Behavioral Assessment Scale (NBAS; Brazelton, 1984) predicted infant outcomes at 18 months of age (Lester, 1984). Others suggest the value of repeated measures (Worobey, 1990). Rather than stability of vulnerabilities, it may be that changes in infant functioning over time are more predictive of later psychopathology. In either case, multiple measures are likely to be more valuable than any single measure. Based on this idea, we have been examining cross-time as well as cross-situation associations of vulnerabilities in infants at risk for the development of depression in relation to their mothers' history of depression (Lusby, Goodman, Bell, & Newport, 2013).

Experiments/Intervention Studies

It is precisely the understanding of mechanisms in the development of psychopathology that will provide key information needed to design increasingly effective preventive interventions. Evidence is mounting in support of the effectiveness of preventive interventions that identify and target common vulnerabilities for the development of psychopathology (Beauchaine, Neuhaus, Brenner, & Gatzke-Kopp, 2008). Further, an understanding of the role of moderators will provide a guide as to where to target these interventions, who is likely to benefit from them, when in development to intervene, and so on. Reliable and valid assessment tools are needed to identify both an individual infant's vulnerabilities and his or her competencies; both would inform the design of targeted interventions, to decrease vulnerabilities and support or enhance competencies. Further, an understanding of the developmental course is essential to identification of precursors, which might serve as triggers for the introduction of interventions. Knowledge of timing of the emergence and course of vulnerabilities will contribute to the likelihood of appropriate timing of interventions. Cicchetti's work to enhance children's strengths, both cognitive–developmental and psychobiological, provides paradigmatic examples of this approach (Cicchetti, Rogosch, & Toth, 2000; Cicchetti, Rogosch, Toth, & Sturge-Apple, 2011). Another example of such work is an intervention to improve parental sensitivity in order to enhance attachment security, which has been found to have small, but significant, effect sizes based on a meta-analytic review (Bakermans-Kranenburg et al., 2003). Work on home-visiting services and other early interventions is similarly promising. More broadly, next steps in this area of study include using knowledge of infant vulnerabilities to design preventive interventions and test the potential to decrease the likelihood of the emergence of psychopathology.

Development/Refinement of Assessment Tools

Progress in research and treatment related to infant vulnerabilities to psychopathology is highly dependent on continuing work on assessment tools. The field will benefit from enhancements of the reliability and validity of methods for identifying vulnerabilities. As discussed earlier in this chapter, refinement of assessment tools will also allow for more targeted interventions, based on the unique vulnerabilities and competencies of each individual.

Cognitive/Perceptual Vulnerabilities

Although infants are not capable of the level of thinking typically associated with cognitive vulnerabilities to depression in adults, an understanding of the development of cognitive vulnerabilities suggests some intriguing possibilities to pursue in future studies of infant vulnerabilities. For older children, we developed a measure of children's perceptions of depression in their mothers (Tully, Goodman, & Brooks-DeWeese, 2005). Creative work is needed to develop such a measure for infants, to understand how they perceive depression in their mothers. For example, in infants, it is possible that attentional tendencies indicate an expectation for particular outcomes. Measures of expectancies or attentional biases are promising, as is eye tracking as a measurement tool.

Summary

In conclusion, while much is known about infant vulnerabilities to the development of psychopathology, there is much more work to be accomplished. This is a sampling of ideas. Longitudinal studies, but also experimental designs, will likely yield the most valuable findings relative to correlational, cross-sectional studies, although the latter play an important foundational role. Also needed is work to refine our theoretical models. Although our models need to take much into account, beyond univariate predictors, statistical approaches are available to answer the interesting and important questions.

ACKNOWLEDGMENTS

I gratefully acknowledge the editorial assistance of Erica Ahlich. The chapter benefited from her keen eye and diligent reference checking.

REFERENCES

Anokhin, A. P., Heath, A. C., & Myers, E. (2006). Genetic and environmental influences on frontal EEG asymmetry: A twin study. *Biological Psychology, 71,* 289–295.

Anthony, E. J. (1974). The syndrome of the psychologically invulnerable child. In E. J. Anthony & C. Koupernik (Eds.), *The child in his family: Children at psychiatric risk* (pp. 529–545). Oxford, UK: Wiley.

Bagner, D., Rodríguez, G., Blake, C., Linares, D., & Carter, A. (2012). Assessment of behavioral and emotional problems in infancy: A systematic review. *Clinical Child and Family Psychology Review, 15*(2), 113–128.

Bakermans-Kranenburg, M. J., van IJzendoorn, I. M. H., & Juffer, F. (2003). Less is more: Meta-analyses of sensitivity and attachment interventions in early childhood. *Psychological Bulletin, 129*(2), 195–215.

Bale, T. L. (2011). Sex differences in prenatal epigenetic programing of stress pathways. *Stress, 14*(4), 348–356.

Bartels, M., Van den Berg, M. P., Sluyter, F., Boomsma, D. I., & de Geus, E. J. C. (2003). Heritability of cortisol levels: Review and simultaneous analysis of twin studies. *Psychoneuroendocrinology, 28,* 121–137.

Bates, J. E., Bayles, K., Bennett, D. S., Ridge, B., & Brown, M. M. (1991). Origins of externalizing behavior problems at eight years of age. In K. H. Rubin & D. J. Pepler (Eds.), *The development and treatment of childhood aggression* (pp. 93–120). Hillsdale, NJ: Erlbaum.

Bazhenova, O. V., Plonskaia, O., & Porges, S. W. (2001). Vagal reactivity and affective adjustment in infants during interaction challenges. *Child Development, 72*(5), 1314–1326.

Beauchaine, T. P. (2012). Physiological markers of emotion and emotion dysregulation in externalizing psychopathology. *Monographs of the Society for Research in Child Development, 77*(2), 79–86.

Beauchaine, T. P., & Gatzke-Kopp, L. M. (2013). Genetic and environmental influences on behavior. In T. P. Beauchaine & S. P. Hinshaw (Eds.), *Child and adolescent psychopathology* (2nd ed., pp. 111–142). Hoboken, NJ: Wiley.

Beauchaine, T. P., Neuhaus, E., Brenner, S. L., & Gatzke-Kopp, L. (2008). Ten good reasons to consider biological processes in prevention and intervention research. *Development and Psychopathology, 20*(3), 745–774.

Beauchaine, T. P., Webster-Stratton, C., & Reid, M. J. (2005). Mediators, moderators, and predictors of 1-year outcomes among children treated for early-onset conduct problems: A latent growth curve analysis. *Journal of Consulting and Clinical Psychology, 73*(3), 371–388.

Belsky, J. (1997). Theory testing, effect-size evaluation, and differential susceptibility to rearing influence: The case of mothering and attachment. *Child Development, 68*(4), 598–600.

Booij, L., Wang, D. S., Levesque, M. L., Tremblay, R. E., & Szyf, M. (2013). Looking beyond the DNA sequence: The relevance of DNA methylation processes for the stress–diathesis model of depression. *Philosophical Transactions of the Royal Society B: Biological Sciences, 368*(1615).

Bornstein, M. H. (2014). Human infancy . . . and the rest of the lifespan. *Annual Review of Psychology, 65*(1), 121–158.

Bornstein, M. H., & Suess, P. E. (2000). Child and mother cardiac vagal tone: Continuity, stability, and concordance across the first 5 years. *Developmental Psychology, 36*(1), 54–65.

Boyce, W. T., & Ellis, B. J. (2005). Biological sensitivity to context: I. An evolutionary-developmental theory of the origins and functions of stress reactivity. *Development and Psychopathology, 17*(2), 271–301.

Brazelton, T. B. (1984). *Neonatal Behavioral Assessment Scale.* Philadelphia: Lippincott.

Briggs-Gowan, M. J., & Carter, A. (2007). Applying the Infant–Toddler Social and Emotional Assessment (ITSEA) and Brief-ITSEA in early intervention. *Infant Mental Health Journal, 28*(6), 564–583.

Broth, M. R., Goodman, S. H., Hall, C., & Raynor, L. C. (2004). Depressed and well mothers' emotion interpretation accuracy and the quality of mother–infant interaction. *Infancy, 6*(1), 37–55.

Brune, M. (2012). Does the oxytocin receptor polymorphism (rs2254298) confer "vulnerability" for psychopathology or "differential susceptibility"?: Insights from evolution. *BMC Medicine, 10*(1), 38.

Calkins, S. D., Dedmon, S. E., Gill, K. L., Lomax, L. E., & Johnson, L. M. (2002). Frustration in infancy: Implications for emotion regulation, physiological processes, and temperament. *Infancy, 3*(2), 175–197.

Carter, A. S., Briggs-Gowan, M. J., Jones, S. M., & Little, T. D. (2003). The Infant–Toddler Social and Emotional Assessment (ITSEA): Factor structure, reliability, and validity. *Journal of Abnormal Child Psychology, 31*(5), 495–514.

Caspi, A., Hariri, A. R., Holmes, A., Uher, R., & Moffitt, T. E. (2010). Genetic sensitivity to the environment: The case of the serotonin transporter gene and its implications for studying complex diseases and traits. *American Journal of Psychiatry, 167*(5), 509–527.

Cicchetti, D. (2013). Annual research review: Resilient functioning in maltreated children—past, present, and future perspectives. *Journal of Child Psychology and Psychiatry, 54*(4), 402–422.

Cicchetti, D., & Rogosch, F. A. (1996). Equifinality and multifinality in developmental psychopathology. *Development and Psychopathology, 8*, 597–600.

Cicchetti, D., Rogosch, F. A., & Toth, S. L. (2000). The efficacy of toddler–parent psychotherapy for fostering cognitive development in offspring of depressed mothers. *Journal of Abnormal Child Psychology, 28*, 135–148.

Cicchetti, D., Rogosch, F. A., Toth, S. L., & Sturge-Apple, M. L. (2011). Normalizing the development of cortisol regulation in maltreated infants through preventive interventions. *Development and Psychopathology, 23*(3), 789–800.

Cicchetti, D., & Schneider-Rosen, K. (1986). An organizational approach to childhood depression. In M. Rutter, C. E. Izard, & P. B. Read (Eds.), *Depression in young people: Developmental and clinical perspectives* (pp. 71–134). New York: Guilford Press.

Cole, P. M., Martin, S. E., & Dennis, T. A. (2004). Emotion regulation as a scientific construct: Methodological challenges and directions for child development research. *Child Development, 75*, 317–333.

Coussons-Read, M. E. (2013). Effects of prenatal stress on pregnancy and human development: Mechanisms and pathways. *Obstetric Medicine: The Medicine of Pregnancy, 6*(2), 52–57.

Crittenden, P. M. (2009). Attachment and psychopathology. In S. Goldberg, R. Muir, & J. Kerr (Eds.), *Attachment theory: Social, developmental, and clinical perspectives* (pp. 367–406). New York: Routledge.

Curtis, W. J., & Cicchetti, D. (2013). Affective facial expression processing in 15-month-old infants who have experienced maltreatment: An event-related potential study. *Child Maltreatment, 18*(3), 140–154.

Cuthbert, B. N., & Kozak, M. J. (2013). Constructing constructs for psychopathology: The NIMH research domain criteria. *Journal of Abnormal Psychology, 122*(3), 928–937.

Dale, L. P., O'Hara, E. A., Schein, R., Inserra, L., Keen, J., Flores, M., et al. (2011). Measures of infant behavioral and physiological state regulation predict 54-month behavior problems. *Infant Mental Health Journal, 32*(4), 473–486.

Davidson, R. J. (1994). Asymmetric brain function, affective style, and psychopathology: The role of early experience and plasticity. *Development and Psychopathology, 6*(4), 741–758.

Davidson, R. J., & Fox, N. A. (1982). Asymmetrical brain activity discriminates between positive and negative affective stimuli in human infants. *Science, 218*, 1235–1237.

Davidson, R. J., & Fox, N. A. (1989). Frontal brain asymmetry predicts infants' response to maternal separation. *Journal of Abnormal Psychology, 98*, 127–131.

Davies, P. T., Sturge-Apple, M. L., Cicchetti, D., Manning, L. G., & Vonhold, S. E. (2012). Pathways and processes of risk in associations among maternal antisocial personality symptoms, interparental aggression, and preschooler's psychopathology. *Development and Psychopathology, 24*(3), 807–832.

Davis, E. P., Glynn, L. M., Schetter, C. D., Hobel, C., Chicz-Demet, A., & Sandman, C. A. (2007). Prenatal exposure to maternal depression and cortisol influences infant temperament. *Journal of the American Academy of Child and Adolescent Psychiatry, 46*(6), 737–746.

de Weerth, C., van Hees, Y., & Buitelaar, J. K. (2003). Prenatal maternal cortisol levels and infant behavior during the first 5 months. *Early Human Development, 74*(2), 139–151.

Degnan, K. A., Hane, A. A., Henderson, H. A., Moas, O. L., Reeb-Sutherland, B. C., & Fox, N. A. (2011). Longitudinal stability of temperamental exuberance and social-emotional outcomes in early childhood. *Developmental Psychology, 47*(3), 765.

Dilalla, L. F., Kagan, J., & Reznick, J. S. (1994). Genetic etiology of behavioral inhibition among 2-year-old children. *Infant Behavior and Development, 17*(4), 405–412.

DiPietro, J. A., Bornstein, M. H., Costigan, K. A., Pressman, E. K., Hahn, C.-S., Painter, K., et al. (2002). What does fetal movement predict about behavior during the first two years of life? *Developmental Psychobiology, 40*, 358–371.

Edward, K. L., Castle, D., Mills, C., Davis, L., & Casey, J. (2015). An integrative review of paternal depression. *American Journal of Mens Health, 9*(1), 26–34.

Egger, H. L., & Angold, A. (2006). Common emotional and behavioral disorders in preschool children: Presentation, nosology, and epidemiology. *Journal of Child Psychology and Psychiatry, 47*(3–4), 313–337.

El-Sheikh, M., Arsiwalla, D. D., Hinnant, J. B., & Erath, S. A. (2011). Children's internalizing symptoms: The role of interactions between cortisol and respiratory sinus arrhythmia. *Physiology and Behavior, 103*(2), 225–232.

Elgar, F. J., Mills, R. S. L., McGrath, P. J., Waschbusch, D. A., & Brownridge, D. A. (2007). Maternal and paternal depressive symptoms and child maladjustment: The mediating role of parental behavior. *Journal of Abnormal Child Psychology, 35*(6), 943–955.

Ellis, B. J., Essex, M. J., & Boyce, W. T. (2005). Biological sensitivity to context: II. Empirical explorations of an evolutionary–developmental theory. *Development and Psychopathology, 17*(2), 303–328.

Finer, L. B., & Kost, K. (2011). Unintended pregnancy rates at the state level. *Perspectives on Sexual and Reproductive Health, 43*(2), 78–87.

Fox, N. A. (1991). If it's not left, it's right: Electroencephalograph asymmetry and the development of emotion. *American Psychologist, 46*(8), 863.

Fox, N. A., Henderson, H. A., Rubin, K. H., Calkins, S. D., & Schmidt, L. A. (2001). Continuity and discontinuity of behavioral inhibition and exuberance: Psychophysiological and behavioral influences across the first four years of life. *Child Development, 72*(1), 1–21.

Fracasso, M. P., Porges, S. W., Lamb, M. E., & Rosenberg, A. A. (1994). Cardiac activity in infancy: Reliability and stability of individual differences. *Infant Behavior and Development, 17*, 277–284.

Frick, P. J. (2004). Integrating research on temperament and childhood psychopathology: Its pitfalls and promise. *Journal of Clinical Child and Adolescent Psychology, 33*(1), 2–7.

Friedman, D., Cycowicz, Y. M., & Gaeta, H. (2001). The novelty P3: An event-related brain potential (ERP) sign of the brain's evaluation of novelty. *Neuroscience and Biobehavioral Reviews, 25*(4), 355–373.

Galéra, C., Côté, S. M., Bouvard, M. P., Pingault, J. B., Melchior, M., Michel, G., et al. (2011). Early risk factors for hyperactivity–impulsivity and inattention trajectories from age 17 months to 8 years. *Archives of General Psychiatry, 68*(12), 1267–1275.

Gamma, F., Goldstein, J. M., Seidman, L. J., Fitzmaurice, G. M., Tsuang, M. T., &

Buka, S. L. (2013). Early intermodal integration in offspring of parents with psychosis. *Schizophrenia Bulletin, 40*(5), 992–1000.

Garmezy, N. (1971). Vulnerability research and the issue of primary prevention. *American Journal of Orthopsychiatry, 41*(1), 101–116.

Gartstein, M. A., & Bateman, A. E. (2008). Early manifestations of childhood depression: Influences of infant temperament and parental depressive symptoms. *Infant and Child Development, 17*(3), 223–248.

Gartstein, M. A., Putnam, S. P., & Rothbart, M. K. (2012). Etiology of preschool behavior problems: Contributions of temperament attributes in early childhood. *Infant Mental Health Journal, 33*(2), 197–211.

Goodman, S. H., & Gotlib, I. H. (1999). Risk for psychopathology in the children of depressed mothers: A developmental model for understanding mechanisms of transmission. *Psychological Review, 106,* 458–490.

Goodman, S. H., Rouse, M., Connell, A., Broth, M., Hall, C., & Heyward, D. (2011). Maternal depression and child psychopathology: A meta-analytic review. *Clinical Child and Family Psychology Review, 14,* 1–27.

Goodman, S. H., & Tully, E. C. (2006). Depression in women who are mothers: An integrative model of risk for the development of psychopathology in their sons and daughters. In C. L. M. Keyes & S. H. Goodman (Eds.), *Women and depression: A handbook for the social, behavioral, and biomedical sciences* (pp. 241–282). New York: Cambridge University Press.

Goodman, S. H., & Tully, E. C. (2009). Recurrence of depression during pregnancy: Psychosocial and personal functioning correlates. *Depression and Anxiety, 26*(6), 557–567.

Gonzalez, A. L. (2010). Attachment insecurity and maternal affective discourse as mediators of emotion dysregulation among toddlers of mothers diagnosed with major depressive disorder. Retrieved from *https://login. proxy.library.emory.edu/login?url=http://search.ebscohost.com/login. aspx?direct=true&db=psyh&AN=2010-99080-443&site=ehost-live.*

Gottesman, I. I., & Gould, T. D. (2003). The endophenotype concept in psychiatry: Etymology and strategic intentions. *American Journal of Psychiatry, 160,* 636–645.

Gottesman, I. I., & Shields, J. (1972). *Schizophrenia and genetics: A twin study vantage point.* New York: Academic Press.

Grant, K. A., McMahon, C., Austin, M. P., Reilly, N., Leader, L., & Ali, S. (2009). Maternal prenatal anxiety, postnatal caregiving and infants' cortisol responses to the still-face procedure. *Developmental Psychobiology, 51*(8), 625–637.

Grigoriadis, S., VonderPorten, E. H., Mamisashvili, L., Tomlinson, G., Dennis, C. L., Koren, G., et al. (2013). The impact of maternal depression during pregnancy on perinatal outcomes: A systematic review and meta-analysis. *Journal of Clinical Psychiatry, 74*(4), e321–e341.

Guerin, D. W., Gottfried, A. W., & Thomas, C. W. (1997). Difficult temperament and behaviour problems: A longitudinal study from 1.5 to 12 years. *International Journal of Behavioral Development, 21*(1), 71–90.

Gunnar, M. R., Brodersen, L., Krueger, K., & Rigatuso, J. (1996). Dampening of adrenocortical responses during infancy: Normative changes and individual differences. *Child Development, 67,* 877–889.

Gunnar, M. R., Porter, F. L., Wolf, C. M., & Rigatuso, J. (1995). Neonatal stress reactivity: Predictions to later emotional temperament. *Child Development, 66,* 1–13.

Gunnar, M. R., & Quevedo, K. M. (2007a). Early care experiences and HPA axis regulation in children: A mechanism for later trauma vulnerability. *Progress in Brain Research, 167,* 137–149.

Gunnar, M. R., & Quevedo, K. M. (2007b). The neurobiology of stress and development. *Annual Review of Psychology, 58,* 145–173.

Haley, D. W., Handmaker, N. S., & Lowe, J. (2006). Infant stress reactivity and prenatal alcohol exposure. *Alcoholism: Clinical and Experimental Research, 30*(12), 2055–2064.

Hammen, C. (2002). Context of stress in families of children with depressed parents. In S. H. Goodman & I. H. Gotlib (Eds.), *Children of depressed parents: Mechanisms of risk and implications for treatment* (pp. 175–202). Washington, DC: American Psychological Association.

Hannesdóttir, D. K., Doxie, J., Bell, M. A., Ollendick, T. H., & Wolfe, C. D. (2010). A longitudinal study of emotion regulation and anxiety in middle childhood: Associations with frontal EEG asymmetry in early childhood. *Developmental Psychobiology, 52*(2), 197–204.

Hayes, L. J., Goodman, S. H., & Carlson, E. (2013). Maternal antenatal depression and infant disorganized attachment at 12 months. *Attachment and Human Development, 15*(2), 133–153.

Henderson, H. A., Fox, N. A., & Rubin, K. H. (2001). Temperamental contributions to social behavior: The moderating roles of frontal EEG asymmetry and gender. *Journal of the American Academy of Child and Adolescent Psychiatry, 40*(1), 68–74.

Hoffman, C., Crnic, K. A., & Baker, J. K. (2006). Maternal depression and parenting: Implications for children's emergent emotion regulation and behavioral functioning. *Parenting: Science and Practice, 6*(4), 271–295.

Hostinar, C. E., Sullivan, R. M., & Gunnar, M. R. (2014). Psychobiological mechanisms underlying the social buffering of the hypothalamic–pituitary–adrenocortical axis: A review of animal models and human studies across development. *Psychological Bulletin, 140*(1), 256–282.

Huizink, A. C., & Mulder, E. J. H. (2006). Maternal smoking, drinking or cannabis use during pregnancy and neurobehavioral and cognitive functioning in human offspring. *Neuroscience and Biobehavioral Reviews, 30*(1), 24–41.

Iacono, W. G., Malone, S. M., & McGue, M. (2003). Substance use disorders, externalizing psychopathology, and P300 event-related potential amplitude. *International Journal of Psychophysiology, 48*(2), 147–178.

Ingram, R. E., & Price, J. M. (2010). *Vulnerability to psychopathology: Risk across the lifespan* (2nd ed.). New York: Guilford Press.

Ivanova, M. Y., Achenbach, T. M., Rescorla, L. A., Harder, V. S., Ang, R. P., Bilenberg, N., et al. (2010). Preschool psychopathology reported by parents in 23 societies: Testing the seven-syndrome model of the Child Behavior Checklist for ages 1.5–5. *Journal of the American Academy of Child and Adolescent Psychiatry, 49*(12), 1215–1224.

Jansen, J., Beijers, R., Riksen-Walraven, M., & de Weerth, C. (2010). Cortisol reactivity in young infants. *Psychoneuroendocrinology, 35*(3), 329–338.

Janson, H., & Mathiesen, K. S. (2008). Temperament profiles from infancy to middle childhood: Development and associations with behavior problems. *Developmental Psychology, 44*(5), 1314–1328.

Jones, N. A., Field, T., Davalos, M., & Pickens, J. (1997). EEG stability in infants/children of depressed mothers. *Child Psychiatry and Human Development, 28,* 59–70.

Jones, N. A., Field, T., Fox, N. A., Lundy, B., & Davalos, M. (1997). EEG activation in 1-month-old infants of depressed mothers. *Development and Psychopathology, 9*(3), 491–505.

Kagan, J., & Snidman, N. (1999). Early childhood predictors of adult anxiety disorders. *Biological Psychiatry, 46*(11), 1536–1541.

Karlén, J., Frostell, A., Theodorsson, E., Faresjö, T., & Ludvigsson, J. (2013). Maternal influence on child HPA axis: A prospective study of cortisol levels in hair. *Pediatrics, 132*(5), e1333–e1340.

Keenan, K. (2000). Emotion dysregulation as a risk factor for child psychopathology. *Clinical Psychology: Science and Practice, 7*(4), 418–434.

Keenan, K., Gunthorpe, D., & Grace, D. (2007). Parsing the relations between SES and stress reactivity: Examining individual differences in neonatal stress response. *Infant Behavior and Development, 30*(1), 134–145.

Kessler, R. C., Berglund, P., Demler, O., Jin, R., Merikangas, K. R., & Walters, E. E. (2005). Lifetime prevalence and age-of-onset distributions of DSM-IV disorders in the National Comorbidity Survey Replication. *Archives of General Psychiatry, 62,* 593–602.

Kofink, D., Boks, M. P., Timmers, H. T., & Kas, M. J. (2013). Epigenetic dynamics in psychiatric disorders: Environmental programming of neurodevelopmental processes. *Neuroscience and Biobehavioral Reviews, 37*(5), 831–845.

Laurent, H. K. (2014). Clarifying the contours of emotion regulation: Insights from parent–child stress research. *Child Development Perspectives, 8*(1), 30–35.

Lavigne, J. V., LeBailly, S. A., Hopkins, J., Gouze, K. R., & Binns, H. J. (2009). The prevalence of ADHD, ODD, depression, and anxiety in a community sample of 4-year-olds. *Journal of Clinical Child and Adolescent Psychology, 38*(3), 315–328.

Lester, B. M. (1984). Data analysis and prediction. In T. B. Brazelton (Ed.), *Neonatal Behavioral Assessment Scale* (2nd ed., pp. 85–96). London: Blackwell Scientific.

Linehan, M. M. (1993). *Cognitive-behavioral treatment of borderline personality disorder.* New York: Guilford Press.

Lonigan, C. J., Phillips, B. M., Wilson, S. B., & Allan, N. P. (2011). Temperament and anxiety in children and adolescents. In W. K. Silverman & A. Fields (Eds.), *Anxiety disorders in children and adolescents: Research, assessment, and intervention* (2nd ed.). Cambridge, UK: Cambridge University Press.

Lovejoy, M. C., Graczyk, P. A., O'Hare, E., & Neuman, G. (2000). Maternal depression and parenting behavior: A meta-analytic review. *Clinical Psychology Review, 20*(5), 561–592.

Luby, J. L., Heffelfinger, A. K., Mrakotsky, C., Brown, K. M., Hessler, M. J., Wallis, et al. (2003). The clinical picture of depression in preschool children. *Journal of the American Academy of Child and Adolescent Psychiatry, 42*(3), 340–348.

Luby, J. L., Mrakotsky, C., Heffelfinger, A., Brown, K., Hessler, M., & Spitznagel, E.

(2003). Modification of DSM-IV criteria for depressed preschool children. *American Journal of Psychiatry, 160*(6), 1169–1172.

Lusby, C. M., Goodman, S. H., Bell, M. A., & Newport, D. J. (2013). Electroencephalogram patterns in infants of depressed mothers. *Developmental Psychobiology, 56*(3), 459–473.

Lusby, C. M., Goodman, S. H., Bell, M. A., & Newport, D. J. (2014). Electroencephalogram patterns in infants of depressed mothers. *Developmental Psychobiology, 56*(3), 459–473.

Marshall, P. J., Bar-Haim, Y., & Fox, N. A. (2002). Development of the EEG from 5 months to 4 years of age. *Clinical Neurophysiology, 113*(8), 1199–1208.

Marshall, P. J., Reeb, B. C., Fox, N. A., Nelson, C. A., III, & Zeanah, C. H. (2008). Effects of early intervention on EEG power and coherence in previously institutionalized children in Romania. *Development and Psychopathology, 20*(3), 861–880.

Masten, A. S. (2001). Ordinary magic: Resilience processes in development. *American Psychologist, 56*(3), 227–238.

Masten, A. S., & Garmezy, N. (1985). Risk, vulnerability, and protective factors in developmental psychopathology. In B. B. Lahey & A. E. Kazdin (Eds.), *Advances in clinical child psychology* (Vol. 8, pp. 1–52). New York: Plenum Press.

Matheny, A. P., Jr. (1989). Children's behavioral inhibition over age and across situations: Genetic similarity for a trait during change. *Journal of Personality, 57*(2), 215–235.

Matthews, S. G., & Phillips, D. I. (2012). Transgenerational inheritance of stress pathology. *Experimental Neurology, 233*(1), 95–101.

McLaughlin, K. A., Fox, N. A., Zeanah, C. H., & Nelson, C. A. (2011). Adverse rearing environments and neural development in children: The development of frontal electroencephalogram asymmetry. *Biological Psychiatry, 70*(11), 1008–1015.

Micali, N., & Treasure, J. (2009). Biological effects of a maternal ED on pregnancy and foetal development: A review. *European Eating Disorders Review, 17*(6), 448–454.

Milhiet, V., Boudebesse, C., Bellivier, F., Drouot, X., Henry, C., Leboyer, M., et al. (2014). Circadian abnormalities as markers of susceptibility in bipolar disorders. *Frontiers in Bioscience (Scholar Edition), 6*, 120–137.

Monroe, S. M., & Simons, A. D. (1991). Diathesis–stress theories in the context of life-stress research: Implications for depressive disorders. *Psychological Bulletin, 110*, 406–425.

Mueller, A., Brocke, B., Fries, E., Lesch, K.-P., & Kirschbaum, C. (2010). The role of the serotonin transporter polymorphism for the endocrine stress response in newborns. *Psychoneuroendocrinology, 35*(2), 289–296.

Murphy, L. B., & Moriarty, A. E. (1976). *Vulnerability, coping and growth from infancy to adolescence.* New Haven, CT: Yale University Press.

Nilsson, E., Hultman, C. M., Cnattingius, S., Olausson, P. O., Bjork, C., & Lichtenstein, P. (2008). Schizophrenia and offspring's risk for adverse pregnancy outcomes and infant death. *British Journal of Psychiatry, 193*(4), 311–315.

O'Donnell, K. J., Bugge Jensen, A., Freeman, L., Khalife, N., O'Connor, T. G., & Glover, V. (2012). Maternal prenatal anxiety and downregulation of placental 11β-HSD2. *Psychoneuroendocrinology, 37*(6), 818–826.

Patterson, G. R. (1982). *Coercive family processes.* Eugene, OR: Castilia.

Patton, G. C., Coffey, C., Carlin, J. B., Olsson, C. A., & Morley, R. (2004). Prematurity at birth and adolescent depressive disorder. *British Journal of Psychiatry, 184*(5), 446–447.

Perez-Edgar, K., Schmidt, L. A., Henderson, H. A., Schulkin, J., & Fox, N. A. (2008). Salivary cortisol levels and infant temperament shape developmental trajectories in boys at risk for behavioral maladjustment. *Psychoneuroendocrinology, 33*(7), 916–925.

Pesonen, A. K., Räikkönen, K., Heinonen, K., Komsi, N., Järvenpää, A. L., & Strandberg, T. (2008). A transactional model of temperamental development: Evidence of a relationship between child temperament and maternal stress over five years. *Social Development, 17*(2), 326–340.

Pluess, M., & Belsky, J. (2013). Vantage sensitivity: Individual differences in response to positive experiences. *Psychological Bulletin, 139*(4), 901.

Porges, S. W. (2007). The polyvagal perspective. *Biological Psychology, 74*(2), 116–143.

Porges, S. W. (2011). *The polyvagal theory: Neurophysiological foundations of emotions, attachment, communication, and self-regulation.* New York: Norton.

Porges, S. W., Doussard-Roosevelt, J. A., Portales, A. L., & Greenspan, S. I. (1996). Infant regulation of the vagal "brake" predicts child behavior problems: A psychobiological model of social behavior. *Developmental Psychobiology, 29*, 697–712.

Porges, S. W., Doussard-Roosevelt, J. A., Portales, L. A., & Suess, P. E. (1994). Cardiac vagal tone: Stability and relation to difficultness in infants and 3-year-olds. *Developmental Psychobiology, 27*(5), 289–300.

Putnam, S. P., & Stifter, C. A. (2005). Behavioral approach–inhibition in toddlers: Prediction from infancy, positive and negative affect components, and relations with behavior problems. *Child Development, 76*, 212–226.

Raposa, E. B., Hammen, C. L., & Brennan, P. A. (2011). Effects of child psychopathology on maternal depression: The mediating role of child-related acute and chronic stressors. *Journal of Abnormal Child Psychology, 39*(8), 1177–1186.

Riese, M. L. (1990). Neonatal temperament in monozygotic and dizygotic twin pairs. *Child Development, 61*(4), 1230–1237.

Rosenblum, K. L., Dayton, C. J., & Muzik, M. (2009). Infant social and emotional development: Emerging competence in a relational context. In C. H. Zeanah (Ed.), *Handbook of infant mental health* (3rd ed., pp. 80–103). New York: Guilford Press.

Ross, L. E., Grigoriadis, S., L., M., Mamisashvili, L., Vonderporten, E. H., Roerecke, M., Rehm, J., et al. (2013). Selected pregnancy and delivery outcomes after exposure to antidepressant medication: A systematic review and meta-analysis. *JAMA Psychiatry, 70*(4), 436–443.

Rothbart, M. K., & Derryberry, D. (1981). Development of individual differences in temperament. In M. E. Lamb & A. L. Brown (Eds.), *Advances in developmental psychology* (Vol. 1, pp. 37–86). Hillsdale, NJ: Erlbaum.

Rothbart, M. K., & Goldsmith, H. H. (1985). Three approaches to the study of infant temperament. *Developmental Review, 5*(3), 237–260.

Rottenberg, J., Clift, A., Bolden, S., & Salomon, K. (2007). RSA fluctuation in major depressive disorder. *Psychophysiology, 44*(3), 450–458.

Rottenberg, J., Wilhelm, F. H., Gross, J. J., & Gotlib, I. H. (2002). Respiratory sinus arrhythmia as a predictor of outcome in major depressive disorder. *Journal of Affective Disorders, 71*(1–3), 265–272.

Rouse, M. H., & Goodman, S. H. (2014). Perinatal depression influences on infant negative affectivity: Timing, severity, and co-morbid anxiety. *Infant Behavior and Development, 37*(4), 739–751.

Rubin, D. H., Althoff, R. R., Ehli, E. A., Davies, G. E., Rettew, D. C., Crehan, E. T., et al. (2013). Candidate gene associations with withdrawn behavior. *Journal of Child Psychology and Psychiatry, 54*(12), 1337–1345.

Rutter, M. (1987). Psychosocial resilience and protective mechanisms. *American Journal of Orthopsychiatry, 57*(3), 316–331.

Rutter, M. (1990). Commentary: Some focus and process considerations regarding effects of parental depression on children. *Developmental Psychology, 26,* 60–67.

Rutter, M. (2007). Gene–environment interdependence. *Developmental Science, 10*(1), 12–18.

Sameroff, A. J. (1975). Transactional models in early social relations. *Human Development, 18,* 65–79.

Sameroff, A. J. (2009). *The transactional model of development: How children and contexts shape each other.* Washington, DC: American Psychological Association.

Sanislow, C. A., Pine, D. S., Quinn, K. J., Kozak, M. J., Garvey, M. A., Heinssen, R. K., et al. (2010). Developing constructs for psychopathology research: Research domain criteria. *Journal of Abnormal Psychology, 119*(4), 631–639.

Sayal, K., Heron, J., Maughan, B., Rowe, R., & Ramchandani, P. (2014). Infant temperament and childhood psychiatric disorder: Longitudinal study. *Child: Care, Health and Development, 40*(2), 292–297.

Schneider, M. L., Moore, C. F., & Kraemer, G. W. (2003). On the relevance of prenatal stress to developmental psychopathology: A primate model. In D. Cicchetti & E. Walker (Eds.), *Neurodevelopmental mechanisms in psychopathology* (pp. 155–186). New York: Cambridge University Press.

Shamir-Essakow, G., Ungerer, J., & Rapee, R. (2005). Attachment, behavioral inhibition, and anxiety in preschool children. *Journal of Abnormal Child Psychology, 33*(2), 131–143.

Shiner, R. L., Buss, K. A., McClowry, S. G., Putnam, S. P., Saudino, K. J., & Zentner, M. (2012). What is temperament now?: Assessing progress in temperament research on the twenty-fifth anniversary of Goldsmith et al. *Child Development Perspectives, 6*(4), 436–444.

Snieder, H., van Doornen, L. J., Boomsma, D. I., & Thayer, J. F. (2007). Sex differences and heritability of two indices of heart rate dynamics: A twin study. *Twin Research and Human Genetics, 10*(2), 364–372.

Sroufe, L. A., Coffino, B., & Carlson, E. A. (2010). Conceptualizing the role of early experience: Lessons from the Minnesota longitudinal study. *Developmental Review, 30*(1), 36–51.

Sroufe, L. A., & Rutter, M. (1984). The domain of developmental psychopathology. *Child Development, 55,* 17–29.

Steptoe, A., van Jaarsveld, C. H. M., Semmler, C., Plomin, R., & Wardle, J. (2009).

Heritability of daytime cortisol levels and cortisol reactivity in children. *Psychoneuroendocrinology, 34*(2), 273–280.

Stifter, C. A., & Fox, N. A. (1990). Infant reactivity: Physiological correlates of newborn and 5-month temperament. *Developmental Psychology, 26*(4), 582.

Talge, N. M., Holzman, C., Wang, J., Lucia, V., Gardiner, J., & Breslau, N. (2010). Late-preterm birth and its association with cognitive and socioemotional outcomes at 6 years of age. *Pediatrics, 126*(6), 1124–1131.

Teerikangas, O. M., Aronen, E. T., Martin, R. P., & Huttunen, M. O. (1998). Effects of infant temperament and early intervention on the psychiatric symptoms of adolescents. *Journal of the American Academy of Child and Adolescent Psychiatry, 37*(10), 1070–1076.

Tharner, A., Dierckx, B., Luijk, M. P. C. M., van Ijzendoorn, M. H., Bakermans-Kranenburg, M. J., van Ginkel, J. R., et al. (2013). Attachment disorganization moderates the effect of maternal postnatal depressive symptoms on infant autonomic functioning. *Psychophysiology, 50*(2), 195–203.

Thibodeau, R., Jorgensen, R. S., & Kim, S. (2006). Depression, anxiety, and resting frontal EEG asymmetry: A meta-analytic review. *Journal of Abnormal Psychology, 115*(4), 715–729.

Tully, E. C., Goodman, S. H., & Brooks-DeWeese, A. (2005). *Measuring children's perceptions of mothers' depression: The CHiPPS measure.* Paper presented at the International Society for Research in Child and Adolescent Psychopathology, New York, NY.

Waters, E., & Sroufe, L. A. (1983). Competence as a developmental construct. *Developmental Review, 3*, 70–97.

Werner, E. E., & Smith, R. (1982). *Vulnerable but invincible: A longitudinal study of resilient youth and children.* New York: McGraw-Hill.

Werner, E. E., & Smith, R. S. (1977). *Kauai's children come of age.* Honoulu: University Press of Hawaii.

Williams, L. R., Degnan, K., Perez-Edgar, K., Henderson, H., Rubin, K., Pine, D., et al. (2009). Impact of behavioral inhibition and parenting style on internalizing and externalizing problems from early childhood through adolescence. *Journal of Abnormal Child Psychology, 37*(8), 1063–1075.

Worobey, J. (1990). Behavioral assessment of the neonate. In J. Colombo & J. W. Fagen (Eds.), *Individual differences in infancy: Reliability, stability, prediction* (pp. 137–161). New York: Erlbaum.

Yaroslavsky, I., Rottenberg, J., & Kovacs, M. (2013). The utility of combining RSA indices in depression prediction. *Journal of Abnormal Psychology, 122*(2), 314.

Zero to Three. (2005). *Diagnostic classification of mental health and developmental disorders of infancy and early childhood, revised (DC:0–3R).* Washington, DC: Author.

PART V

THE FUTURE
OF INFANCY RESEARCH

CHAPTER 18

An Interdisciplinary Biopsychosocial Perspective on Psychological Development

George F. Michel, Emily C. Marcinowski, Iryna Babik,
Julie M. Campbell, and Eliza L. Nelson

The biopsychosocial approach was proposed initially as an alternative to the biomedical approach for the investigation of the origin of abnormal psychological functioning (cf. Engel, 1977). The biomedical approach concentrated on specifically biological sources, such as abnormal genes, injury (particularly brain damage associated with premature birth, perinatal complications, postnatal accidents, or abuse), or exposure to pathogens in order to predict differences in functioning. The biopsychosocial approach added social and societal factors to the biological account. The social factors included not only the influences of parental care, peers, and adult models, but also psychological factors such as personal experiences, memories, and the interrelations among the psychological functions of language, cognition, and emotion. Societal factors included socioeconomic status, the media, formal schooling, and cultural traditions, pressures, and expectations. The biopsychosocial approach proposed that all of these factors should be considered when predicting individual differences in the well-being and psychological functioning of the individual (Borrell-Carrió, Suchman, & Epstein, 2004; Engel, 1977, 1980). Both approaches had the "medical" focus of identifying predictors of subsequent "abnormal" functioning for the purpose of rehabilitation and/or prevention.

Subsequently, the biopsychosocial approach was co-opted as the conceptual frame for all developmental research because it appeared to be a solution to the nature–nurture dilemma. That is, in this approach, both nature and nurture were contributors to development as a result of some pattern of interaction among these factors. Within the biopsychosocial approach, biological, social/psychological, and societal factors could be examined separately (and then combined) to predict individual differences in psychological functioning. We argue that neither the biomedical nor the biopsychosocial approach is particularly developmental. Both focus on predicting functional differences among individuals at a certain period of their development (most often adulthood, although preschool, early school, and teen periods also have received considerable investigation). Seldom are the processes of development traced from a presumed origin toward the manifestation of the particular trait or function of interest. Thus, what appears to be a developmental study does not reveal the influences that directly affect the creation of similarities and differences in the *developmental trajectories* that yield species-typical, group-typical (e.g., culture), or individually unique traits.

Since both approaches attempt to predict particular types of psychological functioning from a specific set of earlier conditions or characteristics (a "development to" approach; Michel & Tyler, 2007b), they miss understanding *how* both "normal" and "abnormal" functioning develops. Moreover, although the biopsychosocial approach promotes a multidisciplinary perspective in research, it fails to provide an interdisciplinary account of human development because the contributions from each discipline often are treated as static predictors, which can interact as somewhat independent factors. It is presumed that the relative contribution of each factor in predicting the outcome describes the magnitude of its role in the development of the trait. However, this multidisciplinary approach misses the interdisciplinary account of how the development of any trait or function occurs under the influence of multiple dynamically changing, interrelated, and mutually influencing factors. These nonlinear coactions are not captured by techniques for measuring statistical, or additive, interactions. In contrast, the "development from" approach (Michel & Tyler, 2007b) treats factors affecting the development and expression of a trait as coactive factors that mutually influence one another during the development of the trait. We propose that an interdisciplinary biopsychosocial framework, which incorporates the "development from" approach, can provide a better account of infant development and its consequences. Therefore, this chapter is a call for the future construction of an expanded biopsychosocial approach that is both developmental and interdisciplinary, and yet continuous with the research reported within this handbook.

Before characterizing this new interdisciplinary biopsychosocial framework, we must describe the differences between a development to and a development from approach to the investigation of developmental phenomena. Then, we identify the strengths and weaknesses of the biomedical approach and compare those with the strengths and weaknesses of the conventional biopsychosocial approach. Finally, we introduce the new interdisciplinary biopsychosocial approach and describe how it builds on the strengths of the other two approaches but corrects their weaknesses and encourages changes in the constructs that are used to characterize psychological development and the procedures used to investigate it.

Development "To" versus Development "From"

From the development to perspective, human (actually, all animals, but we focus on human) behavioral traits are the consequence of some biologically determined propensities (e.g., natural selection of genes that control the development of neuroanatomical mechanisms) interacting with socially and culturally constructed environmental events (e.g., working mothers, literacy, geographic separation of extended families, enculturation). This focuses developmental investigation on seeking the earliest manifestations of the trait and any disrupting factors during development. Such "disruptive factors" are used as explanations for how "abnormal" traits develop. When "biologically determined propensities" are unknown or very complex, biological "markers" of the propensity are sought (e.g., salivary, urine, or blood biochemistry, single-nucleotide polymorphisms, peculiarities of electroencephalogram [EEG]). In the development to approach, experience is unlikely to play a constructive role in the development of any trait; rather, the final product is often presumed to be preset as "encoded," as a "neural module," or as a "prewired program" (Bateson & Mameli, 2007). Experience during development plays either a permissive role (permitting normal development) or a disruptive role (interfering with normal development). Knowing the genetically controlled propensities for particular traits would mean that the experiences of an individual might be controlled to prevent expression or permit expression of those traits relevant to a culturally preferred development.

A development from perspective focuses developmental research on how the transactions of the individual's current phenotypic traits with the individual's current social and physical environment at one phase during development results in the maintenance of those traits, their loss, or their transformation into different traits in the subsequent phase of development. This transaction continues through the lifespan. Modern molecular biology supports this development from perspective by confirming that gene expression is part of a complex system (network) of developmental causes that operate throughout the lifespan to produce phenotypic variability of traits. Information in the genome is intertwined with ecological influences from the environment in different ways and at different periods throughout the lifespan (cf. Gerhart & Kirschner, 1997; Gilbert, 2006; Kirschner & Gerhart, 2006; Raff, 1996; Schlichting & Pigliucci, 1998). Cells are chemical manufacturing plants controlled by an intricate and dynamic set of chemical messengers that travel within and between cells to turn "on" or "off" the expression of specific deoxyribonucleic acid (DNA) sequences and the production and character of cellular structures and products. This layer of bio-chemical reactions that affect DNA expression is called the "epigenome." The transduction of environmental stimuli into neurobiological processes permits "experience" of the individual's social and physical environment to become a part of the epigenome, thus affecting DNA expression (Michel, 2010).

The epigenome plays a major role in heredity, as well as in development and health. These epigenomic processes begin before conception during the formation of germ cells (eggs and sperm) and continue throughout the life-span. Moreover, whereas we inherit our DNA from our parents, we also inherit the environment—including diet (Drake & Walker, 2004; Mennella, Ziegler, Briefel, & Novak, 2006), specific social and physical experiences, and habitat (West, King, & Arberg, 1988). These inherited environments can alter epig-enome activity throughout the lifespan. Such cross-generational communication can range from simply altering the environment for future generations to alter-ing DNA expression through epigenetic inheritance to the setting of cultural goals and ideals. As Fleming and colleagues (2002) have demonstrated, there are multigenerational experiential effects. A mother rat's caregiving affects how her pups, as adults, treat their own offspring. These "grandmother effects" force us to begin the investigation of developmental trajectories before the zygote and not assume that an individual's development begins only at conception.

We propose that a development from approach is capable of accounting both for the expression of psychological patterns specific to the individual and the individual's culture, as well as patterns common to humans, in general, without shifting explanatory constructs or frameworks from individual to soci-ety to culture. Thus, careful analyses of the mechanisms governing developmen-tal trajectories have led to explanations of behavior that incorporate sociocul-tural and physiological information in a synthetic and nonhierarchical manner.

A Biomedical Perspective

Traditionally, the biomedical perspective reflected two misleading notions: (1) reductionism, or the notion that complex phenomena derive from a single pri-mary principle; and (2) mind–body dualism, or the notion that mental phe-nomena are separable from the bodily phenomena (Engel, 1977). Reductionism requires that psychological functions are understood best by reducing them to the functioning of their neural components and these, in turn, would be best understood by reducing them to their gene-controlled biochemical signaling pathways. From a reductionist stance, the psychological functions (language, cognition, emotion, and social aptitude) of an individual are treated as conse-quences of neural circuits created by molecular genetic processes. Accordingly, genes are considered to provide coded information "blueprints" for all human phenotypes (including psychological functions) and the phenotypic development of the individual is a maturational process during which psychological functions unfold or emerge over age according to genetically controlled processes of neural "wiring." The environment (especially in the form of exposure to pathogens, brain damage, and physical abuse) can disrupt this maturational process but ordinarily is benignly permissive for development. Nevertheless, in cases of abnormal development, certain environmental interventions might help to prevent or rehabilitate abnormal functioning.

The weakness of this reductionist perspective has been revealed many times but perhaps Roger Sperry (1965, 1980), Nobel Lauriate in developmental neurobiology, captured it best:

> The molecules of the brain cell [are] obliged to submit to a course of activity in time and space that is largely determined by the overall dynamic and spatial properties of the whole [neural] cell [which does] not have very much to say about when they are going to fire their messages or in what time pattern they will fire them. The flow and timing of [neural activity is] governed largely by properties of the whole cerebral circuit, within which the given cells and fibers are incorporated, and also by the relationship of this circuit system to other circuit systems. Further, the general circuit properties of the whole brain may undergo radical and widespread changes [as a result of] a shifting pattern of central excitation [opening or priming] one group of circuit pathways [having special properties while] closing, repressing, or inhibiting other circuit potentialities. Of course, all of the simpler molecular, cellular, and physiological forces remain present and continue to operate, but these lower level forces and properties have been superseded by those of higher levels of organization. However, proper function in the uppermost levels always depends on normal operation at subsidiary levels. (1965, p. 79)

Although there has been an expansion of neuroscience and molecular biological research in the intervening 50 years, Sperry's characterization of the complexity of causality involved at each of the different levels of organization in the actions of the nervous system from cells to circuits is still appropriate (Michel, 2014; Rose & Rose, 2012).

As Sperry (1980) noted, psychological functioning is dependent on the proper functioning of the biochemistry of neural cells; however, this dependency is not an example of reductionism. Experiential input from social and physical conditions can engender the development of neural systems that can support new psychological functions. In that way, psychological functioning (engagement with the social and physical world of the individual) can constrain neural functioning. Of course, psychological functioning cannot force neural systems to engender phenomena that the system cannot engender. In that way neural functioning constrains psychological functioning. However, there is much more plasticity in development than is usually considered.

Psychological functioning integrates and incorporates influences from the biomechanics of the skeletal–muscular system (e.g., height, weight), the endocrine system (e.g., secretion of protein and steroid hormones), the immune system (e.g., cytokine secretions), and the digestive system (e.g., gut bacteria, digestive system secretions), as well as the nervous system. Moreover, these different systems are mutually coactive. Disruption of the functioning of these components may affect development because, as Kennedy (1992) proposed, psychological functioning (particularly behavior) is the physiology of the whole individual. And this physiology, in turn, is reflective of, and constrained by, the social and physical milieu of that individual. That milieu will be different for each individual. Hence, psychological functioning will be individually different and that difference will permeate every level of organization and functioning of the individual. In turn, that individual's functioning can affect his or her social and physical milieu. Psychological functioning is a collaborative coaction among multiple components and such coaction reduces the number of options possible within each component according to the particular pattern of coaction operative at any period during development.

The valuable aspect of the biomedical perspective is that it recognized the important role of physiology in psychological functions. What it missed was that physiological systems are intimately and collaboratively coactive (Figure 18.1). The nervous system does not interact with the endocrine system—they coact as a neuroendocrine system. Indeed, the immune system coacts with both the nervous and endocrine systems. Also missing is the recognition of biomechanical influences on psychological phenomena (e.g., size, weight, muscle mass). As Figure 18.1 illustrates, when determining the consequences of stressful conditions on the individual's functioning, perceptual systems are involved as well as complex coactions of various neural systems (particularly those involved with symbolic and mnemonic functions) along with the endocrine and immune systems.

Measuring cortisol in blood or saliva does not reveal the way other endocrines and neurotransmitters modulate (enhance and/or decrease) the influence of cortisol on target tissues or the way those target tissues have to be prepared by previous physiological processes prompted by the individual's experience with a social and physical environment. Nor does it reveal that the environment has rhythms that affect the individual's physiological rhythms, the secretion of cortisol, and the sensitivity of target systems to cortisol. There is too much complexity that is hidden by the simple biological marker but which is relevant for understanding the development of the individual's psychological functioning. It is this complexity of causality that is missing from the biomedical perspective that is its greatest weakness. However, there is an approach (developmental psychobiology) that reveals that both of the commonalities of psychological functioning and traits that occur across individuals that reflect social/cultural influences and those that reflect species-typical characters are a consequence of the same causal processes operating during development that produce individual differences (Michel, 2007, 2013b, 2014; Michel & Moore, 1995; Michel & Tyler, 2007a).

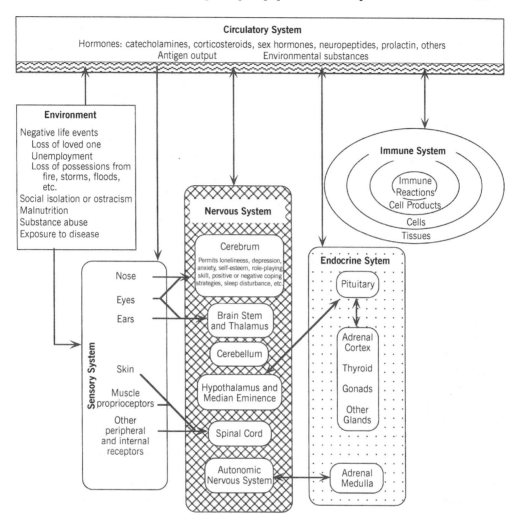

FIGURE 18.1. A schematic of the patterns of relations that exist among the physiological systems of the individual that are affected by stress-inducing situations. The schematic emphasizes the complexity of collaborative coaction among them. The circulatory system permits each system to influence and be influenced by the other systems. From Michel and Moore (1995). Reprinted with permission from MIT Press.

A Biopsychosocial Perspective

The biopsychosocial perspective correctly emphasized that understanding the phenomenon of psychological functioning must involve information acquired from the multiple levels of organization, that comprise the individual, combined with information from the context within which the individual operates. Studying a psychological function by focusing only on the systems of which the individual is composed will fail to capture the full causal network of that function. Psychological functions and traits can be explained successfully only when knowledge of an individual's component systems (e.g., nervous system) is incorporated into knowledge of the systems of which the individual is a component (e.g., society; Bateson, 2005). For research purposes, psychological functions may be studied only on a psychological level, a neural level, or a molecular level, but the knowledge from each of these levels must relate to one another and to the knowledge about the individual's social and physical milieu (which are determined, in part, by the individual's culture and society).

The psychological functions and traits of the individual operate within a complex social and physical milieu of cultural and societal events and conditions (Bronfenbrenner & Morris, 1998). The biopsychosocial perspective captures those important influences, but fails to reveal how such influences come to affect the individual. Obviously, the infant's psychological functioning operates within, and is influenced by Bronfenbrenner's microsystem, but that microsystem is affected by the behavior, appearance, and biomechanics of the infant. Moreover, there is no theory as to how the microsystem is transduced into effective factors that can operate within the infant's physiological systems (see Michel, 2010, for one account). Nor is there any mechanism for how Bronfenbrenner's exosystem and macrosystem can affect each other or the microsystem. Without evidence for how transduction occurs across these different levels of influential factors, the study of development is left with simply identifying "markers" of social, cultural, and familial influences (e.g., socioeconomic status, racism, nationalism, religious sects, patterns of parental care) that may predict differences in the outcome of developmental trajectories. Again, this approach, like the biomedical approach, does not provide an account of the development that permits the use of the same causes for individual differences and social-cultural and species-typical commonalities of psychological functioning.

An Interdisciplinary Biopsychosocial Perspective

Both the biomedical and the biopsychosocial perspectives support multidisciplinary research, but in a very conventional manner. These multidisciplinary research designs incorporate different experts (e.g., from neuroscience, molecular genetics, psychology, education, sociology, and public health) to investigate a societally important psychological function (e.g., school failure). Unfortunately, this conventional approach is similar to the account of the blind men and an elephant. Without strong interdisciplinary expertise, even the best intentions of experts can result only in a hodgepodge account that provides little knowledge about the elephant.

In place of the conventional biopsychosocial perspective, we propose an interdisciplinary biopsychosocial framework that treats an infant's development as a continuous fusion of effects from the social and physical environment, mediated by the sensory, motor, biomechanical properties, and physiognomy of the infant. The fusion of these effects across time governs the trajectory of prenatal and postnatal development. For analytic research purposes, investigators may examine separately biological, psychological, and social properties, and their effects on infant development. However, the eventual explanation of the development of any psychological function or trait must synthesize the knowledge derived from these different investigations into a coherent account of their collaborative coaction. Research must reveal how the transactions of the infant with his or her social and physical environment at each phase of development results in (1) the maintenance of psychological functions, (2) their loss, or (3) their transformation into different functions at subsequent phases (and so on through the lifespan). Adopting an interdisciplinary biopsychosocial perspective for investigating infant development will change conceptual frameworks, research procedures, and data analysis techniques because it requires extensive longitudinal research conducted by researchers with strong interdisciplinary expertise.

Left unspecified in the conventional biopsychosocial (and the biomedical) account are the developmental processes that tie the predictors (or markers) to the manifestation of psychological functions or traits. Construction of path models with measures of societal and biological factors as mediating or moderating contributors to the predictive correlation between earlier and later developing psychological functions is not an account of how the later function developed from the earlier function. Detailed trajectory descriptions and analyses are needed to identify how different sorts of interventions, occurring at different points in development, can shift the trajectory to a societally more appropriate path (Figure 18.2). Of course, modeling complex processes can be a daunting challenge when only parts of the model can be feasibly tested empirically with any one investigation. Therefore, the new interdisciplinary biopsychosocial perspective for understanding developmental phenomena requires long-term systematic and programmatic research projects, not conventional hypothesis-testing studies (Kagan, 2013).

Implications for Research Procedures

Infancy (roughly the first 18 postnatal months) represents the continuation and the consequences of prenatal developmental processes. Since birth involves the expansion of the individual's physical and social milieu, it also contributes to the formation of developmental processes essential for setting the trajectories of further development that likely affect the psychological functioning of adults. Of course, infancy can be a focus of research that has little relevance to developmental issues and questions. Because infants are especially vulnerable to many potential dangers to their survival, infants may manifest specific ontogenetic

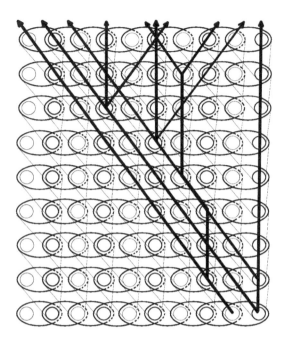

FIGURE 18.2. Development is a continuous transformation throughout the lifespan. At the lowest level of this figure, coaction of different genomes (dark and light smaller circles) with their environments (larger ellipses) results in the manifestation of certain phenotypes (second level). Trajectory analysis reveals the transitions during development, which affect phenotypic development. Such analyses identify when the coaction of individuals with their environments results in changes in trajectory, and this prompts investigation into the mechanisms for such change. Copyright 2014 by G. F. Michel. Reprinted with permission.

adaptations (Michel & Moore, 1995; Oppenheim, 1984) that relate to particular problems of infancy, but may not contribute to future developmental consequences other than to ensure that the infant has a future. For this chapter, we focus on infancy as a phase in development and do not address issues of ontogenetic adaptation (see Michel & Moore, 1995, about ontogenetic adaptations).

An interdisciplinary biopsychosocial approach begins with longitudinal designs that provide *detailed observations of a developmental phenomenon* in quasi-natural settings in order to identify developmental processes before undertaking further manipulative or comparative investigations (Kagan, 2013). Not only will this distinguish ontogenetic adaptions from development, but also investigation will not be biased by looking for the presence of adult functions in the infant (a problem of the "development to" approach; Michel & Tyler, 2007b). The psychological function of interest must be precisely defined so that potential differences in its character across development may be identified. Without precise descriptions, a function can appear not to develop because the description fails to detect changes in mechanisms or processes involved in the manifestation of the function. For example, the mechanisms underlying performance in number comprehension tasks that rely on differential looking times for visually presented groupings of items in young infants may be quite different from the mechanisms involved in number symbol manipulation of preschool-age children. Failure to identify those mechanisms represents a failure to discover both how the infant's ability (sensitivity to looking at different groups of items) developed and how that ability is related to the child's ability.

Initial descriptive knowledge of infant development requires *longitudinal designs* in order to identify and characterize similarities and differences in the developmental patterns and pathways (trajectories) among individuals. However, in order to identify patterns of stability and change in development, these longitudinal designs must have a sufficient number of assessments to reveal the shape of the developmental trajectory. The frequency of data collection can influence the shape of the observed developmental trajectory and, as a result, change the description of the developmental pattern (e.g., Ferre, Babik, & Michel, 2010; Michel, Nelson, Babik, Campbell, & Marcinowski, 2013). Also, selecting the time period between descriptive assessments is critical to what may be discovered about the trajectory (Adolph & Robinson, 2008). For some psychological functions, weekly or daily assessments may provide a description of the function's development that reveals a different pattern in the trajectory from that which becomes apparent with monthly assessments (Michel et al., 2013). Unless the infant's development is being tracked into childhood, too few assessments during infancy leave the developmental trajectory underspecified for effective causal modeling.

Age (time) may be used as part of the description of development, however, not as a part of any explanation of development (Michel & Tyler, 2005; Tyler, 2006). Development is a process. Time (age) is an intrinsic aspect of the description of that process for any ability, trait, or character. Time (age) cannot explain how any ability, trait, or character (1) may remain stable across age in the face of environmental fluctuation, (2) may be enhanced or diminished across age, or (3) may change fundamentally across age. All of these aspects of the developmental process require identification of the necessary and sufficient conditions responsible for their occurrence. Removing age as an explanation of development fundamentally alters the construct of the critical period such that it prompts the investigation of those factors that initiate and end the period, and this permits discovery of factors that are nonintuitively related to the development of a trait that may, nonetheless, alter the trajectory at other points in development.

With the description of trajectories, the investigator can begin to seek *which factors are responsible for stability* and *which factors are responsible for the change in a trajectory* at particular phases of development. Indeed, some factors might facilitate development at certain phases, but hinder it at others. Again, investigations of the factors promoting change and maintaining stability require examination of the ways that the component systems of the individual relate to the individual's social and physical context. Development is a historical and serially ordered process. Past events and functioning affect current functioning, that, in turn, affects future functioning, and so on. Development is a pattern of morphological and physiological phenotypes, which is both individually specific and characterized by species typicality (cf. Gilbert & Epel, 2009; Michel & Tyler, 2007a, for details about how species typicality may be achieved). Consequently, developmental research should reveal the factors creating and governing the serial order of the trajectories and the processes that produce both change and stability of that order over time and across individuals (Michel & Moore, 1995). The conceptual changes required by the interdisciplinary biopsychosocial perspective affect the description of development and the concepts of environment, experience, learning, critical periods, and human nature (among others).

Learning, Experience, and Environment

Too often, these three concepts are used interchangeably. Although learning is an aspect of experience and experience involves environmental influences, these three concepts represent important differences in how they operate during development (see Michel, 2010). *Learning* involves increasing or decreasing the frequency with which specific behaviors will occur or how specific behaviors are associated either with specific stimuli or with the consequences of other behaviors. In all cases of learning, there must be a nascent system upon which learning can lead to further development. Left unknown is how this initial nascent system develops. Although processes of conditioning, practice, training, observation, and imitation can be aspects of experience and contribute to the development of specific psychological functions, they cannot account for the development of the nascent systems upon which these processes depend. The use (via learning processes) of these nascent systems often improves their efficiency or the competence with which they operate, extends or restricts their range of use, converts a vaguely specified system into one that is more precise or detailed, or alters the stimuli that can activate the system. Thus, learning can expand the relation of a psychological function to new stimuli and other functions, and it can facilitate the manifestation and/or maintenance of the function once developed. However, other factors must operate for the developmental construction of a psychological function. Here we are in agreement with critiques of the learning theory approach to all psychological development (e.g., Buller, 2005).

In contrast to learning, *experience* represents the manner by which certain environmental factors influence the developmental construction of functions (e.g., induction; Gottlieb, 1992). Experience operates only through the transduction of environmental influences into physiological processes that, in turn, may affect the developmental organization and operations of the nervous system and other physiological systems. Transduction requires specific sensory mechanisms that permit certain physical forces (e.g., chemical, mechanical, electromagnetic) to be converted into physiological processes that affect neural transmission. Experiential influences require that the sensory systems respond to physical forces and affect neural activity. Thus, experience is an embodied character of the individual.

During infancy, the sensory systems are developing from states of relative insensitivity to physical stimuli to states of increasing sophistication in the character of their sensitivity. However, even their activation during primitive states of sensitivity contributes both to their own developing sensitivity and to their influence on the nervous system. Because of changes in their developmental states, the capabilities of responding to physical forces and of affecting neural activity differ for different sensory transducers at various points during the individual's development. Moreover, the development of feedback mechanisms (in part provoked by sensory activity) to sensory systems contributes to the development of their sophistication in processing complex physical stimuli (involving temporal and spatial patterns). Thus, experiential influences can contribute to the development of the nascent systems upon which learning depends.

Failure to recognize what a sensory system can or cannot do at any point during development can lead to both over- and underestimation of the capabilities of the individual at that point. Different mechanisms may accomplish similar functions, but the mechanisms may differ strikingly in (1) the means by which they achieve the function; (2) the function's robustness in response to perturbation; and (3) the range of options available for producing variations of the function, some of which may result in shifts in the developmental trajectory. Auditory stimulation, extensive or insufficient contact, and light stimulation can affect the development of many of the infant's perceptual and other psychological functions (e.g., social relations), sometimes by affecting hormonal secretion as well as neural activity. Even the sensory feedback generated by the infant's own actions contributes to the development of sensorimotor programs and, perhaps, hemispheric specialization for information processing (Michel et al., 2013).

At each phase of development, the individual exhibits specific behavioral abilities in coaction with its social and physical environments that can "scaffold" the manifestation of the abilities. The behavior of the individual also provides specific kinds of stimulation that become, in turn, experiences that influence the individual's further development. These "circular relationships of self-stimulation" (Schneirla, 1957, p. 86) are an important source of psychological development. For analytic purposes, it may be important to consider the individual and his or her environment as separate; however, for the individual, there is no separation. Thus, stimulation from three sources (self-stimulation, self-generated stimulation, and externally generated stimulation) can provide embodied experiences that construct the nascent systems important for the development of psychological functions. Although different, all three types of stimulation operate on the developing system in the same manner. That is, for stimuli to act as experiences in the individual's development, they must be embodied, or in other words, they must be transduced into cellular processes that can affect physiological functioning. Thus, as far as the individual's component systems are concerned, the source of the stimulation is irrelevant.

Environmental influences on development (which must be distinguished from experiential influences because they operate without sensory transduction) can be divided into two (not mutually exclusive) types: (1) those environmental factors that are external to the organismic boundary (epidermis in humans) of the individual (e.g., foods, electromagnetic radiations, pollutants, pathogens), and (2) any factor in a cell (or that can enter cells) that is not DNA but can affect DNA activity (e.g., hormones, neurotransmitters, various proteins, certain parasites and viruses). These factors can influence development by directly or indirectly affecting cellular processes (as part of the epigenome). For example, prenatal and postnatal nutritional status can affect the development of the infant via its influence on cellular metabolism and its impact on the production of growth hormones. Moreover, the nutritional status during the development of the infant's grandparents can affect the infant's development in many ways. These cross-generation effects involve epigenetic processes whereby expression of the DNA in the grandparents' germ cells is altered by their nutritional status and passed on to their offspring, and so on.

In addition to environmental, experiential, and learning contributions to the development of the infant, researchers have to consider *self-organizational processes* in the development of the individual's anatomical/physiological systems. These self-organizational processes contribute to the organization of cell types and cellular relations essential for organ formation and many aspects of sense organs and neural development (cf. Hoffmann, 2012). In part, these contribute to the development of the nascent structures upon which systems involved in psychological functioning develop. Although disruptions of DNA functioning can alter the course of the developmental self-organization of these systems, they are not guided in their organization by DNA expression. Rather, the DNA is part of the necessary conditions within which their self-organization can emerge (Gilbert & Epel, 2009).

Too often, psychologists mistakenly believe that genes (DNA) contain information that specifies the predisposition for psychological traits ("the loaded gun") and the environment affects the extent of their manifestation ("pulling the trigger"). Hence, the developmental manifestation of a trait was considered a consequence of gene–environment interaction. This prompted studies designed to examine gene × environment interactions. However, such studies do not reveal the influences that directly create the developmental trajectories that tie genetic and environmental markers to differences in the manifestation of psychological traits (Michel, 2010, 2014).

Critical Periods

The conventional concept "critical" or "sensitive period" assumes that normal development depends on certain experiences occurring during a particular time window. Abnormal development arises when these experiences do not occur during this time or when unusual experiences occur during this period. Moreover, the concept implies that rehabilitation of abnormal development is severely limited once the time has passed. Because the "description" and the "explanation" of development are different, the interdisciplinary biopsychosocial perspective requires more investigations into the "how" of development rather than further investigation of whether or not there are critical or sensitive periods in the development of sensory, motor, cognitive, or socioemotional traits and abilities. Only by focusing on the mechanisms of development can ways of "correcting" developmental trajectories, even during later phases, be identified (see Michel, 2012, for examples).

Human Nature

Infant research revealed many abilities that do not appear to be acquired through learning. The typical response to such observations is to consider the abilities to be the products of biological evolution (e.g., Bloom, 2013) and to label them as "human nature." These abilities are sometimes described as innate or core abilities. However, the concept of innate has many different implications that need not relate to one another and can lead to conceptual confusion (Lehrman, 1970; Michel & Moore, 1995). The investigation of normally occurring stimuli and behaviors in a natural setting is important for revealing the developmental origins of species typicality. Thus, the development of a behavior pattern may appear "innate" and constant in all or nearly all individuals of a species (species-typical) because natural selection combined with the individual's developmental processes to assure the compatibility of the interaction of the individual with the species-typical environment. Gottlieb (1992) and others (e.g., Lehrman, 1970; Michel & Moore, 1995; Schneirla, 1966) argued that only systematic developmental investigations can reveal the contributions of the species-typical environment to the manifestation of species-typical psychological functions.

Moreover, what is selected during evolution is not a specific state of the individual's system, but rather mechanisms and processes that can produce a range of states in response to a range of conditions. The adaptability of the individual creates a range of alternative phenotypes (the norm of reaction; Schlichting & Pigliucci, 1998) on which selection can operate. The norm of reaction is a theoretical construct to prevent investigators from confusing some limited set of observed developmental functions with some intrinsic limit-setting conditions. The phenotypic norm of reaction for any individual genotype can be known only after it has developed in all combinations of conditions and durations of exposure to each of those combinations of conditions. Thus, developmental processes harbor an unknown range of variability. Basing evolution on the variability in developmental trajectories (revealed by systematic investigation) eliminates the teleology inherent in the "development to" evolutionary explanations and permits random mutations to eventually help stabilize, but not solidify, the development of existing phenotypes.

Since the individual is an organized system, delaying or accelerating the rate of development among different features or traits (heterochrony) can ramify to affect the development and expression of other features. Heterochrony across the development of traits is considered a fundamental source for the production of new patterns of organization upon which natural selection can operate (de Beer, 1930; Gould, 1977). Distinctly different individuals can emerge from alterations in the relative rate of development among specific features or traits. Indeed, maintaining or failing to maintain a trait beyond its typical developmental time frame can have ramifications on the development and functional organization of other traits because the individual is a coherent system. It is these developmental mechanisms that create the variability in development that marks the character of human nature and upon which natural selection operates (Michel, 2013a). However, since natural selection is differential reproductive success, only those traits that demonstrably affect reproduction and are reliably transmitted across generations can come under natural selection pressure, which will be delimited by the developmental options available (Gilbert & Epel, 2009).

Future Directions and Caveats

Investigation of infant development must begin with detailed descriptive data collected from direct observation of the infant's behavior that identify behavior and experiences directly, and not via parental reports or standardized tests (Kagan, 2013). Perhaps the common neglect of detailed observational data (Kagan, 2013) derives in part from the conventional wisdom that only randomized experimental designs can capture causal links among variables. However, historical phenomena such as human development can derive causality from model construction and testing (much as it is done in modern cosmology and physics). Since infant development is a complex process with multiple influences and individual variations in trajectory, observational data must document the correlations among many variables. Fortunately, modern statistical programs permit translation of the correlations among many variables into a model that represents a causal hypothesis (Shipley, 2000). Building these models begins with correlations among observational data (typically represented by a "directed graph"; Pearl, 2000) in which variables are connected by lines (a path analysis). This graph models a causal hypothesis. Competing hypotheses can then be constructed and *new data must be collected* that will permit adjudication among these competing hypotheses using either standard methods of statistical analysis, or more modern techniques that compare competing models using criteria derived from information or Bayesian theory.

Developmental research traditionally investigates relations between biological "markers" and psychological outcomes by connecting a modern neuroscience procedure (e.g., EEG, functional magnetic resonance imaging [fMRI], genomewide association studies [GWAS], magnetoencephalography [MEG], near-infrared spectroscopy [NIRS], salivary cortisol) with a modern procedure for assessing infant psychological functioning (e.g., attachment, behavioral inhibition, face recognition, phoneme discrimination, stranger anxiety). Adding a biological marker (e.g., salivary cortisol, EEG data) or a social marker (e.g., a measure of social class or of exposure to parental abuse) to a psychological study does not meet the requirements of an interdisciplinary investigation. Indeed, even knowledge of all research on the use of cortisol as a marker of adrenal functioning (or stress) is not equivalent to understanding how cortisol functions in concert with other hormones, other systems, circadian and other rhythmic cycles, immune function, and neural activity. That is the kind of *biological expertise* that is needed for comprehending how environmental conditions can become "stressors" for parents that, in turn, can produce differences in parental care that affect infant development.

Employing a measure of socioeconomic status or of exposure to certain forms of media is not the same as understanding how social status and institutions affect the organization of social relations, or how media is structured and disseminated among the populace. The latter is the kind of *social expertise* that needs to be combined with biological expertise for comprehending how these factors can become "stressors" for parents that, in turn, can produce differences in parental care that affect infant development. Also, it is important to determine how these macro-, exo-, and microsystems are transduced into factors that can affect the infant's development. An interdisciplinary biopsychosocial perspective requires that researchers acquire expertise in two or three systems within which the individual functions. Only then will they effectively relate the causes operating within and across each system. In this way, several experts can combine their overlapping expertise so as to achieve the more synthetic integration proposed by Bateson (2005).

Conclusions

One prevailing message of this chapter is a plea to study *the processes of development*, rather than predictors and outcomes. Development is a complicated process, resulting from multiple levels of influences, including traditionally biological (e.g., cellular processes, systemic physiology), psychological (e.g., behavioral organization, problem solving, self-differentiation), and social (e.g., habitat, cultural traditions, familial dynamics) factors (a biopsychosocial perspective).

Instead of studying these levels in isolation or seeking simple "markers" for each level, infant behavior should be viewed as emerging from a history of *all* of these continuously changing influences throughout infancy. A simple predictor-outcome study, even with markers of social, biological, or psychological characteristics treated as potential mediating or moderating factors cannot capture the pattern in an infant's developmental trajectory. For developmental theory, it is the specific character of these trajectories that signify later developmental consequences. Since each infant experiences a unique environment and age (time) cannot act upon the infant, grouping and comparing infants by age will not reveal the processes contributing to development.

Moreover, in contrast to a multidisciplinary approach, interdisciplinary knowledge facilitates comprehension of the ways that various levels fuse to shape the trajectory of the infant's development. Working with this perspective places greater emphasis on the "development from" approach (Michel & Tyler, 2007b) that requires the investigator to focus on identifying how various factors affect earlier functions so that they give rise to later functions. Therefore, we propose that an interdisciplinary biopsychosocial framework can guide future developmental research toward a richer understanding of infant development.

REFERENCES

Adolph, K. E., & Robinson, S. R. (2008). In defense of change processes. *Child Development, 79*(6), 1648–1653.

Bateson, P. (2005). The return of the whole organism. *Journal of Biosciences, 30*(1), 31–39.

Bateson, P., & Mameli, M. (2007). The innate and the acquired: Useful clusters or a residual distinction from folk biology? *Developmental Psychobiology, 49*(8), 818–831.

Bloom, P. (2013). *Just babies: The origins of good and evil.* New York: Crown.

Borrell-Carrió, F., Suchman, A. L., & Epstein, R. M. (2004). The biopsychosocial model 25 years later: Principles, practice, and scientific inquiry. *Annals of Family Medicine, 2*(6), 576–582.

Bronfenbrenner, U., & Morris, P. A. (1998). The ecology of developmental process. In W. Damon (Series Ed.) & R. M. Lerner (Vol. Ed.), *Handbook of child psychology: Vol. 1. Theoretical models of human development* (5th ed., pp. 993–1028). New York: Wiley.

Buller, D. J. (2005) *Adapting minds: Evolutionary psychology and the persistent quest for human nature.* Cambridge, MA: MIT Press.

de Beer, G. (1930). *Embryology and evolution.* Oxford, UK: Clarendon Press.

Drake, A. J., & Walker, B. R. (2004). The intergenerational effects of fetal programming: Non-genomic mechanisms for the inheritance of low birth weight and cardiovascular risk. *Journal of Endocrinology, 180*(1), 1–16.

Engel, G. L. (1977). The need for a new medical model: A challenge for biomedicine. *Science, 196*, 129–136.

Engel, G. L. (1980). The clinical application of the biopsychosocial model. *American Journal of Psychiatry, 137*, 535–544.

Ferre, C. L., Babik, I., & Michel, G. F. (2010). Development of infant prehension handedness: A longitudinal analysis during the 6- to 14-month age period. *Infant Behavior and Development, 33*, 492–502.

Fleming, A. S., Kraemer, G. W., Gonzalez, A., Lovic, V., Rees, S., & Melo, A. (2002). Mothering begets mothering: The transmission of behavior and its neurobiology across generations. *Pharmacology Biochemistry and Behavior, 73*(1), 61–75.

Gerhart, J., & Kirschner, M. (1997). *Cells, embryos, and evolution: Toward a cellular and developmental understanding of phenotypic variation and evolutionary adaptability.* Malden, MA: Blackwell Science.

Gilbert, S. F. (2006). The generation of novelty: The province of developmental biology. *Biological Theory, 1*(2), 209–212.

Gilbert, S. F., & Epel, D. (2009). *Ecological developmental biology.* Sunderland, MA: Sinauer.

Gottlieb, G. (1992). *Individual development and evolution: The genesis of novel behavior.* New York: Oxford University Press.

Gould, S. J. (1977). *Ontogeny and phylogeny.* Cambridge, MA: Harvard University Press.

Hoffmann, P. M. (2012). *Life's ratchet: How molecular machines extract order from chaos.* New York: Basic Books.

Kagan, J. (2013). Equal time for psychological and biological contributions to human variation. *Review of General Psychology, 17*, 351–357.

Kennedy, J. S. (1992). *The new anthropomorphism.* Cambridge, UK: Cambridge University Press.

Kirschner, M. W., & Gerhart, J. C. (2006). *The plausibility of life: Resolving Darwin's dilemma.* New Haven, CT: Yale University Press.

Lehrman, D. S. (1970). Semantic and conceptual issues in the nature–nurture problem. In L. R. Aronson, E. Tobach, D. S. Lehrman, & J. S. Rosenblatt (Eds.), *Development and evolution of behavior* (pp. 17–52). San Francisco: Freeman.

Mennella, J. A., Ziegler, P., Briefel, R., & Novak, T. (2006). Feeding infants and toddlers study: The types of foods fed to Hispanic infants and toddlers. *Journal of the American Dietetic Association, 106*, 96–106.

Michel, G. F. (2007). Doing what comes naturally: The role of self-generated experience in behavioral development. *European Journal of Developmental Science, 1*(2), 155–164.

Michel, G. F. (2010). The roles of environment, experience, and learning in behavioral development. In K. Hood, C. Halpern, G. Greenberg, & R. Lerner (Eds.), *Handbook of Developmental Science, Behavior and Genetics* (pp. 123–165). Malden, MA: Wiley.

Michel, G. F. (2012). Using knowledge of development to promote recovery of function after brain damage. *Developmental Psychobiology, 54*(3), 350–356.

Michel, G. F. (2013a). The concept of homology in the development of handedness. *Developmental Psychobiology, 55*(1), 84–91.

Michel, G. F. (2013b). The role of developmental psychobiology in the unification of psychology. *Review of General Psychology, 17*, 210–215.

Michel, G. F. (2014). A developmental psychobiological approach to human development. *Review of Human Development, 11*, 37–49.

Michel, G. F., & Moore, C. L. (1995). *Developmental psychobiology: An interdisciplinary science.* Cambridge, MA: MIT Press.

Michel, G. F., Nelson, E. L., Babik, I., Campbell, J. M., & Marcinowski, E. C. (2013). Multiple trajectories in the developmental psychobiology of human handedness. In R. M. Lerner & J. B. Benson (Eds.), *Embodiment and epigenesis: Theoretical and methodological issues in understanding the role of biology within the relational developmental system* (Part B: Ontogenetic Dimensions, pp. 227–260). New York: Academic Press.

Michel, G. F., & Tyler, A. N. (2005). Critical period: A history of the transition from questions of when, to what, to how. *Developmental Psychobiology, 46*(3), 156–162.

Michel, G. F., & Tyler, A. N. (2007a). Can knowledge of developmental processes illuminate the evolution of parental care? *Developmental Psychobiology, 49*(1), 33–44.

Michel, G. F., & Tyler, A. N. (2007b). Developing human nature: "Development to" vs. "Development from." *Developmental Psychobiology, 49*(8), 788–799.

Oppenheim, R. W. (1984). Ontogenetic adaptations in neural and behavioral development: Toward a more "ecological" developmental psychobiology. In H. F. R. Prechtl (Ed.), *Continuity of neural functions from prenatal to postnatal life* (pp. 16–29). Philadelphia: Lippincott.

Pearl, J. (2000). *Causality.* Cambridge, UK: Cambridge University Press.

Raff, R. A. (1996). *The shape of life.* Chicago: Chicago University Press.

Rose, H., & Rose, S. (2012). *Genes, cells, and brains: The Promethean promises of the new biology.* Brooklyn, NY: Verso.

Schlichting, C. D., & Pigliucci, M. (1998). *Phenotypic evolution: A reaction norm perspective.* Sunderland, MA: Sinauer Associates.

Schneirla, T. C. (1957). The concept of development in comparative psychology. In D. B. Harris (Ed.), *The concept of development* (pp. 78–108). Minneapolis: University of Minnesota Press.

Schneirla, T. C. (1966). Behavioral development and comparative psychology. *Quarterly Review of Biology, 41*, 283–302.

Shipley, B. (2000). *Cause and correlation in biology.* Cambridge, UK: Cambridge University Press.

Sperry, R. W. (1965). Mind, brain and humanist values. In J. R. Platt (Ed.), *New views of the nature of man* (pp. 71–92). Chicago: University of Chicago Press.

Sperry, R. W. (1980). Mind–brain interaction. *Neuroscience, 5*, 195–206.

Tyler, A. N. (2006). When is a description not an explanation: A response to Armstrong, et al. (2006). *Developmental Psychobiology, 48*(4), 332–335.

West, M. J., King, A. P., & Arberg, A. A. (1988). The inheritance of niches. In E. M. Blass (Ed.), *Handbook of Behavioral Neurobiology* (Vol. 9, pp. 41–62). New York: Plenum Press.

Author Index

Subject Index

Note: *f* or *t* following a page number indicates a figure or a table.

469